R E V I E W   O F

OPHTHALMOLOGY

REVIEW OF
OPHTHALMOLOGY

Neil J. Friedman, MD
Adjunct Clinical Associate Professor
Department of Ophthalmology
Stanford University School of Medicine, Stanford
Private Practice
Mid-Peninsula Ophthalmology Medical Group
Palo Alto, California

Peter K. Kaiser, MD
Director, Clinical Research Center
Cole Eye Institute
The Cleveland Clinic Foundation
Cleveland, Ohio

William B. Trattler, MD
Volunteer Assistant Professor of Ophthalmology
Bascom Palmer Eye Institute
University of Miami Medical School, Miami
Private Practice
Center for Excellence in Eye Care
Miami, Florida

ELSEVIER
SAUNDERS

ELSEVIER
SAUNDERS

The Curtis Center
170 S Independence Mall W 300E
Philadelphia, Pennsylvania 19106

NOTICE

Ophthalmology is an ever-changing field. Standard safety precautions must be followed, but as new research and clinical experience broaden our knowledge, changes in treatment and drug therapy may become necessary or appropriate. Readers are advised to check the most current product information provided by the manufacturer of each drug to be administered to verify the recommended dose, the method and duration of administration, and contraindications. It is the responsibility of the licensed prescriber, relying on experience and knowledge of the patient, to determine dosages and the best treatment for each individual patient. Neither the publisher nor the author assumes any liability for any injury and/or damage to persons or property arising from this publication.

The Publisher

Library of Congress Cataloging-in-Publication Data
Friedman, Neil J.
 Review of ophthalmology/Neil J. Friedman, Peter K. Kaiser, William B. Trattler.—1st ed.
  p. ; cm.
 Includes index.
 ISBN 0-7216-8776-8
 1. Ophthalmology. 2. Eye—Diseases. I. Kaiser, Peter K. II. Trattler, William B.
III. Title.
 [DNLM: 1. Eye Diseases. 2. Ophthalmology. WW 140 F9116r 2005]
 RE46.F844 2005
 617.7—dc22

                2004050809

Acquisitions Editor: Paul Fam
Developmental Editor: Joanie Milnes
Publishing Services Manager: Tina Rebane
Project Manager: Norm Stellander
Design Manager: Ellen Zanolle

Printed in China

Last digit is the print number: 9 8 7 6 5 4 3 2 1

Preface

The extent and breadth of knowledge required to master the field of ophthalmology can be intimidating. This is especially apparent during the first few years of training, when residents are expected to know almost every esoteric fact, yet there is barely time between clinic, surgery, call, and research to read and assimilate the plethora of textbooks and literature. Later in one's career, especially with the trend toward subspecialization, it is common to lose familiarity with much of the information acquired about various disorders, particularly those that are rare.

The purpose of this book is to bring together in one text the majority of critical information that we are expected to know during training in an easy-to-digest fashion. Whether studying for a test or reviewing a once-known but now forgotten topic, a review book is an efficient and easily accessible tool for achieving such a goal. The various review manuals that already exist are primarily tomes of multiple-choice-style questions with an accompanying section containing answers and explanations. Although this method of study is very effective, we have personally found an outline format with a sampling of review questions to be more helpful.

The chapters of this text are organized into common subspecialties of ophthalmology that we all encounter. The limitation of such a classification scheme is that in order to be comprehensive, some overlap among different sections is inevitable. We have done our best to produce concise, easy-to-read chapters with minimal duplication of material. In addition, we have included tables and mnemonics where appropriate to help the reader learn and retain critical information. The findings of many of the important clinical ophthalmology studies are also reviewed.

The nature of any review book is that it is for review; it is not a primary text and should not serve as one. The illustrations were selected to highlight anatomic details, common ophthalmic tests, and examples of classic histopathology and clinical findings. These pictures were purposely kept to a minimum, as this book is not meant to be an atlas of disease. We have attempted to provide a wide selection of references for each chapter so that the reader may pursue further study of a given topic. It is our hope that this book will serve as a practical review guide for all ophthalmologists, as well as one that will enable the doctor in training to develop a broad foundation in ophthalmology.

Neil J. Friedman, MD
Peter K. Kaiser, MD
William B. Trattler, MD

Acknowledgments

This book has been a team effort involving the help and support of colleagues, friends, and family, and as such there are numerous people to whom we owe our thanks.

First, we are grateful to our colleagues and students at the following institutions across the country for sharing their limitless knowledge and wisdom: the Bascom Palmer Eye Institute, the Cole Eye Institute, the Scheie Eye Institute, and the Stanford University Department of Ophthalmology. We would especially like to thank the following individuals for their critical review of specific chapters: Maria Braun, MD; Lloyd Clark, MD; Chris Engelman, MD; Lilia Fannin, MD; Anne Fung, MD; Louis Kasner, MD; Danny Lin, MD; Maria Portellos, MD; Brad Simons, MD, PhD; Kimberly Guo Yen, MD; and Michael Yen, MD.

For their expertise and helpful suggestions, we also owe a debt of gratitude to our editorial and publishing staff: Natasha Andjelkovic, Paul Fam, Joanie Milnes, Norm Stellander and everyone in their dedicated departments, who transitioned in the midst of the project yet kept it running seamlessly.

And as always, we are most appreciative of the unwavering support and love of our families: Alan, Diane, Lisa, Jill, Ali, Jeremy, Henry, Marcia, Meredith, Peter, Anafu, Christine, Maureen, PJ, and Stephanie.

Contents

CHAPTER 1

Optics

PROPERTIES OF LIGHT

Light behaves as waves and as particles (photons)

Speed is directly proportional to wavelength (λ) and frequency (v): $v = \lambda v$

In any given medium, speed of light is constant ($v_{vacuum} = c = 3.0 \times 10^{10}$ cm/sec); therefore, wavelength and frequency are inversely proportional

Light slows down in any substance other than air or vacuum, amount of slowing depends on medium; frequency of light remains unchanged, but wavelength changes (becomes shorter) (Figure 1-1)

Energy is directly proportional to frequency and inversely proportional to wavelength: $E = hv = h(c/v)$

Index of refraction (n): ratio of speed of light in a vacuum to speed of light in specific material ($n = c/v$)

Air = 1.00, water = 1.33, aqueous and vitreous = 1.33, cornea = 1.37, crystalline lens = 1.42, polymethyl methacrylate (PMMA) = 1.49, glass = 1.52

Interference: overlapping of light waves; may be constructive or destructive

Constructive: peaks of 2 waves overlap, resulting in maximum intensity at that wavelength

Destructive: peak of 1 wave overlaps with trough of another, obliterating both waves

EXAMPLE: antireflective coatings (destructive interference, 1/4 wavelength apart); interference filters (allow only green light out of the eye during fluorescein angiography); laser interferometry (retinal function test; OCT)

Coherence: ability of 2 light beams to cause interference (large white source has a coherence close to zero)

EXAMPLE: optical coherence tomography (OCT)

Polarization: each light wave has an electrical field with a particular orientation

Nonpolarized light: electrical field of each wave has a random orientation

Polarized light: all electrical fields have same orientation

EXAMPLE: Haidinger's brushes (polarizing filter rotated in front of blue background produces rotating image like a double-ended brush or propeller; type of entopic phenomenon; test of macular function), Titmus stereo testing, polarized microscopy, polarizing sunglasses

Diffraction: bending of light waves around edges; change in direction of light wave is related to wavelength (the shorter the wavelength, the less the change in direction); amount of diffraction is related to size of aperture (the smaller the aperture, the greater the diffraction); interference of new waves with original rays forms a diffraction pattern

EXAMPLE: Airy disc (diffraction pattern produced by a small, circular aperture; occurs when pupil size is <2.5 mm; diameter of central disc increases as pupil size decreases); pinhole (reduces refractive error and improves vision by increasing depth of focus, but limited by diffraction; optimal size is 1.2 mm; may correct for up to 3D; smaller aperture limits visual acuity; squinting is method of creating a natural pinhole to improve vision; pinhole can also improve vision in eyes with corneal or lenticular irregularities; pinhole can reduce vision in eyes with retinal disorders)

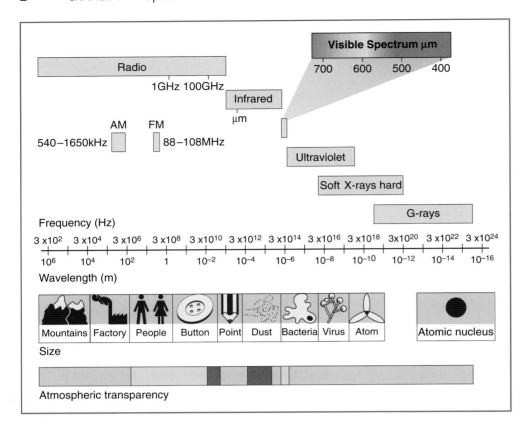

Figure 1-1. The electromagnetic spectrum. The pictures of mountains, people, buttons, viruses, and so forth, are used to produce a real (i.e., visceral) feeling of the size of some of the wavelengths. (From Miller D, Burns SK: Visable light. In Yanoff M, Duker JS [eds]: *Ophthalmology*, 2nd ed, St. Louis, Mosby, 2004.)

Scattering: disruption of light by irregularities in light path; shorter wavelengths scatter to a greater extent

> **EXAMPLE**: Opacity (corneal scar or cataract) scatters light, causing glare and image degradation; in atmosphere, scattering involves particles (Rayleigh scattering) and blue light (scattered to the greatest extent; therefore, sky appears blue)

Reflection: bouncing of light off optical interfaces; the greater the refractive index difference between the 2 media, the greater the reflection; also, varies with angle of incidence

> **EXAMPLE**: Asteroid hyalosis (asteroids reflect light back into examiner's eye, creating glare; patient is asymptomatic)

Transmission: percentage of light penetrating a substance (%T); can vary with wavelength

Absorption: expressed as optical density (OD) = log 1/T

Illumination: measure of incident light

Luminance: measure of reflected or emitted light (lumen/m²); apostilb = diffusing surface with luminance of 1 lumen/m² (used in Humphrey and Goldmann visual field testing)

> **EXAMPLE**: contrast sensitivity is ability to detect small changes in luminance

Laser: **l**ight **a**mplification by **s**timulated **e**mission of **r**adiation; excited material releases photons of same wavelength and frequency; process is amplified so that released photons are in phase (constructive interference); produces monochromatic, coherent, high-intensity polarized light; power can be increased by increasing energy or decreasing time (P = E/t); Q-switching and mode-locking (types of shutters that synchronize light phase) are methods of increasing laser power by compressing output in time

REFRACTION

Light changes direction when it travels from one material to another of different refractive index (e.g., across an optical interface); direction of refraction is toward the normal when light passes from a medium with a lower index of refraction to a medium with a higher one, and away from the normal when light passes from a more dense to a less dense medium (higher refractive index materials are more difficult for light to travel through, so light takes a shorter path [closer to the normal]); light does not deviate if it is perpendicular to interface (parallel to the normal) (Figure 1-2).

Snell's law: n sin (i) = n' sin (r); n = refractive index of material; i = angle of incidence (measured from the

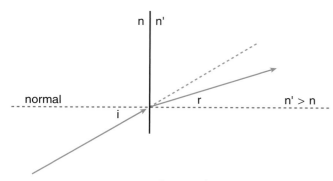

Figure 1-2. Refraction of light ray.

normal); r = angle of refraction (measured from the normal)

Critical angle: angle at which incident light is bent exactly 90° away from the normal (when going from medium of higher to lower n) and after which all light is reflected

> **EXAMPLE**: Glass/air interface has a critical angle of 41°; critical angle of cornea = 46.5°

Total internal reflection: angle of incidence exceeds critical angle, so light is reflected back into material with higher index of refraction; $n \sin (i_c) = n' \sin (90°)$; $\sin (i_c) = (n'/n) \times 1$

> **EXAMPLE**: Gonioscopy lens is necessary to view angle structures owing to total internal reflection of the cornea

PRISMS

Prisms displace and deviate light (because surfaces are nonparallel); light rays are deviated toward base; image is displaced toward apex.

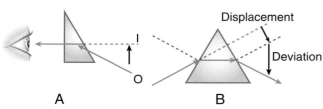

Figure 1-3. A, Displacement of image toward apex. **B**, Displacement and deviation of light by prism.

Prism diopter (PD, Δ): displacement (in cm) of light ray passing through a prism, measured 100 cm (1 m) from prism

> **EXAMPLE**: 15 prism diopters = ray displaced 15 cm at a distance of 1 m ($1\Delta = 1$ cm displacement/1 m); $1° \approx 2^{\Delta}$ (this approximation is useful for angles smaller than 45°)

Angle of minimum deviation: total angle of deviation is least when there is equal bending at both surfaces of prism

Plastic prisms are calibrated by angle of minimum deviation: back surface parallel to frontal plane

Glass prisms are calibrated in **Prentice position**: back surface perpendicular to visual axis

Prism placed in front of the eye creates a phoria in the direction of the base

> **EXAMPLE**: Base-out prism induces exophoria; to correct, use prism with apex in the opposite direction

Apex is always pointed in direction of deviation: base-out for esotropia, base-in for exotropia, base-down for hypertropia

Stacking prisms is not additive; 1 prism in front of each eye is additive

Risley prism: 2 right-angle prisms positioned back to back, which can be rotated to yield variable prism diopters from 0 to 30$^{\Delta}$; used to measure prismatic correction for tropias

Fresnel prisms: composed of side-by-side strips of small prisms; prism power is related to apex angle, not the size of the prism; available as lightweight, thin press-on prism to reduce base thickness of the spectacle prism; disadvantage is reflection and scatter at prism interface, causing decreased visual acuity

Prismatic effect of lenses: spectacles induce prism; all off-axis rays are bent toward or away from axis, depending on lens vergence

A   B

Figure 1-4. A, Plus lenses act like 2 prisms base to base. **B**, Minus lenses act like 2 prisms apex to apex.

Perceived movement of fixation target when lens moves in front of the eye:
> **Plus lenses** produce **"against" motion** (target moves in opposite direction from lens)
> **Minus lenses** produce **"with" motion** (target moves in same direction as lens)

Amount of motion is proportional to the power of the lens

Prismatic effect of glasses on strabismic deviations: $2.5 \times D = \%$ difference; minus lenses make deviation appear larger ("minus measures more"); plus lenses decrease measured deviation

Prentice's rule: prismatic power of lens = Δ = hD (h = distance from optical axis of lens [cm], D = power of lens [D])

Prismatic power of a lens increases as one moves farther away from optical center (vs power of prism, which is constant)

> **EXAMPLE:** Reading 1 cm below optical center:
> OD − 3.00; OS + 1.00 + 3.00 × 90
>
> OD: prism power = 1 cm × 3D = 3^Δ BD (base-down)
> OS: prism power vertical meridian: 1 cm + 1D = 1^Δ BU (base-up) (Note: power of cylinder in 90° meridian is zero)
> Net prismatic effect = 4^Δ (either BD over OD, or BU over OS)

Treatment of vertical prismatic effect of anisometropia:
1. Contact lenses (optical center moves with eyes)
2. Lower optical centers of lenses (reduce amount of induced prism)
3. Prescribe slab-off prism (technique of grinding lens [done to the more minus of the 2 lenses] to remove base-down prism [to reduce amount of induced prism])
4. Single vision reading glasses

Prismatic effect of bifocal glasses:

Image jump: produced by sudden prismatic power at top of bifocal segment; not influenced by type of underlying lens; as line of sight crosses from optical center of lens to bifocal segment, image position suddenly shifts up owing to base-down prismatic effect of bifocal segment (more bothersome than image displacement; therefore, choose segment type to minimize image jump)

Image displacement: displacement of image by total prismatic effect of lens and bifocal segment; minimized when prismatic effect of bifocal segment and distance lens are in opposite directions

Prismatic effect of underlying lens:
Hyperopic lenses induce base-up prism, causing image to move progressively downward in downgaze
Myopic lenses induce base-down prism, causing image to move progressively upward in downgaze

Prismatic effect of bifocal segment:
Round top (acts like base-down prism): maximum image jump; image displacement less for hyperope than for myope
Flat top (acts like base-up prism): minimum image jump; image displacement more for hyperope than for myope
Executive type or progressive lenses: no image jump (optical centers at top of segment)

Plus lens: choose round top

Minus lens: choose flat top or executive type
(For myopes, image jump is very difficult to ignore because it is in same direction as image displacement; so, avoid round tops in myopes)

Chromatic effects: prismatic effect varies with wavelength
Shorter wavelengths are bent farther, causing chromatic aberration
White light shines through prism: blue rays closer to base (bend farthest), red rays closer to apex
In the eye, blue rays come to focus closer to lens than do red rays; difference between blue and red is 1.5 to 3D

Duochrome test: red and green filters create 0.5 D difference; use to check accuracy of refraction
If letters on red side are clearer, focal point is in front of retina (eye is "fogged" or myopic)
If letters on green side are clearer, focal point is behind retina (eye is overminused or hyperopic)
Technique: start with red side clearer and add minus sphere in 0.25 D steps until red and green sides are equal (focal point on retina); works in colorblind patients because it is based on chromatic aberration rather than color discrimination

Vector addition of prisms: prismatic deviations in different directions are additive, based on pythagorean theorem ($a^2 + b^2 = c^2$)

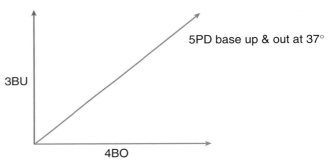

Figure 1-5. Addition of base-up (BU) and base-out (BO) prisms.

VERGENCE

The amount of spreading of a bundle of light rays (wavefront) emerging from a point source

Direction of light travel must be specified (by convention, left to right)

Convergence (converging rays): plus vergence; rare in nature; must be produced by an optical system

Divergence (diverging rays): minus vergence

Parallel rays: zero vergence

Diopter: unit of vergence; reciprocal of distance (in meters) to point at which rays intersect; reciprocal of focal length of lens

Lens: adds vergence to light (amount of vergence = power of lens [in diopters])
Plus (convex) lens adds vergence; minus (concave) lens subtracts vergence

Basic lens formula: U + D = V (U = vergence of light entering lens; D = power of lens; V = vergence of light leaving lens)

Power of a spherical surface in a fluid: $D_s = (n' - n)/r$

(n' − n = difference in refractive indices; r = radius of curvature of surface [in meters])

EXAMPLE: Power of corneal surface: back = −5.7 D; front = +52.9 D (front: n' = 1.37, n = 1.00; back: n' = 1.33, n = 1.37; r = 0.007)

Power of a thin lens immersed in fluid: $D_{air}/D_{fluid} = (n_{lens} - n_{air})/(n_{lens} - n_{fluid})$

Refracting power of a thin lens is proportional to difference in refractive indices between lens and medium

Objects and images:

Object rays: rays that define the object; always on incoming (left) side of lens

Image rays: rays that define the image; always on outgoing (right) side of lens

Objects and images can be on either side of lens: real if on same side as respective rays; virtual if on opposite side from rays (locate by imaginary extension of rays through lens)

If object is moved, image moves in same direction relative to light

Adding power to system also moves image: plus power pulls image against light; minus power pushes image with light

Lenses:

Real (thick) lenses: (Figure 1-6)

6 CARDINAL POINTS: 2 principal planes (H and H'); 2 nodal points (N and N'); 2 focal points (F and F')

Refraction occurs at principal planes (U is measured from H; V is measured from H')

Focal lengths are also measured from principal planes

Nodal points coincide with principal planes (exception: if different refractive media are on opposite sides of the lens, then nodal points are both displaced toward the medium with the higher refractive index)

Central ray: passes through both nodal points (tip of object to N, across to N'; then, emerges parallel to original direction)

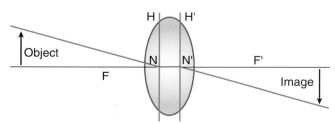

Figure 1-6. Conjugate points of real lens: each pair of object-image points in an optical system is conjugate; if direction of light is reversed, position of object and image is exactly reversed.

MENISCUS LENSES: difference between anterior and posterior curvature determines power

Steeper anterior curvature = convergent lens (+ power); principal planes displaced anteriorly

Steeper posterior curvature = divergent lens (− power); principal planes displaced posteriorly

Power of lens is measured at posterior surface (posterior vertex power)

Conjugate points: each pair of object-image points in an optical system is conjugate; if direction of light is reversed, position of object and image is exactly reversed

Conjugate planes:

EXAMPLE: Slide and viewer's retina (image of slide is formed on retina of each person in audience, and very faint image of each person's retina is projected on the screen), direct ophthalmoscope (patient's retina and examiner's retina are conjugate; indirect ophthalmoscope (3 conjugate planes [patient's retina, aerial image plane, examiner's retina]; any object placed at far point [aerial image] will be imaged sharply in focus on patient's retina)

Ideal (thin) lenses: special case of thick lens; as lens gets thinner, principal planes move closer together; in an ideal lens, principal planes overlap at optical center

2 FOCAL POINTS:

PRIMARY (F): object point for image at infinity (point on optical axis at which object is placed so parallel rays emerge from lens)

SECONDARY (F'): image point for object at infinity (point on optical axis at which incident parallel rays are focused)

FOCAL LENGTH: distance between lens and focal points; reciprocal of lens power (f = 1/D)

EXAMPLE: Focal length of +20 D lens is 1/20 = 0.05 meter

NODAL POINT (N): point through which light ray passes undeviated; located at center of thin lens (**optical center**)

RAY TRACING: use to determine image size, orientation, and position

3 PRINCIPAL RAYS:

1. Central ray: undeviated ray passing from tip of object through nodal point of lens (or center of curvature of mirror) to tip of image; gives size and orientation of image (form similar triangles; thus, sizes of object and image are in same ratio as their distances from the lens)
2. Ray from tip of object through F emerges from lens parallel to optical axis
3. Ray from tip of object parallel to optical axis emerges from lens and passes through F' (Figure 1-7)

Lens effectivity: function of lens power and distance from desired point of focus; depends on vertex distance and refractive index of media in which lens is placed ($D_{air} = [n_{IOL} - n_{air}]/[n_{IOL} - n_{aqueous}] \times D_{aqueous}$); moving a lens forward away from eye increases effec-

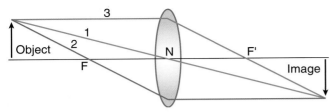

Figure 1-7. Three principal rays of ideal lens.

tive plus power, so plus lens becomes stronger and minus lens becomes weaker; when vertex distance decreases, a more plus lens is required to maintain the same distance correction (i.e., as desired point of focus is approached, more plus power is needed); the more powerful the lens, the more significant is the change in position

Vertex distance conversion:
1. Focal point of original lens = far point
2. Distance of new lens from far point = required focal length of new lens
3. Power of new lens = reciprocal of new focal length

EXAMPLE: +12.50 D spectacle lens at vertex distance of 13 mm; calculate contact lens (CL) power:

1. +12.50D lens has focal point of 0.08 m = 8 cm = far point
2. Distance of new lens (CL) from far point is 8 cm − 13 mm = 67 mm = required focal length of CL
3. Power of CL = 1/0.067 m = +15 D

Approximation: $D_2 = D_1 + S(D_1)^2$ (S = vertex distance in meters)

Pure cylindrical lens: power only in 1 meridian (perpendicular to axis of lens); produces focal line parallel to axis

Spherocylindrical lens: power in 1 meridian greater than other
  Spherical equivalent: average spherical power of a spherocylindrical lens; equal to sphere plus 1/2 the cylinder; places circle of least confusion on retina
  Conoid of Sturm: 3-dimensional envelope of light rays refracted by a circular spherocylindrical lens; consists of: vertical line → vertical ellipse → circle (of least confusion) → horizontal ellipse → horizontal line (Figure 1-8)
  Circle of least confusion: circular cross section of conoid of Sturm, which lies halfway (dioptrically) between the 2 focal lines at which image is least blurred; dioptrically calculated by spherical equivalent
  Interval of Sturm: distance between anterior and posterior focal lines

Cylinder transposition: converting cylinder notation (plus → minus; minus → plus)
  New sphere = old sphere + old cylinder
  New cylinder = magnitude of old cylinder but with opposite power
  New axis = change old axis by 90°

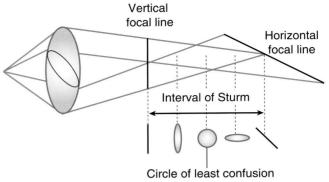

Figure 1-8. Conoid of Sturm.

EXAMPLE: +3.00 +1.50 × 45 → +4.50 −1.50 × 135

Power cross diagram: depicts 2 principal meridians of lens with the power acting in each meridian (90° from axis), rather than according to axis.

Figure 1-9. Various lens notations.

Combining cylinders at oblique axis: complex calculation; therefore, measure with lensometer

Power of cylinder at oblique axis: power of the cylinder +1.00 × 180° is +1.00 @ 90°; +0.75 @ 60°; +0.50 @ 45°; +0.25 @ 30°; 0 @ 0°

EXAMPLE

JACKSON CROSS CYLINDER: special lens used for refraction to determine cylinder power and orientation; combination of plus cylinder in 1 axis and minus cylinder of equal magnitude in axis 90° away; spherical equivalent is zero

(**e.g.**: $-1.00 + 2.00 \times 180$)

Therefore, does not change the position of the circle of least confusion with respect to the retina; normally, have 0.25 D cross cylinder in phoroptor; if patient's acuity is 20/40 or worse, must use larger power cross cylinder so patient can discriminate difference

TIGHT SUTURE AFTER CATARACT OR CORNEAL SURGERY: steepens cornea in meridian of suture, inducing astigmatism

Aberrations

Lenses behave ideally only near optical axis; peripheral to this paraxial region, aberrations occur

Spherical: shape-dependent aberration; periphery of lens has increasing prismatic effect; thus, peripheral rays refracted farther than paraxial ones, producing a blur interval along the optical axis

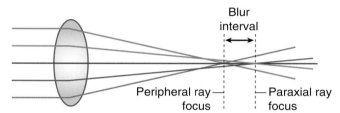

Figure 1-10. Spherical aberration.

Produces bull's-eye retinoscopic reflex

Reduce by avoiding biconvex lens shape; use plano-convex, meniscus, or aspheric lens surface

Eye has 3 mechanisms for reducing spherical aberration of lens:
1. Smaller pupil size eliminates a greater number of peripheral rays
2. Cornea progressively flattens in periphery
3. Nucleus of crystalline lens has higher index of refraction

Coma: comet-shaped image deformity from off-axis peripheral rays

Curvature of field: spherical lens produces curved image of flat object

Astigmatism of oblique incidence: tilting spherical lens induces astigmatism (oblique rays encounter different curvatures at front and back lens surfaces)

EXAMPLE: pantoscopic tilt (amount of induced sphere and cylinder depends on power of lens and amount of tilt)

Distortion: differential magnification from optical axis to lens periphery alters straight edges of square objects; shape of distortion is opposite of shape of lens (plus lens produces **pincushion** distortion; minus lens produces **barrel** distortion); effect increases with power of lens

Chromatic: light of different wavelengths is refracted by different amounts (shorter wavelengths are bent farther; chromatic interval between blue and red is 1.5 to 3.0 D)

EXAMPLE: at night with Purkinje shift, chromatic aberration moves focal point of eye anteriorly, producing myopia

MAGNIFICATION

Transverse (linear or lateral): magnification of image size (away from optical axis); must be able to measure object and image size; ratio of image height to object height (or image distance to object distance); if image is inverted, magnification is negative $M_L = I/O$

Axial: magnification of depth; magnification along optical axis; equal to square of transverse magnification $M_{Ax} = M_L^2$

Angular: magnification of angle subtended by an image with respect to an object; useful when object or image size cannot be measured

EXAMPLE: moon gazing with telescope

$M_A = xD = D/4$ (standardized to 25 cm [1/4 m], the near point of the average eye)

EXAMPLE: with direct ophthalmoscope, eye acts as simple magnifier of retina: $M_A = 60/4 = 15\times$ magnification

Size of image seen through glasses:

Shape factors: for any corrective lens, an increase in either front surface curvature or lens thickness will increase the image size (therefore, equalize the front surface curvatures and lens thickness for the 2 lenses)

FRONT SURFACE CURVATURE: every D of change will change image size by 1/2% (magnification decreases as plus power decreases)

CENTER THICKNESS: every mm of change in thickness will change image size by 1/2% (magnification decreases as lens thickness decreases)

Power factors:

VERTEX POWER (refractive power): minus power lenses produce smaller images than do plus lenses

VERTEX DISTANCE: an increase in vertex distance will increase the magnification of plus lenses and decrease the magnification (increase the minification) of minus lenses

PLUS LENS: every millimeter increase in vertex distance will increase magnification by 0.1% per diopter of lens power

MINUS LENS: every millimeter increase in vertex distance will decrease magnification by 0.1% per diopter of lens power

Spectacle lens changes retinal image size by 2% per diopter of power at 12 mm vertex distance

Anisometropia: difference in power between the 2 eyes; every 1 D produces approximately 2% of aniseikonia

Aniseikonia: difference in image size between eyes from unequal magnification of correcting lenses

Up to 6% to 7% is usually well tolerated; corresponds to approximately 3 D of spectacle anisometropia; children can adjust to much larger degrees

> **EXAMPLE**: unilateral aphakia: 25% enlargement with spectacle lens; 7% with contact lens; 2.5% with IOL

Knapp's rule: when proper corrective lens is positioned at anterior focal point of eye, retinal image size will be equal in both eyes, no matter what the degree of anisometropia (applies only to axial ametropia)

Telescopes: magnify objects by increasing angle that object subtends on retina

> *Astronomical telescope* (Keplerian): combination of 2 plus lenses; focal points coincide in intermediate image plane; distance between lenses is sum of focal lengths; use higher power as eyepiece; inverted image.

Objective (+)   +10D   Eyepiece (+)   +20D

15cm

f_o = 10cm f_e = 5cm

Figure 1-11. Astronomical telescope.

> *Galilean telescope*: combination of a weak plus lens (objective) and a strong minus lens (eyepiece); distance between lenses is difference of focal lengths; erect image (e.g., surgical loupe).

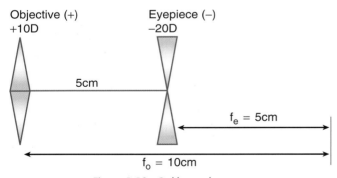

Objective (+)   +10D   Eyepiece (−)   −20D

5cm

f_e = 5cm

f_o = 10cm

Figure 1-12. Galilean telescope.

Angular magnification is same for both telescopes (power of eyepiece/power of objective): $M_A = -D_e/D_o$

Accommodation through telescope = $A_T = A_N(M_A^2)$ (A_N = normal accommodation)

> **EXAMPLE**: for monocular aphakia, overcorrect aphakic CL by +3.00 D; then, correct induced myopic error with spectacle of −3.00 D. This produces an inverse Galilean telescope

system that results in significantly smaller magnification difference between the 2 eyes than occurs with a CL alone

MIRRORS

Law of reflection: angle of incidence = angle of reflection (measured from the normal)

Objects and images: real if located on left side of mirror, virtual if on right side (inside) of mirror

Focal length: 1/2 the radius of curvature (f = r/2)

Reflecting power: reciprocal of focal length ($D_r = -1/f = -2/r$)

Convex: positive radius of curvature (r); adds minus vergence; produces virtual, erect, minified image ("VErMin")

> **EXAMPLE**: rear view mirror; cornea (reflecting power of cornea = −1/f = −2/r = −2/0.0077 = −260 D [much stronger than refracting power])

Concave: negative r; adds plus vergence; image can be virtual or real, erect or inverted, magnified or minified, depending on object location with respect to center of curvature of mirror:

> At twice focal length (center of curvature): real, inverted, same size
> Between center and focal length: real, inverted, magnified
> At focal length: at infinity
> Inside focal length: virtual, erect, magnified

Plano: no change in vergence; image is virtual, erect, same size; field of view is double the size of the mirror

> **EXAMPLE**: dressing mirror needs to be only half of body length to provide view of entire self

Central ray: passes through center of curvature of mirror, not center of mirror

Primary and secondary focal points coincide

Purkinje-Sanson images: 4 images from reflecting surfaces of eye

1. Front surface of cornea (image of object at infinity is located at focal point of mirror = 1/−260 = −3.85 mm; thus, this is a virtual, erect, minified image 3.85 mm posterior to front surface of cornea)

> **EXAMPLE**: keratometry (see figure 1-25)

2. Back surface of cornea (virtual, erect, minified image)
3. Front surface of lens (virtual, erect, minified image)
4. Back surface of lens (real, inverted, minified image)

(If patient has intraocular lens [IOL], Purkinje-Sanson images 3 and 4 are taken from front and back surfaces of the IOL, respectively; these are useful in assessment of mild degrees of pseudophacodonesis)

EYE AS OPTICAL SYSTEM

Model Eye

Gullstrand studied the eye's optical system and, based on average measurements (power = +58.64 D; F = 17.05 mm), he created a simplified model: the **"reduced"** or **"schematic" eye**: power = +60 D; F = 17 mm; F′ = 22.6 mm

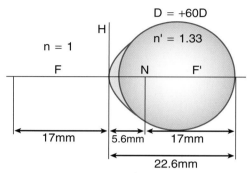

Figure 1-13. Schematic eye.

$$\frac{\text{Object height}}{\text{Image height}} = \frac{\text{Distance from nodal point}}{17\,\text{mm}}$$

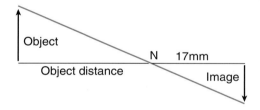

EXAMPLE: calculate the diameter of the blind spot projected 2 meters in front of the eye
(ON = 1.7 mm tall, thus by similar triangles: 1.7/17 = X/2000; X = 2000(1.7/17) = 200 mm)

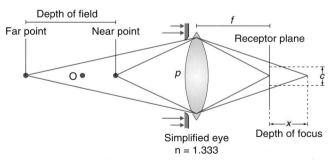

Figure 1-14. A model eye with a single refraction surface. (From Miller D, Magnante PC: Optics of the normal human eye. In Yanoff M, Duker JS [eds]: *Ophthalmology*, 2nd ed, St Louis, Mosby, 2004.)

Vision Measurements

Minimum visible: presence or absence of stimulus; depends on amount of light striking photoreceptors

Minimum discriminable: resolving power of eye; depends on ability to detect differences in light intensity

Minimum separable: smallest angle at which 2 separate objects can be discriminated; detection of a break in a line

Vernier acuity: spatial discrimination; ability to detect misalignment of 2 lines (8 seconds of arc; smaller than diameter of photoreceptor)

Snellen acuity: based on angle that smallest letter subtends on retina; each letter subtends 5 minutes of arc at a specific distance (represented by the denominator [i.e., 20/40 letter subtends 5 minutes at 40 feet, 20/20 letter subtends 5 minutes at 20 feet]; the numerator is the testing distance); each stroke width and space subtends 1 minute

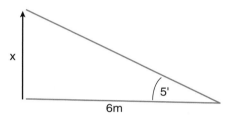

EXAMPLE: calculate the size of a 20/20 letter at 20 ft (6 m): tan = opposite/adjacent; tan 1′ = 0.0003 therefore, tan 5′ = 0.0015 = x/6000; x = 8.7 mm

Figure 1-15. Calculation of Snellen letter size.

ETDRS Chart: 5 letters per line; space between letters is equal to size of letter on that line; geometric proportion of optotype height (changes in 0.1 log unit increments)

Near acuity: must record testing distance

Acuity testing in children: optokinetic nystagmus (OKN), CSM (central, steady, maintain), preferential looking, Allen pictures, HOTV (letter symbols used in pediatric visual acuity testing), visual evoked potential (VEP)

Factors other than disease that reduce measured visual acuity: uncorrected refractive error, eccentric viewing, decreased contrast, smaller pupil size, older age

Legal blindness (in US): VA = 20/200 or worse or VF < 20° in better-seeing eye

Visual acuity is influenced by pupil size: larger pupil limits vision owing to spherical and chromatic aberrations; smaller pupil limits vision owing to diffraction; optimal pupil size is 3 mm

Laser inferometer: helium neon laser beam is split and projected onto retina, producing interference fringes; spacing of fringes can be varied; retinal function is estimated by narrowest fringes discernible

Contrast sensitivity: ability to detect changes in luminance

Refractive Error

Secondary focal point (F′) of eye is not located on retina (accommodation must be completely relaxed) (Figure 1-16)
- **Emmetropia**: focal point on retina
- **Myopia**: focal point in front of retina
- **Hyperopia**: focal point behind retina
  - Total hyperopia = manifest hyperopia (absolute and facultative) + latent hyperopia (exposed with cycloplegia)

Axial vs refractive:
- **Axial myopia**: length of eye too long (refractive power normal)
- **Refractive myopia**: refractive power too strong (length normal)
- **Axial hyperopia**: length too short (refractive power normal)
- **Refractive hyperopia**: refractive power too weak (length normal)

Far point: farthest-away eye can see clearly with accommodation completely relaxed (turn light around, start at retina, and trace rays backward through optics of eye; point at which rays intersect is far point)
- **Myopia**: far point is centimeters to infinity in front of eye
- **Hyperopia**: far point is behind eye (virtual far point)

Astigmatism: produces 2 focal lines rather than a single focal point (Table 1-1)
- **Classification**: corneal or lenticular; regular (symmetric [mirror image axis between eyes] or asymmetric) or irregular
- **"With-the-rule"**: cornea is steepest in vertical meridian; axis of plus cylinder is 90° (±20°); usually young patients (elastic lids press on top and bottom of cornea)

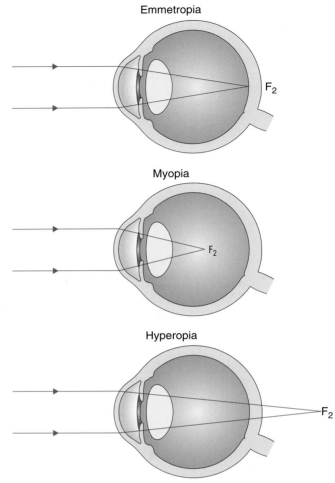

Figure 1-16. Emmetropia, myopia, and hyperopia. In emmetropia, the far point is at infinity and the secondary focal point (F$_2$) is at the retina. In myopia, the far point is the front of the eye, and the secondary focal point (F$_2$) is in the vitreous. In hyperopia, the secondary focal point (F$_2$) is located behind the eye. (Modified with permission from Azar DT, Strauss L: Principles of applied clinical optics. In Albert DM, Jakobiec FA [eds]: *Principles and Practice of Ophthalmology*, vol 6, 2nd ed, Philadelphia, WB Saunders, 2000.)

"Against-the-rule": cornea is steepest in horizontal meridian; axis of plus cylinder is 180° (±20°); older patients

Correction of ametropia: choose lens with focal point that coincides with far point of patient's eye

Table 1–1. **Classification of Astigmatism**

Type	Location of focal lines	Corrective lens	
Compound myopic	Both in front of retina	−sph −cyl; −sph +cyl	(−sphere regardless of notation)
Simple myopic	1 in front, 1 on retina	−sph +cyl; plano −cyl	(−sphere or plano)
Mixed	1 in front, 1 behind	−sph +cyl; +sph −cyl	(−sphere or +sphere depending on notation)
Simple hyperopic	1 on retina, 1 behind	+sph −cyl; plano +cyl	(+sphere or plano)
Compound hyperopic	Both behind retina	+sph +cyl; +sph −cyl	(+sphere regardless of notation)

Acquired hyperopia:
  Decreased effective axial length: retrobulbar tumor, choroidal tumor, central serous chorioretinopathy
  Decreased refractive power: lens change (posterior lens dislocation, aphakia, diabetes), drugs (chloroquine, phenothiazines, antihistamines, benzodiazepines), poor accommodation (tonic pupil, drugs, trauma), flattening of cornea (contact lens), intraocular silicone oil

Acquired myopia:
  Increased lens power: osmotic effect (diabetes, galactosemia, uremia, sulfonamides), nuclear sclerotic cataracts, anterior lenticonus, change in lens position or shape (medication [miotics]), anterior lens dislocation, excessive accommodation)
  Increased corneal power: keratoconus, congenital glaucoma, CL-induced corneal warpage
  Increased axial length: congenital glaucoma, posterior staphyloma, after scleral buckle, retinopathy of prematurity (ROP)

Night myopia: increased myopia in dark
  Pupil dilation: spherical aberration, irregular astigmatism uncovered
  Purkinje shift: spectral sensitivity shifts toward shorter wavelengths at lower light levels, and chromatic aberration moves the focal point anteriorly
  Dark focus: no accommodative target in dark; therefore, tend to overaccommodate for distance and underaccommodate for near
  Length of refraction lane: shorter than 20 feet produces 1/6 D undercorrection (add minus 0.25 D to final refraction)

Acquired astigmatism: lid lesion (tumor, chalazion, ptosis), pterygium, limbal dermoid, corneal degenerations and ectasias, surgery (corneal, cataract), lenticular, CB tumor

Accommodation

Eye gains plus power when crystalline lens becomes more convex

Accommodation response can be described as:

Amplitude of accommodation: total dioptric amount eye can accommodate
  Near point: only for emmetropes
  Prince rule: combines reading card with a ruler calibrated in centimeters and diopters to measure amplitude of accommodation

  Technique: place +3.00 D lens in front of distance correction to bring far point to 1/3 mm (33 cm); then, measure how near patient can read and convert into diopters; subtract far point from near point to determine amplitude
  Method of spheres: fixate on reading target (e.g., 40 cm), successively increase minus sphere until print blurs, then increase plus sphere until blurring occurs again; absolute difference between the spheres is the amplitude of accommodation

  EXAMPLE: range of −4.00 D to +2.00 D = amplitude of 6 D

Range of accommodation: distance between far point and near point; measured with tape measure or accommodative rule
  Far point: point on visual axis conjugate to retina when accommodation is completely relaxed
  Near point: point on visual axis conjugate to retina when accommodation is fully active
    FOR MYOPIA: near point = amount of myopia + amplitude of accommodation
    FOR HYPEROPIA: near point = difference between amplitude of accommodation and amount of hyperopia

Presbyopia: loss of accommodation with age; becomes symptomatic in early 40s with asthenopic symptoms and need for reading glasses

Theories of Accommodation:
  Helmholtz: zonular tension decreases, lens becomes more spherical, focusing power increases; presbyopia is due to loss of lens elasticity
  Tscherning-Schachar: equatorial zonular tension increases, lens diameter increases, central lens steepens, focusing power increases; lens grows throughout life, decreasing the working distance between lens and ciliary body; presbyopia is due to decreased ciliary muscle effectivity

Donder's Table (average accommodative amplitudes for different ages) (Table 1-2)
  Up to age 40, accommodation decreases by 1 D every 4 years (starting at 14 D at age 8)
  At age 40, accommodation is 6.0 D (±2 D)
  Between ages 40 and 48, accommodation decreases by 1.5 D every 4 years
  Above age 48, accommodation decreases by 0.5 D every 4 years

Conditions that cause asthenopia (eye fatigue with sustained near effort): hypothyroidism, anemia, pregnancy, nutritional deficiencies, chronic illness

Table 1–2. **Donder's Table**

Age:	8	12	16	20	24	28	32	36	40	44	48	52	56	60	64	68
Accommodation (D):	14	13	12	11	10	9	8	7	6	4.5	3	2.5	2	1.5	1	0.5

Premature presbyopia (subnormal accommodation): debilitating illness, diphtheria, botulism, mercury toxicity, head injury, CN3 palsy, Adie's tonic pupil, tranquilizers; treat with reading add, base-in prism (helps convergence)

Color Vision

3 components of color: hue, saturation, brightness

Hue: main component of color perception; depends on which wavelength is perceived as dominant

Saturation: richness of color; vivid colors are saturated; adding white desaturates color (paler) but does not change hue

Brightness: sensation produced by retinal illumination; filters decrease brightness

> **EXAMPLE**: yellow light; correct mixture of green and red also results in yellow; mixing 2 complements produces white; add white light to yellow, still yellow

Bezold-Brucke phenomenon: as brightness increases, most hues appear to change
  At low intensities, blue-green, green, and yellow-green appear greener; at high intensities, they appear bluer
  At low intensities, reds and oranges appear redder; at high intensities, they appear yellower
  Exception: blue of 478 nm, green of 503 nm, and yellow of 578 nm do not change with changes in intensity

Abney effect: as white is added to any hue, desaturating it, the hue appears to change slightly in color; all colors (except yellow) appear yellower

Luminosity curve: illustrates sensitivity to different wavelengths
  Constructed by asking observer to increase luminance of lights of various wavelengths until they appear equal in brightness to a yellow light of fixed luminance
  Light-adapted eye: yellow, yellow-green, and orange appear brighter than blues, greens, and reds; peak sensitivity = 555 nm
  Dark-adapted: peak sensitivity = 505 nm (blue)

Afterimages: after a color is stared at for 20 seconds, it begins to fade (desaturate)
  Then, with gazing at white background, the complement of the color appears (afterimage)
  > **EXAMPLE**: red is perceived when a greater number of red cones are stimulated than green or blue cones; after 20 seconds, red cones fatigue (cannot regenerate pigment fast enough), so color fades; when white background is looked at, there is a relatively greater response by green and blue cones; therefore, a blue-green afterimage is seen (complement of red)

Color Perception: white wall appears white because white paint reflects all photons equally well

Charcoal appears black because it absorbs most of the light that strikes it

Blue flower appears blue because it best absorbs red, yellow, and green; blue is absorbed least, so a greater number of blue photons are reflected

Green leaf appears green because chlorophyll absorbs blue and red and reflects green

Incandescent/tungsten light emits a relatively greater number of photons of longer (red) wavelength than shorter (blue) wavelength; conversely, fluorescent light emits a relatively greater number of blue and green wavelengths; therefore, a purple dress may appear redder under incandescent light and bluer under fluorescent light

PRESCRIBING GLASSES

Use cycloplegia in children and hyperopes to uncover full refractive error

Infants average 2 D of hyperopia; myopic shift between ages 8 and 13; most adults are emmetropic

Children: give full cycloplegic refraction

Table 1–3. **Guidelines for prescribing glasses for children**

Hyperopia:	≥+5D
Anisometropia	≥1.5D
Myopia:	
Up to age 1	≥−5D
Ages 1–6	≥−3D
Age >6	≥−1D
Anisometropia	≥3D
Astigmatism:	
Up to age 1	≥3D
Ages 1–6	≥2D
Age >6	≥1D
Anisometropia	≥1.5D

Adults: give manifest refraction; may not accept full astigmatic component, so if cylinder is decreased, adjust sphere to keep spherical equivalent constant; be careful about changing axis

Minus cylinder grinding: placing astigmatic correction on rear surface (closer to eye) is optically preferable
  Astigmatic dial: 12 spokes corresponding to clock hours are projected on screen; spokes parallel to principal meridians of eye's astigmatism are sharp (corresponding with focal lines of conoid of Sturm); the others are blurred

Match base curves: when prescribing new glasses, keep base curve same as that of old lenses

    Geneva lens clock: measures base curve of lens; direct dioptric power of convex, concave, or aspheric lens surface is read on the dial of the clock; calibration is based on the refractive index of crown glass (1.523)

Binocular balance: equally controls accommodation in both eyes (visual acuity must be equal)

    Methods:

1. *Prism dissociation*: 3^Δ BU over one eye and 3^Δ BD over the other (use Risley prism in phoroptor)
2. *Balanced fogging*: fog both eyes and alternate cover until equally fogged
3. *Duochrome test*: red-green balance both eyes (vision must be 20/30 or better)

Bifocal add: place segments as high as practical in relation to optical centers of the distance lenses

    Measure accommodation: perform monocularly, then binocularly

    Near point of accommodation (use refractive correction)

    Accommodative amplitude (use Prince rule)

    Determine accommodative requirement for near vision task

    EXAMPLE: reading at 40 cm = 2.5 D

    Hold 1/2 of measured accommodative amplitude in reserve to prevent asthenopic symptoms

    EXAMPLE: Prince rule measures 2.0 D of amplitude; thus, 1.0 D is available to patient

    Power of add is difference between accommodation (1.0 D) and total amount of accommodation required (2.5 D)

    With calculated add in front of distance correction, measure accommodative range (near point to far point of accommodation); if range is too close, reduce add in steps of 0.25 D until correct range found

Kestenbaum's rule: used to estimate strength of plus lens required to read newspaper print without accommodation

    Add power = reciprocal of best distance acuity

    Reciprocal of add power = working distance (in meters)

    EXAMPLE: 20/80 vision; add = 80/20 = +4.00 D; working distance = 1/4 (0.25 m)

Aphakic Spectacles: disadvantages include magnification of 25%, altered depth perception, pincushion distortion, ring scotoma (prismatic effect at edge of lens causes visual field loss of 20%), "jack-in-the-box" phenomenon (peripherally invisible objects suddenly appear when gaze is shifted)

CONTACT LENSES (CL)

Toric lens: lenses with different radii of curvature in each meridian

    Front toric: anterior surface with 2 different radii of curvature, posterior surface spherical; corrects lenticular astigmatism

    Back toric: cylinder on back surface only; corrects corneal astigmatism

    Bitoric: minus cylinder on posterior surface, plus cylinder on anterior surface; corrects corneal and lenticular astigmatism

Ballasted lens: heavier base to orient lens by gravity; 2 types

    Prism: 1.5 to 2^Δ BD prism added

    Truncated: flat along inferior edge

Sagittal depth/apical height: distance between back surface of lens center and a flat surface

Radius of curvature (base curve): curvature of posterior lens surface for a given diameter; the shorter the radius of curvature, the greater the sagittal depth (the steeper the lens)

Overall diameter: for a given base curve, increasing diameter increases the apical vault

    EXAMPLE: to tighten a lens, reduce radius of curvature or increase diameter

Oxygen transmission: DK (relative gas permeability) value; D = diffusion coefficient; K = solubility of oxygen in material; oxygen transmissibility = DK/L (L = lens thickness)

Accommodative demand: depends on magnification, which varies with different lens powers and vertex distances

    Hyperopes: decreased accommodative demand when CL are worn compared with spectacles (presbyopic symptoms appear earlier with spectacles)

    Myopes: increased accommodative demand when CL are used (presbyopic symptoms appear earlier with CL). In high myopia, spectacles induce base-in prism with near convergence, lessening requirement for convergence

Fitting rigid CL: SAM-FAP rule ("steeper add minus, flatter add plus")

    Fit steeper than corneal surface (forms a plus tear meniscus between cornea and CL, which alters required power of CL). Therefore, need to subtract power (add minus) at end of calculation; for each diopter, the base curve is made "steeper than K"; subtract 1D from the final CL power; if lens is fit flatter than K, a minus tear meniscus is formed, so must add plus power

    Remember, a rigid lens with base curve of 44 D does not have a power of 44 D; rather, the radius of the CL's central posterior curve is equal to the radius of curvature of a cornea with a calculated power of 44 D

Power calculation: if trial lens not available for over-refraction

1. Measure refraction and keratometry
2. Choose base curve steeper than low K (usually +0.50 D steeper to form a tear lens; tear lens prevents apical touch)
3. Convert refraction to minus cylinder form and zero vertex distance; disregard the cylinder (minus cylinder is formed by the tears)
4. Power of CL is sphere from refraction adjusted for tear lens (subtract +0.50); "SAM-FAP"

Evaluating fit:

Soft lens: evaluate movement (poor movement = too tight [too steep], excessive movement = too flat); choose power based on spherical equivalent

Rigid lens: assess fluorescein pattern

Figure 1-17. Fluorescein pattern of corneal contact lens fitted 1 D steeper than "flat K." Note the central clearance. (From White P, Scott C: Contact lenses. In Yanoff M, Duker JS [eds]: *Ophthalmology*, London, Mosby, 1999.)

Figure 1-18. Fluorescein pattern of corneal contact lens fitted "on K." Note the central alignment. (From White P, Scott C: Contact lenses. In Yanoff M, Duker JS [eds]: *Ophthalmology*, London, Mosby, 1999.)

Figure 1-19. Fluorescein pattern of corneal contact lens fitted 1 D flatter than "flat K." Note the central touch. (From White P, Scott C: Contact lenses. In Yanoff M, Duker JS [eds]: *Ophthalmology*, London, Mosby, 1999.)

LOW VISION AIDS

Kestenbaum's rule: estimates strength of plus lens required to read newspaper print without accommodation.

Near devices:

High bifocal add or single vision reading glasses (up to +20 D): large field of view but short reading distance

Magnifiers: handheld (up to +20 D; small field of view) or stand (up to +50 D; bulky)

Loupes: long working distance but small field of view

Electronic displays: high magnification but expensive

Distance devices:

Telescopes: restricted field of view

INTRAOCULAR LENSES (IOL)

Formulas for IOL calculation (see Chapter 10)

Empiric: derived from clinical studies by regression analysis

1ST GENERATION: SRK, Gills-Lloyd

2ND GENERATION: SRK II, Thompson-M, Donzis

Theoretical: derived from optics by vergence formulas

1ST GENERATION: Binkhorst I, Fyodorov, Colenbrander

2ND GENERATION: Binkhorst II, Shamas

3RD GENERATION: Hoffer Q, Holladay 1, SRK/T

4TH GENERATION: Holladay 2

Newer-generation theoretical formulas are the most accurate

A rough estimation of lens power can be quickly obtained with the SRK formula:

IOL power for emmetropia = $P = A - 2.5L - 0.9K$

A = A constant (related to lens type)

L = axial length in mm; 1 mm error = 2.5 D error in IOL power

K = average keratometry value in D; 1.0 D error ≈ 1.0 D error in IOL power

Lens position is important: 1 mm error = 1.0 D change in power

Calculate IOL power for refractive target other than emmetropia: $D_{IOL} = P - (R/1.5)$ (R = desired refractive error)

IOL power for a different lens = original IOL power ± difference in A constants

EXAMPLE: if instead of +20.0 D IOL with A constant of 118, want to use a different style IOL with A constant of 118.5, equivalent power of the new IOL is +20.5 D

OPHTHALMIC INSTRUMENTS

Direct ophthalmoscope: coaxial light and lenses to neutralize patient and examiner refractive errors, so retinas become conjugate; examiner uses optics of patient's eye as simple magnifier ($M_A = 60/4 = 15\times$); field of view ~7°

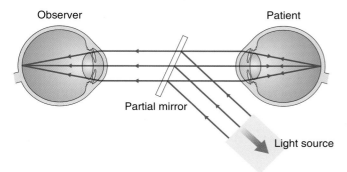

Figure 1-20. Optics of the direct ophthalmoscope. By using a mirror (either half-silvered or with a central aperture), the directions of the light of observation and the light incident to the patient are made concentric (coaxial). (From Miller D, Thall EH, Atebara NH: Ophthalmic instrumentation. In Yanoff M, Duker JS [eds]: *Ophthalmology*, 2nd ed, St. Louis, Mosby, 2004.)

Indirect ophthalmoscope: enlarged field of view (25°) with stereopsis by adding condensing lens between patient and examiner; binocular eyepiece reduces interpupillary distance to 15 mm (~4×); $M_A = D_{eye}/D_{lens} = 60/20 = 3\times$; $M_{Ax} = 3^2 = 9$, but eyepiece reduces depth 4×; therefore $M_{Ax} = 9/4 = 2.25\times$

→ Entering illumination beam
← Exiting observation beam

Figure 1-21. Theoretical optics of the indirect ophthalmoscope. The illumination beam enters a small part of the pupil and does not overlap with the observation beam; this minimizes bothersome reflection and backscatter. (From Miller D, Thall EH, Atebara NH: Ophthalmic instrumentation. In Yanoff M and Duker JS [eds]: *Ophthalmology*, 2nd ed, St. Louis, Mosby, 2004.)

Retinoscope: instrument to objectively measure refractive state of eye

- The blurred image of the filament on the patient's retina is considered a new light source returning to examiner's eye. By observing the characteristics of the reflex, examiner can determine patient's refractive error.
- If examiner is at far point of patient's eye, all light rays emanating from patient's pupil pass through retinoscope and examiner's pupil, and patient's pupil will appear uniformly illuminated (neutralization)
- If far point is between examiner and patient (myopic), reflex moves in direction opposite to retinoscope sweep ("against" motion)
- If far point is behind examiner (hyperopia), reflex has "with" motion
- Use correcting lens to determine point of neutralization
- Correct for working distance to obtain patient's final refraction (add reciprocal of working distance to final finding)
- If poor, irregular retinoscopic reflex, try contact lens overrefraction or stenopeic slit refraction

Slit-lamp biomicroscope: illumination and magnification allow stereo viewing of ocular structures; illumination and viewing arms have common pivot point

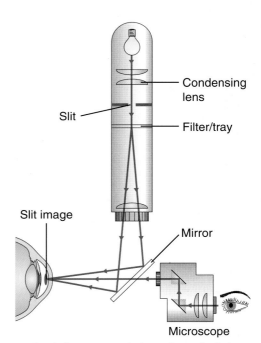

Figure 1-22. The slit lamp. Some slit lamps bring the light to a sharp focus within the slit aperture, and the light within the slit is focused by the condensing lens onto the patient's eyes. The observation system of a modern slit lamp has many potential reflecting surfaces—antireflection coatings on these surfaces help loss of light. (Modified from Spalton DJ, Hitchings RA, Hunter PA: *Atlas of Clinical Ophthalmology*, New York, Grower Medical, 1985.)

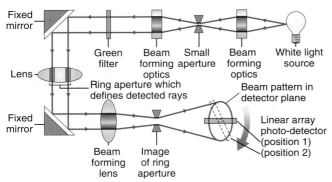

Figure 1-23. The lensometer resembles an optical bench. The movable illuminated target sends light to the field lens, with the target in the end-point position. Because the focal point of the field coincides with the position of the unknown lens, all final images are of the same size. (From Miller D, Thall EH, Atebara NH: Ophthalmic instrumentation. In Yanoff M, Duker JS [eds]: *Ophthalmology*, 2nd ed, St. Louis, Mosby, 2004.)

Figure 1-24. Optics of a typical automated lensometer. Parallel light strikes unknown lens. The refracted light rays (which are confined to a pencil beam within an annulus) ultimately strike an array of electronic photoreceptors. (From Miller D, Thall EH, Atebara NH: Ophthalmic instrumentation. In Yanoff M, Duker JS [eds]: *Ophthalmology*, 2nd ed, St. Louis, Mosby, 2004.)

Lensometer: measures power of spectacle or CL using telescope to detect neutralization point; distance measurement is determined from back vertex power; add measurement is taken from front vertex power; prism measurement is derived from displacement of target pattern (Figures 1-23 and 1-24)

Keratometer: measures curvature of anterior corneal surface based on power of reflecting surface; measures only 4 paracentral points 3 mm apart; doubling of image prevents interference from eye movements (Figure 1-25)

Applanation tonometry: direct measure of IOP as force/area with split-field prism; at applanated diameter of 3.06 mm, corneal resistance to deformation and attractive force of tear surface tension cancel each other

A- and B-scan ultrasonography: measure acoustic reflectivity of interfaces to provide 2-dimensional picture of ocular structures

Ocular coherence tomography (OCT): measures optical reflectivity to provide cross-sectional image of ocular structures

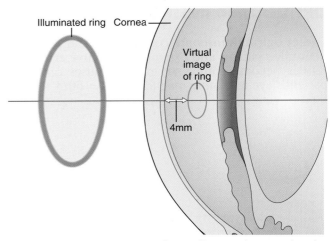

Figure 1-25. Keratometer principle. An illuminated ring is placed in front of the cornea, which acts as a convex mirror and produces a virtual image of the ring approximately 4 mm behind the cornea. (From Miller D, Thall EH, Atebara NH: Ophthalmic instrumentation. In Yanoff M and Duker JS [eds]: *Ophthalmology*, 2nd ed, St. Louis, Mosby, 2004.)

EQUATIONS

Vergence formula:
$$U + D = V$$
U = object vergence, D = lens power, V = image vergence

Lens power (diopters):
$$D = 1/f$$
f = focal length (meters)

Snell's law:
$$n \sin(i) = n' \sin(r)$$
n = refractive index, i = angle of incidence, r = angle of refraction

Prismatic power:
$$\Delta = \frac{\text{image deflection (cm)}}{\text{meters}} = 100 \tan(\beta)$$
β = angle of deviation

Prentice's rule:
$$\Delta = hD$$
h = distance from optical axis (cm), D = lens power

Reduced schematic eye (calculations of retinal image size):
$$\frac{I}{17\,mm} = \frac{O}{X}$$
I = retinal image size, O = object size, X = distance to object

Spherical equivalent = sphere + (cylinder/2)

Refracting power of a spherical surface:
$$D_s = \frac{n' - n}{r}$$
n'= refractive index to right
n= refractive index to left

r = radius of curvature of surface (m)
(+ = convex; − = concave)

Reflecting power of a spherical mirror:

$$D_r = \frac{-1}{f} = \frac{-2}{r}$$

f = focal length of mirror
r = radius of curvature of mirror
(− = convex; + = concave)

Power of a thin lens immersed in fluid:

$$\frac{D_{air}}{D_{aqueous}} = \frac{n_{IOL} - n_{air}}{n_{IOL} - n_{aqueous}}$$

Power of lens at new vertex distance:
$D_2 = D_1 + S(D_1)^2$
D_1 = original dioptric power of lens
D_2 = new dioptric power
S = difference in location (meters)

Linear magnification:
$M_L = I/O$
I = image distance or height
O = object distance or height

Axial magnification:
$M_{ax} = (M_L)^2$

Angular magnification:
$M_A = xD$
x = distance, D = dioptric power of lens
Simple magnifier:
$M_A = D/4$ (divide by 4 because distance set as
reading distance of 0.25 m)

EXAMPLE: 1× magnifier = +4 lens; 2× magnifier = +8 lens

Telescope (Galilean and astronomical):
$M_A = -D_e/D_o$
D_e = power of eyepiece
D_o = power of objective

Total accommodation through telescope:
$A_T = A_N(M_A)^2$
A_N = normal accommodation required
M_A = telescope magnification

IOL power (SRK):
P = A − 2.5 L − 0.9 K
A = A constant for type of IOL, L = axial length,
K = average keratometry value

AC/A ratio (accommodative converge/accommoda-tion): (see Chapter 5, Strabismus)
Normal = 3:1 to 5:1 (expressed as PD of deviation
per D of accommodation)
Calculations:
Heterophoria method: measure deviation with
fixation target at 6 m and at 1/3 m

$$AC/A = \frac{\text{deviation at near} - \text{deviation at distance}}{\text{accommodative demand}} + PD$$

PD = interpupillary distance (cm)

Lens gradient method: stimulate accommodation by measuring deviation with target at 6 m, then remea-suring with −1 D sphere in front of both eyes; or, relax accommodation by measuring deviation with target at 1/3 m, then remeasuring with +3 D sphere in front of both eyes

$$AC/A = \frac{\text{deviation with lens} - \text{deviation without lens}}{\text{lens power}}$$

Review Questions *(Answers start on page 355)*

1. Prince's rule is helpful in determining all of the following except
   a. amplitude of accommodation
   b. near point of accommodation
   c. far point of accommodation
   d. accommodative convergence

2. A myope who pushes his spectacles closer to his face and tilts them is
   a. decreasing effectivity, increasing cylinder
   b. decreasing effectivity, decreasing cylinder
   c. increasing effectivity, decreasing cylinder
   d. increasing effectivity, increasing cylinder

3. The Prentice position refers to
   a. glass prism perpendicular to visual axis
   b. glass prism in frontal plane
   c. plastic prism perpendicular to visual axis
   d. plastic prism in frontal plane

4. The purpose of Q-switching a laser is to
   a. increase energy, increase power
   b. decrease energy, increase power
   c. decrease energy, decrease power
   d. increase energy, decrease power

5. A 50-year-old woman with aphakic glasses wants a new pair of spectacles to use when applying make-up. How much power should be added to her distance correction so that she can focus while sitting 50 cm in front of her mirror?
   a. −2.00 D
   b. −1.00 D
   c. +1.00 D
   d. +2.00 D

6. How far from a plano mirror must a 6-ft-tall man stand to see his whole body?
   a. 2 feet
   b. 3 feet
   c. 6 feet
   d. 12 feet

7. A 33-year-old woman with a refraction of −9.00 +3.00 × 90 OD at vertex distance 10 mm and keratometry readings of 46.00@90/43.00@180 is fit for a rigid gas-permeable (RGP) contact lens 1 D steeper than flattest K. What power lens is required?
   a. −5.00 D
   b. −6.00 D
   c. −7.00 D
   d. −8.00 D

8. What is the size of a 20/60 letter on a standard 20-ft Snellen chart (tangent of 1 minute of arc = 0.0003)?
   a. 9 mm
   b. 15 mm
   c. 18 mm
   d. 27 mm

9. A Galilean telescope with a +5 D objective and a –20 D eyepiece produces an image with what magnification and direction?
   a. 4×, erect
   b. 4×, inverted
   c. 100×, erect
   d. 100×, inverted

10. An object is placed 33 cm in front of an eye. The image formed by reflection from the front surface of the cornea (radius of curvature equals 8 mm) is located
    a. 4 mm in front of cornea
    b. 4 mm behind cornea
    c. 8 mm in front of cornea
    d. 8 mm behind cornea

11. A convex mirror produces what type of image?
    a. virtual, inverted, magnified
    b. real, inverted, minified
    c. real, erect, magnified
    d. virtual, erect, minified

12. In general, the most bothersome problem associated with bifocals is
    a. image jump
    b. image displacement
    c. induced prism
    d. anisophoria

13. A refraction with a stenopeic slit gives the following measurements: +1.00 at 90° and –2.00 at 180°. The corresponding spectacle prescription is
    a. –2.00 + 1.00 × 90
    b. –2.00 + 1.00 × 180
    c. –2.00 + 3.00 × 180
    d. +1.00 + 3.00 × 90

14. A point source of light is placed 1/3 of a meter to the left of a +7 D lens. Where will its image come to focus?
    a. 25 cm to the right of the lens
    b. 25 cm to the left of the lens
    c. 10 cm to the right of the lens
    d. 10 cm to the left of the lens

15. What is the equivalent sphere of the following cross cylinder: –3.00 × 180 combined with +0.50 × 90?
    a. –1.00
    b. –1.25
    c. –1.50
    d. –1.75

16. What is the size of a letter on a standard 20-ft Snellen chart if it forms an image of 1/2 mm on a patient's retina?

    a. 59 cm
    b. 30 cm
    c. 25 cm
    d. 18 cm

17. The image of a distant object is largest in which patient?
    a. aphake with contact lens
    b. hyperope with spectacles
    c. emmetrope
    d. myope with spectacles

18. What type of image is produced if an object is placed in front of a convex lens within its focal length?
    a. erect and real
    b. erect and virtual
    c. inverted and real
    d. inverted and virtual

19. What is the correct glasses prescription if retinoscopy performed at 50 cm shows neutralization with a plano lens?
    a. –2.00
    b. –1.50
    c. plano
    d. +2.00

20. An anisometropic patient experiences difficulty while reading with bifocals. Which of the following is not helpful for reducing the induced phoria?
    a. dissimilar segments
    b. slab-off lens
    c. progressive lenses
    d. fresnel "press-on" prisms

21. A Geneva lens clock is used to measure what?
    a. thickness
    b. power
    c. index of refraction
    d. base curve

22. What is the induced prism when a 67-year-old woman reads 10 mm below the upper segment optical center of her bifocals, which measure +2.50 + 1.00 × 90 OD and –1.50 + 1.50 × 180 OS add +2.50 OU
    a. 4.0 prism diopters
    b. 3.5 prism diopters
    c. 2.5 prism diopters
    d. 2.0 prism diopters

23. The optimal size of a pinhole for measuring pinhole visual acuity is approximately
    a. 2.50 mm
    b. 2.00 mm
    c. 1.25 mm
    d. 0.75 mm

24. A person looking at an object 5 m away through a 10^Δ prism placed base-in over the right eye would see the image displaced
    a. 20 cm to the right
    b. 50 cm to the right

c. 20 cm to the left
d. 50 cm to the left

25. Calculate the soft contact lens power for a 40-year-old hyperope who wears +14.00 D glasses at a vertex distance of 11 mm.
    a. +15.00 D
    b. +16.00 D
    c. +17.00 D
    d. +18.00 D

26. After cataract surgery, a patient's refraction is −0.75 + 1.75 × 10, in what meridian should a suture be cut to reduce the astigmatism?
    a. 180°
    b. 100°
    c. 90°
    d. 10°

27. What is the appropriate correction in the IOL power if the A constant for the lens to be implanted is changed from 117 to 118?
    a. decrease IOL power by 1.0 D
    b. increase IOL power by 1.0 D
    c. decrease IOL power by 0.5 D
    d. increase IOL power by 0.5 D

28. An IOL labeled with a power of +20 D has a refractive index of 1.5. If this lens were removed from the package and measured with a lensometer, what power would be found?
    a. +10 D
    b. +13 D
    c. +30 D
    d. +59 D

29. The total cylindrical power of a 0.50 D cross cylinder is
    a. plano
    b. 0.25 D
    c. 0.50 D
    d. 1.00 D

30. To minimize image displacement in a hyperope, the best type of bifocal segment style is
    a. flat top
    b. progressive
    c. round top
    d. executive

31. The logMAR equivalent to 20/40 Snellen acuity is
    a. 0.4
    b. 0.3
    c. 0.2
    d. 0.1

SUGGESTED READINGS

American Academy of Ophthalmology: Optics, Refraction, and Contact Lenses, vol 3. San Francisco, AAO, 2004.

Benjamin WJ: Borish's Clinical Refraction. Philadelphia, WB Saunders, 1998.

MacInnes BJ: Ophthalmology Board Review: Optics and Refraction. St. Louis, Mosby, 1994.

Milder B, Rubin ML, Weinstein GW: The Fine Art of Prescribing Glasses Without Making a Spectacle of Yourself. Gainesville, Triad Scientific Publications, 1991.

Rubin ML: Optics for Clinicians. Gainesville, Triad Scientific Publications, 1993.

CHAPTER 2

Pharmacology

OSMOTICS: alter tonicity

INCREASE pH: increases nonionized (lipid soluble) form of drug, increasing corneal penetration (pH of tears = 7.4)

INCREASE VISCOSITY: viscous additives (methylcellulose, polyvinyl alcohol) increase contact time and therefore penetration

INCREASE CONTACT TIME: gels and oil-based ointment formulations (mineral oil, petrolatum); must be able to release drug

Therapeutic index: method of comparing potency of different antibiotics. A measure of relative effective (therapeutic) concentration of antibiotic at target site against a target organism.

Inhibitory quotient:

$$IQ = \frac{\text{concentration of drug in tissue}}{\text{minimum inhibitory concentration (MIC)}}$$

The most potent antibiotic has the lowest MIC (or highest IQ).

OCULAR PHARMACOLOGY

Pharmacodynamics: the study of the biochemical and physiologic effects of drugs and their mechanisms of action.

Pharmacokinetics: the study of the factors that determine the relationship between drug dosage and the change in concentration over time in a biological system.

Bioavailability: amount of drug absorbed (penetration into ocular tissues)

Depends on concentration, rate of absorption, tissue binding, transport, metabolism, and excretion

Methods of improving bioavailability:

INCREASE CONCENTRATION: limited by solubility and tonicity (hypertonicity causes reflex tearing, which dilutes and washes drug from the eye)

SURFACTANTS: surface-active agents alter cell membranes, increasing permeability of the corneal epithelium

ROUTES OF ADMINISTRATION

Topical: absorption related to corneal penetration

1 drop = 50 µL

Conjunctival cul-de-sac holds only 10 µL (20% of drop)

Drop diluted by reflex tearing and normal tear turnover: only ~50% of drug that reaches the cul-de-sac is present 4 minutes later (10% of drop)

Corneal barriers to penetration:

TIGHT JUNCTIONS (epithelium and endothelium): limit passage of hydrophilic drugs

STROMA (water rich): limits passage of lipophilic drugs

Methods of increasing absorption:

1. Add surfactants (disrupts epithelial integrity; e.g., benzalkonium chloride, topical anesthetic).
2. Promote punctal occlusion (decreases drainage).
3. Close eyelid after drops are placed.

4. Increase lipid solubility of drug (increases pH).
5. Increase frequency of drops.

Topical medications have systemic adverse effects because the drugs bypass hepatic "first-pass" metabolism (cul-de-sac → nasolacrimal duct → mucosa → bloodstream)

Examples of other delivery systems:

PRODRUG: dipivalyl epinephrine (propine; prodrug of epinephrine, less toxicity)

OINTMENT: drugs that have better uptake in ointment form, including tetracycline, chloramphenicol, and fluoromethalone

SUSTAINED RELEASE GEL: pilocarpine (Pilopine HS; decreased dosing)

INSERT: pilocarpine (Ocusert; membrane-controlled system; slow release over 1 week); hydroxypropyl cellulose (Lacrisert; artificial tears in slow-release pellet); collagen shield (bandage contact lens presoaked in antibiotic)

Subconjunctival/sub-Tenon's: increases duration and concentration, bypasses conjunctival and corneal barriers, avoids systemic toxicity; useful if poor compliance

Retrobulbar/peribulbar: used for anesthesia; alcohol or chlorpromazine (to kill pain fibers and ON in blind, painful eye)

Intraocular: direct ocular effects; beware toxicity (particularly from preservatives) retinal tear, RD, endophthalmitis; used intraoperatively and in retinal diseases including macular edema, CMV retinitis, CNV, endophthalmitis

Systemic: must cross blood-ocular barrier (blood-aqueous for anterior segment, blood-retinal for posterior segment); penetrance is improved with decreased molecular size, decreased protein binding, and increased lipid solubility

Concentration

1% solution = 1 g/100 mL = 10 mg/mL

> EXAMPLE: How much atropine is contained in 5 mL of a 2% solution?
> 2% = 2 g/100 mL = 20 mg/mL = 100 mg in 5 mL

ANESTHETICS

Mechanism: reversible blockade of nerve fiber conduction (block sodium channels); pH dependent (less effective at low pH [inflamed tissue])

Structure: 2 classes; do not necessarily have allergic cross-reactivity

Ester: hydrolyzed by plasma cholinesterase and metabolized in liver; cocaine, tetracaine, proparacaine, procaine, benoxinate

Amide: longer duration and less systemic toxicity; metabolized in liver; lidocaine, mepivacaine, bupivacaine

Topical: disturb intercellular junction of corneal epithelium (increase permeability)

Proparacaine (Ophthaine): 10- to 30-minute duration, corneal toxicity; may cause allergic dermatitis (also common with atropine and neomycin); does not necessarily have allergic cross-reactivity with tetracaine

Tetracaine (Pontacaine): similar to proparacaine but longer duration and more toxic to corneal epithelium

Benoxinate: similar to proparacaine; combined with fluorescein (Fluress) for tonometry

Cocaine: greatest epithelial toxicity; excellent anesthesia, sympathomimetic effect (test for Horner's syndrome)

Parenteral: may be used with epinephrine (1:100,000) to increase duration by preventing systemic absorption; also decreases bleeding; hyaluronidase (Wydase) 150 IU increases tissue penetration but decreases duration

Toxicity: hypotension, convulsions, nausea, vomiting

Lidocaine (Xylocaine): 1-hour duration (2 hours with epinephrine); used for local anesthesia/akinesia

Procaine (Novocain): 30- to 45-minute duration

Mepivacaine (Carbocaine): 2-hour duration

Bupivacaine (Marcaine): 6-hour duration

General: all agents decrease IOP except ketamine, chloral hydrate, N_2O, and ether

Malignant hyperthermia: rare, autosomal dominant condition that occurs after exposure to inhalation agents (most commonly halothane) or succinylcholine; more common in children and males

Interference with oxidative phosphorylation causes hypermetabolic crisis

FINDINGS: tachycardia (1st sign), tachypnea, unstable BP, arrhythmias, cyanosis, sweating, increased temperature, muscle contractions; later, heart failure and DIC develop; laboratory tests show respiratory and metabolic acidosis and increased K, Mg, myoglobin, CPK, hypoxemia, hypercarbia, myoglobinuria

SCREENING: elevated CPK, muscle biopsy/contracture test, platelet bioassay (decreased ATP in platelet exposed to halothane)

TREATMENT: stop anesthesia, hyperventilate, give sodium bicarbonate, cool patient (iced saline IV and lavage; surface cooling), mannitol and furosemide (Lasix), dantrolene (prevents release of calcium from sarcoplasmic reticulum), procainamide, insulin

PROGNOSIS: 50% to 60% mortality

AUTONOMIC SYSTEM

Sympathetic

Extensive system for mass response ("fight or flight")
Synapses near cord (superior cervical ganglion)
Long postganglionic nerves

Adrenergic receptors:
  α_1: smooth muscle contraction (arteries [decrease aqueous production by reducing ciliary body blood flow], iris dilator, Müller's muscle)
  α_2: feedback inhibition, ciliary body (decreases production and/or increases outflow)
  β_1: cardiac stimulation
  β_2: pulmonary and GI smooth muscle relaxation, ciliary body/trabecular meshwork (increase aqueous production, increase outflow facility)

Neurotransmitter: acetylcholine (ACh) at preganglionic terminal, epinephrine and norepinephrine (NE) at postganglionic terminal
  Monoamine oxidase (MAO) breaks down NE in nerve terminal; blocked by MAO inhibitors
  Catechol-O-methyltransferase (COMT) breaks down NE in effector cell
  Reserpine prevents storage of NE in nerve terminal
  Cocaine, tricyclics block reuptake of NE by nerve terminal (thus, potentiate its action)
  Hydroxyamphetamine increases release of NE from nerve terminal

Parasympathetic

More limited system for discrete response (homeostatic)
Synapses near end organ (ciliary ganglion)
Short postganglionic nerves

Cholinergic receptors:
  Nicotinic: somatic motor and preganglionic autonomic nerves (extraocular muscles, levator, orbicularis [outside eye])
  Muscarinic: postganglionic parasympathetic nerves (iris sphincter, ciliary muscle [inside eye])

Neurotransmitter: acetylcholine (ACh)
  Acetylcholinesterase (AchE) breaks down ACh

Cholinergic Drugs

Direct-acting agonists: act on end organ; therefore, do not need intact innervation; cause shallowing of AC; disruption of blood-aqueous barrier, miosis, brow ache, and decrease in IOP
  Acetylcholine (miochol: very short-acting, unstable, used intracamerally), methacholine, carbacholine (carbachol; direct and indirect acting), pilocarpine (less potent than ACh, but resistant to AChE; no miosis if IOP >40 mm Hg)

Table 2–1. **Autonomic system responses**

Organ/Function	Sympathetic (fight/flight)	Parasympathetic (homeostasis)
HR	Increase	Decrease
BP	Increase	Decrease
GI motility	Decrease	Increase
Bronchioles	Dilate	Constrict
Bladder	Constrict	Dilate
Vessels	Constrict	Dilate
Sweat	Decrease	Increase
Pupils	Dilate	Constrict
Eyelids	Elevate	Normal

Indirect-acting agonists: anticholinesterases (AChE); strongest agents; cause miosis and decrease in IOP.
  Reversible: physostigmine (eserine; treat lid lice), edrophonium (Tensilon; for diagnosis of myasthenia gravis), carbacholine
  Irreversible: echothiophate (phospholine iodide; treat glaucoma and accommodative ET; may cause iris cysts and subcapsular cataracts), isofluorophate (very long-acting, not used clinically), demecarium
  Adverse effects: cataract, RD, blocks metabolism of succinylcholine (prolonged respiratory paralysis) and ester anesthetics, can mimic acute abdomen (GI effects); antidote is pralidoxime (PAM) or atropine

Muscarinic antagonists: anticholinergics; cause deepening of AC, stabilization of blood-aqueous barrier, mydriasis, and cycloplegia
  Atropine (1- to 2-week duration; most allergenic), scopolamine (Hyoscine; 1 week duration; greater CNS toxicity than atropine), homatropine (1- to 3-day duration), cyclopentolate (Cyclogyl; 24-hour duration; beware CNS side effects with 2% solution, especially in children), tropicamide (Mydriacyl; 4- to 6-hour duration)
  Toxicity: mental status changes, hallucinations, tachycardia, urinary retention, dry mouth/skin, fever
  Antidote: physostigmine (1 to 4 mg IV)

Nicotinic antagonists:
  Nondepolarizing agents: gallamine, pancuronium; do not cause muscle contraction
  Depolarizing agents: succinylcholine, decamethonium; cause muscle contraction and elevated IOP; contraindicated for ruptured globe (EOM contraction can cause extrusion of intraocular contents)

Adrenergic Drugs

Sympathomimetics: may cause mydriasis, vasoconstriction, decreased IOP

> **Direct-acting α-agonists**: epinephrine, phenylephrine, dipivefrin, clonidine, apraclonidine, brimonidine, methyldopa, naphazoline (Naphcon), oxymetazoline (Afrin), tetrahydrozoline (Visine)
>
> **Direct-acting β-agonists**: epinephrine, isoproterenol, terbutaline, dopamine, albuterol
>
> **Indirect-acting agonists**: cocaine, hydroxyamphetamine (Paradrine), ephedrine

Sympatholytics: may cause decreased IOP

> **General blockers**: guanethidine, bethanidine, protriptyline, 6-hydroxydopamine
>
> **α-blockers**: thymoxamine, dibenamine, phentolamine, prazosin, labetalol, dapiprazole (Rev-Eyes; miosis)
>
> **β-blockers**: timolol, levobunolol, betaxolol, metipranolol, carteolol, propranolol, metoprolol, atenolol, nadolol, pindolol

OCULAR HYPOTENSIVE (GLAUCOMA) MEDICATIONS

β-Blockers

Mechanism: reduce aqueous production (inhibit Na^+/K^+ pump)

Loss of effectiveness over time due to downregulation of β-receptors (long-term drift)

Adverse effects: bradycardia, heart block, bronchospasm, impotence, lethargy, depression, headache, rarely diarrhea and hallucinations, alopecia, dermatitis; may mask hypoglycemia

Nonselective (β_1 and β_2): timolol (Timoptic), levobunolol (Betagan), metipranolol (Optipranolol), carteolol (Ocupress)

> 10% do not show a therapeutic effect; inhibit lipoprotein lipase (break down chylomicrons and VLDL) and cholesterol acyltransferase (incorporate cholesterol into HDL); may cause decreased HDL levels
>
> Carteolol has intrinsic sympathomimetic activity

Cardioselective ($\beta_1 \gg \beta_2$): betaxolol (Betoptic)
Fewer pulmonary adverse effects

> **Indications**: patients with pulmonary problems who cannot tolerate nonselective β-blocker; often used for normal tension glaucoma; may not cause as much vasoconstriction of vessels supplying ON

α₂-Agonists

Aproclonidine (Iopidine), **brimonidine** (Alphagan-P)

> **Mechanism**: reduce aqueous production

> **Adverse effects**: allergy, superior lid retraction, dry mouth, blanching of conjunctival vessels, miosis, lethargy, headache

Dipivefrin (Propine): prodrug of epinephrine (converted into epinephrine in cornea by esterases), lower concentration and increased solubility vs epinephrine (penetrates cornea 17× better); thus, less toxicity and fewer adverse effects

> **Mechanism**: improves aqueous outflow, slightly reduces aqueous production
>
> **Adverse effects**: allergy, CME in aphakia, hypertension, tachycardia (fewer systemic adverse effects than epinephrine)

Epinephrine: 1% to 2% is equivalent to propine 0.1%; 3 salt forms: hydrochloride, borate, bitartrate (1st two are equivalent, 2% bitartrate is equivalent to 1% hydrochloride or borate)

> **Mechanism**: improves aqueous outflow, slightly reduces aqueous production
>
> **Adverse effects**: allergy, CME in aphakia (reversible), hypertension, tachycardia, arrhythmias, adrenochrome (black) deposits in conjunctiva

Miotics

Mechanism: increase aqueous outflow (contraction of ciliary muscle opens trabecular meshwork), decrease uveoscleral outflow

Pilocarpine: acetylcholine agonist; peak action at 2 hours, 8-hour duration

> Beware for treatment of angle-closure: causes shallowing of AC and narrowing of angle, but miosis pulls peripheral iris away from angle, balancing out the other effects
>
> **Adverse effects**: headache, accommodative spasm, miosis (dimming, reduction of vision), myopia (forward shift of lens-iris diaphragm), pupillary block, follicular conjunctivitis, dermatitis, rarely retinal tear
>
> **Other effects**: breakdown of blood-aqueous barrier, reduction of uveoscleral outflow

Carbachol: acetylcholine agonist and acetylcholinesterase inhibitor; stronger effect and longer duration of action; poor corneal penetration; needs corneal surface disrupter (benzalkonium chloride)

> **Miostat**: intraocular formulation used during surgery for pupillary miosis

Echothiophate (phospholine iodide): cholinesterase inhibitor; 3-week duration; also used in accommodative esotropia

> **Adverse effects**: greater orbicularis, ciliary, and iris muscle spasm; cataracts in adults (therefore, use only in aphakic or pseudophakic patients); iris cysts in children (proliferation of iris pigment epithelium; phenylephrine prevents cyst formation); decreased serum pseudocholinesterase

activity (can accentuate succinylcholine effects during general anesthesia)

Carbonic Anhydrase Inhibitors

Mechanism: decrease bicarbonate formation in ciliary body epithelium; bicarbonate formation is linked to Na^+ and fluid transport, so CAIs reduce aqueous production

Carbonic anhydrase catalyzes the reaction: $CO_2 + H_2O \leftrightarrow H_2CO_3$

Amount of carbonic anhydrase is 100× that needed for aqueous production; so, >99% must be inhibited to achieve IOP decrease

Sulfonamide derivative (do not administer to patients with sulfa allergy)

Oral: acetazolamide (Diamox; PO/IV), methazolamide (Neptazane; PO; more lipid soluble, less toxicity)
  Adverse effects: metabolic acidosis (IV administration causes greater metabolic acidosis), kidney stones (reduced excretion of urinary citrate or magnesium), hypokalemia (especially when used with other diuretics; very dangerous with digoxin), paresthesias (hands/feet/lips), GI upset, diarrhea, lethargy, loss of libido, metallic taste, aplastic anemia, Stevens-Johnson syndrome; transient myopia

Topical: dorzolamide (Trusopt), brinzolamide (Azopt)
  Adverse effects: metallic taste, paresthesias, malaise, weight loss, depression, skin rash, corneal edema

Prostaglandin Analogues/Prostanoids

Mechanism: increase uveoscleral outflow

Latanaprost (Xalatan), **bimatoprost** (Lumigan), **travoprost** (Travatan), **unoprostone** isopropyl (Rescula): prostaglandin $F_{2\alpha}$ analogs
  Adverse effects: flu-like symptoms, hyperemia, eyelash growth, iris pigmentation (increases number of melanosomes), CME, reactivation of HSV keratitis

Hyperosmotic Agents

Mechanism: low-molecular weight substances that increase serum osmolality to draw fluid out of eye (reduces vitreous volume)

Adverse effects: headache, thirst, nausea, vomiting, diarrhea, diuresis, dizziness; IV agents can cause subarachnoid hemorrhage

Urea (IV; 30% solution): not commonly used; extravasation causes tissue necrosis

Mannitol (Osmitrol; IV; 20% solution): most potent; may exacerbate congestive heart failure

Glycerin (Osmoglyn; PO; 50% solution): may cause hyperglycemia in diabetics (metabolized by liver into glucose)

Isosorbide (Ismotic; PO): not metabolized (can be used in diabetics); secreted 95% unchanged in urine

Other hyperosmotic agents: used topically for corneal edema
  Glycerin (Ophthalgan; topical; 100% solution): used to clear corneal edema for examination or laser procedure
  Muro 128 (hypertonic saline; topical; drops or ointment; 2.5% or 5% solution): used to reduce epithelial edema of cornea, especially in treatment of recurrent erosions

Order of Allergy

Greatest to least: iopidine > epinephrine > propine > brimonidine > β-blocker > pilocarpine

ANTI-INFLAMMATORY DRUGS

The Inflammatory Pathway: (Figure 2-1)

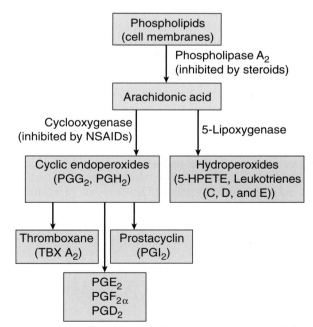

Figure 2-1. The inflammatory pathway. NSAIDs, nonsteroidal anti-inflammatory drugs; PG, prostaglandin; 5-HPETE, 5-hydroperoxy-eicosatetraenoic acid.

Nonsteroidal Antiinflammatory Drugs (NSAIDs)

Mechanism: inhibit cyclooxygenase pathway

Classes:
  Salicylates: ASA, diflunisal, salicylamide
  Acetic acids: indomethacin, diclofenac (Voltaren), sulindac, etodolac, ketorolac (Acular, Toradol)

Phenylalkanoic acids: ibuprofen, suprofen (Profenal), flurbiprofen (Ocufen), naproxen, fenoprofen, ketoprofen

Cyclooxygenase-2 inhibitors: celebrex, vioxx

Indications:

Prevent miosis during intraocular surgery: Profenal, Ocufen

Allergic conjunctivitis, corneal pain, postsurgical inflammation, CME: Voltaren, Acular

Scleritis, uveitis: oral agents

Steroids

Mechanism: anti-inflammatory and immunosuppressive by inhibiting release of arachidonic acid, inhibiting release of lysosomal enzymes, preventing macrophage migration, interfering with lymphocyte function, decreasing fibroblast activity, inhibiting neovascularization, and reducing capillary permeability

Preparations:

Phosphate: hydrophilic; poor penetration of intact corneal epithelium (improved penetration with epithelial defect)

Alcohol: biphasic; penetrate intact cornea

Acetate: more biphasic; best corneal penetration

Potency: increased by 1-2 double bond, 9 fluorination, 6 methylation, O at C11; IOP elevation from deoxygenation at C21 (Table 2-2 and Table 2-3)

Derivatives of progesterone (weaker): FML, medrysone

Subconjunctival/sub-Tenon's injection: produces higher ocular concentration and longer duration; beware in IOP responder

Other routes of administration: oral, IV, intraocular Oral dose of 7.5 mg dexamethasone results in intravitreal concentration of therapeutic levels

Table 2–2. Relative potencies of steroids

Steroid	Relative Potency
Hydrocortisone	1 (the standard)
Cortisone	0.8
Prednisone	4
Prednisolone	5
Dexamethasone	25–30
Betamethasone	25–30
Fluoromethalone	40–50
Triamcinolone	4
Fluocinolone	240

Table 2–3. Common ophthalmic steroids

Generic Name	Trade Name
Topical	
Prednisolone acetate 1%	Pred Forte, Econo Pred
Fluoromethalone acetate 0.1%	Flarex
Dexamethasone alcohol 0.1%	Maxidex
Fluoromethalone alcohol 0.1%	FML
Prednisolone phosphate 1%	Inflamase
Dexamethasone phosphate 1%	Decadron
Subconjunctival	
Dexamethasone phosphate	Decadron
Methylprednisolone acetate	Solumedrol, Depomedrol
Prednisolone acetate	Durapred
Triamcinolone acetonide	Kenalog
Betamethasone	Celestone

Indications: conjunctivitis, keratitis, scleritis, uveitis, hyphema, CME, macular edema, CNV, endophthalmitis

Adverse effects:

Systemic: adrenal insufficiency, hyperglycemia, hypertension, hypokalemia, peptic ulcers, delayed wound healing, superinfection, emotional lability, psychosis, growth retardation, muscle atrophy, osteoporosis, aseptic necrosis of the hip, hirsutism, weight gain, cushingoid appearance, pseudotumor cerebri

Ocular: cataracts (PSC), elevated IOP, delayed wound healing/corneal re-epithelialization, secondary infections

IOP-elevating potential: dexamethasone > prednisolone > fluoromethalone > hydrocortisone > tetrahydrotriamcinolone > medrysone (after 6 weeks of dexamethasone therapy, 42% have IOP >20 mm Hg; 6% have IOP >31)

Steroids with less IOP elevating potential: fluoromethalone (FML), rimexolone (Vexol), loteprednol (Lotemax, Alrex)

ANTIALLERGY MEDICATIONS

Antihistamines/Vasoconstrictors (over-the-counter)

Naphazoline hydrochloride/pheniramine maleate (OcuHist, Opcon-A, Naphcon-A), **Naphazoline hydrochloride/antazoline phosphate** (Vasocon-A): vasoconstrictor naphazoline temporarily removes redness, but can cause rebound redness with chronic use

Mast Cell Stabilizer

Cromolyn (Crolom; Opticrom): reduces permeability of mast cell plasma membrane, preventing release of histamine; reduces phosphodiesterase activity (facilitator of mast cell degranulation); inhibits activation of neutrophils, monocytes, and eosinophils; does not interfere with binding of antigen to previously sensitized cells; no antihistamine activity therefore useful for chronic allergies, not for acute symptomatic relief

H₁-Blockers + Mast Cell Stabilizers + NSAID

Nedocromil (Alocril), **Pemirolast** (Alamast), **Ketotifen** (Zaditor), **Azelastine** (Optivar), **Epinastine** (Elestat): triple-action drugs are effective against itch, less on redness

Mast Cell Stabilizer + Eosinophil Suppressor

Lodoxamide (Alomide): 2500 times more potent than cromolyn; also inhibits eosinophil activation

H₁-Blockers (antihistamines)

Levocabastine (Livostin), **Emedastine** (Emadine): pure H₁-specific receptor antagonists; bind to histamine receptors (inhibit itching and hyperemia)

H₁-Blocker + Mast Cell Stabilizer

Olopatadine (Patanol): stabilizes mast cells and binds to H₁ receptors (inhibits itching); binds to H₂ receptors at low level (inhibits hyperemia)

IMMUNOSUPPRESSIVE AGENTS

Cytotoxic Antimetabolites

Inhibit purine ring biosynthesis

Methotrexate: folate analogue; inhibits folate metabolism; inhibits synthesis of deoxythymidine monophosphate nucleotide; inhibits enzyme dehydrofolate reductase; inhibits T-cell function
  Adverse effects: leukopenia, thrombocytopenia, hepatotoxicity, lung or renal toxicity; teratogenic; periorbital edema, hyperemia

Azathioprine (Imuran): purine analogue

Cytotoxic Alkylating Agents

Create cross-linkage between DNA strands, resulting in inhibition of transcription of mRNA and prevention of DNA synthesis

Chlorambucil (Leukeran): interacts with 7-guanine of DNA, resulting in strand breakage or cross-linkage
  Adverse effects: sterility, bone marrow suppression

Cyclophosphamide (Cytoxan):
  Adverse effects: hemorrhagic cystitis (oral > IV), sterility, bone marrow suppression
  Prevent hemorrhagic cystitis with high water intake (IV or oral)

Cytostatic Anti-Inflammatories

Steroids (see earlier)

Immune Modulator

Cyclosporine: blocks production of IL-2 and IL-2 receptors, inhibits proliferation of lymphocytes, inhibits T-cell activation and recruitment, interferes with production of IL-2 by T cells, prevents formation of IL-2 receptors by T cells; natural product of fungi
  Indications:
    TOPICAL: necrotizing scleritis, Sjögren's syndrome/dry eye syndrome, ligneous conjunctivitis, atopic keratoconjunctivitis
    SYSTEMIC: Mooren's ulcer, uveitis in Behçet's or sympathetic ophthalmia, prevention of corneal transplant rejection; also used in OCP and thyroid-related ophthalmopathy
  Adverse effects (systemic administration only): renal toxicity (renal tubular atrophy, interstitial fibrosis), hypertension, paresthesia, elevated ESR, hypertrichosis, hepatotoxicity, hyperuricemia

Others

Colchicine: inhibits leukocyte migration; prevents recurrence of Behçet's

Oncolytic agents:
  Antineoplastics: bleomycin, dactinomycin, mitomycin (topically in glaucoma, corneal and pterygium surgery), daunorubicin, doxorubicin
    ADVERSE EFFECTS: anemia, SJS syndrome, decreased vision, conjunctivitis, tearing
  Alkylating agents: busulfan, carmustine, chlorambucil, cyclophosphamide
    ADVERSE EFFECTS: rare
  Vinca alkaloids: vincristine, vinblastine
    ADVERSE EFFECTS: diplopia, nystagmus, ptosis, CN palsies
  Antiestrogen: tamoxifen
    ADVERSE EFFECTS: corneal opacities, retinopathy

Heavy metals: cisplatin
  ADVERSE EFFECTS: papilledema, optic neuritis
Antimetabolites: methotrexate, 5-fluorouracil (topically in glaucoma surgery)
  ADVERSE EFFECTS: periorbital edema, conjunctival hyperemia, photophobia, tearing; corneal epithelial erosions

ANTI-INFECTIVE DRUGS

Antibiotics

Inhibitors of Intermediary Metabolism

Sulfonamides: static; sulfacetamide, sulfadiazine, sulfisoxizole, sulfamethoxazole; resistance is problem
  Mechanism: inhibit folic acid synthesis
  Spectrum: Gram-positives and Gram-negatives; also, toxoplasmosis, *Chlamydia*, *Actinomyces*, *Pneumocystis*
  Indications: blepharitis, conjunctivitis, toxoplasmosis
  Adverse effects: allergy (SJS syndrome), transient myopia
  Pyrimethamine (Daraprim):
    ADVERSE EFFECTS: bone marrow depression (anemia, thrombocytopenia; prevent with use of folinic acid [Leucovorin])
  Dapsone:
    INDICATIONS: OCP, leprosy
    CONTRAINDICATIONS: patients allergic to sulfa or with G6PD deficiency

Trimethoprim: blocks next step in folate metabolism; often combined with sulfamethoxazole (Bactrim)
  Spectrum: Gram-positives and Gram-negatives (*Staphylococcus*, *Streptococcus*, *Serratia*, *Proteus*, *Haemophilus*, *Enterobacter*, *Escherichia coli*, *Klebsiella*)
  Indications: conjunctivitis

Inhibitors of Cell Wall Synthesis

β-Lactams (cidal)

Penicillins (PCN): least toxic; variable protein binding
  Adverse effects: allergy, diarrhea
  Penicillin G:
    SPECTRUM: *Streptococcus* and non–penicillinase-producing *Staphylococcus*, *Neisseria*, *Treponema pallidum*
    INDICATIONS: syphilis
  Isoxazolyl PCNs: penicillinase-resistant; methicillin, nafcillin, oxacillin, cloxacillin, dicloxacillin
    SPECTRUM: extended to *Staphylococcus aureus*
  Amino PCNs: broader spectrum; ampicillin, amoxicillin
    SPECTRUM: Gram-positives (except Staph), *Neisseria*, *Haemophilus*, *Proteus*, *Shigella*, *Salmonella*, *Listeria*, *Escherichia coli*
    INDICATIONS: preseptal cellulitis

Carboxy PCNs: anti-pseudomonal; carbenicillin, ticarcillin
    SPECTRUM: extended to Gram-negatives (*Pseudomonas* and Enterobacteriaceae) and anaerobes (*Bacteroides*)
  Ureido PCNs: anti-pseudomonal; piperacillin, mezlocillin, azlocillin
    SPECTRUM: extended to Gram-negatives (*Pseudomonas* and Enterobacteriaceae) and anaerobes (*Bacteroides*)
  β-Lactamase Inhibitors: combined with PCNs to increase spectrum of activity; clavulanate (amox/clavulanate = Augmentin), sulbactam (amp/sulbactam = Unasyn)

Cephalosporins: more resistant to β-lactamases; 20% cross-react with PCN-allergic patients
  1st generation: cefazolin (Ancef, Kefzol), cephalexin (Keflex), cephalothin (Keflin), cefaclor (Ceclor)
    SPECTRUM: Gram-positives (Staph, Strep) and some Gram-negatives
    INDICATIONS: cefazolin for keratitis, endophthalmitis
  2nd generation: cefamandole (Mandol), cefonicid (Monocid), cefotetan (Cefotan), cefoxitin (Mefoxin), cefuroxime (Zinacef)
    SPECTRUM: better Gram-negative but less Gram-positive, anaerobic (cefoxitin, cefotetan), *Haemophilus influenzae* and *Neisseria* (cefuroxime)
  3rd generation: cefoperazone (Cefobid), cefotaxime (Claforan), ceftazidime (Tazidime), ceftizoxime (Cefizox), ceftriaxone (Rocephin), moxalactam (Moxam)
    SPECTRUM: even better Gram-negative, *Pseudomonas* (ceftazidime)

Monobactams (aztreonam): aerobic Gram-negatives

Carbapenems (imipenem): β-lactamase resistant; very broad activity (almost all Gram-positives, Gram-negatives, and anaerobes); does not cover methicillin-resistant *Staphylococcus aureus* (MRSA)

Non β-Lactams (cidal)

Polymyxin B: basic peptides; act as detergents and disrupt cell membrane
  Spectrum: Gram-negatives (*Haemophilus*, *Enterobacter*, *Escherichia coli*, *Klebsiella*, *Pseudomonas*)
  Indications: conjunctivitis (combined with trimethoprim [Polytrim])

Bacitracin: polypeptides; often used in combination with neomycin or polymyxin to broaden activity
  Spectrum: Gram-positives, *Neisseria*, *Haemophilus*, *Actinomyces*
  Indications: blepharitis, conjunctivitis

Vancomycin: glycopeptide
  Spectrum: very good for Gram-positives; staph (including MRSA), strep (including PCN- resist-

ant strains), *Bacillus*, *Propionibacterium acnes*, *Clostridium difficile*
Indications: keratitis, endophthalmitis
Adverse effects: systemic administration is associated with ototoxicity and nephrotoxicity

Inhibitors of Protein Synthesis

Aminoglycosides: cidal; inhibit 30S ribosome; poor GI absorption
Gentamycin (better for *Serratia*), tobramycin (better for *Pseudomonas*), amikacin (best for *Pseudomonas* and *Mycobacterium*; less nephrotoxic than gent), streptomycin (TB, *S viridans*), neomycin (*Acanthamoeba*; allergy common), paromomycin (*Acanthamoeba*), kanamycin
Spectrum: Gram-negative bacilli and some staph (gent and tobra are active against *S aureus* and *S epidermidis*)
Indications: conjunctivitis, keratitis, endophthalmitis
Adverse effects: systemic administration is associated with ototoxicity and nephrotoxicity, allergy

Spectinomycin: cidal; inhibits 30S ribosome; not an aminoglycoside; used for *Neisseria*

Tetracyclines: static; inhibit 30S ribosome; take on empty stomach (chelates calcium, antacids; iron, causing decreased absorption)
Tetracycline, doxycycline, minocycline, meclocycline
Spectrum: Gram-positive and Gram-negative, *Chlamydia*, *Rickettsia*, *Mycoplasma*
Indications: prophylaxis and treatment of ophthalmia neonatorum, *Chlamydia*; also rosacea, meibomianitis, scleral melting (due to anti-inflammatory and anticollagenolytic properties)
Adverse effects: GI upset, phototoxic dermatitis, tooth discoloration in children, teratogenic, nephrotoxicity and hepatotoxicity, decreased prothrombin activity (potentiates Coumadin)

Macrolides: static; inhibit 50S ribosome
Erythromycin, azithromycin, clarithromycin
Spectrum: Gram-positives and a few Gram-negatives, *Chlamydia*, *Mycoplasma*, *Legionella*
Indications: blepharitis, conjunctivitis, *Chlamydia*
Adverse effects: GI upset

Chloramphenicol: static; inhibits 50S ribosome
Spectrum: Gram-positives and Gram-negatives, anaerobes, *Chlamydia*, *Rickettsia*, *Mycoplasma*, spirochetes
Adverse effects: risk of aplastic anemia and reversible bone marrow suppression

Clindamycin: static; inhibits 50S ribosome
Spectrum: Gram-positives and anaerobes, toxoplasmosis
Indications: toxoplasmosis

Adverse effects: may cause pseudomembranous colitis (due to overgrowth of *C difficile*; treat with vancomycin or metronidazole)

Others

Fluoroquinolones: cidal; analogues of nalidixic acid; inhibitors of genetic replication; inhibit DNA gyrase (topoisomerase II) and topoisomerase IV; low resistance
2nd generation: ciprofloxacin (Ciloxan), ofloxacin (Ocuflox), norfloxacin (Chibroxin)
3rd generation: levofloxacin (Quixin)
4th generation: gatifloxacin (Zymar), moxifloxacin (Vigamox)
Spectrum: aerobic Gram-negatives and some Gram-positives (*Haemophilus influenzae*, *Pseudomonas*, Enterobacteriaceae, *S aureus*); also, *Chlamydia*, *Rickettsia*, *Mycoplasma*, and *Mycobacterium*. 4th generation agents have extended spectrum with enhanced activitiy against Gram-positives, fluoroquinolone-resistant organisms, and atypical mycobacteria
Indications: conjunctivitis, keratitis, surgical prophylaxis; prophylaxis in penetrating trauma (oral cipro achieves high levels in vitreous)
Adverse effects: GI upset; cartilage damage in children

Anti-TB Agents

Isoniazid: cidal; inhibits cell wall synthesis of mycobacteria
Adverse effects: hepatotoxicity, vitamin B$_6$ deficiency

Rifampin: inhibits RNA polymerase of mycobacteria
Adverse effects: hepatotoxicity, turns body fluids orange-red

Pyrazinamide: unknown mechanism; analogue of nicotinamide
Adverse effects: hepatotoxicity, gout

Ethambutol: chelates metals
Adverse effects: may cause optic neuropathy

Fumagillin: treatment of microsporidia keratoconjunctivitis

Antivirals

Mechanism: static; inhibit genetic replication; most are nucleotide analogues

Topical: treatment of HSV keratitis
Idoxuridine (Stoxil): can cause follicular conjunctivitis, corneal epitheliopathy, punctal stenosis
Vidarabine (Vira-A): adverse effects less severe than IDU
Trifluorothymidine (Viroptic): inhibits thymidylate synthetase (virus-specific enzyme); best tolerated

Systemic:
  Acyclovir (Zovirax; guanosine analogue; activated only by thymidine kinase (virus-specific enzyme)), *valacyclovir* (Valtrex; prodrug of acyclovir), *penciclovir, famciclovir* (Famvir; prodrug of peniclovir)
    INDICATIONS: treatment of HSV and VZV
    ADVERSE EFFECTS: may cause GI upset; high doses can cause nephrotoxicity and neurotoxicity
  Ganciclovir (Cytovene): treatment of CMV
    ADVERSE EFFECTS: bone marrow suppression (cannot use with AZT)
  Foscarnet (Foscavir): treatment of CMV
    ADVERSE EFFECTS: nephrotoxicitiy, less myelosuppression

Antifungals

Mechanism: disrupt cell membranes

Classification:
  Yeasts: form pseudohyphae; *Candida, Cryptococcus*
  Molds: filamentous; form hyphae
    SEPTATE: *Fusarium, Aspergillus, Penicillium, Curvularia, Paecilomyces, Phialophora*
    NONSEPTATE: *Phycomycetes, Rhizopus, Mucor*
  Dimorphic fungi: grow as yeast or mold; *Histoplasma, Blastomyces, Coccidioides*

Polyenes: bind to ergosterol
  Amphotericin B: systemic
    SPECTRUM: broad (especially *Candida*; also, *Cryptococcus, Blastomyces, Histoplasma, Coccidioides*, mucormycosis; not as good for *Aspergillus, Fusarium*)
    INDICATIONS: keratitis, endopthalmitis (IVDA, immunosuppression, hyperalimentation)
    ADVERSE EFFECTS: fever, hypotension, headache, phlebitis, GI upset, nephrotoxicity, anemia
  Natamycin: topical only; too toxic for IV use, toxic to retina intravitreally
    SPECTRUM: filamentous fungi (especially *Aspergillus, Fusarium*), not as good for *Candida*; not effective against *Mucor* (nonseptate, branching hyphae)
    INDICATIONS: keratitis (removal of epithelium improves penetration)

Azoles: inhibit ergosterol synthesis; second-line agents to amphotericin; also used for *Acanthamoeba*
  Adverse effects: GI upset, headache, rash
  Imidazoles:
    MICONAZOLE (topical, IV, intravitreal): broad spectrum (filamentous fungi and yeast)
      ADVERSE EFFECTS: may cause corneal erosions, anemia
    KETOCONAZOLE (topical, oral): broad spectrum
      ADVERSE EFFECTS: reversible hepatotoxicity
    CLOTRIMAZOLE (oral): good for *Aspergillus*

ADVERSE EFFECTS: hepatotoxicity
  Triazoles: safer
    ITRACONAZOLE (oral): broad spectrum
    FLUCONAZOLE

Antimetabolites: most fungi are resistant, except *Cryptococcus* and some *Candida*
  Flucytosine: converted to 5-FU, disrupts DNA synthesis
    ADVERSE EFFECTS: myelosuppression, nausea, vomiting, diarrhea

Antiamoebics

Mechanism: cidal (amoebae and cysts); cationic surface-active properties; interfere with cell membranes and inhibit enzymes

Indications: topical for *Acanthamoeba* keratitis

Biguanides: polyhexamethylene biguanide (PHMB), chlorhexidine; first-line agents, less corneal toxicity

Diamidines: propamidine (Brolene), hexamidine; synergistic effect with biguanides, corneal toxicity

Antihelmintics

Mebendazole, thiabendazole, albendazole: inhibit glucose uptake and microtubule synthesis
  Adverse effects: GI upset

Pyrantel pamoate: neuromuscular junction blocker
  Adverse effects: nausea, vomiting, headache, rash

Diethylcarbamazine: enables phagocytosis of microfilaria

Ivermectin: increases GABA release paralyzing microfilaria
  Adverse effects: fever, headache, rash

Praziquantel: causes calcium loss, paralyzing worm
  Adverse effects: GI upset, fever

MISCELLANEOUS

Aminocaproic acid (Amicar): synthetic amino acid similar to lysine
  Mechanism: antifibrinolytic; stabilizes blood clot, delays lysis, decreases secondary hemorrhages
  Indications: hyphema
  Contraindications: hypercoagulable states, pregnancy, renal disease, liver disease, patients at risk for MI, pulmonary embolism, CVA
  Adverse effects: nausea, vomiting, diarrhea, hypotension, rash

Botulinum toxin (Botox): neurotoxin that blocks release of acetylcholine from nerve terminal; paralyzes muscle (1 to 3 months)
  Indications: blepharospasm, hemifacial spasm, strabismus

Adverse effects: ptosis, diplopia, exposure keratopathy

Fluorescein dye: IV for fluorescein angiography

Adverse effects: nausea, vomiting, dizziness, headache, dyspnea, hypotension, skin necrosis, phototoxic reactions, anaphylaxis

Indocyanine green dye: IV for ICG angiography; contraindicated in patients allergic to iodine

Adverse effects: GI upset, hypotension, urticaria, anaphylaxis

OCULAR TOXICOLOGY

Anticholinergics (atropine, scopolamine, donnatal): toxicity causes flushing, agitation, tachycardia, somnolence, dry mouth, dry eye, mydriasis, cycloplegia, blurry vision, angle-closure; increased sensitivity in albinism, Down's syndrome, and neonates

Antihistamines (diphenhydramine): dry eye, mydriasis, cycloplegia, blurry vision

Antibiotics:
  Aminoglycosides: intraocular administration may cause macular infarction (IVFA: pruned tree appearance of retinal vasculature)
  Chloramphenicol: optic neuropathy; peripheral neuritis can precede visual complaints by 1 to 2 weeks
  Penicillin and tetracycline: pseudotumor
  Sulfonamides: conjunctivitis, transient myopia
  Isoniazid, rifampin, ethambutol: optic neuropathy

Antimalarials (chloroquine/hydroxychloroquine): cornea verticillata, fine pigmentary macular changes (bull's-eye maculopathy); patients may complain of halos around lights; visual acuity usually unchanged; dose related

Quinine: overdose can result in acute visual loss (to NLP), tinnitus, weakness, confusion

Barbiturates (phenobarbital): nystagmus, diplopia, ptosis, conjunctivitis

Phenothiazines (chlorpromazine, thioridazine): pigmentary retinopathy, corneal deposits, cataracts

Table 2–4. **Ocular Toxicology**

Ocular Structure	Effect	Drug
Extraocular muscles	Nystagmus, diplopia	Anesthetics, sedatives, anticonvulsants, propranolol, antibiotics, phenothiazines, pentobarbital, carbamazepine, MAO inhibitors
Lid	Edema	Chloral hydrate
	Discoloration	Phenothiazines
	Ptosis	Guanethidine, propranolol, barbiturates
Conjunctiva	Hyperemia	Reserpine, methyldopa
	Allergy	Antibiotics, sulfonamides, atropine, antivirals, glaucoma medications
	Discoloration	Phenothiazines, chlorambucil, phenylbutazone
Cornea	Keratitis	Antibiotics, phenylbutazone, barbiturates, chlorambucil, steroids
	Deposits	Chloroquine, amiodarone, tamoxifen, indomethacin, gold
	Pigmentation	Vitamin D
Increased IOP	Open angle	Anticholinergics, caffeine, steroids
	Narrow angle	Anticholinergics, antihistamines, phenothiazines, tricyclic antidepressants, Haldol
Lens	Opacities/cataract	Steroids, phenothiazines, ibuprofen, allopurinol, long-acting miotics
	Myopia	Sulfonamides, tetracycline, Compazine, autonomic antagonists
Retina	Edema	Chloramphenicol, indomethacin, tamoxifen, carmustine
	Hemorrhage	Anticoagulants, ethambutol
	Vascular damage	Oral contraceptives, oxygen, aminoglycosides, talc, carmustine, interferon
	Pigmentary degeneration	Phenothiazines, indomethacin, nalidixic acid, ethambutol, Accutane, chloroquine, hydroxychloroquine
Optic nerve	Neuropathy	Ethambutol, isoniazid, sulfonamides, digitalis, imipramine, streptomycin, busulfan, cisplatin, vincristine, chloramphenicol, disulfiram
	Papilledema	Steroids, vitamin A, tetracycline, phenylbutazone, amiodarone, nalidixic acid, isotretinoin

Tricyclic antidepressants: mydriasis, cycloplegia, dry eye, angle-closure

Dilantin: diplopia, nystagmus, papilledema

Gold: deposits in inferior corneal stroma and anterior lens capsule (chrysiasis)

Talc: multiple tiny yellow-white glistening particles scattered through posterior pole with macular edema, venous engorgement, hemorrhages, arterial occlusion, retinal nonperfusion, and peripheral NV

Amiodarone: cornea verticillata, occasionally anterior subcapsular opacities

Digoxin: changes in color vision (xanthopsia [yellow vision]), scotomas

Diuretics (hydrochlorothiazide): xanthopsia, transient myopia

Viagra: decreased retinal blood flow by up to ~30%; blue vision

Carmustine: retinal infarction, RPE changes, arterial occlusions, hemorrhages, macular edema, glaucoma, optic neuritis, INO

Narcotics (opiates): miosis

NSAIDs (indomethacin): corneal deposits, diplopia, optic neuritis, pigmentary macular changes; may have changes in vision, dark adaptation, and visual fields

Corticosteroids: posterior subcapsular cataracts, increased IOP, delayed wound healing, infections, pseudotumor cerebri

Oral contraceptives: dry eye, vascular occlusions, perivasculitis, optic neuritis, pseudotumor cerebri

Tamoxifen: deposits in cornea and macula, may have macular edema

Isotretinoin: impairment of dark adaptation

Interferon: reversible vaso-occlusive disease

Review Questions *(Answers start on page 357)*

1. Which antibiotic results in the highest intravitreal concentration when administered orally?
   a. ciprofloxacin
   b. penicillin
   c. bactrim
   d. clindamycin

2. Which anesthetic agent would most interfere with an intraocular gas bubble?
   a. isoflurane
   b. propofol
   c. pentathol
   d. nitrous oxide

3. Which of the following is not an adverse effect of CAIs?
   a. death
   b. paresthesias
   c. iris cysts
   d. Stevens-Johnson syndrome

4. Which β-blocker has the least effect on β_2 receptors?
   a. levobunolol
   b. betaxolol
   c. carteolol
   d. timolol

5. Which drug has the least effect on uveoscleral outflow?
   a. atropine
   b. Xalatan
   c. pilocarpine
   d. Trusopt

6. Which enzyme is inhibited by steroids?
   a. cyclooxygenase
   b. phospholipase A_2
   c. lipoxygenase
   d. endoperoxidase

7. Which of the following steroid formulations has the best corneal penetrability?
   a. prednisolone acetate
   b. dexamethasone phosphate
   c. prednisolone phosphate
   d. dexamethasone alcohol

8. Adverse effects of foscarnet include all of the following except
   a. seizures
   b. infertility
   c. electrolyte abnormalities
   d. myelosuppression

9. Which glaucoma medication is not effective when IOP is >60 mm Hg?
   a. Diamox
   b. timoptic
   c. pilocarpine
   d. Iopidine

10. Which medicine is not associated with OCP-like conjunctival shrinkage?
    a. phospholine iodide
    b. pilocarpine
    c. epinephrine
    d. timoptic

11. Which β-blocker is β_1-selective?
    a. carteolol
    b. timolol
    c. betaxolol
    d. levobunolol

12. The most appropriate treatment for neurosyphilis is
    a. penicillin G
    b. erythromycin
    c. penicillin VK
    d. tetracycline

13. The correct mechanism of action of botulinum toxin is
    a. prevents release of acetylcholine
    b. blocks acetylcholine receptors
    c. inhibits reuptake of acetylcholine
    d. it is an acetylcholinesterase inhibitor

14. Fluoroquinolones are least effective against
    a. *Klebsiella*
    b. *H influenzae*
    c. anaerobic cocci
    d. *Serratia*

15. Hydroxychloroquine toxicity depends most on
    a. patient age
    b. cumulative dose
    c. patient race
    d. daily dose

16. Calculate the amount of cocaine in 2 mL of a 4% solution
    a. 2 mg
    b. 8 mg
    c. 20 mg
    d. 80 mg

17. NSAIDs block the formation of all of the following substances except
    a. thromboxane
    b. leukotrienes
    c. prostaglandins
    d. prostacyclin

18. Systemic effects of steroids may include all of the following except
    a. papilledema
    b. hirsutism
    c. potassium depletion
    d. renal tubular acidosis

19. Which drug does not produce decreased tear production?
    a. pilocarpine
    b. Benadryl
    c. timoptic
    d. atropine

20. Natamycin is a
    a. diamine
    b. imidazole
    c. polyene
    d. aminoglycoside

21. Which glaucoma medicine does not decrease aqueous production?
    a. Iopidine
    b. pilocarpine
    c. Diamox
    d. timoptic

22. β-Blockers may cause all of the following except
    a. constipation
    b. impotence
    c. alopecia
    d. depression

23. Idoxuridine may cause all of the following except
    a. filamentary keratitis
    b. punctal stenosis
    c. corneal hypesthesia
    d. nonhealing epithelial erosion

24. Which of the following antifungal agents has the broadest spectrum against yeast-like fungi?
    a. miconazole
    b. natamycin
    c. ketoconazole
    d. amphotericin

25. All of the following medications are combination antihistamine and mast cell stabilizers except
    a. Alomide
    b. Zaditor
    c. Optivar
    d. Patanol

SUGGESTED READINGS

Doughty M: Ocular Pharmacology and Therapeutics: A Primary Care Guide. Philadelphia, Butterworth-Heinemann, 2001.

Fraunfelder FT, Fraunfelder FW, Randall JA: Drug-Induced Ocular Side Effects, 5th edition. Philadelphia, Butterworth-Heinemann, 2001.

Fraunfelder FT, Roy FH: Current Ocular Therapy, 5th edition. Philadelphia, WB Saunders, 2000.

Grant WM, Schuman JS: Toxicology of the Eye, 4th edition. Springfield, Ill, Charles C. Thomas, 1993.

Greenbaum S: Ocular Anesthesia. Philadelphia, WB Saunders, 1997.

Physicians' Desk Reference for Ophthalmic Medicines. Montvale, NJ, Medical Economics, 2003.

Zimmerman TJ: Textbook of Ocular Pharmacology. Philadelphia, Lippincott-Raven, 1997.

CHAPTER 3

Embryology/ Pathology

Embryology

Formation of eye: embryonic plate → neural plate → optic pits → optic vesicles → optic cups (Figures 3-1 and 3-2)

Embryonic plate:
1. Ectoderm (forms eye and brain): neural ectoderm, surface ectoderm, and neural crest
2. Mesoderm
3. Endoderm

Optic pit: forms at day 23 of gestation

Optic vesicle: anterolateral outpouching of primitive brain stem; evaginates on day 25 and becomes the globe

Optic vesicle induces the lens placode at day 27

Abnormalities of evagination: may result in anophthalmia, cyclopia (synophthalmia), congenital cystic eye, congenital nonattachment of the retina. Apical forebrain lesions such as synophthalmia are associated with arrhinencephaly, proboscis, ethmocephaly, trisomy 13

Optic cup: develops embryologically as an anterolateral evagination of the forebrain

Inner layer becomes the retina

Outer layer becomes the retinal pigment epithelium

Potential space between the two becomes the subretinal space (which was the cavity of the neural tube and optic vesicle)

Cells at anterior margin of optic cup form the posterior pigment epithelium of the iris

Cells between the future iris and the future retina form the ciliary body

Embryonic fissure: on undersurface of optic cups; closes on day 33 allowing pressurization of globe

Closure occurs first in midzone/equator, then extends posteriorly and anteriorly

Serves as portal for mesoderm to enter eye (i.e., hyaloid artery)

Coloboma: failure of closure of embryonic fissure; sporadic or AD; typical (located in inferonasal quadrant) or atypical (located elsewhere)

May involve retina and choroid (associated with basal encephalocoele, cleft palate, and CHARGE syndrome), iris, and/or optic nerve.

An eyelid coloboma is not related to closure of embryonic fissure

Microphthalmos with cyst: small, abnormal eye with cystic expansion extending posteriorly into orbit

Arises in area of and external to a choroidal coloboma; cyst usually contains dysplastic neuroectodermal tissue and may not directly connect with the eye

Optic pit: considered an atypical coloboma; associated with basal encephalocele

Hyaloid artery: enters through embryonic fissure and forms vasa hyaloidea propria (blood supply to primary vitreous) (Figure 3-3)

Intravitreal portion regresses by $8^{1}/_{2}$ months; intraneural portion becomes central retinal artery

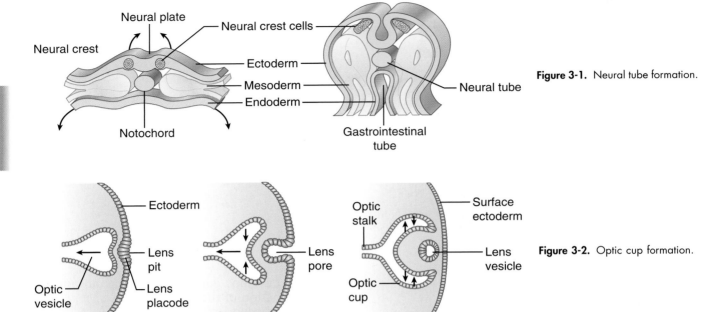

Figure 3-1. Neural tube formation.

Figure 3-2. Optic cup formation.

Posterior tunica vasculosa lentis supplies the posterior lens

Retinal vascular development begins during 16th week: mesenchymal cells next to hyaloid artery form capillary network, then form arteries and veins. Vessels grow centrifugally from optic disc, reach nasal ora serrata during 8th month and temporal ora 1 to 2 months later

3% of normal neonates have a patent hyaloid artery

Remnants of hyaloid vasculature system:

BERGMEISTER'S PAPILLAE: at optic nerve head; glial sheath of Bergmeister envelops posterior 1/3 of hyaloid artery and begins to atrophy during 7th month; epipapillary veil results if it does not fully regress

PERIPAPILLARY LOOP: vascular loop extending from optic nerve head; risk of artery obstruction or vitreous hemorrhage

MITTENDORF'S DOT: small opacity on posterior lens capsule at which hyaloid artery is attached to posterior tunica vasculosa lentis

PERSISTENT PUPILLARY MEMBRANE: thin iris strands bridging pupil; may attach to anterior lens capsule; remnants of anterior tunica vasculosa lentis

Primitive epithelial papillae: cells from inner layer of optic cup at superior end of embryonic fissure, which becomes the optic disc

Ganglion cell axons grow through

Myelination starts centrally, reaching chiasm at 7½ months and lamina cribrosa at birth; complete approximately 1 month after birth

Inner limiting membrane of Elschnig: covers ON, contiguous with ILM

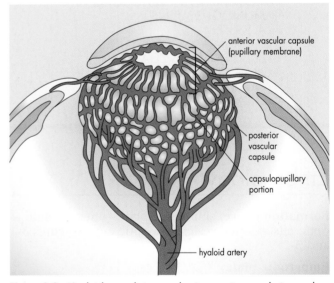

Figure 3-3. Hyaloid vasculature and primary vitreous during embryologic ocular development. (From Dass AB, Trese MT: Persistent hyperplastic primary vitreous. In Yanoff M, Duker JS [eds]: *Ophthalmology*, London, Mosby, 1999.)

ON may show deceptively exaggerated cupping because nerve fibers posterior to lamina cribrosa are incompletely myelinated at birth

ON hypoplasia is associated with DeMorsier's syndrome; 13% have pituitary abnormalities

Vitreous: produced by lens, retina, and walls of hyaloid artery; contains mesenchymal cells

Primary vitreous: formed by hyaloid vascular system (vasa hyaloidea propria, which includes hyaloid canal, hyaloid vessels, and posterior

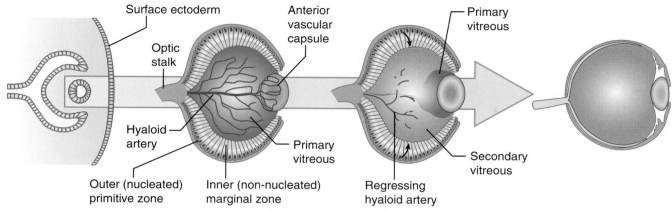

Surface ectoderm

Optic stalk

Anterior vascular capsule

Primary vitreous

Hyaloid artery

Primary vitreous

Regressing hyaloid artery

Secondary vitreous

Outer (nucleated) primitive zone

Inner (non-nucleated) marginal zone

Figure 3-4. Posterior segment development.

portions of tunica vasculosa lentis); eventually replaced by secondary vitreous. Failure to regress causes PHPV

Secondary vitreous: formed by retina

Area of Martegiani: extends from disc into vitreous to become Cloquet's canal

Cloquet's canal: junction of primary and secondary vitreous

Tertiary vitreous: zonule fibers formed from ciliary processes and lens capsule

Berger's space: retrolental space

Retina: neuroectoderm; vascularization begins at 4 months; temporal periphery is last portion to become vascularized

Development of fovea is not complete until 4 or more weeks after birth

Retinal dysplasia: abnormal proliferation of developing retina produces tubular structures with a rosette-like appearance; represents nonspecific response to disorganizing influence during development; associated with maternal LSD ingestion, Patau's syndrome (trisomy 13), microphthalmos, congenital glaucoma, Peter's anomaly, uveal and optic nerve colobomas, cyclopia, and synophthalmia

Choroid: requires RPE for development

Stroma is from neural crest cells

Vascular endothelium is from mesoderm

Vessel walls are from neural crest cells

Sclera: neural crest cells and mesoderm (temporal aspect)

Blue hue at birth due to thinness (see underlying uveal pigment)

Cornea: neural crest cells (2 waves)

1st wave grows between epithelium and lens, forming double layer of corneal endothelium

2nd wave grows between epithelium and endothelium; this zone is rich in hyaluronic acid and collagen fibrils

At 4 months, Descemet's membrane develops

At 5 months, Bowman's membrane develops

Angle: neural crest cells from peripheral cornea differentiate into chamber angle during 7th week

In 4th month, Schlemm's canal forms

In 7th month, angle moves posteriorly

In 8th month, formation is complete; trabecular meshwork appears just before birth

Lens: at 27 days, surface ectoderm adjacent to optic vesicle enlarges to form lens placode (lens plate)

Circular indentation then occurs on lens plate, forming lens pit, which invaginates the wall of the optic vesicle until it closes to form a sphere

Basement membrane of the surface ectoderm forms the surface of the sphere (the lens vesicle) and subsequently becomes the lens capsule

Lens epithelial cells on posterior aspect of this sphere elongate and migrate first (primary lens fibers); these cells fill the core of the lens vesicle at approximately 40 days (embryonal nucleus)

At 7 weeks, anterior cells migrate toward equator and proliferate to form secondary lens fibers that encase the embryonal nucleus and form the Y sutures; Y sutures represent the meeting of embryonal and fetal nuclei (upright anteriorly, inverted posteriorly)

After 3 months, zonules of Zinn (zonular fibers) develop (Figure 3-5)

Summary

3 weeks	Lens placode from surface ectoderm
6 weeks	Lens vesicle; further development requires normal neuroretina
12 weeks	Tunica vasculosa lentis
28–38 weeks	Degeneration of tunica vasculosa lentis

Lens of a newborn is more spherical than that of an adult; therefore, anterior chamber appears shallow

Iris: rim of optic cup grows around lens and forms iris

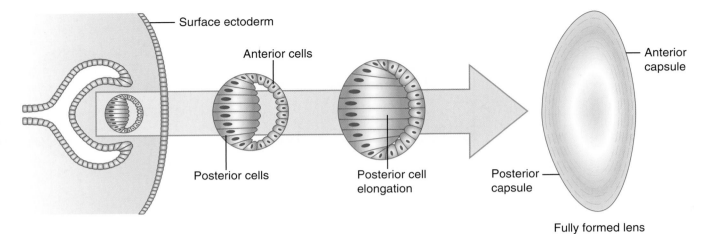

Figure 3-5. Lens development.

Epithelial layers (IPE; anterior pigmented and posterior nonpigmented) are from inner and outer layers of the optic cup (neuroectoderm); forms part of the blood-aqueous barrier

In 7th week, stroma forms from neural crest cells, and tunica vasculosa lentis forms

In 6th month, sphincter and dilator muscles form from neuroectoderm

In 7th month, blood vessels enter iris

In 9th month, tunica vasculosa lentis disappears

Newborn iris is usually gray-blue; development of iris color takes weeks to months, as stromal chromatophores (dendritic melanocytes from neural crest) complete their migration into uvea shortly after birth

Iris dilator muscle is immature, causing relative miosis in infancy

RPE and posterior pigment epithelium of the iris form from the outer layer of the optic cup (have mature coloration because pigment granules develop very early in gestation)

Ciliary body (CB): formation begins in 3rd month; fold in optic cup becomes epithelial layers of ciliary processes

In 4th month, filaments from surface cells form zonules; the major arterial circle of the iris (located in CB), the longitudinal ciliary muscle, and the ciliary processes develop

In 5th month, pars plana develops, and ciliary body stroma and ciliary muscle develop from neural crest cells adjacent to cornea

In 7th month, circular fibers of ciliary muscle differentiate

Patient's age can be determined by analysis of CB cellularity

Nasolacrimal system: at 6 weeks, surface ectoderm is buried in mesoderm, between maxillary and lateral nasal processes

During 3rd month, the cord canalizes

Defects: may result in imperforate valve of Hasner; rarely, absent puncta or canaliculi

Eyelids: at 8 weeks, upper lids form by fusion of medial and lateral frontonasal processes; lower lids by fusion of maxillary processes and medial nasal processes

At 12 weeks, lid folds fuse

At 24 weeks, separation begins from nasal side

Embryologic tissues and their components:

Neural ectoderm: sensory retina, RPE, nonpigmented ciliary body epithelium, pigmented CB epithelium (extension of RPE), iris pigment epithelium, iris sphincter and dilator muscle, optic nerve (neural and glial elements), sympathetic ganglion, lateral geniculate body, ocular pigment granules (RPE, CB, iris pigment epithelium), peripheral nerves related to eye function, erector pili muscle associated with hair follicles of the skin

Surface ectoderm: crystalline lens, corneal and conjunctival epithelium, lid epithelium, lacrimal gland, nasolacrimal system

Surface and neural ectoderm: vitreous, zonules

Neural crest cells: corneal stroma and endothelium, iris stroma, TM, chamber angle, Schlemm's canal, sclera (except temporal portion), sheaths and tendons of extraocular muscles, ciliary muscle (nonpigmented layer of ciliary body), choroidal stroma, melanocytes, meningeal sheaths, orbital bones, connective tissue of orbit, muscular and connective tissue layers of blood vessels

S-100 STAIN: specific for neural crest–derived structures

3 WAVES OF NEURAL CREST CELL MIGRATION (during 7th week): corneal and TM endothelium, keratocytes (corneal stroma), iris stroma

ANTERIOR SEGMENT DISORDERS DUE TO NEURAL CREST ABNORMALITIES:

Period after conception	Event	Period after conception	Event
22nd day	Optic groove appears	3rd month	Differentiation of precursors of rods and cones
25th day	Optic vesicle forms from optic pit		Ciliary body develops
26th day	Primordia of superior rectus, inferior rectus, medial rectus, and inferior oblique appear		Appearance of limbus
			Anterior chamber appears as a potential space
27th day	Formation of lens plate from surface ectoderm		Sclera condenses
	Primordium of lateral rectus appears		Eyelid folds lengthen and fuse
28th day	Embryonic fissure forms	4th month	Formation of retinal vasculature begins
	Cells destined to become retinal pigment epithelium acquire pigmentation		Beginning of regression of hyaloid vessels
			Formation of physiologic cup of optic disc
29th day	Primordium of superior oblique appears		Formation of lamina cribrosa
5th week	Lens pit forms and deepens into lens vesicle		Major arterial circle of iris forms
	Hyaloid vessels develop		Development of iris sphincter muscle
	Primary vitreous develops		Development of longitudinal ciliary muscle and processes of ciliary body
	Osseous structures of the orbit begin to develop		Formation of tertiary vitreous
6th week	Closure of embryonic fissure		Bowman's membrane forms
	Corneal epithelial cells develop interconnections		Canal of Schlemm appears
	Differentiation of retinal pigment epithelium		Eyelid glands and cilia form
	Proliferation of neural retinal cells	5th month	Photoreceptors differentiate
	Formation of secondary vitreous		Eyelid separation begins
	Formation of primary lens fibers	6th month	Cones differentiate
	Development of periocular vasculature		Ganglion cells thicken in macula
	Appearance of eyelid folds and nasolacrimal duct		Differentiation of dilator pupillae muscle
	Ciliary ganglion appears		Nasolacrimal system becomes patent
7th week	Migration of ganglion cells toward optic disc	7th month	Rods differentiate
	Formation of embryonic lens nucleus		Ora serrata forms
	Development of choroidal vessels from periocular mesenchyme		Migration of ganglion cells to form nerve fiber layer of Henle
	Three waves of neural crest migration:		Choroid becomes pigmented
	first wave: formation of corneal and trabecular endothelium		Circular ciliary muscle fibers develop
	second wave: formation of corneal stroma		Myelination of optic nerve
	third wave: formation of iris stroma		Posterior movement of anterior chamber angle
	Formation of tunica vasculosa lentis		Orbicularis muscle differentiation
	Sclera begins to form	8th month	Completion of anterior chamber angle formation
			Hyaloid vessels disappear
		9th month	Retinal vessels reach the temporal periphery
			Pupillary membrane disappears
		After birth	Development of macula

Figure 3-6. Time line of ocular embryogenesis. (From Azar NJ, Davis EA: Embryology in the eye. In Yanoff M, Duker JS [eds]: *Ophthalmology*, 2nd ed, St. Louis, Mosby, 2004.)

ABNORMAL MIGRATION: congenital glaucoma, posterior embryotoxin, Axenfeld-Rieger syndrome, Peter's anomaly, sclerocornea
ABNORMAL PROLIFERATION: ICE syndromes
ABNORMAL TERMINAL INDUCTION: corneal endothelial dystrophies
Mesoderm: blood vessel endothelium, anterior chamber angle outflow apparatus, sclera (small area temporally), extraocular muscles, Schlemm's canal, portion of vitreous
Mesenchyme: primitive connective tissue; originates from neural crest cells and mesoderm (Figure 3-6)

Pathology

MICROBIAL STUDIES

Stains

Gram: bacteria, fungi

Giemsa: *Acanthamoeba*, fungi, and cytology; best for intranuclear inclusion bodies

Acid fast (Ziehl-Neelsen): *Mycobacterium*, *Nocardia*

Periodic acid–Schiff (PAS): fungi

Gomori's methenamine silver: fungi

Calcofluor white: fungi and *Acanthamoeba* (binds to cell wall, visible with fluorescent microscopy)

KOH: fungi

Culture Media

Blood: most bacteria; very good for atypical *Mycobacterium*

Blood agar in 5% to 10% carbon dioxide: *Moraxella*

Chocolate (contains hemin and NAD): *Haemophilus*, *Neisseria*

Thioglycolate: anaerobes

Sabouraud's: fungi

Löwenstein-Jensen: *Mycobacterium tuberculosis, Nocardia*

Loeffler's: *Corynebacteria*

Non-nutrient agar with *E. coli* overgrowth: *Acanthamoeba*

Cytology

Intracytoplasmic basophilic inclusions (Giemsa stain): *Chlamydia*

Intranuclear eosinophilic inclusions (Papanicolaou stain): herpes (Tzanck smear)

TISSUE STAINS

Hematoxylin and eosin (H&E): hematoxylin is specific for nucleic acids within nuclei and stains blue (basophilic); eosin is specific for most cytoplasmic organelles (such as mitochondria) and stains pink (eosinophilic)

Periodic acid–Schiff (PAS): stains basement membrane material magenta (Descemet's, lens capsule, Bruch's membrane, ILM [internal limiting membrane], gutattae, drusen); also stains glycogen, fungi, conjunctival goblet cells (useful for differentiation of corneal from conjunctival epithelium)

Masson trichrome: stains collagen blue and hyaline red; used for granular dystrophy

Congo red: stains amyloid orange; used for lattice dystrophy

Crystal violet: stains amyloid red-purple; used for lattice dystrophy

Alcian blue: stains acid mucopolysaccharide blue; used for macular dystrophy

Colloidal iron: stains acid mucopolysaccharide blue; used for macular dystrophy

Oil red O: stains neutral lipids red-orange in frozen section; must be used on fresh tissue because formalin leaches out lipid

Sudan black: stains phospholipids; myelin in ON

Luxol fast blue: stains myelin blue; demyelinated plaques lose affinity for stain

Bodian: stains nerve fibers black

Mucicarmine: stains mucus pink/red; mucus-secreting adenocarcinomas (i.e., GI, breast)

Verhoeff Van Gieson: stains elastic tissue black

Movat's pentachrome: stains elastic tissue black

Wilder: stains reticulin fibers black

Alizarin red: stains calcium red-orange

von Kossa: stains calcium black

Prussian blue: stains iron (hemosiderin, ferric ions) blue

Fontana-Masson: stains melanin black; used for amelanotic melanoma

S-100 protein: stains nevi, melanomas, schwannomas, neurofibromas, and other heterologous cell lines

Polarizing filters: for evaluating structures or deposits that have a regular molecular structure (amyloid, calcium oxalate crystals), as well as suture granulomas and vegetable foreign bodies

TISSUE FIXATION

Orientation of globe: identify SO (tendinous insertion) and IO (muscular insertion) muscles

Paraffin: embedding process for histologic examination: water is removed, organic solvents leach out lipids; PMMA is dissolved completely; to preserve lipids, fresh or frozen tissue specimens are used; paraffin must be removed before different stains are applied

Glutaraldehyde: for electron microscopy

Formalin and Bouin's fixative: for light microscopy; 10% buffered formalin (formalin = 40% solution of formaldehyde in water); formalin stabilizes protein, lipid, and carbohydrates, and prevents postmortem enzymatic destruction of tissue

Ethyl alcohol: cytology

Fixation Artifacts:
  Lange's fold: fold at ora serrata in newborn eyes probably caused by unequal shrinkage of retinociliary tissues during fixation
  Artifactual RD: common histologic finding, differentiated from true retinal detachment by lack of subretinal fluid, preservation of photoreceptors, and pigment attached to outer surface of rods and cones

A

B

Figure 3-7. A, Artifact RD with no fluid, pigment adherent to photo-receptors, and normal retinal architecture. **B**, True RD with material in subretinal space and degeneration of outer retinal layers. (From Yanoff M, Fine BS: *Ocular pathology*, 5th ed, St. Louis, Mosby, 2002.)

Clefts in corneal stroma: clear spaces within stroma; obliterated in corneal edema

HYPERSENSITIVITY REACTIONS (COOMBS AND GELL CLASSIFICATION)

Type I: anaphylactic/immediate hypersensitivity

EXAMPLE: hay fever, vernal, atopic, GPC

Type II: cytotoxic hypersensitivity

EXAMPLE: OCP, Mooren's ulcer

Type III: immune complex deposition

EXAMPLE: Stevens-Johnson, marginal infiltrates, disciform keratitis, subepithelial infiltrates, Wessely ring, scleritis, retinal vasculitis

Type IV: cell-mediated, delayed hypersensitivity

EXAMPLE: phlyctenule, graft reaction, contact dermatitis, interstitial keratitis, granulomatous disease (TB, syphilis, leprosy)

Type V: stimulating antibody

EXAMPLE: Graves' disease, myasthenia gravis

IMMUNOGLOBULINS

IgG: most abundant; crosses the placenta; binds complement

IgA: second most abundant; monomeric or joined by J chain; important against viral infection; found in secretions

IgM: largest; binds complement; important in primary immune response

IgD: present in newborns

IgE: sensitizes mast cells and tissue leukocytes; role in atopy

HLA (HUMAN LEUKOCYTE ANTIGEN) SYSTEM

Major histocompatibility complex (MHC) proteins found on surfaces of all nucleated cells

In humans, MHC proteins are the human leukocyte antigen (HLA) molecules

Gene loci are located on chromosome 6
> *Class I*: antigen presentation to cytotoxic T cells (CD 8 positive); loci A, B, C
> *Class II*: antigen presentation to helper T cells (CD 4 positive); loci DR, DP, DQ

Table 3-1. HLA Associations

Uveitis	
A29	Birdshot retinochoroidopathy (90%)
B7, DR2	Presumed ocular histoplasmosis syndrome (80%)
B8, B13	Sarcoidosis
B8, B51, DR2, DR15	Intermediate uveitis
B27 (1% to 5% of population)	Adult iridocyclitis (usually unilateral): Reiter's syndrome (75%), ankylosing spondylitis (90%), inflammatory bowel disease (90%), psoriatic arthritis, JRA (subtype V)
B51	Behçet's disease (70%)
DR4	Sympathetic ophthalmia, Vogt-Koyanagi-Harada syndrome
DR15	Pars planitis
DQ7	Acute retinal necrosis (50%)
External Disease	
B5, DR3, DR4	HSV keratitis
B8, DR3	Sjögren's syndrome
B12	Ocular cicatricial pemphigoid
B15	Scleritis
DR3	Thygeson's SPK
Neuro-ophthalmology	
A1, B8, DR3	Myasthenia gravis
B7, DR2	Multiple sclerosis
DR3	Graves' disease

INFLAMMATION

Tissue infiltration by inflammatory cells

Types of Inflammatory Cells

Neutrophils: polymorphonuclear leukocytes (PMNs)
Primary cell in acute inflammation; phagocytosis
Multilobed nucleus
Abscess: focal collection of PMNs
Pus: PMNs and tissue necrosis

Eosinophils:
Allergic and parasite-related reactions ("worms, wheezes, weird diseases"); modulation of mast cell reactions, phagocytosis of Ag-Ab complexes
Bilobed nucleus, granular cytoplasm

Mast cells: tissue basophils
IgE bound to surface; Ag causes degranulation with release of histamine and heparin

EXAMPLE: anaphylaxis, allergic conjunctivitis

Looks like plasma cell

Lymphocytes:
Main cell in humoral and cell-mediated immune reactions
Types: B cells, T cells (helper, suppressor, cytotoxic, killer, null cells)
Scanty cytoplasm

Plasma cells: activated B cells
Synthesis and secretion of antibodies
Eccentric "cartwheel" nucleus, basophilic cytoplasm
Plasmacytoid cell: granular eosinophilic cytoplasm
Russell body: immunoglobulin crystals

Macrophages: histiocytes, monocytes (Figure 3-8)
Primary phagocytic cell; second line of cellular defense; regulation of lymphocytes via Ag presentation and monokine production
Transformation into epithelioid and giant cells
Kidney-shaped nucleus

Epithelioid histiocyte: activated macrophage with vesicular nucleus and eosinophilic cytoplasm; cells resemble epithelium; hallmark of granulomatous inflammation; fuse to form giant cells

Giant cells: 3 types
Langhans': nuclei arranged around periphery in ring/horseshoe pattern

EXAMPLE: TB, sarcoidosis

Touton: midperipheral ring of nuclei; central eosinophilic cytoplasm; nuclei are surrounded by clear zone of foamy lipid

EXAMPLE: JXG

Foreign body: nuclei randomly distributed; surrounds or contains foreign body

Types of Inflammation

Acute:
Suppurative: neutrophils
Nonsuppurative: lymphocytes

Chronic:
Nongranulomatous: lymphocytes and plasma cells
Granulation tissue in reparative phase; exuberant response causes pyogenic granuloma
Granulomatous: epithelioid histiocytes; 3 patterns
DIFFUSE: epithelioid cells distributed randomly against background of lymphocytes and plasma cells

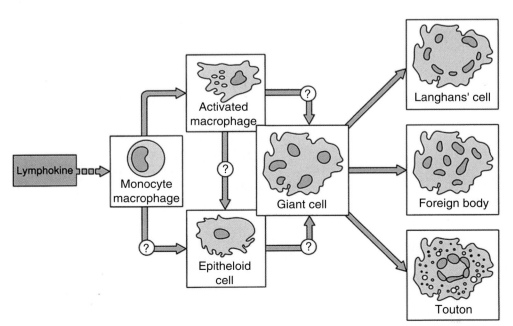

Figure 3-8. Macrophage differentiation. (Modified from Roitt IM, Brostoff J, Male DK: *Immunology*, 2nd ed, London, Gower Medical, 1989.)

EXAMPLE: sympathetic ophthalmia, fungal infection, JXG, lepromatous leprosy

DISCRETE: epithelioid cells form nodules with giant cells, surrounded by rim of lymphocytes and plasma cells

EXAMPLE: sarcoidosis, miliary TB, tuberculoid leprosy

ZONAL: palisaded giant cells surround central nidus

EXAMPLE: phacoantigenic endophthalmitis (phacotoxic uveitis is nongranulomatous); rheumatoid scleritis (nidus = scleral collagen); chalazion

Endophthalmitis: inflammation involving at least one ocular coat and adjacent cavity, sclera is not involved

Panophthalmitis: suppurative endophthalmitis also involving sclera and orbit

Sequelae of Inflammation

Cornea: scarrring

Calcific band keratopathy: basophilic granules in Bowman's membrane

Inflammatory pannus: subepithelial fibrovascular and inflammatory ingrowth with destruction of Bowman's membrane

EXAMPLE: trachoma

Degenerative pannus: fibrous tissue between epithelium and intact Bowman's membrane

EXAMPLE: chronic corneal edema

Anterior chamber: organization of hypopyon; retrocorneal fibrous membranes

Peripheral anterior synechiae (PAS): seclusio pupillae (if 360°)

Pupillary membrane: occlusio pupillae

Lens:

Anterior subcapsular cataract: fibrous plaque beneath folded anterior capsule, secreted by irritated metaplastic anterior epithelial cells

Posterior subcapsular cataract: bladder cells adjacent to capsule

Ciliary body:

Cyclitic membrane: retrolental collagenous membrane attached to ciliary body; contraction leads to detachment of pars plana, ciliary muscle remains adherent to scleral spur attachment; due to organization and scarring of vitreous, metaplastic ciliary epithelium, organized inflammatory residua

Retina:

CME: retinal vascular leakage or Müller cell edema

RPE changes: hypertrophy, hyperplasia, and migration (pseudo–retinitis pigmentosa); fibrous metaplasia (collagen and basement membrane material deposited on Bruch's membrane, contain lacunae of RPE cells [pseudoadenomatous proliferation]); intraocular bone from osseous metaplasia

Reactive gliosis

Phthisis: rectus muscle traction on hypotonous globe causes squared-off appearance; thickened sclera, high incidence of retinal detachment and disorganization, calcareous degeneration of lens

EYELID EPITHELIAL CHANGES

Hyperkeratosis: thickening of the keratin layer; clinically appears as white, flaky lesion (leukoplakia)

Parakeratosis: thickening of the keratin layer with retention of nuclei; indicates shortened epidermal regeneration time; granular layer is thin or absent

Dyskeratosis: keratin formation within the basal cell layer or deeper

Acanthosis: thickening of the squamous cell layer due to proliferation of prickle cells

Acantholysis: loss of cohesion between epidermal cells with breakdown of intercellular junctions, creating spaces within the epidermis; occurs in pemphigus and produces intraepithelial bullae

Dysplasia: disorderly maturation of epithelium with loss of polarity, cytologic atypia, and mitotic figures found above the basilar layer

Mild: <50% epidermal thickness involved

Severe: >50% involved

Carcinoma in situ (CIN): full-thickness replacement of epithelium by malignant cells without invasion through the basement membrane

Squamous cell carcinoma: malignant epithelial cells invade below basement membrane

Anaplasia: cytologic malignancy with pleomorphism, anisocytosis, abnormal nuclei, and mitotic figures

Papillomatosis: proliferation of dermal papillae, causing surface undulation

Pseudoepitheliomatous hyperplasia: inflammatory response with hyperplasia of epithelium, which mimics carcinoma; acanthosis with protrusion of broad tongues of benign epidermis into the dermis

Elastosis: actinic damage; seen as blue staining (normally pink) of superficial dermal collagen with H&E stain; damaged collagen stains with elastic tissue stains but is not susceptible to digestion with elastase (Figure 3-9)

AGING CHANGES

Cornea: Hassal-Henle warts (excrescences and thickenings of Descemet's memrane in corneal periphery)

Ciliary epithelium: hyperplasia and proliferation

Figure 3-9. Elastosis demonstrating basophilic degeneration of conjunctival substantia propria in a pinguecula. (From Yanoff M, Fine BS: *Ocular pathology*, 5th ed, St. Louis, Mosby, 2002.)

Pars plana and pars plicata: clear (teardrop) cysts

Retina: loss of retinal cells and replacement with glial tissue; chorioretinal adhesions and pigmentary lesions in periphery; peripheral microcystoid degeneration (Blessig-Iwanoff cysts): located in outer plexiform layer; bubbly appearance just behind ora serrata; lined by Müller cells; contain mucopolysacharides

WOUNDS

Wound Healing

Cornea: stromal healing is avascular; fibrosis; neutrophils arrive via tears; wound edges swell and glycosaminoglycans (keratan sulfate, chondroitin sulfate) disintegrate at edge of wound; activated fibroblasts migrate across wound and produce collagen and fibronectin; anterior surface re-epithelializes; endothelium migrates and regenerates Descemet's membrane

Sclera: does not heal itself; it is avascular and acellular; ingrowth of granulation tissue from episclera and choroid

Iris: no healing

Retina: scars are produced by glial cells rather than fibroblasts

Wound Complications

Epithelial ingrowth: sheet of multilayered nonkeratinized squamous epithelium over any intraocular surface; may form cyst (free-floating or attached to iris); implanted cells tend to be 2 to 4 cell layers thick and have conjunctival characteristics (more than corneal)

Fibrous downgrowth: proliferating fibroblasts originate from episcleral or corneal stroma; contraction can occur

Hemorrhage:
Corneal blood staining: hemoglobin breakdown products are forced through endothelial cells by increased IOP; Hgb molecules are removed by phagocytic and biochemical processes
Hemosiderosis bulbi: hemosiderin contains iron; can damage essential intracellular enzyme systems
Ochre membrane: hemorrhage that accumulates on posterior surface of detached vitreous
Synchysis scintillans: accumulation of cholesterol within vitreous following breakdown of RBC membranes; angular, birefringent, flat crystalline particles with golden hue located in dependent portions of globe; cholesterol dissolves during preparation of tissues in paraffin; cholesterol clefts are negative image of cholesterol crystals, surrounded by serous fluid

---

BOX 3-1. Differential Diagnostics of Intraocular Calcification

Retinoblastoma
Choroidal osteoma
Choroidal hemangioma
Phthisis
Osseous choristoma

BOX 3-2. Differential Diagnostics of Intraocular Cartilage

PHPV (retrolental plaque)
Medulloepithelioma
Teratoma
Trisomy 13
Complex choristoma of conjunctiva

Figure 3-10. Trisomy 13 demonstrating intraocular cartilage and retinal dysplasia. (Reported in Hoepner J, Yanoff M: *Am J Ophthalmol* 74:729, 1972.)

BOX 3-3. **Collagen**

Type 1: normal corneal stroma; Bowman's membrane (highly disorganized type 1, basal lamina has type 4)
Type 2: vitreous
Type 3: stromal wound healing
Type 4: basement membranes

OCULAR INJURIES

Blunt Trauma

Scleral rupture (weak spots):
1. Limbus (on opposite side from trauma)
2. Posterior to rectus muscle insertions
3. Equator
4. Lamina cribrosa (ON)

Uveal tract is connected to sclera in 3 places:
1. Scleral spur
2. Internal ostia of vortex veins
3. Peripapillary tissue

Cyclodialysis: disinsertion of longitudinal fibers of ciliary muscle from scleral spur

Angle recession: rupture of face of ciliary body; plane of relative weakness at ciliary body face extending posteriorly between longitudinal fibers and more central oblique and circular fibers; oblique and circular muscles atrophy, changing cross-sectional shape of ciliary body from triangular to fusiform

Iridodialysis: disinsertion of iris root from ciliary body

Vossius ring: compression and rupture of iris pigment epithelial cells against anterior surface of lens deposit ring of melanin concentric to pupil

Lens capsule rupture: capsule is thinnest at posterior pole; cataract can form immediately; epithelium may be stimulated by trauma to form anterior lenticular fibrous plaque

Descemet's rupture: causes acute edema (hydrops); due to minor trauma (keratoconus) or major trauma (forceps injury)

Choroidal rupture: often concentric to optic disc; risk of CNVM

Retinal dialysis: retina anchored anteriorly to non-pigmented epithelium of pars plana and reinforced by vitreous base, which straddles the ora serrata; circumferential tear of retina at point of attachment of ora or immediately posterior to vitreous base attachment

Commotio retinae: temporary loss of retinal transparency due to disruption of photoreceptor elements

Penetrating Trauma

Penetration: partial-thickness wound (into)

Perforation: full-thickness wound (through) (globe penetration is due to perforation of the cornea or sclera; globe perforation is a double penetrating injury)

Sequelae of Trauma

Phthisis bulbi:
Atrophia bulbi without shrinkage: initially, size and shape of eye are maintained; with loss of nutrition: cataract develops, retina atrophies and separates from RPE by serous fluid accumulation, synechiae cause increased IOP.
Atrophia bulbi with shrinkage: eye becomes soft due to ciliary body dysfunction; internal structures are atrophic but histologically recognizable; globe becomes smaller with squared-off shape (because of tension of rectus muscles); AC collapses; corneal endothelial cell damage leads to corneal edema and opacification
Atrophia bulbi with disorganization (phthisis bulbi): globe shrinks to average diameter of 16 to 19 mm; most ocular contents are disorganized; calcification of Bowman's layer, lens, retina, and drusen; bone formation in uveal tract

Intraocular Foreign Body

Copper:
≥85%: noninfectious suppurative endophthalmitis
<85% (chalcosis): copper deposits in basement membranes (Kayser-Fleisher ring, sunflower cataract, retinal degeneration)

Steel (contains iron): siderosis bulbi

Organic (vegetable matter): severe granulomatous foreign body response

Chemical Injury

Acid: precipitates proteins; zone of coagulative necrosis acts as barrier to deeper penetration

Alkali: denatures proteins and lyses cell membranes; no effective barrier is created—therefore, deeper penetration; vascular occlusion, ischemia, corneal damage during healing phase due to collagenase released by regenerating tissue

Radiation

Nonionizing: depends on wavelenth
Microwave: cataract
Infrared: true exfoliation of lens capsule (glass-blower's cataract)
Ultraviolet: keratitis (welder's flash)

Ionizing: tissue damage is direct (actively reproducing cells) or indirect (blood vessels); epithelial atrophy and ulceration, dermatitis of eyelids, dysfunction of adnexa, destructive ocular surface disease with keratinization, cataract; retinal necrosis, ischemia, neovascularization, optic atrophy (retina is relatively radioresistant, but retinal blood vessels are vulnerable)

Table 3-2. Most Common Cause of Infections

Endophthalmitis:	
Acute postoperative (<6 wk)	Coagulase-negative *Staphylococcus*
Delayed postoperative	*Propionibacterium acnes*, coagulase-negative *Staphylococcus*
From filtering bleb	*Streptococcus pneumoniae*, *Staphylococcus*, *Haemophilus influenzae*
Post-traumatic	*Staphylococcus* species, *Bacillus cereus*, Gram-negative organisms
Endogenous (IVDA)	*Candida*
Dacryocystitis	*Streptococcus pneumoniae*, *Staphylococcus*
Dacryadenitis	*Staphylococcus*
Canaliculitis	*Actinomyces*
Orbital cellulitis (children)	*Staphylococcus aureus*
Preseptal cellulites	*Staphylococcus aureus*
Angular blepharitis	*Staphylococcus*, *Moraxella*

BOX 3-4. Tumors

Congenital:
  Hamartoma: composed of tissues normally found in that area
    EXAMPLE: hemangioma
  Choristoma: composed of tissues not normally found in that area
    EXAMPLE: choroidal osteoma
Most common primary intraocular tumor: choroidal melanoma
Most common primary intraocular tumor in children: retinoblastoma
Most common lacrimal gland tumor: adenocystic carcinoma
Most common benign orbital tumor in adults: cavernous hemangioma
Most common metastasis to orbit in children: neuroblastoma

Review Questions *(Answers start on page 358)*

1. Which stain is the most helpful in the diagnosis of sebaceous cell carcinoma?
   a. Giemsa
   b. Hematoxylin and eosin
   c. Oil-red-O
   d. Methenamine silver

2. Pagetoid spread is most commonly associated with
   a. malignant melanoma
   b. squamous cell carcinoma
   c. sebaceous cell carcinoma
   d. Merkel cell tumor

3. A melanoma occurring in which of the following locations has the best prognosis?
   a. iris
   b. ciliary body
   c. choroid, anteriorly
   d. choroid, posterior pole

4. Calcification in retinoblastoma is due to
   a. RPE metaplasia
   b. necrosis
   c. hemorrhage
   d. metastasis

5. The type of organism that causes Lyme disease is a
   a. bacillus
   b. spirochete
   c. protozoan
   d. tick

6. Characteristics of ghost cells include all of the following except
   a. khaki colored
   b. rigid
   c. Heinz bodies
   d. biconcave

7. A moll gland is best categorized as
   a. mucin
   b. apocrine
   c. sebaceous
   d. holocrine

8. Which of the following is not a Gram-positive rod?
   a. *Corynebacterium*
   b. *Bacillus*
   c. *Serratia*
   d. *Listeria*

9. Trantas' dots are composed of what cell type?
   a. macrophage
   b. neutrophil
   c. eosinophil
   d. mast cell

10. Types of collagen that can be found in the cornea include all of the following except
    a. I
    b. II
    c. III
    d. IV

11. Lens nuclei are retained in all of the following conditions except
    a. Leigh's syndrome
    b. Lowe's syndrome
    c. rubella
    d. Alport's syndrome

12. Vogt-Koyanagi-Harada syndrome is best described by which type of hypersensitivity reaction?
    a. I
    b. II
    c. III
    d. IV

13. Lacy vacuolization of the iris occurs in which disease?
    a. CVO
    b. diabetes
    c. CRAO
    d. hypercholesterolemia

14. Antoni A and B cells occur in which tumor?
    a. neurilemmoma
    b. meningioma
    c. glioma
    d. neurofibroma

15. Which tumor is classically described as having a "Swiss cheese" appearance?
    a. rhabdomyosarcoma
    b. adenoid cystic carcinoma
    c. benign mixed tumor
    d. meningioma

16. Which iris nodule is correctly paired with its histopathology
    a. Juvenile xanthogranuloma, inflammatory cells
    b. Lisch nodule, neural crest hamartoma
    c. Koeppe nodule, stromal hyperplasia
    d. Brushfield spot, histiocytes and Touton giant cells

17. Which of the following statements is true concerning immunoglobulin
    a. IgG crosses the placenta
    b. IgA binds complement
    c. IgM is present in newborns
    d. IgD is the second most abundant

18. A retinal detachment caused by fixation artifact can be differentiated from a true retinal detachment by all of the following except
    a. a fold at the ora serrata
    b. no subretinal fluid
    c. normal retinal architecture
    d. pigment adherent to photoreceptors

19. Which of the following epithelial changes in the eyelid refers to thickening of the squamous cell layer
    a. parakeratosis
    b. acanthosis
    c. dysplasia
    d. papillomatosis

20. Intraocular hemorrhage may cause all of the following sequelae except
    a. synchysis scintillans
    b. ochre membrane
    c. asteroid hyalosis
    d. hemosiderosis bulbi

21. Intraocular calcification may occur in all of the following except
    a. retinoblastoma
    b. medulloepithelioma
    c. choroidal hemangioma
    d. phthisis

22. The histopathology of which tumor is classically described as a storiform pattern of tumor cells
    a. rhabdomyosarcoma
    b. plasmacytoma
    c. neurilemoma
    d. fibrous histiocytoma

SUGGESTED READINGS

Embryology

Mann I: The Development of the Human Eye. New York, Grune & Stratton, 1964.

Pathology

Apple DJ: Ocular Pathology: Clinical Applications and Self-Assessment, 5th edition. St. Louis, Mosby, 1998.
Char PH: Tumors of the Eye and Ocular Adnexa. Hamilton, Ontario, Canada, BC Decker, 2001.
Eagle RC: Eye Pathology: An Atlas and Basic Text. Philadelphia, WB Saunders, 1999.
Spencer WH: Ophthalmic Pathology: An Atlas and Textbook, 4th edition. Philadelphia, WB Saunders, 1996.
Yanoff M, Fine BS: Ocular Pathology, 5th edition. Philadelphia, Mosby, 2002.

CHAPTER 4

Neuro-ophthalmology

ANATOMY OF THE VISUAL PATHWAY

Optic nerve → chiasm → optic tract → lateral geniculate body → optic radiations → occipital lobe (Figure 4-1)

Optic nerve: composed of 1.2 million nerve fibers; approximately 1.5 mm in diameter, enlarges to 3.5 mm posterior to lamina cribrosa due to myelin sheath; located 3 to 4 mm from fovea; causes absolute scotoma (blind spot) 15° temporal to fixation and slightly below horizontal meridian; approximately 50 mm in length (1 mm intraocular, 25 mm intraorbital, 9 mm canalicular, 15 mm intracranial) (Figure 4-2)

- *Surrounded by 3 layers of meninges*: dura mater (outer layer; merges with sclera), arachnoid layer, pia mater (inner layer, fused to surface of nerve); space between arachnoid and pia contains CSF
- ON runs through annulus of Zinn (ring of tendinous origins of the rectus muscles) and enters the optic canal
- *Optic canal*: 7 mm long and 5 to 7 mm wide; thinnest medially, adjacent to ethmoid and sphenoid sinuses; dura of ON fuses with periosteum of canal
- *Intracranial ON*: above are found the frontal lobe, olfactory tract, and anterior cerebral and anterior communicating arteries; laterally, the internal carotid artery emerges from the cavernous sinus
- *Blood supply* (Figure 4-3)
  - ORBITAL PORTION: ophthalmic artery with meningeal anastomoses
  - INTRACANALICULAR PORTION: pial branches from ophthalmic artery; possibly internal carotid artery (ICA)
  - INTRACRANIAL PORTION: small vessels from ICA, anterior cerebral and anterior communicating arteries

Chiasm: 10 mm above pituitary gland

- *55% of ON fibers cross in chiasm*: nasal retinal fibers cross in chiasm to contralateral optic tract (decussating nasal fibers); temporal fibers remain uncrossed
- *"Knee of von Willebrand"*: inferonasal retinal fibers cross in chiasm and course anteriorly approximately 4 mm into contralateral ON before running posteriorly
- Carotid arteries course on either side of chiasm (Figure 4-4)
- *Blood supply*: ICA; occasionally by anterior cerebral and anterior communicating arteries

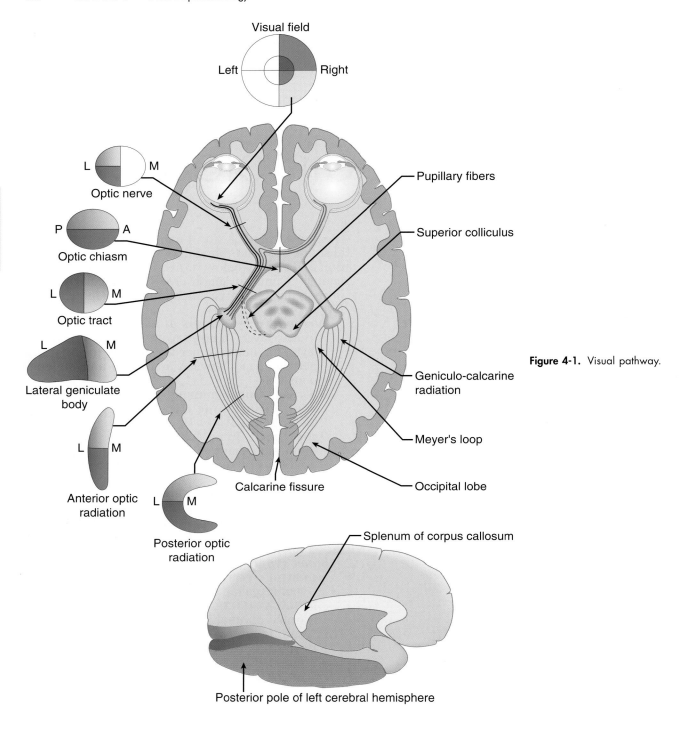

Figure 4-1. Visual pathway.

Optic tract: lower fibers lie laterally (90° rotation of fibers); tract courses laterally around cerebral peduncle

Damage to optic tract results in contralateral relative afferent pupillary defect (RAPD) because 55% of fibers cross (greater quantity of nasal fibers [nasal to foveal]), including the large monocular crescent (which corresponds with the extreme nasal retina)

Special fibers run to the hypothalamus, contributing to neuroendocrine systems that control diurnal rhythms

A major projection leaves the optic tract just before the lateral geniculate body (LGB) to form the brachium of the superior colliculus (also called *optic tectum*)

Superior colliculus: involved in foveation reflexes (receives input from pupillary fibers); injury disrupts eye movements but does not cause visual field (VF) defect

Pupillary fibers pass through brachium of superior colliculus to pretectal area, which innervates both Edinger-Westphal subnuclei of CN3

Optic tract provides retinal input to visual nucleus (pulvinar) in the thalamus

Blood supply: anterior choroidal artery; branches from posterior communicating artery

Lateral geniculate body (LGB): part of the thalamus (Figure 4-5)

Lower fibers lie laterally in optic tract and LGB (90° rotation of fibers)

Crossed fibers (contralateral eye): project to layers 1, 4, and 6

Uncrossed fibers (ipsilateral eye): project to layers 2, 3, and 5

Layers of LGB can also be categorized by neuronal size:

MAGNOCELLULAR NEURONS (M cells): layers 1 and 2; subserve motion detection, stereoacuity, and contrast sensitivity; project to layer 4C alpha of visual cortex

PARVOCELLULAR NEURONS (P cells): layers 3 to 6; subserve fine spatial resolution and color vision; project to layer 4C beta of visual cortex

KONIOCELLULAR NEURONS (K cells): sit in interlaminar zones and superficial layers; receive input from both retinas and the superior colliculus; may modulate information among other pathways

BLOOD SUPPLY: anterior communicating artery and choroidal arteries

Optic radiations: myelinated nerve fibers; connect LGB to occipital cortex

Superior retinal fibers (inferior VF): travel in white matter underneath parietal cortex to occipital lobe

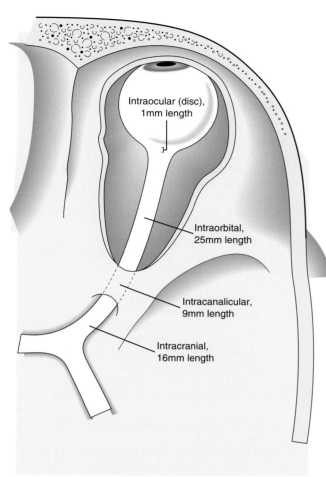

Figure 4-2. The 4 portions of the optic nerve. The lengths are given. (From Sadun AA: Anatomy and physiology. In Yanoff M, Duker JS [eds]: *Ophthalmology*, 2n ed, St. Louis, Mosby, 2004.)

Labels in Figure 4-2:
Intraocular (disc), 1mm length
Intraorbital, 25mm length
Intracanalicular, 9mm length
Intracranial, 16mm length

Figure 4-3. Anterior optic nerve. The sheath and the vascular supply to the intraocular and intraorbital portions are shown. (From Sadun AA: Anatomy and physiology. In Yanoff M, Duker JS [eds]: *Ophthalmology*, 2nd ed, St. Louis, Mosby, 2004.)

Labels in Figure 4-3:
Circle of Zinn–Haller
Short posterior ciliary artery
Optic nerve sheath
Subarachnoid space
Optic nerve
Pial vasculature
Ophthalmic artery
Ophthalmic vein
Central artery and vein
Eye

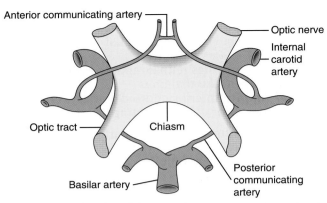

Figure 4-4. Relationship of the optic chiasm, optic nerves, and optic tracts to the arterial circle of Willis. The chiasm passes through the circle of Willis and receives its arterial supply from the anterior cerebral and communicating arteries from above, and the posterior communicating, posterior cerebral, and basilar arteries from below. (Adapted from Reed H, Drance SM: *The Essentials of Perimetry: Static and Kinetic*, 2nd ed, London, Oxford University Press, 1972.)

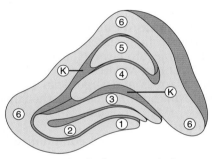

Figure 4-5. Lateral geniculate body section. The layers are numbered from ventral to dorsal in this posterior view. K fibers travel between the lamellae. (From Lawton AW: Retrochiasmal pathways, higher cortical function, and nonorganic visual loss. In Yanoff M, Duker JS [eds]: *Ophthalmology*, 2nd ed, St. Louis, Mosby, 2004.)

Inferior retinal fibers (superior VF): travel around ventricular system into temporal lobe (*Meyer's loop*); Meyer's loop is about 5 cm from tip of temporal lobe; temporal lobe injury causes incongruous homonymous superior quadrantanopia, or a "pie-in-the-sky" VF defect

Macular fibers: travel more centrally than do inferior retinal fibers

Blood supply: middle cerebral arteries

Primary visual cortex (striate cortex, V1, Brodmann's area 17): medial face of occipital lobe, divided horizontally by calcarine fissure

Visual cortex contains a topographic map of the contralateral hemifield; central portion of VF is highly magnified

Macular region is posterior, extending slightly onto lateral aspect of occipital lobe

Peripheral VF is located anteriorly along calcarine fissure

Temporal crescent in each VF (from 55° to 100°) is seen only by nasal retina of ipsilateral eye;

located most anteriorly; only site posterior to chiasm that if injured would cause a monocular VF defect; temporal crescent may also be the only portion of VF spared after occipital lobe damage

Blood supply: middle and posterior cerebral arteries

Visual association areas: areas 18 and 19

Other areas:

Ganglia:
1. **CILIOSPINAL CENTER OF BUDGE**: sympathetic fibers from hypothalamus synapse; located at level C8-T2
2. **SUPERIOR CERVICAL**: 2nd-order sympathetic fibers synapse
3. **CILIARY**: small parasympathetic ganglion; 1 cm from optic foramen between ON and lateral rectus muscle
   RECEIVES 3 ROOTS:
   Long sensory: sensory from cornea, iris, and ciliary body
   Short parasympathetic: motor to ciliary body and iris sphincter
   Sympathetic: conjunctival vasoconstrictor fibers and iris dilator
4. **GENICULATE**: traversed by CN 7; contains cell bodies that provide taste from anterior 2/3 of tongue
5. **SPHENOPALATINE**: parasympathetic fibers to lacrimal gland

Horizontal gaze center: controls gaze to ipsilateral side; located in paramedian pontine reticular formation (PPRF) at level of CN 6 nucleus; projects to ipsilateral CN 6 nucleus and (via medial longitudinal fasciculus [MLF]) to contralateral CN 6 nucleus (Figure 4-6)

Medial Longitudinal Fasciculus (MLF): extends from anterior horn cells of the spinal cord to the thalamus; connects CN 3 nuclei and gaze centers (ipsilateral CN 3 and contalateral CN 6)

Vertical gaze center: originates in frontal eye fields or in superior colliculus; requires bilateral cortical input; projections travel to rostral interstitial nucleus of the MLF (riMLF) located behind red nucleus in midbrain; fibers travel to nuclei of CN 3 and 4 (Figure 4-7)

UPGAZE (lateral portion of riMLF): stimulates CN 3 nucleus (SR and IO)

DOWNGAZE (medial portion of riMLF): stimulates CN 3 nucleus (IR) and CN 4 nucleus

TORSIONAL MOVEMENTS: via interstitial nucleus of Cajal

Glial cells:

OLIGODENDROCYTES: myelination (begins at LGB and reaches lamina cribrosa after birth)

ASTROCYTES: support and nutrition

MICROGLIAL CELLS: phagocytosis

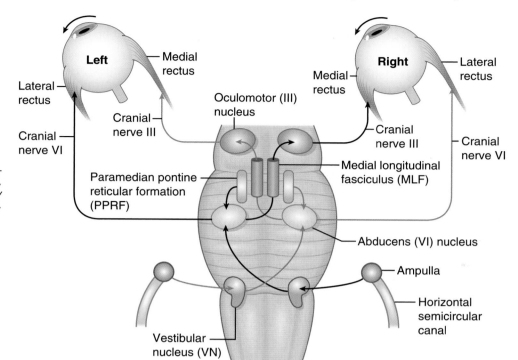

Figure 4-6. Horizontal eye movement pathways. (From Bajandas FJ, Kline LB: *Neuro-Ophthalmology Review Manual*. Thorofare, NJ, Slack, 1988.)

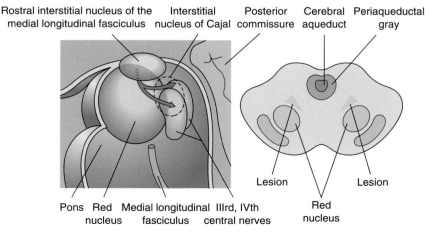

Figure 4-7. Pathways for vertical gaze. Upgaze pathways originate in the rostral interstitial nucleus of the medial longitudinal fasciculus and project dorsally to innervate the oculomotor and trochlear nerves, traveling through the posterior commissure. Lesions to both axon bundles are necessary to produce upgaze paralysis (lesions B or C). Upgaze paralysis is a feature of the dorsal midbrain syndrome as a result of the lesion's effect on the posterior commissure (lesion A). Downgaze pathways also originate in the rostral interstitial nucleus of the medial longitudinal fasciculus but probably travel more ventrally. Bilateral lesions also are needed to affect downgaze and usually are located dorsomedial to the red nucleus. (From Donahue SP, Lavin PJM: Disorders of supranuclear control of ocular motility. In Yanoff M, Duker JS [eds]: *Ophthalmology*, London, Mosby, 1999.)

PHYSIOLOGY

Testing

Color vision tets: Ishihara pseudoisochromatic or Hardy-Rand-Ritter plates; Farnsworth tests
  Congenital defects: usually red/green
  Acquired macular disease: may diminish blue/yellow in early stages (blue cones concentrated in perifoveal ring)
  Fovea has mostly red/green cones, so red/green defects are detected in optic nerve diseases. Perception of red object indicates gross macular function

Photostress recovery test: determine best-corrected vision, shine bright light into eye for 10 seconds, record time for vision to recover within 1 line of best-corrected vision; test each eye separately; invalid for eyes with vision worse than 20/80
  Optic nerve disease: normal recovery time (less than 60 seconds)
  Macular disease: prolonged time (longer than 90 seconds)

Contrast sensitivity: Pelli-Robson chart; Regan contrast sensitivity chart; VectorVision chart

Visually evoked cortical potentials (VEP, VER): measure macular visual function, integrity of primary and secondary visual cortex, and continuity of optic nerve and tract radiations; fovea has large area in occipital cortex, close to recording electrodes; smaller area representing more peripheral retina lies deep within calcarine fissure
  Can measure vision in preverbal infants
  Flash VER: strobe light
  Pattern VER: checkerboard pattern or bar grating (amacrine and ganglion cell layer of retina)
  P100 wave: positive deflection at 100 msec; amplitude is height from peak to trough, latency is time from onset of flash to peak of wave
  Toxic or compressive optic neuropathies: reduction of amplitude more pronounced than prolongation of latency

Figure 4-8. Normal visual evoked cortical response. (Reprinted with permission from Slamovits TL: Basic and clinical science course. Section 12: Retina and Vitreous, San Francisco, American Academy of Ophthalmology, 1993.)

Demyelination: latency is prolonged; amplitude may be only mildly reduced

Amsler grid: tests central 10° of the visual field (held at 14 inches); 10 cm × 10 cm grid composed of 5-mm squares; primarily used to evaluate foveal pathology

Optokinetic nystagmus (OKN): presence suggests visual input is present; slow phase is noted in direction of moving stimulus
  Parieto-occipital area controls slow pursuit, frontal lobe controls saccades
  Pathway in visual association area terminates in ipsilateral pontine gaze center, resulting in pursuit movements to the same side (i.e., right visual association area controls pursuit to the right)

Can use to diagnose functional visual loss
  Normal (symmetric) OKN response: occipital lobe, temporal lobe, LGB, or optic tract lesions do not interfere with pursuit
  Deficient pursuit movements to side of lesion (asymmetric OKN): parietal lobe lesion
  Cogan's dictum (for homonomous hemianopia): asymmetric OKN indicates parietal lobe lesion; symmetric OKN indicates occipital lobe lesion
  Reversal of OKN response: 60% of patients with congenital motor nystagmus
  Dorsal midbrain syndrome: downward moving OKN drum causes convergence-retraction nystagmus
  Congenital ocular motor apraxia: loss of voluntary horizontal gaze (vertical gaze intact); abnormal OKN (fast phase absent); maintained tonic deviation

Red glass test: evaluation of diplopia

Potential acuity meter (PAM): projects image of letter chart onto retina to test macular potential in patients with media opacities

Purkinje vascular phenomena and blue field entopic test: visualization of retinal vasculature; indicates gross retinal function

Visual Field (VF) Defects

Types:
  Blind spot: physiologic due to ON; 15° temporal to fixation and slightly below horizontal midline
  Baring of blind spot: glaucoma, normal patients
  Cecocentral scotoma: involves blind spot and macula (within 25° of fixation); can occur in any condition that produces a central scotoma, dominant optic atrophy, Leber's optic atrophy, toxic/nutritional optic neuropathy, optic pit with serous retinal detachment, optic neuritis
  Central scotoma: unilateral (optic neuritis, compressive lesion of ON, retinal lesion [macular

edema, disciform scar]); bilateral (toxic optic neuropathy, nutritional deficiency, macular lesions)

Arcuate scotoma: glaucoma, optic neuritis, AION, BRAO, BVO, ON drusen

Altitudinal defect: damage to upper or lower pole of optic disc; optic neuritis, AION, hemiretinal artery or vein occlusion

Spiraling of visual field: suggests malingering/ functional visual loss

Pseudo-bitemporal hemianopia (slope and cross-vertical meridian): uncorrected refractive error, tilted optic disc, enlarged blind spot (papilledema), large central or cecocentral scotoma, sector retinitis pigmentosa (nasal quadrant), overhanging lid, coloboma

Binasal defect: most nasal defects due to arcuate scotomas (glaucoma); also, pressure on temporal aspect of ON and anterior angle of chiasm, aneurysm, pituitary adenoma, infarct

Constricted field (ring scotoma): retinitis pigmentosa, advanced glaucoma, thyroid-related ophthalmopathy, ON drusen, vitamin A deficiency, occipital stroke, panretinal photocoagulation, functional visual loss

Neurologic defect: bilateral and respects vertical midline

Localizing VF defects:
Nerve fiber layer: arcuate, papillomacular, temporal wedge

Chiasm: bitemporal hemianopia (junctional scotoma if involving Willebrand's knee)

Optic tract: incongruous homonymous hemianopia

Temporal lobe (Meyer's loop): "pie-in-the-sky" (denser superiorly, spares central)

Parietal lobe: denser inferiorly

Occipital lobe: congruous; ±macular sparing

Neurologic VF defects:
Congruity of VF defect (retrochiasmal lesions): the more congruous the defect, the more posterior the lesion

Superior field: anterior retinal ganglion cells → lateral portion of optic tract → temporal lobe (Meyer's loop) → inferior bank of calcarine fissure

Vision not reduced by unilateral lesion posterior to the chiasm (20/20 acuity with macula-splitting hemianopia)

Chiasm: pituitary tumor, pituitary apoplexy, craniopharyngioma, meningioma, optic nerve glioma, aneurysm, trauma, infection, metastatic tumor, MS, sarcoid

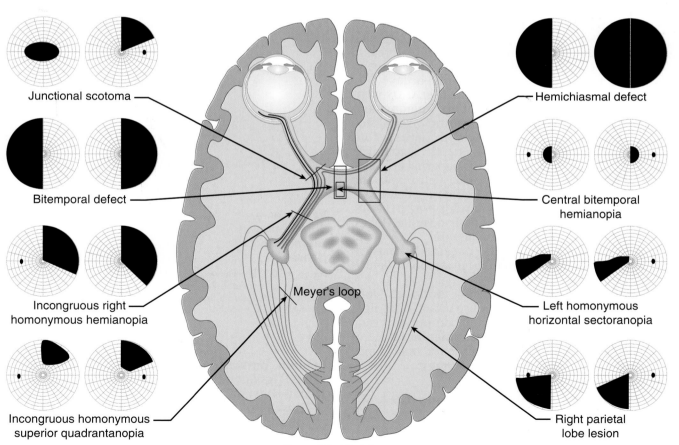

Junctional scotoma

Bitemporal defect

Incongruous right homonymous hemianopia

Incongruous homonymous superior quadrantanopia

Meyer's loop

Hemichiasmal defect

Central bitemporal hemianopia

Left homonymous horizontal sectoranopia

Right parietal lobe lesion

Figure 4-9. VF defects.

ANTERIOR CHIASMAL SYNDROME: lesion at junction of ON and chiasm; involves fibers in Willebrand's knee (contralateral nasal retinal loop); causes **junctional scotoma** (central scotoma in 1 eye and superotemporal defect in the other)

BODY OF CHIASM: bitemporal hemianopia; vision may be preserved

POSTERIOR CHIASM: bitemporal hemianopia; primarily involves crossing macular fibers

LATERAL COMPRESSION (very rare): binasal hemianopia (more commonly caused by bilateral ON or retinal lesions)

Optic tract: posterior sellar or suprasellar lesions; homonymous hemianopia, contralateral RAPD

Retro-LGB lesions: 90% of isolated homonymous hemianopias due to stroke

Optic radiations:

TEMPORAL LOBE (Meyer's loop): **"pie-in-the-sky"** (superior homonymous hemianopia), formed visual hallucinations, seizures

PARIETAL LOBE: inferior homonymous hemianopia, hemiparesis, visual perception difficulty, agnosia, apraxia, OKN asymmetry

GERSTMANN'S SYNDROME: lesion of dominant parietal lobe; acalculia, agraphia, finger agnosia, left-right confusion, associated with inferior homonymous hemianopia if optic radiation involved

Occipital lobe:

HOMONYMOUS HEMIANOPIA WITH MACULAR SPARING: suggests infarct in area supplied by posterior cerebral artery; macular region receives dual supply from both middle cerebral artery and posterior cerebral artery

BILATERAL CONGRUOUS CENTRAL ISLANDS WITH VERTICAL STEP: equivalent to homonymous hemianopia with macular sparing; vertical step does not occur in retinal or optic nerve lesions

CHECKERBOARD FIELD: bilateral incomplete homonymous hemianopias, superior on 1 side and inferior on opposite side (left upper and right lower homonymous quadrant defects)

BILATERAL HOMONYMOUS ALTITUDINAL DEFECTS: infarction or trauma to both occipital lobes, above or below calcarine fissure

MONOCULAR TEMPORAL CRESCENT DEFECT: anterior occipital infarct; far temporal field is seen by only 1 eye

Cortical blindness: bilateral occipital lobe destruction; pupillary response intact, blindsight (rudimentary visual capacity), unformed visual hallucinations, **Riddoch phenomenon** (perceive moving targets but not stationary ones); may deny blindness (**Anton's syndrome**)

Eye Movements under Supranuclear Control

Horizontal gaze center:

Saccades: contralateral frontal eye fields (frontal lobe) → superior colliculus → pontine parame-

dian reticular formation (PPRF) → horizontal gaze center (CN 6 nucleus) → ipsilateral LR and contralateral MR (via MLF)

Smooth pursuit: ipsilateral parieto-occipital lobe → SC → PPRF → horizontal gaze center → ipsilateral LR and contralateral MR (via MLF)

Saccadic system (FEM): generates fast eye movements (refixation); 300° to 700°/sec

Tests: refixation, rotation, calorics, and optokinetic nystagmus (fast saccadic return phase)

Abnormalities: progressive external ophthalmoplegia, myasthenia gravis, Wilson's disease, Huntington's disease, ataxia-telangiectasia, spinocerebellar degeneration, progressive supranuclear palsy, olivopontocerebellar atrophy, Whipple's disease, Gaucher's disease, MS, Pelizaeus-Merzbacher disease

Ocular motor apraxia: failure to initiate a saccade (Figure 4-11)

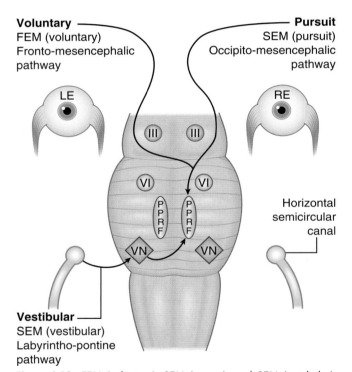

Figure 4-10. FEM (voluntary), SEM (pursuit), and SEM (vestibular). Pathways all converge on PPRF for horizontal eye movements. VN, vestibular nuclei. (From Bajandas FJ, Kline LB: *Neuro-Ophthalmology Review Manual*. Thorofare, NJ, Slack, 1988.)

Smooth pursuit system (SEM): following movements; ipsilateral parieto-occipital junction (horizontal); interstitial nucleus of Cajal (vertical)

Tests: Doll's head, rotation, OKN (pursuit movement)

Abnormalities: demyelination (young patients), microvascular disease (older patients)

Figure 4-11. Composite reminder of the course and lateralization of the 3 conjugate horizontal eye movement pathways. (From Bajandas FJ, Kline LB: *Neuro-ophthalmology Review Manual.* Thorofare, NJ, Slack, 1988, p 55.)

Vergence system: maintains foveal fixation on approaching object; controlled by frontal and occipital lobes, and possibly midbrain

Types: voluntary, accommodative, fusional

Test: look from distance to near

Position maintenance system (vestibulo-ocular reflex [VOR]): maintains specific gaze position during head movements

Teleologically oldest eye movement system; also fastest (shortest latency)

Semicircular canals → CN 8 → vestibular nucleus → contralateral horizontal gaze center → EOMs

Test: calorics; rotation

Abnormalities cause oscillopsia

Nonoptic reflex systems: integrate eye movements with body movements

Normal caloric and Doll's head responses when nuclear and internuclear connections are intact

Calorics: irrigate water into ears and observe induced eye movements; mnemonic COWS (cold opposite, warm same) refers to direction of fast phase of nystagmus in awake patient (jerk nystagmus); in comatose patient, get tonic deviation in opposite direction of mnemonic (sustained slow phase movement only)

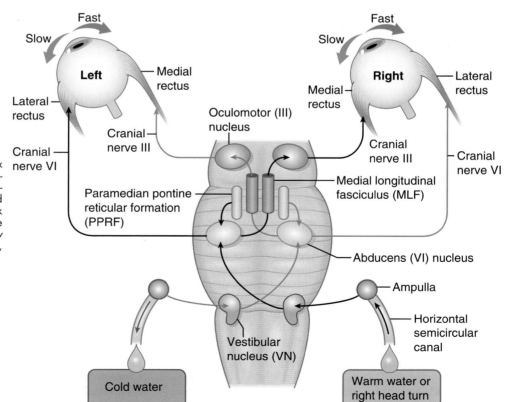

Figure 4-12. Vestibulo-ocular reflex demonstrating right beating nystagmus. Right COWS = cold opposite, warm same. (Calorics should be performed with head back 60°.) (From Bajandas FJ, Kline LB: *Neuro-Ophthalmology Review Manual.* Thorofare, NJ, Slack, 1988.)

Bilateral cold water irrigation produces nystagmus with fast phase upward in awake patient and downward tonic deviation in comatose patient; opposite effects with warm water

PATHWAY: vestibular nuclei → contralateral CN 6 nuclei → ipsilateral LR and contralateral MR (via MLF); no connection to the PPRF

Doll's head (oculocephalic reflex): turn head and observe direction of eye movements; vestibular system moves eyes; use when patient cannot voluntarily move eyes

Eyes should have tonic movement in direction opposite head rotation

INTACT DOLL'S HEAD: supranuclear lesion (cranial nerve pathways to muscles are intact) (i.e., progressive supranuclear palsy)

ABNORMAL DOLL'S HEAD: lesion is infranuclear paresis or restrictive disease (perform forced ductions)

Bell's phenomenon: upward turning of eyes with forced closure of eyelids

INTACT BELL'S PHENOMENON: supranuclear lesion

DIPLOPIA

Types:
Comitant: amount of deviation same in all fields of gaze
Incomitant: amount of deviation varies in different fields of gaze

Etiology:
Monocular: high astigmatism, chalazion or lid mass, corneal abnormality, iris atrophy, polycoria, cataract, subluxed crystalline lens, decentered IOL, posterior capsular opacity, retinal pathology, functional
Binocular: neuropathic (cranial nerve palsies, MS), myopathic (thyroid-related ophthalmopathy, orbital pseudotumor), neuromuscular junction (myasthenia gravis)

DDx:
Supranuclear (due to inadequate convergence): skew deviation, progressive supranuclear palsy, Parkinson's disease, Huntington's disease, dorsal midbrain syndrome
Intermittent: MG, MS, migraine, thyroid-related ophthalmopathy, convergence spasm, decompensated phoria, convergence-retraction nystagmus, ocular myotonia
Vertical: MG, MS, thyroid-related, orbital disease (tumor, trauma, inflammation), CN 3 or CN 4 palsy, Brown's syndrome, skew deviation
Aberrent regeneration: Duane's syndrome, Marcus Gunn jaw-winking syndrome

Restrictive syndromes: IOP elevation > 4 mm Hg when eyes directed into restricted field (thyroid, trauma, inflammatory orbital disease, neoplastic process)

EYE MOVEMENT DISORDERS

Central Disorders (Supranuclear)

Often no symptoms or complaints

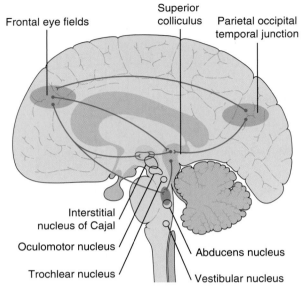

Rostral interstitial nucleus of the medial longitudinal fasciculus
Paramedian pontine reticular formation

Figure 4-13. Supranuclear control of eye movements. The pontine horizontal gaze center (blue) and the vertical gaze center in the midbrain (yellow) receive input from the frontal eye fields to initiate saccades, and from the parietal occipital temporal junction to control pursuit. These gaze centers control ocular motility by synapsing upon the ocular motor nerve nuclei (III, IV, and VI). (From Lavin PJM, Donahue SP: Disorders of supranuclear control of ocular motility. In Yanoff M, Duker JS [eds]: *Ophthalmology*, 2nd ed, St. Louis, Mosby, 2004.)

Ocular Motor Apraxia

Saccadic palsy; impairment of voluntary eye movements with preservation of reflex movements; male > female; congenital or acquired **(Balint's syndrome)**; extensive bilateral cerebral disease involving supranuclear pathways (usually bilateral frontoparietal)

Associations: Gaucher's disease, spinocerebeller degeneration, MR, ataxia-telangiectasia, Wilson's disease, hypoplasia of corpus callosum, hydrocephalus; rarely cerebellar mass lesion (perform MRI)

Findings:
Head thrusting: patient must move head to look at objects; head thrust toward desired direction of gaze results in contralateral slow eye movement so patient must overshoot target; lessens with age; may resolve by age 20; patient may also blink to break fixation
Abnormal OKN: fast phase absent
Abnormal vestibular: rotational nystagmus absent
Normal pursuits

Horizontal Gaze Palsies

Congenital

Must distinguish between supranuclear and infranuclear causes; often abnormality of CN 6 or interneurons; vertical movements usually unaffected

Möbius' Syndrome

Horizontal gaze palsy with CN 6, 7, 8, and 9 palsies (facial diplegia, deafness, abnormal digits)

Acquired

Frontoparietal lesion (stroke, trauma, or infection): tonic deviation of eyes to side of lesion (contralateral area 8 unopposed)

> ***Doll's head testing and calorics***: can turn eyes contralateral to lesion (intact vestibular pathway)

Parieto-occipital lesion: ipsilateral pursuit palsy (cogwheel pursuit)

Tegmental lesion: ipsilateral pursuit and saccadic palsy

Pontine lesion (PPRF): ipsilateral horizontal gaze palsy

Parkinson's disease: reduced blinking, reduced saccades, reduced glabellar reflex suppression, blepharospasm, oculogyric crisis

Huntington's chorea

Metabolic disorders: hyperglycemia, Wernicke's encephalopathy, Wilson's disease

Drug-induced: tricyclic antidepressants, phenytoin, phenothiazines

Pseudogaze palsies: myasthenia gravis, chronic progressive external ophthalmoplegia (CPEO), Duane's syndrome

Internuclear ophthalmoplegia (INO): lesion of MLF; inability to adduct ipsilateral eye with nystagmus of fellow eye; may have skew deviation and upbeat nystagmus (Figure 4-14)

> ***Unilateral***: ischemia, demyelination, tumor, infection (meningitis, encephalitis), trauma, compression
>
> ***Bilateral***: demyelination (most common), trauma, ischemia, infection, Chiari malformation, toxicity (amitriptyline, ethanol, benzodiazepine)
>
> ***Types***:
>
> ANTERIOR (midbrain): preserved convergence
>
> POSTERIOR (pons): impaired convergence (WEBINO = wall-eyed bilateral INO)

One-and-a-half syndrome (Fisher syndrome): lesion of CN 6 nucleus and ipsilateral MLF; causes ipsilateral gaze palsy and INO; only movement is abduction of contralateral eye (with nystagmus); supranuclear lesion therefore converges intact; called paralytic pontine exotropia when patient appears XT (Figure 4-15)

> ***Etiology***: MS, basilar artery occlusion, pontine metastases

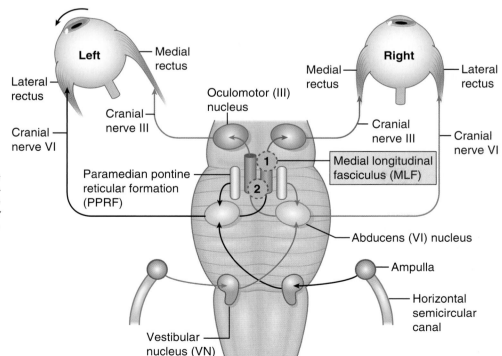

Figure 4-14. 1. Right internuclear ophthalmoplegia (INO) 2. Bilateral INO. (From Bajandas FJ, Kline LB: *Neuro-Ophthalmology Review Manual.* Thorofare, NJ, Slack, 1988.)

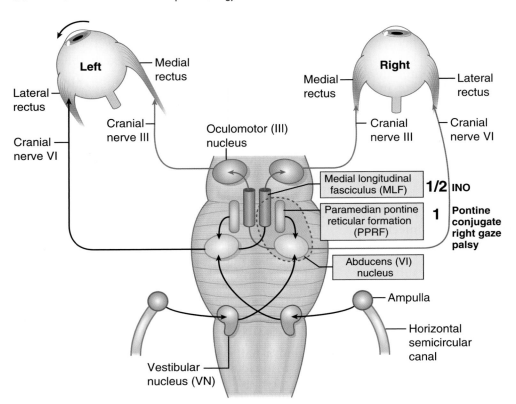

Figure 4-15. Right acute 1¹/₂ syndrome (paralytic pontine exotropia). (From Bajandas FJ, Kline LB: *Neuro-Ophthalmology Review Manual.* Thorofare, NJ, Slack, 1988.)

Vertical Gaze Abnormalities

Parinaud's Syndrome (Dorsal Midbrain Syndrome)

Supranuclear gaze palsy with nuclear CN 3 palsy

Etiology: 90% due to pineal tumor; also, demyelination, infarction, tumor

Findings: supranuclear paresis of upgaze (Doll's head intact), bilateral mid-dilated pupils, convergence-retraction nystagmus on attempted upgaze (synchronous backward jerking movements of both eyes due to co-contraction of horizontal recti), light-near dissociation, vertical OKN, skew deviation, lid retraction (Collier's sign)

Diagnosis: MRI; Hcg level

Treatment: XRT

Progressive Supranuclear Palsy (Steele-Richardson-Olszewski Syndrome)

Progressive vertical (early) and horizontal (late) gaze palsy (downward gaze usually affected first); no Bell's phenomenon; doll's head maneuver gives full ROM, indicating supranuclear nature of disorder; eventually frozen globe to all stimuli, spasm of fixation, decreased blink rate, blepharitis, blepharospasm; occasionally, apraxia of eye opening; also, axial rigidity, dysarthria, and dementia

Skew Deviation

Vertical misalignment of visual axes due to imbalance of prenuclear inputs; comitant or incomitant

Vertical tropia, hyperdeviation usually increases on ipsilateral downgaze, no cyclodeviation; hypodeviated eye usually ipsilateral to lesion, except when associated with INO in which hyperdeviated eye is ipsilateral; may occur with other brain stem symptoms or cerebellar disease

Etiology: brain stem infarct, MS, increased ICP, pseudotumor cerebri, vestibulo-ocular imbalance, cerebellar disease; vertebral-basilar insufficiency may cause transient skew deviation

Treatment: often transient and requires observation only; chronic deviations may be treated with prism spectacles or surgery

Whipple's Disease

Oculomasticatory myorhythmia (vertical eye movements and facial activity similar to myoclonus)

Olivopontocerebellar Atrophy

Hereditary or sporadic; onset early adulthood; unsteady gait, slurred speech, dementia, optic atrophy, retinal degeneration

Eye movements progressively slow in all directions, finally complete external ophthalmoplegia

Pathology: cerebellar and pontine atrophy

Kernicterus

Progressive loss of eye movements

Also, metabolic diseases (maple syrup disease, Wernicke's encephalopathy), drug-induced

Nystagmus

Rhythmic involuntary oscillations of the eyes due to disorder of slow eye movement (SEM) system. Direction named after fast phase (brain's attempt to correct problem), even though abnormality is noted with slow phase

Etiology: abnormal slow eye movement, high gain instability (SEM is working at high gain), vestibular tone imbalance, integrator leak (gaze-evoked nystagmus), OKN abnormality

Characteristics: may be fast or slow, pendular or jerk (designated by direction of rapid phase), unidirectional or multidirectional, symmetric or asymmetric, congenital or acquired
   Gain: eye moves 15° (output) in response to a retinal image position error of 15° (gain = 1)
   Foveation: bring an image onto, or maintain an image on, the fovea
   Frequency: oscillations per second (Hz)
   Amplitude: excursion of oscillation
   Intensity: product of amplitude and frequency
   Null point: position in which intensity of nystagmus is least
   Neutral point: position in which a reversal of the direction of jerk nystagmus occurs

Childhood Nystagmus

Most commonly, congenital, latent, sensory, and spasmus nutans (see Chapter 5, Pediatrics/Strabismus)

Physiologic Nystagmus

Several forms of nystagmus, including end-gaze, optokinetic, caloric, and rotational

Acquired Nystagmus

Pattern helps localize pathology, may have oscillopsia

Bruns'

Combination of gaze-paretic nystagmus when looking toward lesion (fast phase toward the lesion), and vestibular imbalance nystagmus when looking away from lesion (fast phase away from lesion) (i.e., with right-sided lesion: high-amplitude, low-frequency, right-beating nystagmus on right gaze; low-amplitude, high-frequency, left-beating nystagmus on left gaze)

Gaze-paretic component is of high amplitude and low frequency (because of impairment of horizontal gaze mechanism on side of lesion)

Vestibular component is of low amplitude and high frequency, with fast phase away from damaged vestibular nuclei on side of lesion

Due to cerebellopontine angle mass (usually acoustic neuroma or meningioma)

Convergence-Retraction

Co-contraction of lateral recti produces convergence movement (abnormal saccades) on attempted upgaze

Due to periaqueductal gray matter or dorsal midbrain lesion (Parinaud's, pinealoma, trauma, brain stem AVM, MS)

Dissociated

Asymmetric between the 2 eyes (different direction, amplitude, frequency, etc); always pathologic

Due to posterior fossa disease, MS

Downbeat

Eyes drift upward with corrective saccade downward; worsens in downgaze, improves in upgaze; oscillopsia

Due to lesion that affects pathways responsible for downgaze; cervicomedullary junction lesion (Arnold-Chiari malformation, tumor, syrinx: 33%), spinocerebellar degeneration, intoxication, lithium, paraneoplastic cerebellar degeneration, 50% with no identifiable cause

Gaze-Evoked

Nystagmus in direction of gaze, absent in primary position, fast phase toward lesion

Due to extra-axial mass compressing brain stem (acoustic neuroma, cerebellar hemisphere tumor), intoxication

Waveform: exponentially decreasing

Periodic Alternating Nystagmus (PAN)

Changes horizontal direction; jerks right 90 seconds, 5- to 10-second pause, jerks left 90 seconds, repeats; remains horizontal in vertical gaze; usually acquired

Due to disease of vestibulocerebellar system (albinism, cranio-cervico junction lesion [Arnold-Chiari malformation], MS, syphilis, tumor, vascular, dilantin, spinocerebellar degeneration)

Treatment: baclofen; surgery (large recession of all 4 recti muscles)

Seesaw

Vertical and torsional nystagmus with 1 eye rising and intorting while fellow eye falls and excyclotorts, then reverses

Due to suprasellar lesions, CVA, or trauma, or is congenital

MRI: rule out large parasellar tumors expanding into third ventricle

Treatment: baclofen

Upbeat

Eyes drift downward with corrective saccade upward

Due to medullary lesions, midline cerebellar (vermis) lesions, medulloblastoma, cerebellar degeneration, MS

Vestibular

Horizontal, rotary, jerk nystagmus in primary gaze; same in all fields of gaze; slow component is linear; remains horizontal in vertical gaze

Due to vestibular disease, infection (labrynthitis), Meniere's disease, vascular, trauma, toxicity

Peripheral vestibular disease: fast phase toward good side; slow phase toward lesion; associated with tinnitus, vertigo, deafness; fixation inhibits vertigo and nystagmus; direction of Romberg fall changes with head turning

Central vestibular disease: nonlocalizing; no tinnitus or deafness

Voluntary

Unsustainable for longer than 30 seconds; associated with hysteria and malingering

Other Eye Movement Disorders

Ocular Bobbing

Intermittent conjugate rapid downward eye movements followed by slow return to primary position

Often secondary to hemorrhage; patient usually comatose

Ocular Dipping

Opposite of ocular bobbing; intermittent rapid upward eye movements followed by slow return to primary position

Ocular Myoclonus

Vertical pendular nystagmus associated with synchronous palatal (uvula) beating

Due to bilateral pseudohypertrophy of inferior olives in medulla, lesion in myoclonic triangle (red nucleus, ipsilateral inferior olive, contralateral dentate nucleus)

Opsoclonus (Saccadomania)

Rapid, chaotic eye movements in all directions; persists in sleep

Associated with dancing hands and feet

Abnormality of pause cells (normally suppress burst cells of PPRF)

Due to remote effect on cerebellum from metastatic neuroblastoma, occasionally with encephalitis

Waveform: no slow phase; repetitive, random; no intersaccadic interval

Oscillopsia

Illusion of movement in the seen world

Usually occurs in SO myokymia and acquired nystagmus; rarely in congenital nystagmus

Due to vestibulo-ocular reflex abnormality

CRANIAL NERVE PALSIES

Oculomotor Nerve (CN 3) Palsy

Anatomy: nucleus in rostral midbrain; fascicle travels ventrally through midbrain, traversing red nucleus and corticospinal tract in cerebral peduncle; nerve enters subarachnoid space, passes between posterior cerebral and superior cerebellar arteries, then courses lateral to posterior communicating artery and enters lateral wall of cavernous sinus; receives sympathetics from internal carotid plexus; passes through superior orbital fissure and divides into superior (supplies SR and levator) and inferior (supplies IR, MR, IO, iris sphincter, and ciliary muscle) divisions.

Only 1 subnucleus (midline location) supplies both levator palpebrae superioris; fibers from SR subnucleus supply contralateral SR; Edinger-Westphal nucleus supplies both pupils (Figure 4-18)

Types: complete, partial, pupil-sparing

Findings: ptosis, hypotropia, exotropia; may involve pupil (fixed and dilated); may cause pain

7 syndromes:
  Nuclear CN 3 palsy (see Fig. 4-17, ①): extremely rare; contralateral SR paresis and bilateral ptosis; pupil involvement is both or neither
  Fascicle syndromes (see Fig. 4-17, ②): ischemic, infiltrative (tumor), or inflammatory (rare)
    NOTHNAGEL'S SYNDROME: lesion of fascicle and superior cerebellar peduncle that causes ipsilateral CN 3 paresis and cerebellar ataxia
    BENEDIKT'S SYNDROME: lesion of fascicle and red nucleus that causes ipsilateral CN 3 paresis,

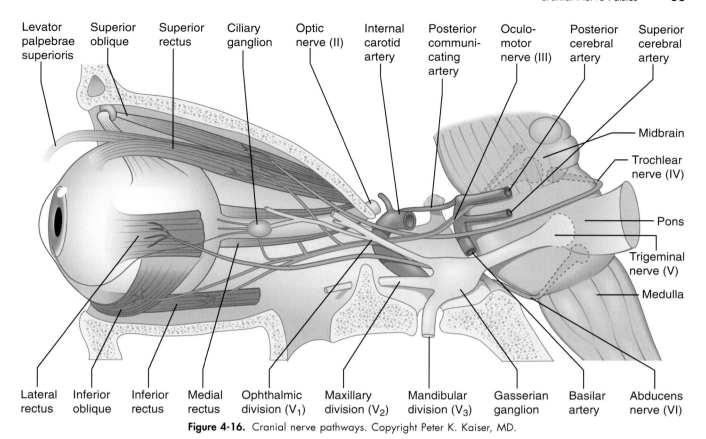

Levator palpebrae superioris | Superior oblique | Superior rectus | Ciliary ganglion | Optic nerve (II) | Internal carotid artery | Posterior communicating artery | Oculo-motor nerve (III) | Posterior cerebral artery | Superior cerebral artery

Midbrain
Trochlear nerve (IV)
Pons
Trigeminal nerve (V)
Medulla

Lateral rectus | Inferior oblique | Inferior rectus | Medial rectus | Ophthalmic division (V$_1$) | Maxillary division (V$_2$) | Mandibular division (V$_3$) | Gasserian ganglion | Basilar artery | Abducens nerve (VI)

Figure 4-16. Cranial nerve pathways. Copyright Peter K. Kaiser, MD.

Levator palpebrae superioris | Superior rectus | Ciliary ganglion | Internal carotid artery | Posterior communicating artery | Red nucleus | Edinger-Westphal nucleus

Corticospinal (pyramidal) tract

Superior colliculus
Inferior colliculus

Inferior oblique | Inferior rectus | Medial rectus | Oculomotor nucleus

Figure 4-17. Seven syndromes of CN 3 palsy. Copyright Peter K. Kaiser, MD.

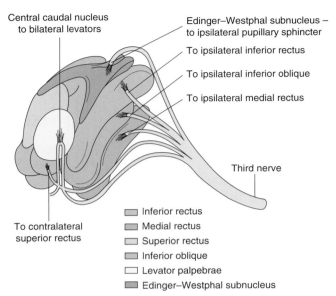

Figure 4-18. Anatomy of the 3rd nerve nucleus. The 3rd nerve nucleus consists of a single, central, caudally located nucleus for the levator palpebrae, paired bilateral subnuclei with crossed projections that innervate the superior recti, and paired bilateral subnuclei with uncrossed projections that innervate the medial recti, inferior recti, and inferior oblique muscles. Parasympathetic input to the ciliary body and iris sphincter arises from the Edinger-Westphal nucleus. (Redrawn from Warwick R: Representation of the extraocular muscles in the oculomotor nuclei of the monkey, *J Comp Neurol* 1953;98:449–503.)

contralateral hemitremor (resting and intentional), and contralateral decreased sensation

WEBER'S SYNDROME: lesion of fascicle and pyrimidal tract that causes ipsilateral CN 3 paresis and contralateral hemiparesis

CLAUDE'S SYNDROME: combination of Nothnagel's and Benedikt's syndromes

Uncal herniation (see Fig. 4-17, ③): supratentorial mass may cause uncal herniation compressing CN 3

Posterior communicating artery (Pcom) aneurysm (see Fig. 4-17, ④): most common nontraumatic, isolated, pupil involving CN 3 palsy; aneurysm at junction of PCom and carotid artery compresses nerve, particularly external parasympathetic pupillomotor fibers; usually painful

Cavernous sinus syndrome (see Fig. 4-17, ⑤): associated with multiple CN palsies (3, 4, V₁, 6) and Horner's; CN 3 palsy often partial and pupil-sparing; may lead to aberrant regeneration

Orbital syndrome (see Fig. 4-17, ⑥): tumor, trauma, pseudotumor, or cellulitis; associated with multiple CN palsies (3, 4, V₁, 6), proptosis, chemosis, injection; ON can appear normal, swollen, or atrophic

After passing through the superior orbital fissure, CN 3 splits into superior and inferior divisions; therefore, CN 3 palsies distal to this point may be complete or partial

Pupil-sparing isolated CN 3 palsy (see Fig. 4-17, ⑦): small-caliber parasympathetic pupillomotor fibers travel in outer layers of nerve closer to blood supply (but more susceptible to damage by compression); fibers at core of nerve are compromised by ischemia; may explain pupil-sparing in 80% of ischemic CN 3 palsies and pupil involved in 95% of compressive CN 3 palsies (trauma, tumor, aneurysm)

ETIOLOGY:

ADULTS: vasculopathic/ischemic (DM, HTN), trauma, giant cell arteritis, occasionally tumor, aneurysm (very rare)

CHILDREN: congenital, trauma, tumor, aneurysm, migraine

14% of PCom aneurysms initially spare pupil

20% of diabetic CN 3 palsies involve pupil

Microvascular CN 3 palsies usually resolve in 3 to 4 months

Myasthenia gravis may mimic CN 3 palsy

Aberrant regeneration: IR and/or MR fibers may innervate levator and/or iris sphincter; sign of previous CN 3 palsy caused by aneurysm or tumor (occasionally trauma); never occurs after vasculopathic injury

Findings:

LID-GAZE DYSKINESIS: lid retracts on downgaze (pseudo–von Graefe's sign) and/or adduction

PUPIL-GAZE DYSKINESIS: more pupillary constriction with convergence than to light (pseudo-Argyll-Robertson pupil) and/or pupillary constriction on downgaze

2 forms:

PRIMARY: no preceding acute CN 3 palsy; insidious development of CN 3 palsy with accompanying signs of misdirection; due to intracavernous lesion (meningioma, aneurysm, neuroma)

SECONDARY: occurs months after CN 3 palsy from trauma, aneurysm (C-C aneurysm), or tumor compression but never after vasculopathic/ischemic lesion

Other causes of CN 3 palsy:

Congenital: variable degrees of aberrant regeneration; 75% have smaller pupil on involved side (due to aberrant regeneration); ptosis and anisocoria

TREATMENT: muscle surgery to straighten eye in primary gaze

Ophthalmoplegic migraine: onset in childhood; positive family history of migraine; paresis of CN 3 occurs as headache abates; usually resolves in 1 month (can be permanent)

Cyclic oculomotor palsy: usually at birth or early childhood; very rare; occurs after complete CN 3 palsy, can be due to diabetic ischemia

FINDINGS: spastic movements of muscles innervated by CN 3 occur at regular intervals for 10 to 30 seconds (spasms of lid elevation, adduction, miosis)

MRI: rule out aneurysm

Workup:

If < age 11: MRI/MRA

If aged 11–45: MRI/MRA and medical workup

If > age 45:

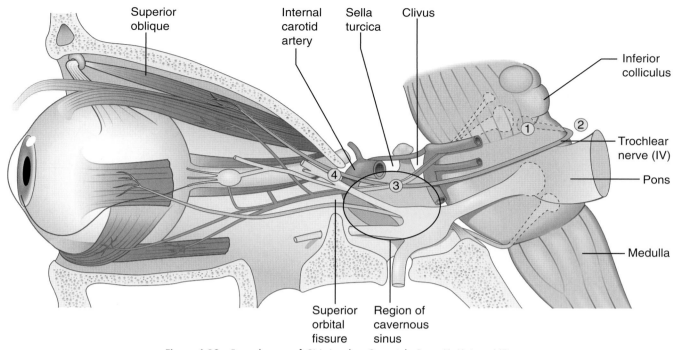

Figure 4-19. 5 syndromes of CN 4 palsy. Copyright Peter K. Kaiser, MD.

WITH PUPIL INVOLVEMENT: MRI/MRA; if normal, cerebral angiography (catheter)

WITH PUPIL-SPARING: usually microvascular; no invasive investigation needed initially; check BP (HTN), blood glucose (DM), ESR, C-reactive protein (giant cell arteritis), CBC, ANA, VDRL, FTA-ABS; if persists >3 months, MRI/MRA with cerebral angiography (aneurysm) if negative

Trochlear Nerve (CN 4) Palsy

Anatomy: nucleus in caudal mesencephalon at level of inferior colliculus; decussates in anterior medullary velum next to aqueduct of Sylvius; fascicle passes between posterior cerebral artery and superior cerebellar artery; nerve travels in lateral wall of cavernous sinus, enters orbit via superior orbital fissure outside annulus of Zinn; innervates superior oblique muscle

Longest intracranial course; only CN that exits dorsally from brain stem; only CN that decussates (except for CN 3 subnucleus that innervates SR); most commonly injured CN following closed head injury (owing to long course)

Etiology: 40% trauma, 30% ischemia, 20% miscellaneous or undetermined, 10% aneurysm

Findings: ipsilateral hypertropia (due to superior rectus overaction)

5 syndromes:

Nuclear/fascicular syndrome (see Fig. 4-19, ①): hemorrhage, infarction, demyelination, trauma; may have contralateral Horner's or INO

Subarachnoid space syndrome (see Fig. 4-19, ②): injury as nerve emerges from dorsal surface of brain stem; trauma (contracoup forces transmitted to brain stem by free tentorial edge), tumor (pinealoma, tentorial meningioma), meningitis, neurosurgical trauma

Cavernous sinus syndrome (see Fig. 4-19, ③): multiple CN palsies (3, 4, V_1, 6) and Horner's

Orbital syndrome (see Fig. 4-19, ④): multiple CN palsies (3, 4, V_1, 6) and Horner's; proptosis, chemosis, injection

Isolated CN 4 palsy:

CONGENITAL: most common; may occur in elderly due to decompensation; large, vertical fusion amplitudes (10–15 prism diopters); check old photos for head tilt

ACQUIRED: acute onset of vertical diplopia; head position (chin down, face turn to opposite side, head tilt to opposite shoulder)

DDx of vertical diplopia: myasthenia gravis, thyroid-related ophthalmopathy, orbital disease (tumor, trauma, inflammation), CN 3 palsy, CN 4 palsy, Brown's syndrome, skew deviation, MS

Diagnosis: Parks-Bielschowsky 3-step test (used for hypertropia due to weakness of a single muscle)

Step 1: Which eye is hypertopic?

LEFT HYPER: paresis of OD elevators (RSR or RIO) or OS depressors (LIR or LSO)

Step 2: Worse on right or left gaze?

If hyper, is worse in left gaze:

Problem with OS muscles that have greatest vertical action during abduction (SR and IR)

Problem with OD muscles that have greatest vertical action during adduction (SO and IO)

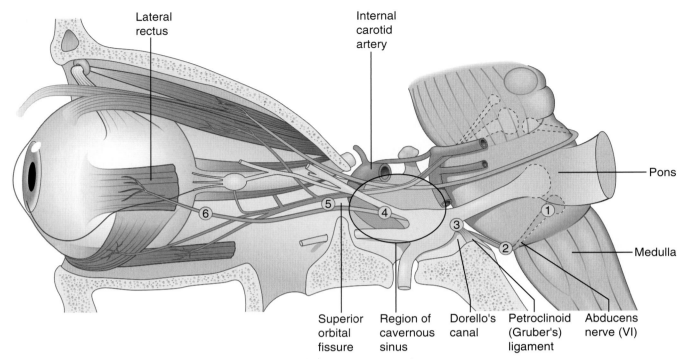

Figure 4-20. 6 syndromes of CN 6 palsy. Copyright Peter K. Kaiser, MD.

SR and IR work best when eye is ABducted
So if left hyper is worse on gaze left: LIR
SO and IO work best when eye is ADducted
So if left hyper is worse on gaze left: RIO
If L hyper is worse on gaze right: RSR or LSO
Step 3: Worse on right or left head tilt?
With head tilt, eyes undergo corrective torsion (with right head tilt, OD intorts and OS extorts)
If 1 of the intorters is the cause of the hyper, then tilting head will worsen hyper on side of head tilt
If worse hyper on left head tilt, problem with left intorters (LSR, LSO) or right extorters (RIR, RIO)

Bilateral CN 4 palsies: usually due to severe head trauma (contusion of anterior medullary velum)
Vertical deviation in primary gaze may or may not be present
RHT in left gaze; LHT in right gaze
Either eye can be hyper on step 3 of 3-step test
V-pattern ET
>10° of torsion with double Maddox rod test

Workup: check BP, blood glucose, CBC, ESR, VDRL, FTA-ABS, ANA; neuroimaging if history of head trauma or cancer, signs of meningitis, young age, other neurologic findings, or isolated palsy that does not improve after 3–4 months

Treatment:
Glasses: occlude lens or prisms for diplopia
Muscle surgery:

KNAPP'S PRINCIPLES FOR CN 4 PALSY: strengthen (tuck) the palsied SO, weaken the antagonist (ipsilateral IO), or weaken the yoke (contralateral IR) to correct hyperdeviation
HARADA-ITO PROCEDURE: anterior and lateral displacement of palsied muscle to correct excyclotorsion

Abducens Nerve (CN 6) Palsy

Anatomy: nucleus in dorsal pons medial to CN 7; travels anterior and lateral to PPRF, then through pyramidal tract, and exits lower pons in pontomedullary groove in subarachnoid space; climbs over clivus (vulnerable to elevated ICP) over petrous ridge, along base of skull, through Dorello's canal, under Gruber's ligament; enters cavernous sinus and then orbit through superior orbital fissure; passes laterally to supply lateral rectus

Second most common CN to be injured following closed head injury

CN 6 lesions occur in conditions that cause increased ICP

6 syndromes:
Brain stem syndromes (see Figure 4-20, ①):
MILLARD-GUBLER SYNDROME: lesion of CN 6 and 7 fascicles and pyrimidal tract causing CN 6 and 7 palsies with contralateral hemiparesis
RAYMOND'S SYNDROME: lesion of CN 6 and pyrimidal tract causing CN 6 palsy and contralateral hemiparesis

FOVILLE'S SYNDROME: lesion of CN 6 nucleus, CN 5 and 7 fascicles, and sympathetics causing ipsilateral 5, 6, and 7 palsies, horizontal conjugate gaze palsy, and ipsilateral Horner's

MÖBIUS' SYNDROME: associated with CN 7 lesion, supernumerary digits, skeletal abnormalities, mental retardation

Subarachnoid space syndrome (see Figure 4-20, ②): increased ICP can cause downward displacement of brain stem with stretching of CN 6 (tethered at exit from pons and Dorello's canal); occurs in 30% of patients with pseudotumor cerebri; also hemorrhage, meningitis, inflammation (sarcoidosis), infiltration (lymphoma, leukemia, carcinoma)

Petrous apex syndrome (see Figure 4-20, ③): portion of CN 6 within Dorello's canal is in contact with tip of petrous pyramid and is susceptible to processes affecting the petrous bone

GRADENIGO'S SYNDROME: localized inflammation or extradural abscess of petrous apex (mastoiditis) following otitis media; CN 6 palsy with ipsilateral decreased hearing, facial pain, and facial paralysis

PSEUDO-GRADENIGO'S SYNDROME: various etiologies

NASOPHARYNGEAL CA: obstruction of Eustachian tube can cause serous otitis media, can invade cavernous sinus causing CN 6 palsy

CEREBELLOPONTINE ANGLE TUMOR: CN 5, 6, and 7 palsies; decreased hearing, papilledema

PETROUS BONE FRACTURE: may have CN 5, 6, 7, or 8 lesions, hemotympanum, Battle's sign (bruising over mastoid bone), CSF otorrhea

BASILAR ANEURYSM

CLIVUS CHORDOMA

Cavernous sinus syndrome (see Figure 4-20, ④):

ETIOLOGY: trauma, vascular (diabetes, migraine, aneurysms, AV fistula), tumor, inflammation, granuloma

FINDINGS: CN 3, 4, V₁, Horner's, ON, chiasm, and pituitary involvement

Orbital syndrome (see Figure 4-20, ⑤):

ETIOLOGY: trauma, tumor, orbital pseudotumor, cellulitis

FINDINGS: proptosis, chemosis, conjunctival injection; may have ON edema or atrophy; CN V₁ may be involved

Isolated CN 6 palsy (see Figure 4-20, ⑥):

CHILDREN: often postviral (resolves over weeks), associated with otitis media; consider tumor (pontine glioma), trauma

ADULTS: vasculopathic, undetermined, MS, tumor (nasopharyngeal CA, cavernous sinus meningioma, chordoma), trauma, temporal arteritis, syphilis

Pseudo–CN 6 palsy: thyroid-related ophthalmopathy, convergence spasm, strabismus, medial wall fracture, myasthenia gravis, orbital myositis, Miller Fisher syndrome

Workup:

Congenital: usually resolves by 6 weeks

Acquired: same as for CN 4 palsy; consider LP and Tensilon test

Trigeminal Nerve (CN 5) Palsy

Anatomy: nerve emerges from ventral pons; passes below tentorium to ganglion; divides into 3 divisions

Ophthalmic (V₁): passes through lateral wall of cavernous sinus; divides into lacrimal, frontal, and nasociliary nerves

Maxillary (V₂): passes through lateral wall of cavernous sinus; exits cranium through foramen rotundum

Mandibular (V₃): exits cranium through foramen ovale (Figure 4-21)

Supplies sensory to face and eye, motor to muscles of mastication

Trigeminal neuralgia (tic doloureaux): due to compression of CN 5 at root (superior cerebellar artery aneurysm or tumor); facial pain involves entire CN 5 division; lasts seconds; 95% unilateral; usually involves maxillary or mandibular distribution, ophthalmic distribution alone is rare

Diagnosis: neuroimaging

Treatment: medical (carbamazepine) or surgical (radiofrequency destruction of trigeminal ganglion through foramen ovale)

Facial Nerve (CN 7) Palsy

Anatomy: passes around CN 6 nucleus; exits brain stem ventrally at cerebellopontine angle; enters internal auditory canal (of petrous portion of temporal bone) with nervus intermedius and cochlear and vestibular nerves; enters facial nerve canal; exits temporal bone via stylomastoid foramen; branches in parotid gland. Supplies facial muscles and lacrimal and salivary glands; posterior 2/3 of tongue; external ear sensation; dampens stapedius

Lacrimal gland innervation (parasympathetic): originates in superior salivatory nucleus, fibers leave brain with nervus intermedius (glossopalatine) and travel with CN 7 through geniculate ganglion, emerges from petrous portion of sphenoid bone as greater superficial petrosal nerve; enters pterygoid canal and enters sphenopalatine ganglion, where primary parasympathetic fibers synapse and second-order fibers join zygomatic nerve, which sends a branch to lacrimal gland.

Frontal lobe (precentral motor cortex) → CN 7 nucleus in pons (controls voluntary movements of face); upper face innervation is bilateral (from both CN 7 nuclei), lower face innervation is from ipsilateral CN 7 nucleus (Figure 4-22)

Supranuclear palsy: lesion in precentral gyrus of cerebral cortex results in contralateral paralysis of

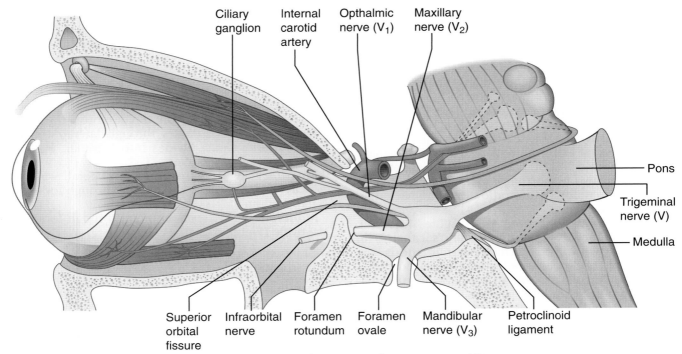

Figure 4-21. CN 5 pathway. Copyright Peter K. Kaiser, MD.

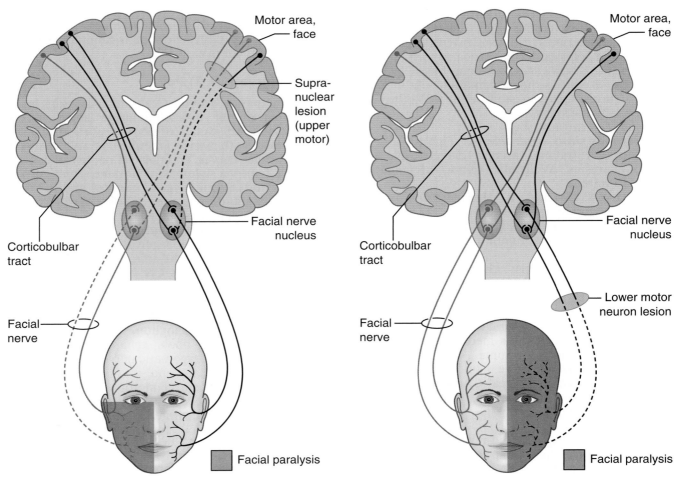

Figure 4-22. Facial weakness due to upper and lower motor neuron lesions. (From Bajandas FJ, Kline LB: *Neuro-Ophthalmology Review Manual.* Thorofare, NJ, Slack, 1988.)

volitional facial movement involving lower face more severely than upper

Emotional and reflex movements (smiling, spontaneous blinking) are preserved (extrapyramidal)

Brain stem lesion (pons): ipsilateral facial weakness involving both upper and lower face; due to tumor, vascular causes

Associated with CN 5 and 6 palsies, lateral gaze palsy, cerebellar ataxia, and contralateral hemiparesis

With CN 5 palsy: cerebellopontine angle tumors, infratemporal fossa tumors

With CN 6 palsy: brain stem injury or injury near anteromedial portion of temporal bone (Gradenigo's syndrome)

Peripheral CN 7 lesion: acute unilateral facial nerve palsy is most common cranial neuropathy

Bell's palsy: idiopathic facial nerve palsy; may be preceded by preauricular or mastoid pain

Facial weakness progressing to paralysis over months

Associated with progressive twitching or facial spasm; suggests neoplasm; most common between ages 15 and 45; 10% have positive family history

TREATMENT: consider oral steroids

PROGNOSIS: 70% have complete recovery in 6 weeks; 85% will fully recover; 10% recurrence (ipsilateral or contralateral)

POOR PROGNOSTIC SIGNS: complete facial paralysis at presentation, impairment of lacrimation, advanced age; if incomplete recovery, aberrant regeneration is common

Trauma: fracture of temporal bone

FINDINGS: hearing loss, vertigo, hemotympanum, perforated tympanic membrane, Battle's sign (bruising over mastoid bone)

Delayed onset or incomplete paralysis usually due to nerve contusion or swelling

Complete facial paralysis immediately after head trauma suggests nerve transection

BIRTH TRAUMA WITH FORCEPS: congenital CN 7 lesion; tends to resolve

Infection:

RAMSAY-HUNT SYNDROME: herpes zoster oticus (HZV infection of outer ear and nerves of inner auditory canal); 20% have sensorineual hearing loss and dizziness

Preauricular or mastoid pain precedes facial paralysis by 1 to 3 days; associated with a vesicular rash of outer ear or on tympanic membrane

TREATMENT: acyclovir and prednisone

PROGNOSIS: poor; only 10% recovery in patients with complete paralysis; 66% recovery with partial paralysis

May develop postherpetic neuralgia

Also HIV, Lyme disease, otitis media, malignant otitis externa (usually elderly diabetics; can progress to cellulitis of inner ear canal and osteomyelitis of temporal bone; usually caused by *Pseudomonas*)

Sarcoidosis: infiltration of CN 7, usually at parotid gland

Erosive cholesteatoma: pressure on segment of CN 7 that travels through middle ear

Tumor: most intracranial and bone tumors that cause facial paralysis are benign (including acoustic neuroma, meningioma, glomus tumors [triad of facial paralysis, pulsatile tinnitus, and hearing loss]); tumors of parotid gland are usually malignant (adenoid cystic carcinoma)

Guillain-Barré syndrome (Miller Fisher variant): facial diplegia can occur with ophthalmoplegia and ataxia; absent deep tendon reflexes; CSF protein elevated with normal cell count

Melkersson-Rosenthal syndrome: recurrent facial paralysis with chronic facial swelling and lingua plicata (furrowing of tongue); unilateral or bilateral; occurs in childhood or adolescence

Aberrant facial innervation:

MARCUS-GUNN JAW WINKING: activation of muscles of mastication induces orbicularis oculi contraction

CROCODILE TEARS: lacrimation evoked by chewing

Other findings: lacrimation (damage to greater superficial petrosal nerve), impaired stapedius muscle reflex (damage to stapedial nerve), impaired taste (damage to chorda tympani nerve), swelling of parotid gland or cervical lymphatics (suggests malignant tumor or inflammatory condition of parotid [sarcoidosis, TB])

Disorders of CN 7 overactivity:

Benign essential blepharospasm: frequent bilateral blinking proceeds to involuntary spasms and forceful contractures of orbicularis; may cause functional blindness; unknown etiology; usually affects women over age 50; absent during sleep

TREATMENT: botulinum toxin (Botox) injections, rarely surgery (orbicularis myomectomy)

Hemifacial spasm: unilateral contractions of facial muscles; usually due to vascular compression of CN 7 at brain stem; rarely caused by tumor; present during sleep

Facial myokymia: fasciculations of facial muscles; if multifocal and progressive, consider MS

Eyelid myokymia: benign fasciculations of eyelid

Multiple CN Palsies

CN 3, 4, and 5: due to lesion of brain stem, cavernous sinus, and/or superior orbital fissure

DDx: AV fistula, cavernous sinus thrombosis, metastases to cavernous sinus, skin malignancy with perineural spread to cavernous sinus, meningioma, mucormycosis, HZV, Tolosa-Hunt syndrome, mucocele, nasopharyngeal CA, carcinomatous meningitis, pituitary apoplexy (headache with bilateral signs and decreased vision)

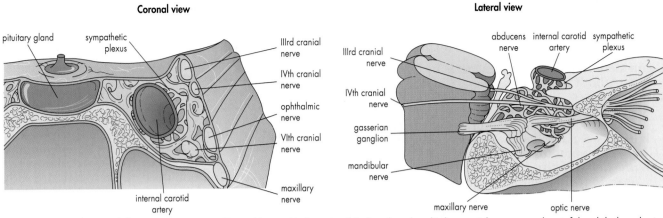

Figure 4-23. Anatomy of the cavernous sinus. (From Moster M: Paresis of isolated and multiple cranial nerves and painful ophthalmoplegia. In Yanoff M, Duker JS [eds]: *Ophthalmology*, London, Mosby, 1999.)

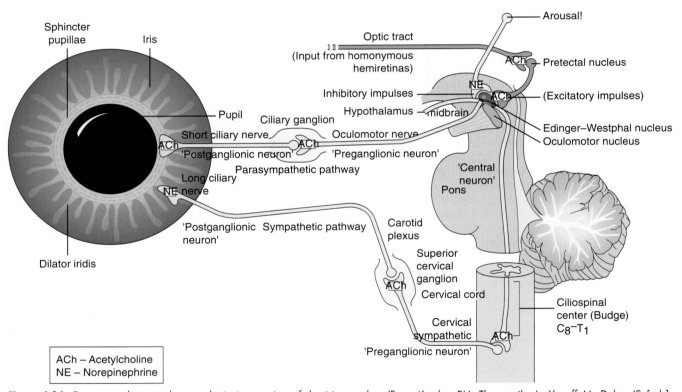

Figure 4-24. Parasympathetic and sympathetic innervation of the iris muscles. (From Kardon RH: The pupils. In Yanoff M, Duker JS [eds]: *Ophthalmology*, 2nd ed, St. Louis, Mosby, 2004.)

Herpes zoster ophthalmicus: CN 3, 4, and 6 palsies occur in about 15%; pain and skin eruption in trigeminal distribution, decreased corneal sensation, pupil may be involved (tonic pupil)

> *Hutchinson's rule*: if tip of nose involved (nasociliary nerve), eye will probably (but not always) be involved

Mimics of multiple cranial nerve palsies: MG, CPEO, orbital lesions (thyroid, pseudotumor, tumor), progressive supranuclear palsy, Guillain-Barré syndrome

PUPILS

Innervation (Figure 4-24)

Iris Sphincter

Parasympathetic innervation from Edinger-Westphal nucleus

Pathway of pupillary light reflex: optic nerve → chiasm (fibers split) → optic tract → pretectal nucleus (synapse) → cross to both EW nuclei (synapse) →

travel via CN 3 though subarachnoid space and cavernous sinus, then travel in inferior division of CN 3 to ciliary ganglion → postganglionic fibers travel via short ciliary nerves to ciliary body and iris sphincter

Iris Dilator

Sympathetic innervation

Pathway: posterior hypothalamus → down spinal cord → synapse in ciliospinal center of Budge (C8-T2 level) → second-order neuron ascends sympathetic chain → over apex of lung → synapse at superior cervical ganglion → third-order neuron ascends with ICA and joins CN 6 in cavernous sinus → enters orbit via long ciliary nerve (through superior orbital fissure next to CN V_1) to iris dilator and Müller's muscle

Disorders

Relative Afferent Pupillary Defect (RAPD; Marcus-Gunn Pupil)

Large retinal lesion, asymmetric optic nerve disease, chiasm lesion, optic tract lesion (contralateral RAPD)

No RAPD: cataract, acute papilledema, amblyopia, refractive error, functional visual loss, lesions posterior to lateral geniculate body

Light-Near Dissociation

Pupil does not react to light but near response intact

Etiology: syphilis (Argyll-Robertson), Adie's pupil, familial dysautonomia (Riley-Day), Parinaud's syndrome, RAPD, physiologic, severe retinal disease, aberrant regeneration of CN 3, diabetes, myotonic dystrophy, encephalitis, alcoholism, HZO

Abnormal Light and Near Response

Pharmacologic, trauma, CN 3 palsy

Anisocoria

Pupils of unequal size

Miosis: small pupil
  DDx: Horner's syndrome, pharmacologic (pilocarpine, brimonidine, narcotics, insecticides), Argyll-Robertson pupil, diabetes, spasm of near reflex, senescence

Mydriasis: large pupil
  DDx: CN 3 palsy, Adie's tonic pupil, pharmacologic (mydriatics, cycloplegics, cocaine), trauma
  Both Horner's and Adie's are examples of denervation hypersensitivity (sympathetic tone loss in Horner's, parasympathetic tone loss in Adie's)

Horner's Syndrome

Sympathetic lesion causing ptosis, miosis, and anhidrosis; anhidrosis often present in both first- and second-order lesions; may also have facial numbness, diplopia, and vertigo; may have mild inverse ptosis of lower lid, dilation lag; anisocoria most pronounced in dim light; congenital (forceps injury, shoulder dystocia); can cause iris heterochromia (ipsilateral lighter iris)

Preganglionic: from hypothalamus to superior cervical ganglion
  First-order neuron (central Horner's): hypothalamus to spinal cord level C8-T2 (Ciliospinal center of Budge)
    ETIOLOGY:
      MIDBRAIN: neuron located near CN 4 nucleus in dorsolateral tegmentum; lesion at this level (usually ischemia) causes Horner's and superior oblique palsy
      PONS: near CN 6 nucleus; ischemia, tumor, demyelination, polio, syringomyelia, and inflammation, Foville's syndrome (lesion of CN 5, 6, and 7 and Horner's)
      MEDULLA: lateral medullary syndrome of Wallenberg (stroke of vertebral artery or PICA causing lateral medullary infarction; lesion of CN 9, 10, and 11; Horner's, vertigo, cerebellar signs, ipsilateral decreased pain/temperature sensation of face, contralateral decreased pain/temperature sensation of trunk and limbs)
      VERTEBROBASILAR STROKES AND VERTEBRAL ARTERY DISSECTION
      CERVICAL DISC DISEASE: arthritis, demyelination, inflammation, tumors
      SYRINGOMYELIA: spinal cord cavities surrounded by gliosis involving spinothalamic tracts; causes ipsilateral loss of pain/temperature sensation but preservation of touch; muscle wasting and weakness (especially small hand muscles); Charcot's arthropathy (35%)
  Second-order neuron: majority of preganglionic Horner's; ciliospinal center of Budge to superior cervical ganglion
    ETIOLOGY: mediastinal or apical tumor (neuroblastoma [most common], Pancoast's), thyroid disease, neurofibroma, pneumothorax, cervical infections, upper respiratory tract tumors, brachial plexus syndromes, carotid artery dissection, aneurysm, trauma

Postganglionic: superior cervical ganglion to iris dilator
  Third order neuron: anhidrosis limited to ipsilateral forehead
    ETIOLOGY:
      INTERNAL CAROTID ARTERY DISSECTION: TIA, stroke, neck pain, amaurosis, dysacusia, bad taste in mouth

LESIONS INVOLVING MECKEL'S CAVE OR CAVERNOUS SINUS: associated with CN 3, 4, V$_1$, V$_2$, and 6 palsies

TRIGEMINAL HERPES ZOSTER

HEADACHE SYNDROMES: migraine, cluster headaches, Raeder's syndrome (middle-aged men with Horner's and daily unilateral headaches)

TUMOR OF PAROTID GLAND, NASOPHARYNX, SINUSES

TRAUMA

Diagnosis: pharmacologic testing

Cocaine test: topical cocaine (4%, 10%) blocks reuptake of norepinephrine (NE), causing pupil dilation

Determines presence of Horner's syndrome

Functioning neuron will release NE, and pupil will dilate

ABNORMAL RESULT: no pupil dilation

Hydroxyamphetamine 1% (Paradrine) test: releases NE from nerve terminal

Distinguishes between preganglionic and postganglionic lesions

POSITIVE IN PREGANGLIONIC LESIONS: pupil dilates because postganglionic neuron is intact

NEGATIVE IN POSTGANGLIONIC LESIONS: pupil does not dilate because neuron does not have NE

Treatment: ptosis surgery to shorten Müller's muscle (Putterman procedure [conjunctival–Müller's muscle resection], Fasanella-Servat procedure [tarsoconjunctival resection])

Adie's Tonic Pupil

Dilated, tonic pupil due to postganglionic parasympathetic pupillomotor damage; 90% women; 20 to 40 years of age; 80% unilateral

Findings: initially, pupil is dilated and poorly reactive; later becomes miotic; segmental contraction of pupil (vermiform movements); light-near dissociation with slow (tonic) redilation after near stimulus

Adie's syndrome: Adie's pupil and decreased deep tendon reflexes; orthostatic hypotension

Pathology: loss of ganglion cells in ciliary ganglion, degenerated axons in short ciliary nerves

DDx: HZV, giant cell arteritis, syphilis, orbital trauma, diabetes, alcoholism, and dysautonomia associated with cancer and amyloidosis

Diagnosis: dilute pilocarpine (0.125%) or mecholyl 2.5% will constrict the tonic pupil but not the normal pupil; false-positive test can occur in CN 3 palsy

Argyll-Robertson Pupil

Bilateral small, irregular pupils with light-near dissociation caused by tertiary syphilis

Hutchinson's Pupil

Unilateral dilated, poorly reactive pupil in comatose patient due to ipsilateral supratentorial mass causing displacement of hippocampal gyrus (uncal herniation) entrapping CN 3; pupillomotor fibers travel in peripheral portion of nerve and are susceptible to early damage from compression

Simple Anisocoria

Most common cause of relative difference (<1 mm) between pupils; occurs in up to 20% of general population

OCULAR MUSCLE DISORDERS

Ophthalmoplegia

Static

Agenesis of extraocular muscles, congenital fibrosis syndrome, congenital myopathies

Progressive

Chronic Progressive External Ophthalmoplegia (CPEO)

Mitochondrial disease, several types

Kearns-Sayre syndrome: ophthalmoplegia with ptosis, retinal pigment degeneration, heart block

Oculopharyngeal Dystrophy (AD)

Onset in 5th to 6th decade; French-Canadian ancestry; progressive dysphagia followed by ptosis; most develop CPEO

Pathology: vacuolar myopathy

Myotonic Dystrophy (AD)

Mapped to chromosome 19; myotonia of peripheral muscles; worsens with cold, excitement, fatigue

Findings: Christmas tree cataract (presenile cataract with polychromatic subcapsular cortical crystals), mild pigmentary retinopathy, ptosis, lid lag, light-near dissociation, miotic pupils, may develop ocular hypotony

Other findings: myotonia, testicular atrophy, frontal baldness, cardiac abnormalities (myopathy, conduction defects), bilateral facial weakness, insulin resistance, mental retardation

Diagnosis: ERG (low voltage), EMG (myotonic discharge)

Inflammatory Disorders

Thyroid-related ophthalmopathy, orbital pseudo-tumor, amyloidosis

Others

Vitamin E deficiency, muscle tumors

Episodic

Familial periodic paralysis, trauma, ischemia, vasculitis, disorders of neuromuscular junction (myasthenia gravis, Eaton-Lambert syndrome, organophosphate poisoning, botulism)

Myasthenia Gravis (MG)

Weakness of voluntary muscles due to autoimmunity to motor end plates (antibodies block ACh receptors), hallmark is fatigability; 90% have eye symptoms, 50% present with eye symptoms; females > males; onset aged 15 to 50; 80% with ocular presentation will develop generalized disease; 15% spontaneously resolve.

Neonatal form: transplacental transfer of ACh receptor antibody

Congenital form: genetic defect in ACh receptor

Types:
  Ocular: consists of ptosis and extraocular weakness only
  Systemic: other skeletal muscles involved; 5% of patients develop Graves' disease

Associations: thymic hyperplasia (70%), thymoma (occurs in 10% of MG patients; 30% of people with thymoma have MG), other autoimmune diseases (rheumatoid arthritis, lupus, thyroid disease)

Drugs that exacerbate MG: steroids, antibiotics (aminoglycosides, clindamycin, erythromycin), β-blockers, D-penicillamine, phenytoin, curare, methoxyflurane, lidocaine

Findings: asymmetric ptosis, seesaw ptosis ("curtaining"; when more ptotic lid is lifted, other lid falls owing to Hering's law), Cogan's lid twitch (when patient looks from downgaze to primary position, lid will overshoot), facial muscle weakness, ophthalmoplegia, pseudo-INO, nystagmus (on extreme gaze)

Other findings: jaw weakness, dysphagia, dysarthria, dyspnea, muscle bulk usually preserved until late

DDx: Myotonic dystrophy, CPEO, involutional ptosis, toxins (snake, arthropod, bacteria [botulism])
  Eaton-Lambert syndrome: paraneoplastic syndrome consisting of profound proximal muscle pain and weakness, dysarthria, dysphagia; associated with small cell lung cancer
    MECHANISM: impaired presynaptic release of ACh; 50% demonstrate specific antibodies against presynaptic voltage-gated calcium channels
    DIAGNOSIS: muscle strength and reflexes are enhanced with exercise; no improvement with edrophonium
    EMG: increased muscle action potentials with repeated nerve stimulation

Diagnosis:
  Tensilon test (edrophonium [IV]; AChE inhibitor that prolongs action of ACh, resulting in stronger muscle contraction): positive 80% to 90% of the time, but high false-negative rate; may cause bradycardia—therefore, give test dose of 1 to 2 mg first; other adverse effects include sweating, nausea, vomiting, salivation, fever, elevated IOP; antidote is atropine sulfate (0.5 mg); alternative test is neostigmine methylsulfate (Prostigmine [IM]: useful in children and adults without ptosis, requires longer observation period [20–45 minutes])
  ACh receptor antibody: 3 types (binding Ab, blocking Ab, modulating Ab); 50% sensitive in ocular MG, 80% sensitive in general MG, 90% positive in MG with thymoma, 99% specific; seronegative MG due to antigen excess, ocular-specific Ab, Ab against other components of ACh receptor
  EMG: fatigue with repetitive nerve stimulation; single-fiber EMG is best
  Photos: check old photos; morning versus evening for variability in lid position
  Rest test: rest with eyes closed for 30 minutes; positive if improvement in ptosis occurs
  Ice test: neuromuscular transmission improves in cold; therefore, apply ice pack for 2 minutes; positive if improvement occurs
  Others: chest CT/MRI, thyroid function and lupus tests

Treatment: mestinon (AChE inhibitor), steroids, plasmapheresis, IV gamma globulin, cyclosporine, azothioprine, thymectomy (33% resolve, 33% improve, 33% no benefit); prism spectacles and consider surgery for stable strabismus (>6–12 months)

Primary Overaction Syndromes

Convergence Spasm

Miosis with increasing esodeviation

Superior Oblique Myokymia

Episodic repetitive firing of SO causes intermittent oscillopsia, shimmering vision, and vertical and/or torsional diplopia; chronic; unknown etiology; treat with carbamazepine (tegretol) or propranolol; consider simultaneous weakening of ipsilateral SO and IO

Ocular Neuromyotonia

Failure of muscle to relax; occurs after radiation therapy to parasellar lesions; may affect CN 3 or 6; diagnose by having patient look in direction of action of muscle (up and in for CN 3, laterally for CN 6); treat with carbamazepine (Tegretol)

Oculogyric Crisis

Bilateral tonic supraduction of eyes and neck hyperextension due to acute effect of phenothiazine overdose; also described with postinfectious Parkinson's disease

EYE MOVEMENTS IN COMA

Normal Eye Movements and Pupils

Bilateral cerebral depression

Limited Eye Movements and Normal Pupils

Metabolic, drugs

Horizontal Limitation

Eyes straight: pontine damage

Eyes deviated to side: cerebral damage

Bilateral horizontal limitations (gaze palsy, INO, CN 6 palsy): pontine damage

Ipsilateral horizontal deviation with contralateral limb weakness: basal ganglia damage

Contralateral horizontal deviation without limb weakness: cerebellar lesions

Vertical Limitation

Eyes straight: midbrain or pretectal damage

Upward deviation: hypoxic encephalopathy (severe cerebellar damage), lithium toxicity, phenothiazine overdose, heatstroke

Downward deviation (more common and more ambiguous than upward deviation): pretectal, metabolic, thalamic hemorrhage; tentorial herniation; pineal tumors; meningitis; hepatic encephalopathy

Vertical-gaze paresis and bilateral CN 3 palsy: midbrain damage

Total Ophthalmoplegia

Midbrain stroke, pituitary apoplexy, meningitis

Skew Deviation

Posterior fossa dysfunction

Bilateral Lid Retraction

Pretectal dysfunction

Nystagmus

Upbeat (structural), downbeat (hypoxic, Arnold-Chiari malformation, toxic [lithium], paraneoplastic), convergence-retraction (dorsal midbrain)

Calorics

Water irrigated into ear produces nystagmus; direction of nystagmus (fast phase) is COWS (cold opposite, warm same); jerk nystagmus in awake patient; tonic deviation in comatose patient in opposite direction of mnemonic; bilateral cold water irrigation produces upbeat nystagmus in awake patient; downward tonic deviation in comatose patient

OPTIC NERVE

Developmental Anomalies

(see Chapter 5, Pediatrics/Strabismus)

Optic Disc Swelling

Nerve fibers anterior to lamina cribrosa swell due to obstruction of axoplasmic flow at level of lamina choroidalis or lamina scleralis

Orthograde transport (ganglion cells to LGB): slow component = 2 mm/day; fast component = 500 mm/day

Retrograde transport (LGB to ganglion cells)

Mechanism: ischemia, inflammation, increased intracranial pressure, compression

Findings: elevated hyperemic nerve head (3 diopters = 1 mm), blurred disc margins, loss of physiologic cup, peripapillary NFL edema, chorioretinal folds, dilated/tortuous veins, peripapillary flame-shaped hemorrhages, exudates, cotton wool spots (NFL infarcts)

Chronic swelling may cause Paton's lines (radial or concentric folds of peripapillary retina), gliosis, high water marks, pale disc, disc pseudodrusen, attenuated vessels, vision loss

DDx of optic disc edema/pseudoedema: papilledema, ischemic optic neuropathy, optic neuritis, CRVO, diabetic papillitis, malignant hypertension, neuroretinitis (cat-scratch disease), infiltration of the optic disc (sarcoidosis, tuberculosis, leukemia, metastases), optic disc drusen, optic nerve head tumors (astrocytic hamartoma, gliomas, capillary hemangioma), orbital disease/compressive optic neuropathy (thyroid-related ophthalmopathy, orbital pseudotumor, orbital mass), inflammatory diseases (syphilis, APMPPE, VKH), Leber's hereditary optic neuropathy

Papilledema

Disc edema due to increased intracranial pressure

Findings: disc edema (may be asymmetric); loss of spontaneous venous pulsations (absent in 20% of normals); transient visual obscurations; diplopia (due to unilateral or bilateral CN 6 palsies); normal color vision, acuity, and pupils; enlarged blind spot on VF; headache, nausea, vomiting
  Chronic cases: pale atrophic nerve, arteriolar attenuation, poor vision, VF loss

DDx: intracranial tumor (posterior fossa in children), meningitis, carcinomatous meningitis, pseudotumor cerebri (IIH)

Diagnosis: check blood pressure; brain CT/MRI, if no mass, perform lumbar puncture (measure opening pressure)

Idiopathic Intracranial Hypertension (IIH; Pseudotumor Cerebri)

Papilledema with normal neuroimaging and CSF

90% female, mean age = 33 years old; associated with obesity

Findings: headache, nausea, vomiting, optic disc edema (may be asymmetric), transient visual obscurations, photopsias, VF defect (enlarged blind spot, constriction, or arcuate scotoma), retrobulbar pain, pulsatile intracranial noises; may have visual loss, positive RAPD, diplopia (CN 6 palsy)
  In children: irritability; no disc swelling if fontanelles open

Associations: endocrine disorder (Addison's; steroid withdrawal), chronic obstructive lung disease, thrombosis of dural sinus (trauma, childbirth, middle ear infection, hypercoagulable state); use of steroids, birth control pills, vitamin A, tetracycline, nalidixic acid, isotretinoin; may be exacerbated with pregnancy

DDx: (see optic disc swelling above)

Diagnosis: normal brain MRI, elevated CSF pressure with normal composition (diagnosis of exclusion)

Treatment:
  No vision loss: headache treatment and weight loss
  Mild vision loss: acetazolamide (Diamox), furosemide, weight loss
  Advanced VF loss: ON sheath decompression, serial lumbar punctures (temporary relief), lumbar-peritoneal shunt

Optic Neuritis

Inflammation of optic nerve; idiopathic or associated with systemic disease; most common optic neuropathy in people <45 years old; female preponderance

Findings: acute unilateral visual loss (can evolve over first week, then spontaneous improvement over weeks [70% regain 20/20]), ocular pain exacerbated by eye movements, decreased color vision and contrast sensitivity, positive RAPD, VF defect (50% diffuse, 20% central scotoma, rarely altitudinal), optic nerve appears normal or swollen (35%), disc pallor late

Other findings:
  Pulfrich phenomenon: motion of pendulum appears elliptical due to altered depth perception from delayed conduction in the demyelinated nerve
  Uhthoff's symptom: worsening of symptoms with heat or exercise; present in 50% after recovery
  Phosphenes: flashes of light induced by eye movements or sound
  Auditory clicks: CN 7 innervates stapedius, and patient hears click with effective transmission

DDx: idiopathic, multiple sclerosis (MS), syphilis, sarcoidosis, Lyme disease, Wegener's granulomatosis, SLE, Devic's syndrome (bilateral optic neuritis and transverse myelitis)
  Controlled High-risk Avonex Multiple Sclerosis Prevention Study (CHAMPS): randomized trial of interferon beta-1a (Avonex) for the prevention of MS after acute demyelinating episode and abnormal MRI
    3-YEAR RESULTS: risk of MS lower and fewer MRI lesions in treatment group

MAJOR CLINICAL STUDY

Optic Neuritis Treatment Trial (ONTT)

Objective: to evaluate the role of corticosteroids in the treatment of unilateral optic neuritis

Methods: patients with unilateral optic neuritis were randomly assigned into 3 treatment groups:
  1. *IV steroids*: 250 mg IV methylprednisolone qid × 3 days, followed by oral prednisone (1 mg/kg/day) × 11 days
  2. *Oral steroids*: prednisone (1 mg/kg/day) × 14 days
  3. *Oral placebo*: 14 days

Results:
  IV steroids: more rapid recovery of visual acuity at 2 weeks; did not reduce risk of subsequent attacks; decreased incidence of MS at 2 years vs placebo, but no difference at 3 years
  Oral prednisone: associated with higher rate of new attacks in either eye at 1 year; highest relapse rate of optic neuritis at 5 years (41% vs 25% for IV and placebo groups)
  Brain MRI: periventricular white matter lesions were associated with MS
    Lesions in 50% of patients with first attack of optic neuritis

5-YEAR RESULTS: 30% risk of developing MS regardless of treatment group
WITH NO LESIONS: 16% developed MS
3 OR MORE LESIONS: 51% developed MS
Increased risk of developing MS if previous neurologic symptoms (regardless of MRI status)
10-YEAR RESULTS:
WITH NO LESIONS: 22% developed MS
WITH ≥1 LESION: 56% developed MS
If normal MRI, no previous neurologic findings or fellow eye involvement: decreased risk of MS if optic neuritis was painless, if disc swelling was present and vision loss was only mild
No patients developed MS who had normal MRI with peripapillary hemorrhage or macular exudates
Abnormal MRI: 43% progress to MS by 3 years; progression to MS at 1 year was 7.5% with IV steroids, 14.7% with oral steroids, and 16.7% with placebo

Conclusions:
In general, about 30% develop MS within 4 years and 38% develop MS by 10 years (risk is higher in women than men)
Consider treating optic neuritis with IV steroids; do not initiate treatment with oral steroids
Regardless of MRI status, there is a higher risk of developing MS if the patient has previous neurologic symptoms or a history of optic neuritis in the fellow eye

Optic Neuropathies

Anterior Ischemic Optic Neuropathy (AION)

Infarction of optic nerve head just posterior to lamina cribrosa due to inadequate perfusion by posterior ciliary arteries; results in acute visual loss

2 forms: arteritic (giant cell arteritis); nonarteritic (ischemic)

Findings: decreased color vision and acuity, positive RAPD, VF loss (altitudinal or arcuate defects most common, central scotomas also occur), unilateral optic disc edema (often involving 1 sector), contralateral disc appears crowded (small C/D ratio)

Arteritic: due to giant cell (temporal) arteritis (inflammatory vasculopathy affecting medium-sized to large vessels) affecting the posterior ciliary arteries; female > male (2 : 1); aged >55 years; may have amaurosis fugax or diplopia
Other findings: scalp tenderness, jaw or tongue claudication, polymyalgia rheumatica (PMR), fever, malaise, anorexia, weight loss, anemia, headache, tender temporal artery, neck pain, brain stem stroke (due to involvement of vertebral artery)
Pathology: granulomatous inflammation with epithelioid cells, lymphocytes, giant cells; disruption of internal elastic lamina and proliferation of intima with aneurysm formation

Figure 4-25. Arteric AION demonstrating vasculitis of all coats of temporal artery with giant cells. (Courtesy of MM Rodrigues. From Yanoff M, Fine BS: *Ocular Pathology*, 5th ed, St. Louis, Mosby, 2002.)

Diagnosis: elevated ESR (for men > [age/2]; for women > [(age +10)/2]; may be normal in 10%), C-reactive protein (above 2.45 mg/dL), low hematocrit (anemia of chronic illness), FA (patchy choroidal filling, nonperfusion), temporal artery biopsy (inflammation in artery wall with disruption of internal elastica lamina, skip lesions [specimen at least 3 cm], perform within 2 weeks of steroid treatment)
Treatment (emergent): steroids (prednisone 60–120 mg orally; consider IV initially) to prevent fellow eye involvement (65% risk of involvement of fellow eye without treatment; usually affected within 10 days)

Nonarteritic (ischemic): no associated symptoms; usually aged 50–75 years; associated with microvascular disease (diabetes, hypertension) and collagen vascular disorders; recurrence in same eye is rare; 25% to 40% risk of fellow eye involvement; normal ESR
Treatment: none
ISCHEMIC OPTIC NEUROPATHY DECOMPRESSION TRIAL (IONDT): optic nerve sheath fenestration is not effective
Smokers had earlier mean onset (age 64) than nonsmokers (age 70)
43% of control patients regained 3 or more lines of vision at 6 months (vs 34% of those having surgery)
Surgery had higher risk of loss of 3 lines of vision (24% vs 12% with observation)

Pseudo–Foster-Kennedy syndrome: AION is most frequent cause of unilateral disc edema and contralateral optic atrophy

Retrobulbar Optic Neuropathy (Posterior Ischemic Optic Neuropathy)

Rare; usually bilateral; occurs with severe anemia and hypotension (i.e., major blood loss from surgery, trauma, GI bleed, dialysis); associated with medications (antibiotics [ethambutol, isoniazid, sulfonamides, chloramphenicol], anticancer drugs [cisplatin, vincristine, busulfan])

Findings: disc swelling may occur if ischemic process extends anteriorly

Treatment: treat acute cause (prompt reversal of hypotension, blood transfusion)

Compressive Optic Neuropathy

Intraorbital, intracanalicular, or intracranial (prechiasmal)

Etiology: ON tumor, pituitary tumor or apoplexy, thyroid-related ophthalmopathy

Findings: slow progressive vision loss, decreased color vision, positive RAPD, VF defect (central scotoma that extends to periphery), proptosis; disc may be normal, pale, or swollen; may have endocrine abnormalities (parachiasmal lesions), chemosis and restricted motility (thyroid)

Diagnosis: orbit CT/MRI

Infiltrative Optic Neuropathy

Etiology: leukemia, lymphoma, multiple myeloma, plasmacytoma, metastatic carcinoma (breast and lung most common), sarcoidosis, TB, cryptococcus, toxoplasmosis, toxocariasis, CMV, coccidiomycosis

Findings: disc may appear grayish-white with associated hemorrhages; mass may be visible

Toxic/Nutritional Optic Neuropathy

Painless symmetric progressive vision loss

Etiology: ethanol, methanol, digoxin, ethambutol, chloramphenicol, isoniazid, rifampin, lead toxicity, tobacco-alcohol amblyopia, thiamine and B_{12} deficiency

Findings: decreased vision (20/200 or worse), VF loss (cecocentral scotomas), disc hyperemia then pallor

Traumatic Optic Neuropathy

ON contusion or compression due to trauma

Findings: decreased vision, VF defects, positive RAPD

CT scan: rule out canal fracture, orbital hematoma, ON hematoma

Treatment: lateral canthotomy for tense orbit, drain subperiosteal hematoma
> *IV steroids* (methylprednisolone): 30-mg/kg loading dose, then 5.4 mg/kg/hr × 48 hours
> If vision improves, switch to 80 mg oral, and taper by 20 mg every 2–3 days; if vision worsens on oral steroids, restart high-dose IV and consider surgical decompression of canal

> Consider surgical decompression of optic canal if no response to steroids after 48 hours
> If no improvement in vision after 3 days, stop steroids

Hereditary Optic Neuropathy

(see Chapter 5, Pediatrics/Strabismus)

Optic Atrophy

Pale white appearance of ON head caused by injury to any part of pathway from retinal ganglion cells to LGB

Etiology: optic neuropathy, optic neuritis, glaucoma, CRAO, tumors, aneurysms

Pathology: increased number of astrocytes (gliosis) within nerve; normal parallel architecture of glial columns seen in sagittal sections is lost; widened space between nerve and meninges; loss of myelin; thickened pial septa

ON Tumors

ON Glioma

Low-grade astrocytoma: usually in children aged <10 years

"Benign" but 14% mortality rate (highest with hypothalamus involvement)

10% to 50% have neurofibromatosis (15% of patients with NF have ON gliomas)

50% intraorbital, 50% intracranial
> **Findings**: vision loss, strabismus, nystagmus, disc edema or atrophy; may have proptosis (intraorbital ON glioma); can spread to chiasm and contralateral ON
> **MRI**: fusiform thickening and kinking of ON

Figure 4-26. Glioma demonstrating central necrosis. (From Yanoff M, Fine BS: *Ocular Pathology*, 5th ed, St. Louis, Mosby, 2002.)

Malignant ON glioma (glioblastoma multiforme): occurs in adults

Painful vision loss; becomes bilateral; death in 3–9 months

ON Meningioma

Derived from outer arachnoid; may arise from ectopic nests of meningeal cells; female > male (3 : 1)

Findings: triad of decreased vision, optic atrophy, optociliary shunt vessels; also proptosis, ON edema, retinal vascular occlusions

Sphenoid wing meningioma: fullness of temporal orbital fossa and orbit

Pathology: psammoma bodies and whorls of concentrically packed spindle cells

Figure 4-27. Meningioma demonstrating proliferation of meningothelial cells. (From Yanoff M, Fine BS: *Ocular Pathology*, 5th ed, St. Louis, Mosby, 2002.)

CT/MRI: railroad track sign (dye accumulation in periphery of nerve)

CHIASM COMPRESSION

Chiasm anatomy: location with respect to pituitary gland
   Prefixed: chiasm is forward; tumor will compress the optic tracts
   Normal: chiasm is aligned with pituitary; tumor will compress chiasm
   Postfixed: chiasm is behind; tumor will compress optic nerves

Etiology: pituitary tumor (most common), pituitary apoplexy, craniopharyngioma, meningioma, glioma, aneurysm, trauma, infection, metastasis, MS, sarcoidosis

VF defects: central scotoma, bitemporal hemianopia, incongruous homonymous hemianopia, junctional scotoma (ipsilateral central scotoma with contralateral superotemporal defect due to lesion at junction of ON and chiasm)

DDx of bitemporal VF defect: sector retinitis pigmentosa, coloboma, tilted disc

Pituitary Tumor

Most commonly chromophobe (often prolactinoma); can also secrete ACTH (Cushing's disease); basophil can secrete ACTH; eosinophil can secrete GH (acromegaly); secreting tumors usually present with endocrine dysfunction, except prolactin-secreting tumor in males (presents with signs of chiasmal compression); 30% nonsecreting (present with vision loss)

Findings: VF defect (bitemporal hemianopia), hormone imbalance, optic atrophy

Diagnosis: X-ray shows large pituitary fossa, double floor sign, bony erosion

Treatment: dopamine antagonist (bromocriptine) for prolactinoma, hormone replacement, transsphenoidal surgery for nonsecreting tumor, XRT

Meningioma

Derived from meningothelial cells of arachnoid; often at sphenoid ridge; occurs in adults, especially middle-aged women

Tuberculum sellae meningioma: compression of optic nerve just before chiasm, may cause unilateral VF defect
   Findings: optic atrophy, hyperostosis

Pathology: whorled cellular pattern; may see psammoma bodies

Pituitary Apoplexy

Acute hemorrhage and expansion of a pituitary tumor, usually secondary to ischemic necrosis

Findings: headache, decreased vision, ocular motility disturbance; progresses to NLP and complete ophthalmoplegia

Sheehan's Syndrome

Panhypopituitarism in pregnancy due to hemorrhage

Craniopharyngioma

Usually causes compression of chiasm from above and behind; occurs in children and young adults

Findings: initial damage to upper nasal fibers (inferior bitemporal field defect); later, upper temporal defect papilledema, optic atrophy

MRI: calcification

DDx of calcification of sella turcica: craniopharyngioma, supraclinoid aneurysm, meningioma, AV malformation, glioma of chiasm (very rare), chordoma (extremely rare)

Glioma

Occurs in children and adults; may extend into both optic nerves causing bilateral vision loss with complicated bilateral VF defects

Aneurysm

ICA and anterior cerebral artery; middle-aged adults; present with vision loss, ophthalmoplegia

Subfrontal Mass Lesion

Slow progressive asymmetric bilateral visual loss, late optic nerve pallor

Other Chiasmal Lesions

MS, trauma, basal meningitis, sphenoid sinus mucocele or carcinoma

RETROCHIASMAL DISORDERS

Cause homonymous VF defects (See Figure 4-9)

Cogan's Dictum: causes homonymous hemianopia

With asymmetric OKN = parietal lobe lesion (usually mass)

With symmetric OKN = occipital lobe lesion (usually infarction)

Optic Tract

Vascular, craniopharyngioma extending posteriorly

Findings: incongruous homonymous hemianopia, bilateral optic atrophy (bowtie appearance), contralateral RAPD

LGB

Very rare

Findings: incongruous homonymous hemianopia or congruous homonymous sectoranopia (sectoral optic atrophy), normal pupils

Temporal Lobe

Glioma, vascular

Findings: "Pie-in-the-sky" VF defect (inferior macular fibers do not travel as far anteriorly into Meyer's loop)

Other findings: déjà vu symptoms, foul odors; may have formed visual hallucinations

Parietal Lobe

Gioma, meningioma, metastases, middle cerebral artery thrombosis

Findings: affect fibers from superior retina first (contralateral inferior homonymous quadrantanopia) or contralateral inferior homonymous hemianopia denser inferiorly; spasticity of conjugate gaze (tonic deviation of eyes to opposite side of parietal lesion); OKN asymmetry (nystagmus dampened when stimuli moved in direction of damaged parietal lobe); may have contralateral motor paresis

Gerstmann's syndrome: lesion of dominant parietal lobe (inferior homonymous hemianopia, acalculia, agraphia, finger agnosia, left-right confusion)

Occipital Lobe

Vascular (90%), tumors, trauma

Findings:
   Central homonymous hemianopia (periphery spared): fibers from macula terminate at tip of occipital lobes
   Macula sparing: fibers from retinal periphery terminate on mesial surface of occipital lobe (supplied by PCA)
   Temporal crescent: homonymous hemianopia with sparing of far temporal periphery (supplied by nasal retina and travels to most anterior portion of mesial surface of contralateral occipital lobe)

Other findings: unformed visual hallucinations, paliopia (perseveration in homonymous field), prosopagnosia (inability to recognize faces; bilateral medial occipitotemporal lesion), Riddoch phenomenon (ability to perceive moving objects but not stationary ones)

Disconnection syndrome: dominant occipital lobe and splenium of corpus collosum; usually due to posterior artery stroke (right homonymous hemianopia with alexia [cannot read] but not agraphia [can write])

CORTICAL LESIONS

Cause disorders of visual integration

Visual information from LGB goes to primary visual cortex (V1) of both occipital lobes; further processing occurs in areas V2–V5

To read, information travels from visual cortex to angular gyrus in parietal lobe of dominant hemisphere (usually on left side). Visual information from right hemifield is transmitted directly from left occipital lobe to ipsilateral angular gyrus, and information from left hemifield is transmitted through splenium of corpus callosum to contralateral angular gyrus

Disorders

Alexia

Inability to read despite normal vision

Pseudoalexia

Can be caused by inability to read, hemianopias with split fixation, and expressive (Broca's) or conduction aphasias

Alexia with Agraphia (Inability to Write)

Parietal lesions involving angular gyrus

Alexia without Agraphia

Large left occipital lesions that also disrupt fibers crossing in splenium of corpus callosum from right occipital cortex to left angular gyrus; information from left VF cannot travel to left parietal lobe (angular gyrus); patient is blind in right visual field, can see and write but not read

Dyslexia

Central nervous system problem in which letters appear reversed; male > female (3 : 1). Visual training does not improve academic abilities of dyslexic or learning disabled children

Visual Neglect

Patient ignores 1 side of visual space

Visual Extinction

Patient ignores 1 side of visual space when presented with simultaneous stimuli to both visual fields; occurs more often with right parietal lesions

Visual Agnosia

Bilateral lesions of occipitotemporal area; inability to recognize objects by sight, although can recognize by touch, language, and intellect

Anomia

Inability to name objects

Prosopagnosia

Bilateral infero-occipital lesions; inability to recognize faces

Cerebral Achromatopsia

Unilateral or bilateral lesion in infero-occipital area; loss of color vision in opposite hemifield

DISORDERS DURING PREGNANCY

Occur more commonly with eclampsia and preeclampsia

Conditions: CSR, hypertensive retinopathy, Purtscher's-like retinopathy, RD, cerebral venous thrombosis, CRAO, carotid cavernous fistula, Sheehan's syndrome (postpartum pituitary infarct causing panhypopituitarism; secondary hemorrhage can cause CN 2–6 palsies)

Conditions that worsen during pregnancy: uveal melanoma, pituitary adenoma, meningioma, DM, Graves' disease, orbital and choroidal hemangiomas

Conditions that improve during pregnancy: multiple sclerosis, optic neuritis, sarcoidosis, lupus

Migraines: may improve or worsen

Preeclampsia: transient visual loss in 50%, cerebral blindness in 1% to 5%; ischemic cerebrovascular complication risk increases 13× during pregnancy and postpartum due to hypercoagulable state
> *Arterial abnormalities*: occur in 60% to 90%; most common during 2nd and 3rd trimesters and first week postpartum
> *Venous abnormalities*: during first 6 weeks postpartum (venous sinus thrombosis presents with headache and papilledema)

BRAIN TUMORS

Foster-Kennedy Syndrome

Frontal lobe mass (usually olfactory or sphenoid ridge meningioma) causing anosmia (loss of smell), ipsilateral optic atrophy (tumor compression), and contralateral ON edema (elevated ICP)

Pseudo–Foster-Kennedy syndrome: bilateral AION (pale nerve from old AION and fellow nerve edema from new AION)

Cerebellopontine Angle Tumors

Usually acoustic neuroma; associated with neurofibromatosis; peripheral CN 7 lesion (orbicularis weakness, inability to wrinkle forehead), CN 6 lesion, CN 5 lesion (decreased corneal sensation), nystagmus (vestibular to contralateral side, gaze paretic to ipsilateral side)

Posterior Fossa Tumors

Cause most severe papilledema because encroach on cerebral aqueduct and 4th ventricle with rapid rise in ICP

Metastases

In order of frequency at autopsy: melanoma, lung, breast, renal, colorectal, ovarian

Table 4-1. Classification of Brain Tumors

By origin:	
Glial (gliomas)	Astrocytoma
Neuronal	Neuroblastoma, medulloblastoma
Connective tissue	Sarcoma
Lymphoreticular	Primary (non-Hodgkin's) CNS lymphoma
Blood vessels	Hemangioma, angioma
Bone	Osteoma
Neural crest	Meningioma (arachnoid cells), primary CNS melanoma
Congenital rests:	
Notochord	Chordoma
Adipose cells	Lipoma
Ectodermal derivatives	Craniopharyngioma, teratoma, dermoid
Glands:	
Pituitary gland	Adenoma
Pineal gland	Pineocytoma, pineoblastoma, germ cell tumors
By age:	
<20 years old	CNS tumors are second most common type of malignancy (leukemia is first); approximately 66% located in posterior fossa; gliomas of cerebellum, brain stem, optic nerve; pinealomas; primitive neuroectodermal tumors; craniopharyngiomas
20–60 years old	Meningiomas, gliomas of cerebral hemispheres, pituitary tumors
>60 years old	Malignant gliomas, metastases

HEADACHES

(Figure 4-28)

Migraines

Etiology: cerebral vasospasm; slow-moving concentric wave of suppressed electrical activity

Types:

Common (without aura): male = female; any age; little or no prodrome; throbbing headache, photophobia, nausea

Classic (with aura) (20%): male = female; any age; trigger factors; visual prodrome followed by hemicranial pain, nausea, vomiting, dizziness, photophobia

Scintillating scotoma (5–30 minutes, half visual field; may have macropsia, micropsia, hallucinations, achromatopsia); may have tingling on 1 side of face and/or ipsilateral hand; rarely, hemiparesis, vertigo, mood changes, distortion of hearing and smell

Complicated: hemiplegic or hemiparetic; mostly children

OPHTHALMOPLEGIC: headache and recurrent paresis of 1 or more ocular motor nerves (usually CN 3)

May last longer than 1 week; rarely, permanent ophthalmoplegia

Childhood: brief attacks of nausea/vomiting; usually no headache

Acephalgic (migraine equivalent): aura without headache

Most common after age 40; history of migraines with or without aura; rule out TIA

Retinal: temporary scotoma or monocular blindness; headache may precede or occur within an hour

Examination during attack reveals venous constriction

Migraine infarction: focal signs persist for longer than 1 week; corresponding lesion on neuroimaging

Status migrainosus: attack lasting longer than 72 hours (with or without treatment); continuous headache or intermittent with interruptions at less than 4 hours

Precipitating factors:

Diet: tyramine (bananas, avocado, yogurt, aged cheese), phenylethylamine (chocolate, cheese, wine), sodium nitrite (preservatives, food coloring, processed meats and fish), monosodium glutamate (Chinese food, processed meats, frozen dinners, canned soup), caffeine, alcohol, artificial sweeteners

Lifestyle: excessive sleep, fasting or dieting, exertion, fatigue, stressful events, depression

Hormonal: supplemental estrogen, menses, oral contraceptives, ovulation

Environmental: sun exposure, loud noise, bright lights, glare, flickering lights, strong odors

Treatment:

General: alter diet, lifestyle, hormonal and environmental factors

Abortive: ice pack, cold shower, exercise, massage, local scalp pressure; analgesics; oral ergotamine or dihydroergotamine (DHE); antiemetics; sumatriptan ([Imitrex], serotonin agonist; works on peripheral trigeminal nerve terminals that supply pain-sensitive vascular and meningeal structures; also causes constriction of certain intracranial blood vessels; oral and injectable forms; 83% obtain relief within 4 hours, 45% have recurrence 24 hours later; adverse effects include flushing or tingling, chest pain)

Sinusitis

Tension

1 kg

Migraine

Trigeminal neuralgia

Figure 4-28. Location of pain for the common headache syndromes. (From Weinstein JM: Headache and facial pain. In Yanoff M, Duker JS [eds]: *Ophthalmology*, London, Mosby, 1999.)

Cluster

most frequent site

less frequent site

least frequent site

Prophylactic: consider if attacks occur once every 2 months or more often, if severity limits normal activity, or if acute therapies have failed or are contraindicated

β-BLOCKERS: reduce frequency of attacks by half (in 70% of patients)

TRICYCLIC ANTIDEPRESSANTS: amitriptyline, nortriptyline, imipramine, and doxepin

SEROTONIN REUPTAKE INHIBITORS: fluoxetine

CALCIUM CHANNEL BLOCKERS: decrease frequency of attacks, do not affect severity

Tension Headaches

Dull, persistent pain like tight band around head

Cluster Headaches

Severe, unilateral, orbital, supraorbital, and/or temporal pain lasting from 15 minutes to 3 hours; may awaken patient from sleep; usually occur in men 30 to 40 years of age; more common in smokers; attacks occur in groups and last weeks or months

Findings (ipsilateral): conjunctival injection, lacrimation, nasal congestion, rhinorrhea, forehead/facial sweating, miosis, ptosis, and/or eyelid edema; may develop postganglionic Horner's syndrome

Glossopharyngeal Neuralgia

Unilateral pain in region of larynx, tongue, tonsil, and ear; may have hoarseness and coughing; can be stimulated by swallowing or pungent tastes

Treatment: carbamazepine, baclofen, phenytoin

Carotidynia

Pain arising from cervical carotid artery, radiates to ipsilateral face and ear; rule out carotid dissection

Temporomandibular Joint (TMJ) Syndrome

Unilateral ear or preauricular pain, radiates to temple, jaw, or neck; worse with chewing

Findings: limitation of normal jaw movement, audible click on jaw opening

Other Causes of Headache/Facial Pain

Acute: subarachnoid hemorrhage, meningitis, encephalitis, focal scalp inflammation, sinusitis, dental disease, acute uveitis, acute glaucoma, scleritis, HZV, cervical spondylitis, giant cell arteritis

Recurrent: asthenopia, cerebral aneurysm or angioma, severe hypertension

Chronic: muscle tension, depression, cerebral tumor, pituitary or nasopharyngeal tumor, metastatic carcinoma, Paget's disease, increased intracranial pressure, chronic subdural hemorrhage, postherpetic neuralgia, trigeminal neuralgia (tic doulourex), Costen's syndrome (temporomandibular osteoarthritis)

VISUAL DISTURBANCES

Functional Visual Loss

Diagnosis of exclusion; trick patient with visual tests

Bottom-up acuity: start with 20/20 line and slowly progress up chart

Deception of eye tested: fogging with Phoroptor; trial frame with 2 high-power cylinders of opposite sign in same axis (so net power is zero), then spin 1 of the cylinders thus fogging good eye; red-green glasses used with duochrome filter of projection chart (red letters are seen with eye behind red lens)

Stereoacuity: minimum amount of acuity is needed to distinguish different stereo images

Binocular integrated multicolored vision assessment test (BIMVAT): red and blue filters placed over near correction in trial frame; blue filter over "bad" eye, then show letters made up of orange, brown, and blue components (orange components seen through blue filter but not red filter); some letters designed so that they can be read as 2 different letters (e.g., P or R) depending on what components are seen, so any letter with all orange components read correctly was read by the "bad" eye

Visual field testing: spiral field

With complete blindness: OKN, signature (truly blind patients can do this without difficulty), touch nose or other finger (patient may mistake this for a visual task and be unable to perform), ERG

Transient Visual Loss

Visual Obscurations

Last seconds; occur in papilledema (change in posture or eye movement) or optic disc drusen

Amaurosis Fugax

Monocular loss or dimming of vision lasting 2 to >30 minutes; commonly due to carotid or cardiac disease, also occurs in temporal arteritis, vertebrobasilar insufficiency (bilateral), hypotension, hyperviscosity (anticardiolipin), migraine, eclampsia; brief episodes may indicate impending CRAO

Uhthoff's Phenomena

Blurring of vision with activity or heat; due to optic neuritis

Scintillating Scotoma

Ocular migraine

Whiteout of Vision or "Chicken-Wire" Pattern

Occipital ischemia

Gradual Peripheral Constriction of Vision with Visual Phenomena

Cerebrovascular disease or occipital migraine

Other Visual Phenomena

Visual Hallucinations

Release hallucinations (Charles Bonnet syndrome): formed (faces, objects) or unformed (flashes of light); occur in areas of absent vision; usually continuous and variable; common in ARMD and patients with large VF defects; associated with lesions anywhere in visual pathway; stop with eye movement

Ictal hallucinations: stereotyped, paroxysmal visual hallucinations; unformed (occipital lobe lesion) or formed (associated with strange odor; temporal lobe lesion)

Palinopsia: abnormal perseveration of visual images; occurs with evolving lesions, more commonly in right hemisphere

Phosphenes

Unstructured flashes of light

Photopsias

Structured geometric figures

VASCULAR DISORDERS

Cerebral Aneurysm

Occurs in 5% of population; rarely symptomatic before age 20; associated with hypertension

Risk factors: HTN, AV malformation, coarctation of the aorta, polycystic kidney disease, fibromuscular dysplasia, Marfan's syndrome, Ehlers-Danlos syndrome

Types: fusiform or saccular ("berry"; most common at arterial bifurcations; 90% supratentorial; >10 mm have highest risk of rupture)

Location:

Internal carotid artery (85%): main trunk (PCA, ophthalmic artery, cavernous sinus), anterior communicating artery, MCA trifurcation, anterior cerebral artery

Basilar artery (5%)

Vertebral artery (5%)

Findings:

Anterior communicating artery: ON compression, chiasm compression, paraplegia

Origin of posterior communicating artery: sudden-onset severe headache, complete CN 3 palsy

Bifurcation of middle cerebral artery: hemiparesis, aphasia

Bifurcation of internal carotid artery: ON compression, chiasm compression, hemiparesis

Subarachnoid hemorrhage: neurosurgical emergency; severe headeache ("worst headache of life"), nausea, vomiting, stiff neck; **Terson's syndrome** (vitreous and subarachnoid hemorrhages [when ICP in ON sheath exceeds ocular venous pressure])

Sentinal bleed: headache with transient neurologic symptoms before major rupture

Diagnosis:

Cerebral arteriogram: 4-vessel study of both carotid and vertebral arteries

MRI: detects aneurysms >5 mm in size

MRA: can detect 3-mm aneurysm

CT scan: acutely to screen for subarachnoid and intraparenchymal bleed; unacceptable screen for unruptured aneurysms (if negative, perform LP to determine presence of subarachnoid blood)

Treatment:

Medical (symptomatic, unruptured): stabilize, lower ICP with hyperventilation and mannitol; prevent vasospasm with calcium channel blockers and blood volume expansion; control blood pressure

Surgery: clip aneurysm; if unable, may need to ligate feeding artery

Prognosis: risk of bleed is 1%/yr

30% mortality at time of rupture; if untreated, 33% mortality at 6 months; survivors have neurologic deficits

Rebleed risk is highest in first 24 hours; untreated patients have 25% risk of rebleed during first 2 weeks

Vasospasm is major cause of morbidity and death; 30% within first 2 weeks, highest risk between days 4 and 10

Arteriovenous Malformation (AVM)

Congenital, may be familial; symptoms usually before age 20; 90% supratentorial, 70% cortical, 20% deep, 10% in posterior fossa or dura mater; 6% have intracranial aneurysm

Findings: intracranial bleed (50%), sometimes with subarachnoid hemorrhage; neurologic symptoms before bleed (50%) (seizures, headaches, other neurologic deficits); may hear bruit

Cortical AVM in occipital lobe: visual symptoms and migraines

Hemispheric AVM: can get homonymous hemianopia

Brain stem AVM: diplopia, nystagmus, gaze palsy, pupil abnormality

Diagnosis:

CT scan: hemorrhage; calcified AVMs visible on plain x-ray

MRI: better for small AVMs

Cerebral angiogram: demonstrate anatomy

Treatment: resection, ligation of feeding vessel, embolization, stereotactic radiosurgery

Prognosis: 20% mortality when bleeding begins; rebleed rate is 2.5%/yr

Carotid Artery Dissection

Intracranial or extracranial

Etiology:

Trauma: blunt (head, neck), carotid artery compression, hanging, manipulative neck therapy, surgery, carotid artery cannulation during angiography

Spontaneous: fibromuscular dysplasia, Marfan's syndrome, Ehlers-Danlos, polycystic kidney disease, syphilis, atherosclerosis, moyamoya, idiopathic

Findings:

Traumatic: ipsilateral headache and ophthalmic signs, contralateral neurologic deficits; may hear bruit

Symptoms can be delayed (weeks to months); severe cases can present with cerebral ischemia and coma

Spontaneous: transient or permanent neurologic defects; amaurosis fugax, monocular visual loss, or ipsilateral Horner's syndrome; intracranial extension may cause CN palsies, diplopia, tongue paralysis, facial numbness

Visual loss from embolic occlusion of ophthalmic artery, central retinal artery, or short posterior ciliary arteries

Rarely, ocular ischemia from reduced blood flow

Diagnosis: MRI

Treatment: controversial

Vertebrobasilar Dissection

40% of all dissecting aneurysms; basilar more common than vertebral

General findings: headache, neck pain, signs of brain stem and cerebellar dysfunction

Basilar artery dissection: ocular motor palsies, progresses to coma and death

Vertebral artery dissection (various presentations): fatal brain stem infarction (usually young adults); subarachnoid hemorrhage; aneurysmal dilation with brain stem and lower cranial nerve signs from mass effect; chronic dissection with recurrent TIAs, strokes, and subarachnoid hemorrhages

Vertebrobasilar Insufficiency (VBI)

Posterior circulation ischemia; vertebrobasilar system (vertebral, basilar, posterior cerebral arteries) supplies occipital cortex and areas involved with ocular motility in brain stem and cerebellum

Etiology: thrombus, emboli, hypertension, arrhythmias, arterial dissection, hypercoagulable state, subclavian steal syndrome

Findings: ataxia, vertigo (may also have tinnitus, deafness, or vomiting), dysarthria, dysphagia, hemiparesis, hemiplegia, drop attack (patient suddenly drops to ground without warning, no loss of consciousness), bilateral dimming of vision lasting seconds to minutes, photopsias, homonymous VF loss without other neurologic findings

Cerebral blindness/cortical blindness: bilateral occipital lobe lesions; pupils react normally; may deny blindness (**Anton's syndrome**)

Cerebral Venous and Dural Sinus Thrombosis

Occlusion of cortical and subcortical veins produces neurologic symptoms; most commonly, cavernous sinus, lateral sinus, and superior sagittal sinus

Etiology: inflammation (Behçet's, SLE), infection, trauma, invasion of vessel wall by tumor (leukemia, lymphoma, meningioma), altered blood flow (hypoperfusion, hematologic disorders, venous emboli, hypercoagulability, oral contraceptives, pregnancy, sickle cell disease, protein C or S deficiency, antithrombin III deficiency, lupus anticoagulant)

Cavernous sinus thrombosis: aseptic or septic (infection of sinus or face; rarely otitis or orbital cellulitis)
  Findings: usually unilateral; orbital congestion, lacrimation, chemosis, eyelid swelling, ptosis, proptosis, ophthalmoplegia (CN 6 most common); may have corneal anesthesia, facial numbness, Horner's syndrome
  Other findings: headache, nausea, vomiting, somnolence, fever, chills, evidence of meningitis or sepsis
  Treatment: antibiotics, anticoagulants, corticosteroids, surgery

Lateral sinus thrombosis: usually septic from chronic otitis media

Findings: CN 6 palsy most common (severe facial pain [Gradenigo's syndrome] if compressed against petroclinoid ligament), papilledema
  Other findings: symptoms of infection, neck pain, tenderness of ipsilateral jugular vein, retroauricular edema; may have facial weakness

Superior sagittal sinus (SSS) thrombosis: usually aseptic
  Aseptic: occurs during pregnancy, immediately postpartum, or with oral contraceptives; risk factors include vasculitis and systemic inflammatory disorders
  Septic: most commonly from meningitis; also paranasal sinus infection, pulmonary infection, tonsillitis, dental infection, pelvic inflammatory disease, and otitis media
  Findings:
    THROMBOSIS OF ANTERIOR THIRD OF SINUS: mild symptoms
    THROMBOSIS OF POSTERIOR SINUS: may cause pseudotumor cerebri (headaches and papilledema; consider in pseudotumor that occurs in thin patients), seizures, altered mental status, focal neurologic signs; may be fatal from brain hemorrhage and herniation
  Treatment: anticoagulation, fibrinolytic agents, ICP-lowering agents

Diagnosis: CT, MRI, MRA (venous phase)

INTRACRANIAL ARACHNOID CYST

Congenital malformation: CSF-filled cyst most commonly in middle cranial fossa (Sylvian fissure)

Findings: seizures, headaches, CN palsy, exophthalmos, hydrocephalus (compression of foramen of Munroe, aqueduct, or 4th ventricle), increased intracranial pressure, papilledema

Cyst rupture may cause subdural hematoma

Treatment: fenestration, shunt

NEURO-OPHTHALMIC MANIFESTATIONS OF AIDS

CNS Lymphoma

High-grade B-cell non-Hodgkin's lymphoma; second most common malignancy in AIDS

Findings: diplopia (from CN 3, 4, 6 involvement; may have disc swelling from infiltration of orbit and optic nerve)

Progressive Multifocal Leukencephalopathy (PML)

Papovavirus destroys oligodendrocytes; gray matter relatively spared; can affect central visual pathway and ocular motor fibers

Findings: ataxia, altered mental status, dementia, hemiparesis, focal neurologic defects

Diagnosis: MRI (demyelination; usually parieto-occipital areas, typically involves subcortical white matter with focal or confluent lesions; may see focal enhancement with contrast)

Treatment: none; death common within 6 months

Review Questions *(Answers start on page 358)*

1. The visual field defect most characteristic of optic neuritis is
   a. altitudinal
   b. central
   c. centrocecal
   d. arcuate

2. Which cranial nerve is most prone to injury in the cavernous sinus?
   a. 3
   b. 4
   c. 5
   d. 6

3. Which of the following agents is least toxic to the optic nerve?
   a. isoniazid
   b. dapsone
   c. methanol
   d. ethambutol

4. Seesaw nystagmus is produced by a lesion located in which area?
   a. chiasm
   b. posterior fossa
   c. suprasellar
   d. cervicomedullary junction

5. What is the location of a lesion that causes an ipsilateral Horner's syndrome and a contralateral CN 4 palsy?
   a. midbrain
   b. pons
   c. cavernous sinus
   d. orbit

6. The least useful test for functional visual loss is
   a. confrontation VF
   b. OKN
   c. HVF
   d. tangent screen at 1 m and 2 m

7. Optociliary shunt vessels may occur in all of the following conditions except
   a. chronic glaucoma
   b. CVO
   c. meningioma
   d. ischemic optic neuropathy

8. Which is not a symptom of pseudotumor cerebri?
   a. diplopia
   b. entoptic phenomena
   c. visual obscurations
   d. headache

9. A 63-year-old woman reports sudden onset of jagged lines in the right peripheral vision. She has experienced 3 episodes in the past month, which lasted approximately 10 to 20 minutes. She denies headaches and any history or family history of migraines. The most likely diagnosis is
   a. vertebrobasilar insufficiency
   b. occipital AVM
   c. migraine variant
   d. posterior vitreous detachment

10. A 60-year-old man with optic disc swelling in the right eye and left optic atrophy most likely has
    a. ischemic optic neuropathy
    b. left sphenoid ridge meningioma
    c. Leber's hereditary optic neuropathy
    d. left optic nerve glioma

11. Which of the following findings may not be present in a patient with an INO?
    a. dissociated horizontal nystagmus
    b. limitation of adduction
    c. absent convergence
    d. abnormal abduction saccades

12. A paradoxical pupillary reaction is not found in which condition?
    a. achromatopsia
    b. albinism
    c. Leber's congenital amaurosis
    d. optic nerve hypoplasia

13. Inheritance of Leber's optic neuropathy is
    a. sporadic
    b. autosomal dominant
    c. mitochondrial DNA
    d. X-linked recessive

14. An OKN strip moved to the left stimulates what part of the brain?
    a. right frontal, left occipital
    b. right frontal, right occipital
    c. left frontal, left occipital
    d. left frontal, right occipital

15. The smooth pursuit system does not involve the
    a. PPRF
    b. prestriate cortex
    c. occipital motor area
    d. frontal motor area

16. Dorsal midbrain syndrome is not associated with
    a. absent convergence
    b. gaze palsy
    c. light-near dissociation
    d. nystagmus

17. The location of Horner's syndrome is best differentiated by which drug?

a. cocaine
b. paredrine
c. pilocarpine 0.125%
d. pilocarpine 1%

18. The blood supply to the prelaminar optic nerve is
    a. meningeal arteries
    b. ophthalmic artery
    c. short posterior ciliary arteries
    d. central retinal artery

19. Optic nerve hypoplasia is associated with all of the following except
    a. paradoxical pupillary response
    b. midline abnormalities
    c. maternal ingestion of LSD
    d. spasmus nutans

20. A lesion in the pons causes
    a. anisocoria
    b. miosis
    c. light-near dissociation
    d. mydriasis

21. Which of the following syndromes is characterized by abduction deficit and contralateral hemiplegia?
    a. Foville's
    b. Gradenigo's
    c. Millard-Gubler
    d. Weber's

22. All of the following are features of progressive supranuclear palsy except
    a. hypometric saccades
    b. loss of oculovestibular reflex
    c. full motility with doll's head maneuver
    d. limitation of downgaze

23. Pituitary apoplexy is characterized by all of the following except
    a. nystagmus
    b. facial numbness
    c. headache
    d. diplopia

24. Which of the following is most likely to produce a junctional scotoma?
    a. craniopharyngioma
    b. multiple sclerosis
    c. pituitary adenoma
    d. meningioma

25. All of the following are characteristics of an optic tract lesion except
    a. APD
    b. decreased vision
    c. homonymous hemianopia
    d. optic nerve pallor

26. The saccade system does not involve the
    a. occipital motor area
    b. premotor cortex
    c. frontal motor area
    d. PPRF

27. A 22-year-old man sustains trauma resulting in a transected left optic nerve. Which of the following is true regarding the right pupil?
    a. It is larger than the left pupil.
    b. It is smaller than the left pupil.
    c. It is equal in size to the left pupil.
    d. It reacts consensually.

28. Characteristics of spasmus nutans include all of the following except
    a. spontaneously disappears within 3 years
    b. may mimic chiasmal glioma
    c. begins before 1 year of age
    d. signs present during sleep

29. A congenital CN 4 palsy can be distinguished from an acquired palsy by
    a. vertical fusional amplitude >10 prism diopters
    b. incyclotropia of 5°
    c. excyclotropia of 5°
    d. spontaneous head tilt to the opposite side

30. Characteristics of a diabetic CN 3 palsy may include all of the following except
    a. pain
    b. spontaneous recovery within 90 days
    c. sluggish pupillary response
    d. aberrant regeneration

31. A CN 3 lesion may cause all of the following except
    a. contralateral ptosis
    b. ipsilateral ptosis
    c. bilateral ptosis
    d. no ptosis

32. Optic nerve drusen is associated with all of the following except
    a. RP
    b. CRAO
    c. CME
    d. CNV

33. A lesion causing limited upgaze with an intact Bell's phenomenon is located where?
    a. supranuclear
    b. nuclear
    c. tract
    d. cavernous sinus

34. An acute subarachnoid hemorrhage due to a ruptured aneurysm may produce all of the following except
    a. ptosis
    b. orbital hemorrhage
    c. vitreous hemorrhage
    d. afferent pupillary defect

SUGGESTED READINGS

American Academy of Ophthalmology: Neuro-ophthalmology, vol 5. San Francisco, AAO, 2004.
Burde RM, Savino PJ, and Trobe JD: Clinical Decisions in Neuro-ophthalmology, 3rd edition. Philadelphia, Mosby, 2002.

Kline LB, Bajandas F: Neuro-ophthalmology Review Manual, 5th edition. Thorofare, NJ, Slack, 2001.

Liu GT, Volpe NJ, and Galetta S: Neuro-ophthalmology Diagnosis and Management. Philadelphia, WB Saunders, 2001.

Loewenfeld IE, Lowenstein O: The Pupil Anatomy: Physiology and Clinical Applications, 2nd edition. Philadelphia, Butterworth-Heineman, 1999.

Milder B, Rubin ML, and Weinstein GW: The Fine Art of Prescribing Glasses Without Making a Spectacle of Yourself. Gainesville, Fla, Triad Scientific Publications Co, 1991.

Miller NR: Walsh & Hoyt's Clinical Neuro-ophthalmology, 5th edition. Baltimore, Lippincott Williams and Wilkins, 1999.

Walsh TJ: Neuro-ophthalmology: Clinical Signs and Symptoms, 4th edition. Baltimore, Williams and Wilkins, 1997.

CHAPTER 5

Pediatrics/Strabismus

Pediatrics

ANATOMY

At birth, diameter of eye is 66% that of adult eye

Eye enlarges until 2 years of age, then further growth in puberty (Table 5-1)

Infants have variable levels of astigmatism

Majority of children are hyperopic; increases up to 7 years of age, then diminishes

Eye color darkens during first few months of life

Dilator pupillae poorly developed at birth

Fovea matures during first few months of life

Myelinization of optic nerve completed shortly after birth

PHYSIOLOGY

Visual acuity levels (see Strabismus section)
    Documented by visual evoked potentials in infancy and preferential looking tests in first months of life
    Premature infants reach landmarks later

Decreased vision in infants and children
    History: family history, complications in pregnancy, perinatal problems
    Examination: visual response (assess each eye independently), pupillary reactions (paradoxical response suggests achromatopsia, CSNB, ON hypoplasia), ocular motility (strabismus, nystagmus, torticollis), cycloplegic refraction, fundus examination
    Additional tests: optokinetic response, forced preferential looking, electroretinogram (ERG), visual evoked response (VEP, VER), ultrasonography, imaging studies
    Differential diagnosis of infant with poor vision and normal ocular structures:
    Leber's congenital amaurosis, achromatopsia, blue cone monochromatism, congenital stationary night blindness, albinism, optic nerve hypoplasia, optic atrophy, congenital infection (TORCH syndrome), cortical visual impairment (due to extensive occipital lobe damage), delay in visual maturation

ORBITAL DISORDERS

Congenital Anomalies

Anophthalmos

Bilateral absence of eye due to failure of primary optic vesicle to form; extremely rare

Findings: hypoplastic orbits

Table 5-1. Changes in ocular measurements with age

Ocular Dimensions	Infant	Adult
Axial length	17 mm	24 mm
Corneal diameter	9.5–10.5 mm	12 mm
Corneal radius of curvature	6.6–7.4 mm	7.4–8.4 mm
Scleral thickness	Half of adult	

Buphthalmos

Large eye due to increased intaocular pressure in congenital glaucoma

Cryptophthalmos

Failure of differentiation of lid and anterior eye structures

Partial or complete absence of the eyebrow, palpebral fissure, eyelashes, and conjunctiva

Attenuation of the levator, orbicularis, tarsus, and conjunctiva

Often associated with severe ocular defects

Microphthalmos

Small, disorganized eye

Disruption of ocular development occurs after budding of optic vesicle

Usually unilateral

Microphthalmos with Cyst

Due to failure of embryonic fissure to close

Usually blue mass of lower lid

Associated with congenital rubella, congenital toxoplasmosis, maternal vitamin A deficiency, maternal thalidomide ingestion, trisomy 13, trisomy 15, and chromosome 18 deletion

Nanophthalmos

Small eye with normal features

Normal-sized lens and thickened sclera

Associated with hyperopia and angle-closure glaucoma

Increased risk of choroidal effusion during intraocular surgery

Infections

Preseptal Cellulitis

Infection anterior to orbital septum; spares globe

Largest risk factor is recent skin trauma

Most common organism: *Staphylococcus aureus*

Findings: lid edema, erythema, and pain; may have fever; may progress to orbital cellulitis

Treatment: systemic antibiotics (IV in severe cases, children <5 years old, and failed oral treatment)

Orbital Cellulitis

Infection posterior to orbital septum; involves globe

Most common cause of proptosis in children

Usually secondary to sinusitis (ethmoid sinus is most common)

Associated with subperiosteal abscesses

Etiology: extension of infection from periorbital structures, sinusitis, dacryocystitis, dacryoadenitis, endophthalmitis, dental infections, intracranial infections, trauma or previous surgery, endogenous (bacteremia with septic embolization)

Organisms: *S. aureus* (most common organism in children), *Streptococcus pneumoniae*, fungi (Phycomycetes, most aggressive)

Findings: fever, decreased vision, positive RAPD, proptosis, restriction of ocular motility, pain on eye movement, periorbital swelling, chemosis, optic disc swelling

CT scan: diagnosis, localization, and involvement of adjacent structures

Treatment: IV antibiotics, surgical drainage

Complications: subperiosteal abscess, cavernous sinus thrombosis, or intracranial extension causing blindness or death

Benign Lesions

Dermoid Cyst (Choristoma)

Arises from dermal elements (neural crest origin)

Lined by keratinizing epithelium with dermal appendages

Most common orbital tumor in childhood

Usually located in superotemporal quadrant near brow, often adjacent to bony suture

Often filled with keratin

Generally do not enlarge after 1 year of age

May induce bony erosion

Rupture can cause intense inflammatory reaction

CT scan: well circumscribed with bony molding

Treatment: complete excision, remove en bloc because contents may cause granulomatous inflammation

Epidermoid Cyst (Choristoma)

Arises from epidermal elements

Lined by epidermis only (no dermal appendages)

Usually filled with keratin

Rupture can lead to an acute inflammatory process

Lipodermoid

Solid tumor usually located beneath the conjunctiva over lateral surface of globe

May appear similar to prolapsed orbital fat, prolapsed lacrimal gland, or lymphoma

Usually no treatment is needed

Difficult to excise completely

Teratoma

Rare, cystic tumor arising from 2 or more germinal layers

Usually composed of ectoderm along with either endoderm or mesoderm (or both)

Can cause dramatic proptosis at birth

Rarely malignant

Capillary Hemangioma

Most common benign tumor of the orbit in children

Often manifests in the first few weeks of life and enlarges over the first 6 to 12 months, with complete regression by age 5 to 8 in 80% of cases

Spontaneous involution over the next few years

Predilection for the superior nasal quadrant of the orbit and medial upper eyelid

Female > male (3 : 2)

Diffuse irregular mass of plump endothelial cells and small vascular channels

High-flow lesion

Findings:
    Strawberry nevus: skin involvement; appears as red, irregularly dimpled, elevated surface; blanches with direct pressure (port wine stain does not blanch)
    Orbital location: can present with proptosis; bluish appearance of eyelids and conjunctiva

Pathology: numerous blood-filled channels lined by endothelium; little contribution from larger vessels or stroma; unencapsulated

Figure 5-1. Capillary hemangioma demonstrating abnormal proliferation of blood vessels and endothelial cells. (From Yanoff M, Fine BS: *Ocular Pathology*, 5th ed, St. Louis, Mosby, 2002.)

CT/MRI scan: well-circumscribed lesion

Treatment: required if tumor causing ptosis or astigmatism with resultant anisometropia, strabismus, or amblyopia. Options include observation, intralesional steroid injection, systemic steroids, interferon, laser, radiation, or excision

Complications:

High-output congestive heart failure can occur with multiple visceral capillary hemangiomas

Respiratory compromise with subglottic hemangiomas
    Eyelid involvement may cause: ptosis with occlusion amblyopia, astigmatism and anisometropia with refractive amblyopia, strabismus with strabismic amblyopia
    Kassabach-Merritt syndrome: consumptive coagulopathy with platelet trapping, resulting in thrombocytopenia and cardiac failure; acute hemorrhage is possible; mortality approximately 30%

Lymphangioma

Rare, lymphatic-filled choristoma

Often superonasal

Appears in first decade of life

Involves the eyelids, conjunctiva, and deeper orbital tissues

Lesion waxes and wanes, but does not involute

Findings: acute pain, proptosis (often increasing with upper respiratory infection), bluish hue to overlying lid, may hemorrhage into channels (chocolate cyst)

Pathology: lymph-filled vascular channels lined by endothelium; unencapsulated

Figure 5-2. Lymphangioma demonstrating lymph-filled spaces, some with blood. (From Yanoff M, Fine BS: *Ocular Pathology*, 5th ed, St. Louis, Mosby, 2002.)

CT scan: may show layered blood in a lobular, cystic mass with infiltrative pattern

MRI: infiltrating pattern with indistinct margins

Treatment: observation (spontaneous regression common); rarely surgical evacuation because complete excision difficult and recurrence common

Complications: anisometropia, amblyopia, strabismus

Varix

Most common vascular abnormality

Dilations of preexisting venous channels

Findings: proptosis (increases with crying or straining; can occur when head is in a dependent position), orbital hemorrhage (especially after trauma), motility disturbance (usually restricted upgaze), disc swelling, optic atrophy

Radiograph: phlebolith present in 30% of cases

Treatment: surgery
  Indications: cosmetic, severe proptosis, optic nerve compression, pain; surgery is often difficult because of intertwining of normal structures and direct communication with cavernous sinus

Fibrous Dysplasia

Tumor of fibrous connective tissue, cartilage, and bone

Progressive disease of childhood and young adulthood

Monostotic (in young adults) or polyostotic

Orbital involvement: usually monostotic; frontal (most common), sphenoid, and ethmoid bones; causes unilateral proptosis during first 2 decades of life

Polyostotic: multiple bones involved; can cause narrowing of optic canal and lacrimal drainage system

Albright's syndrome: polyostotic fibrous dysplasia, short stature, premature closure of epiphysis, precocious puberty, and hyperpigmented macules
  Findings: diplopia, proptosis, headaches, facial asymmetry, decreased visual acuity (compromised optic canal), hearing loss (compromised external ear canal)
  Pathology: normal bone replaced by immature woven bone and osteoid in a cellular fibrous matrix, stroma of the bone is highly vascularized, no osteoblasts present

Neurofibroma

Hamartoma

18% have neurofibromatosis (NF) type 1

Nearly all adults with NF 1 have neurofibromas

Plexiform neurofibroma: most commonly involves the upper lid; tortuous, fibrous cords infiltrate orbital tissues

Nodular: firm and rubbery consistency

Findings: often involves eyelid or causes proptosis, may cause glaucoma

Pathology: well-circumscribed, nonencapsulated proliferation of Schwann cells, perineural cells, and axons; stains with S-100 (specific for neural crest–derived structures) (Figure 5-3)

Treatment: surgical excision

Optic Nerve Glioma (Grade I Astrocytoma)

Considered pilocytic astrocytoma of the juvenile type

Slow-growing hamartoma derived from interstitial cells, astroglia, and oligodendroglia

Usually does not metastasize

Usually appears during first decade of life

Associated with neurofibromatosis (25% to 50%)

Figure 5-3. Neurofibroma demonstrating proliferation of Schwann cells. (From Yanoff M, Fine BS: *Ocular Pathology*, 5th ed, St. Louis, Mosby, 2002.)

Findings: unilateral proptosis, loss of vision, strabismus, and papilledema; may develop retinal vascular occlusions, optociliary shunt vessels; orbital tumors may cause chorioretinal folds, optic disc swelling, or atrophy; chiasmal tumors may cause pituitary or hypothalamic dysfunction, and nystagmus and head nodding from compression of 3rd ventricle

Pathology: circumscribed astrocytic tumor from neural crest tissue, glial hypercellularity, Rosenthal fibers, myxomatous, arachnoid hyperplasia; reactive meningothelial hyperplasia may occur, which can lead to a false diagnosis of meningioma

CT scan: fusiform enlargement of ON, "RR track" appearance (pathognomonic), enlargement of optic foramen, bony erosion

Treatment: observation; consider surgery if tumor spreads posteriorly into the chiasm

Prognosis: in adults, tumor is malignant with death occurring in 6 to 12 months; better prognosis in children or in adults with neurofibromatosis

Orbital Pseudotumor (Idiopathic Orbital Inflammation [IOI])

Idiopathic inflammatory disorder of orbit

Commonly bilateral with episodic recurrence

Findings: decreased vision, diplopia, red eye, headache; acute, painful presentation in children; resembles orbital cellulitis

Other findings: constitutional symptoms in 50%

Treatment: systemic steroids

Graves' Disease

(occasionally occurs in adolescents; see Chapter 6, Orbit/Lids/Adnexa)

Malignant Neoplasms

Rhabdomyosarcoma

Most common primary orbital malignancy of children

Most common soft tissue malignancy of childhood

Most common mesenchymal tumor of orbit

Malignant spindle cell tumor with loose myxomatous matrix

Average age at diagnosis is 8 years old (90% before age 16)

Cell of origin is an undifferentiated, pluripotent cell of the soft tissue

Does *not* originate from the extraocular muscles

Unilateral; tends to involve superonasal portion of orbit

More common in males (5 : 3)

Aggressive local spread through orbital bones

Hematogenous spread to lungs and cervical lymph nodes

Most common location for metastasis is chest

Findings: rapidly progressive proptosis, reddish discoloration of eyelid; may have ptosis; later develop tortuous retinal veins, choroidal folds, and optic nerve edema

4 types:
  Embryonal: most common (70%), usually occurs in children; tumor appears circumscribed, but often there is microscopic evidence of invasion of nearby structures
    PATHOLOGY: elongated spindle cell with central hyperchromatic nucleus, eosinophilic granular cytoplasm; cells arranged in parallel palisading bands; obvious cross-striations are rare (Figure 5-4)
  Botryoid: subtype of embryonal; can occur in anterior orbit, embryonal rhabomyosarcoma abutting a mucosal surface, multiple polypoid masses protruding from hollow viscera
  Pleomorphic: least common, usually occurs in adults, rare involvement of orbit, most differentiated, best prognosis
    PATHOLOGY: dense spindle cell arrangement with enlarged cells containing hyperchromatic nuclei, deeply eosinophilic cytoplasm; may see cross-striations on microscopic examination
  Alveolar: poorest prognosis, usually found in inferior orbit, generally arise in extremities (adolescents)
    PATHOLOGY: dense cellular proliferations of loosely cohesive small round cells separated by connective tissue septa; lack of cohesiveness may explain metastatic potential

A

B

Figure 5-4. A, Embryonal type demonstrating primitive rhabdomyoblasts. **B**, Cross-striations in cytoplasm of some cells. (From Yanoff M, Fine BS: *Ocular Pathology*, 5th ed, St. Louis, Mosby, 2002.)

CT scan: well-circumscribed orbital mass with possible extension into adjacent orbital bones or sinuses, bony destruction

A-scan ultrasound: orbital mass with medium internal reflectivity

Treatment: urgent biopsy, radiation (100% local control with 6000 cGy; 30% mortality due to metastases), chemotherapy for any microscopic metastases, surgical debulking

Prognosis: with chemotherapy and XRT, 3-year survival = 90%; cure rate close to 100% with localized orbital tumor; 60% if invasion of adjacent structures
> ***Tumors arising in the orbit, bladder, and prostate***: 77% disease-free survival at 2 years
> ***Intrathoracic tumors***: worst prognosis, 24% disease-free survival at 2 years

Neuroblastoma

Most frequent metastatic orbital tumor of childhood

Usually originates in adrenal gland or sympathetic ganglion chain, also mediastinum or neck

40% develop orbital metastases

Average age of presentation with metastatic neuroblastoma to orbit is 2 years old

Spontaneous regression is rare

Findings: sudden proptosis and periorbital ecchymosis (raccoon eyes); may have ipsilateral Horner's syndrome and opsoclonus (better prognosis)
> ***Paraneoplastic syndrome associated with metastatic neuroblastoma***: opsoclonus (saccadomania; random, rapid eye movements in all directions that disappear during sleep)

Pathology: sheets of indiscrete round cells with scant cytoplasm and high mitotic figures, areas of tumor necrosis; can have bony invasion; usually positive for neuronal markers (synaptophysin and neuron-specific enolase)

Figure 5-5. Neuroblastoma. (Case presented by Dr. E. Torcynski at the meeting of the Eastern Ophthalmic Society, 1994. From Yanoff M, Fine BS: *Ocular Pathology*, 5th ed, St. Louis, Mosby 2002.)

CT scan: bony destruction

Treatment: chemotherapy and local XRT

Prognosis: poor if age of onset over 1 year and metastases to bone; however, metastases to just liver, bone marrow, or spleen can be associated with a survival rate as high as 84%

Accounts for 15% of all childhood-related deaths

In adults, neuroblastoma usually metastasizes to the uveal tract

Ewing's Sarcoma

Second most frequent metastatic tumor to orbit

Primary intermedullary malignancy of bone; originates in long bones of extremities or axial skeleton

Frequently metastasizes to bone and lungs

Occurs in 2nd to 3rd decade of life

Findings: acute proptosis, hemorrhage, and inflammation from tumor necrosis

Treatment: chemotherapy

Granulocytic Sarcoma ("Chloroma")

Patients with myelogenous leukemia may present with orbital signs before hematologic evidence of leukemia

Findings: proptosis, may have subcutaneous periocular mass

Pathology: infiltration of involved tissues by leukemic cells

Treatment: radiotherapy, chemotherapy

Histiocytosis X

Group of disorders resulting from abnormal proliferation of histiocytes (Langerhans' cells) that may involve orbit

Spectrum of disease, from isolated bone lesions with excellent prognosis (eosinophilic granuloma) to systemic spread with rapid death (Letterer-Siwe disease)

Children under age 2 with multifocal disease have a poor prognosis (50% survival rate)

Findings: most frequent orbital presentation is lytic defect of orbital roof causing progressive proptosis

Pathology: granulomatous histiocytic infiltrate, Birbeck granules (central, dense core and thick outer shell), stains positively for S-100 and vimentin

Eosinophilic granuloma:
  Benign, local, solitary bone lesion
  Most likely to involve superior temporal bony orbit in childhood or adolescence
    CT SCAN AND X-RAY: sharply demarcated osteolytic lesions
    TREATMENT: incision and curettage, intralesional steroids, or radiotherapy

Hand-Schüller-Christian disease:
  Triad of proptosis, lytic skull defects, and diabetes insipidus
  More aggressive
  Multifocal bony lesions; frequently involves orbit, usually superolaterally
    TREATMENT: systemic steroids and chemotherapy
    PROGNOSIS: good

Letterer-Siwe disease:
  Most severe and malignant
  Progressive and fatal
  Multisystem involvement
  Rarely ocular/orbital involvement
    TREATMENT: systemic steroids and chemotherapy

Burkitt's Lymphoma

Primarily affects the maxilla in black children, with secondary invasion of the orbit

Related to Epstein-Barr virus infection

Findings: proptosis and bony destruction

Pathology: malignant B cells, "starry sky" appearance due to histiocytes interspersed among uniform background of lymphocytes

CRANIOFACIAL DISORDERS

Structural development of head and face occur during 4th to 8th week of gestation

Ocular motility disturbances occur in 75% of patients with craniofacial disorders

Craniofacial cleft syndromes: 1 or more facial fissures fail to close during the 6th to 7th week of gestation

Ocular complications:
  Corneal exposure from proptosis or lid defects
  Refractive errors from lid anomalies
  Ocular motility disturbances, most commonly exotropia
  Papilledema and optic atrophy from increased ICP or fibrous dysplasia involving optic canal
  Ocular anomalies from embryogenesis

Syndromes

Treacher-Collins Syndrome (Mandibulofacial Dysostosis)

Hypoplasia of the midface

Associated with dental and ear abnormalities, microtia, micrognathia, hypoplastic malar bones, and low sideburns

Findings: lateral lid defects, absent lateral canthal tendon, absent medial lashes, antimongoloid slant, ectropion, poorly developed puncta and meibomian glands.

Goldenhar's Syndrome (Oculoauriculovertebral Dysplasia)

Abnormalities of the 1st and 2nd brachial arches

Findings: limbal dermoids and dermolipomas

Other findings: hypoplastic facial bones, pretragal auricular appendages, vertebral abnormalities

Can also have lower lid colobomas and/or fistulas between the mouth and ear

Also associated with Duane's syndrome

Hypertelorism

Findings: increased interpupillary distance due to increased distance between medial orbital walls

Associated with blepharophimosis, frontal meningoceles, encephaloceles, meningoencephaloceles, and fibrous dysplasia

Craniosynostoses

Premature closure of bony sutures; inhibits growth of the cranium perpendicular to the axis of the suture; growth can continue parallel to the suture

Findings: hypertelorism; proptosis can also occur

Plagiocephaly: premature closure of one half of the coronal sutures
  Skull develops normally on one side and is underdeveloped on the other side (resulting in a flattened face)
  Other findings: midfacial hypoplasia, proptosis, telecanthus, V pattern XT, oral and dental abnormalities, and respiratory problems

Crouzon's Syndrome (Craniofacial Dysostosis) (AD or Sporadic)

Absence of forward development of the cranium and midface

Multiple combinations of suture closure can occur

Findings: proptosis, V-pattern exotropia, nystagmus, hypertelorism; shallow orbits; optic atrophy (in 25% to 50%; due to narrowing of optic canal, kinking or stretching of optic nerve)

Other findings: mental retardation, hypoplasia of maxilla, parrot's beak nose, high arched palate, external auditory canal atresia, anodonia

Apert's Syndrome (AD)

Crouzon's plus syndactyly

Anterior megalophthalmos

Associated with increased paternal age

Pfeiffer's Syndrome (AD)

Findings: hypertelorism and pointy head; may have shallow orbits, syndactyly, and short digits

Carpenter's Syndrome (AR)

Severe mental retardation

Involvement of sagittal, lambdoidal, and coronal sutures

Median Facial Cleft Syndrome

Findings: hypertelorism, exotropia

Other findings: medial cleft nose, lip, palate; widow's peak; cranium bifidum occultum

Waardenburg's Syndrome (AD)

Findings: lateral displacement of inner canthi/puncta, confluent eyebrows, heterochromia iridis, fundus hypopigmentation

Other findings: sensorineural deafness, white forelock

Hemifacial Microsomia

Findings: upper lid coloboma, strabismus

Other findings: facial asymmetry with microtia, macrostomia, mandibular anomalies, orbital dystopia, ear tags, vertebral anomalies

Hallermann-Streiff Syndrome

Sporadic

Findings: bilateral cataracts, glaucoma

Other findings: mandibular hypoplasia, beaked nose

Pierre Robin Sequence

Findings: retinal detachment, congenital glaucoma and/or cataracts, high myopia

Other findings: micrognathia, glossoptosis, cleft palate

Associated with Stickler's syndrome

Fetal Alcohol Syndrome

Findings: short palpebral fissures, telecanthus, epicanthal folds, comitant strabismus, optic disc anomalies; may have high myopia, anterior segment anomalies

Other findings: thin vermilion border of upper lip, variable mental retardation, small birth weight and height, cardiovascular and skeletal abnormalities

LID DISORDERS

Ablepharon

Absence of lids

Ankyloblepharon

Partial or complete fusion of lid margins; usually temporal, often bilateral

Often autosomal dominant

Associated with craniofacial abnormalities

Can be secondary to thermal or chemical burns, inflammation, ocular cicatricial pemphigoid, Stevens-Johnson syndrome

Blepharophimosis

Horizontally and vertically shortened palpebral fissures with poor levator function

Absent lid crease

May be part of autosomal dominant syndrome (chromosome 3q) with ptosis, telecanthus, epicanthus inversus, lower lid ectropion, hypoplasia of nasal bridge and superior orbital rim, anteverted ears, hypertelorism

Treatment: surgical correction requires multiple procedures

Coloboma

Embryologic cleft involving lid margin; unilateral or bilateral; partial or full thickness

Ranges from notch to absence of entire lid

Upper lid: usually medial third, not associated with systemic abnormalities, usually full thickness

Lower lid: usually lateral third, associated with other abnormalities (Treacher-Collins, Goldenhar's syndrome), usually partial thickness

May have exposure keratitis

Treatment: method of surgical repair depends on size of defect (see section on lid avulsion)

Congenital Blepharoptosis

Droopy eyelid; 75% unilateral; nonhereditary

Rarely causes amblyopia

Associated with blepharophimosis syndrome (AD)

Myogenic most common

Etiology:
  Myogenic:
    Dysgenesis of levator muscle
    Fibroadipose tissue in muscle belly
    Poor levator function, loss of lid crease, eyelid lag, sometimes lagophthalmos
  Aponeurotic:
    Rare, possibly due to birth trauma
    Good eyelid excursion, high or indistinct lid crease

  Neurogenic:
    Congenital CN 3 palsy
    Marcus Gunn jaw-winking (aberrant connections between motor division of CN 5 and levator muscle; jaw movements cause elevation of ptotic lid)

Congenital Horner's Syndrome

Ptosis, miosis, anhydrosis

May cause amblyopia

Treatment: surgical repair (levator resection), severe cases require frontalis sling

Congenital Ectropion

Eversion of eyelid margin due to vertical shortage of anterior lamella

Etiology: inclusion conjunctivitis, anterior lamella inflammation, Down's syndrome

Associated with blepharophimosis syndrome

Treatment: usually not required; otherwise, treat like cicatricial form

Congenital Entropion

Inversion of eyelid margin

Etiology: lid retractor dysgenesis, tarsal plate defects, shortening of posterior lamella

Usually involves lower eyelid

Treatment: may require surgical repair

Congenital Tarsal Kink

Upper eyelid bent back and open with complete fold of tarsal plate

May cause corneal abrasion and exposure keratopathy

Distichiasis

Partial or complete accessory row of eyelashes growing from or posterior to meibomian orifices

Due to improper differentiation of pilosebaceous units

Usually well tolerated, but trichiasis may develop

Treatment: lubrication, cryoepilation, surgical epilation

Epiblepharon

Pretarsal skin and orbicularis override the lid margin, causing a horizontal fold of tissue to push cilia vertically; no entropion

Most common among Asians

Usually occurs in lower lid and resolves spontaneously

Rarely requires surgery (excision of skin and muscle for significant trichiasis)

Epicanthus

Medial canthal vertical skin folds

Due to immature facial bones or redundant skin

Usually bilateral

Produces pseudoesotropia

4 types:
   Epicanthus tarsalis:
      Fold most prominent in upper eyelid
      Commonly associated with Asian eyelid
   Epicanthus inversus:
      Fold most prominent in lower eyelid
      Associated with blepharophimosis syndrome
   Epicanthus palpebralis:
      Fold is equally distributed in upper and lower eyelids
   Epicanthus supraciliaris:
      Fold arises from eyebrow and extends to lacrimal sac

Euryblepharon

Horizontal widening of palpebral fissure due to inferior insertion of lateral canthal tendon

Associated with ectropion of lateral third of lid

Poor lid closure with exposure keratitis

Treatment: lubrication, may require surgical repair with resection of excess lid, lateral canthal tendon repositioning, and vertical eyelid lengthening

Microblepharon

Vertical shortening of lids

May have exposure keratitis

Telecanthus

Widened intercanthal distance due to long medial canthal tendons

Associated with fetal alcohol, Waardenburg's, and blepharophimosis syndromes

Treatment: surgery with transnasal wiring

LACRIMAL DISORDERS

Developmental Anomalies

Atresia of lacrimal puncta: ranges from thin membrane over punctal site to atresia of canaliculus

Supernumerary puncta: no treatment needed

Lacrimal fistula: usually located inferonasal to the medial canthus

Dacryocystocele

Cystic swelling of lacrimal sac accompanies obstruction of lacrimal drainage system above and below the sac

Presents at birth as bluish swelling inferior and nasal to medial canthus

Infection (dacryocystitis) develops if condition does not resolve spontaneously
   Common organisms: *Haemophilus influenzae* (less common now that children are vaccinated against *H. flu*), *Streptococcus pneumoniae, Staphylococcus, Klebsiella, Pseudomonas*

Treatment: digital massage, lacrimal probing, or surgical decompression (for dacryocystitis)

Nasolacrimal Duct Obstruction (NLDO)

Up to 5% of infants have obstruction of the NLD, usually due to membrane covering valve of Hasner

Most open spontaneously within 4 to 6 weeks of birth; 1/3 bilateral

Findings: tearing, discharge; may develop dacryocystitis or conjunctivitis

Digital pressure over lacrimal sac producing mucoid reflux indicates obstruction of nasolacrimal duct

May have a dacryocystocele (dilated lacrimal sac), or amniotic fluid or mucus trapped in tear sac

Treatment: lacrimal sac massage, topical antibiotic, probing and irrigation by 13 months of age (95% cure); consider turbinate infracture and silicone intubation if probing unsuccessful; DCR after multiple failures

CONJUNCTIVAL DISORDERS

Ocular Melanocytosis

Unilateral excessive pigment in uvea, sclera, and episclera

Increase in number of normal melanocytes

More common among Caucasians

Findings: slate grey appearance of sclera, darkened appearance of fundus

When associated with pigmentation of eyelid skin, called nevus of Ota (congenital oculodermal melanocytosis; more common among African Americans and Asians; malignant potential only in Caucasians)

Other findings: heterochromia iridis due to diffuse nevus of uvea; may develop glaucoma (due to melanocytes in trabecular meshwork), rarely uveal, orbital, or meningeal melanoma

Pathology: spindle-shaped pigment cells in sub-epithelial tissue

Conjunctivitis

Ophthalmia Neonatorum

Conjunctivitis within first month of life

Papillary conjunctivitis (no follicular reaction in neonate due to immaturity of immune system)

Etiology:
  Chemical: caused by silver nitrate 1% solution (Crede's prophylaxis); occurs in first 24 hours, lasts 24 to 36 hours (therefore, prophylaxis is now with erythromycin or tetracycline ointment)
    FINDINGS: usually bilateral, bulbar injection with clear watery discharge
    No treatment necessary
  N. gonorrheae: days 1–2; can occur earlier with premature rupture of membranes
    FINDINGS: severe purulent discharge, chemosis, eyelid edema; can be hemorrhagic; may develop corneal ulceration or perforation
    DIAGNOSIS: Gram's stain (Gram-negative intra-cellular diploccocci)
    TREATMENT: IV ceftriaxone × 7 days; bacitracin ointment topically
    High incidence of chlamydia coinfection; therefore, also use oral erythromycin syrup and treat mother and sexual partners
  Other bacteria: days 4–5; *Staphylococci, Streptococci, Haemophilus* (less common now that children are vaccinated against *H. flu*), *Enterococci*
    TREATMENT: bacitracin, erythromycin, or gentamicin ointment; fortified antibiotics for *Pseudomonas*
  HSV: days 5–14; type 2 in 70%
    FINDINGS: serous discharge, conjunctival injection, keratitis; may have vesicular lid lesions
    Can have systemic herpetic infection
    DIAGNOSIS: conjunctival scrapings with multi-nucleated giant cells; cultures take 5–7 days
    TREATMENT: viroptic q2h × 1 week, acyclovir 10 mg/kg IV tid × 10 days
  Chlamydia (neonatal inclusion conjunctivitis): days 5–14; most common infectious cause of neonatal conjunctivitis
    FINDINGS: acute, mucopurulent, papillary (no follicles until 3 months of age); may have pseudomembranes
    Associated with pneumonitis, otitis, naso-pharyngitis, gastritis
    PATHOLOGY: intracytoplasmic inclusions on Giemsa stain

TREATMENT: topical erythromycin, oral erythromycin syrup × 2–3 weeks (125 mg/kg/day qid) to prevent pneumonitis (onset 3–13 weeks later); treat mother and sexual partners with doxycycline 100 mg bid × 1 week (do not use in nursing mothers)
Rule out concomitant *Gonococcus* infection

DDx: trauma, foreign body, corneal abrasion, congenital glaucoma, NLDO, dacryocystitis

Prophylaxis: tetracycline 1% or erythromycin 0.5% ointment at birth

Vernal Keratoconjunctivitis

Form of seasonal (warm months), allergic conjunctivitis

Male > female (2 : 1); onset by age 10 years old, lasts 2–10 years, usually resolves by puberty

Associated with atopic dermatitis (75%) or family history of atopy (66%)

Limbal vernal: more common among African Americans

Symptoms: intense itching, photophobia, pain

Findings: large upper tarsal papillae (cobblestones), minimal conjunctival hyperemia, Horner-Trantas' dots (elevated white accumulations of eosinophils at limbus), limbal follicles (gelatinous nodules at limbus), copious ropy mucus; may have pseudomembrane, keratitis, micropannus, shield ulcer (central oval epithelial defect with white fibrin coating); high levels of histamine and IgE in tears

Pathology: chronic papillary hypertrophy, epithelial hypertrophy then atrophy, conjunctiva contains many mast cells, eosinophils, and basophils

Treatment: topical allergy medication; consider topical cyclosporine

Ligneous

Rare, bilateral, pseudomembranous conjunctivitis in children; commonly young girls

Acute onset, chronic course

Etiology: appears to be exaggerated response to tissue injury following infection, surgery, or trauma

Findings: unilateral or bilateral highly vascularized, raised, friable lesion; with continued inflammation, a white, thickened avascular woody (ligneous) mass appears above the neovascular membrane, usually on palpebral conjunctiva; easily removed but bleeds; may recur

Process affects all mucuos membranes (mouth, vagina, etc)

Pathology: acellular eosinophilic hyaline material (immunoglobulins, primarily IgG), granulation tissue, cellular infiltration (T cells, mast cells, eosinophils)

Treatment: complete excision (expect significant bleeding); any remaining portion of lesion results in rapid recurrence because retained lesion acts as physical barrier to topical medications; ENT evaluation before surgery to ensure respiratory tract not involved because many require general anesthesia

> *Postexcision*: topical steroids every hour; hyaluronidase, acetylcysteine, and α-chymotrypsin every 4 hours; topical antibiotic; topical cyclosporine 2% (applied to surgical bed with sterile cotton-tipped applicator); oral prednisone (1 mg/kg/day); daily débridement of any recurrence

Kawasaki's Disease (Mucocutaneous Lymph Node Syndrome)

Systemic childhood inflammatory disease/vasculitis with prominent mucocutaneous manifestations

Occurs in children <5 years old

More common among individuals of Japanese descent

Epidemics suggest exposure to causal agent; siblings have 10× increased risk

More than 50% of familial cases occur within 10 days after onset of 1st case

Diagnostic criteria (requires 5 of 6): fever, bilateral conjunctivitis (90%), mild bilateral nongranulomatous uveitis (80%), rash, cervical lymphadenopathy, oral lesions (fissures, strawberry tongue), lesions of extremities (edema, erythema, desquamation)

Associated with polyarteritis

Treatment: aspirin; systemic steroids contraindicated (increased risk of coronary artery aneurysm)

Prognosis: 0.3% mortality

Complications: 15% develop coronary arteritis (can lead to coronary artery aneurysm or myocardial infarction)

Tumors

Epibulbar Osseous Choristoma

Hard mass, composed of mature bone

Usually located on bulbar conjunctiva (superotemporal fornix)

Does not enlarge

Not associated with other osteomas

No malignant potential

Treatment: observe or excise

Complex Choristoma

May contain cartilage, ectopic lacrimal gland tissue, smooth muscle, sweat glands, sebaceous glands, hair

Isolated or associated with linear nevus sebaceous syndrome

Ectopic Lacrimal Gland

Fleshy, vascularized tumor with raised translucent nodules

Usually extends into corneal stroma

Mild growth during puberty

Pathology: lacrimal gland parenchyma

Treatment: excision

CORNEAL DISORDERS

Anterior Megalophthalmos

Large anterior segment of eye

Associations: Marfan's syndrome, mucolipidosis type II, Apert's syndrome

Findings: high myopia and astigmatism; enlarged cornea, lens, iris, and ciliary ring; iris transillumination defects, lens dislocation, cataract

Congenital Corneal Staphyloma

Protuberant corneal opacity due to intrauterine keratitis

Findings: atrophic iris adheres to back of markedly thickened, scarred, and vascularized cornea; lens may be adherent to posterior cornea; cornea may perforate

Cornea Plana (AD or AR)

Mapped to chromosome 12q

Associations: sclerocornea, microcornea, and angle-closure glaucoma

Findings: flat cornea with curvature equal to that of sclera (usually 20–30 D), diffuse scarring and vascularization; may have coloboma, cataract, sclerocornea, shallow AC, refractive error

Pathology: thickened epithelium, absent basement membrane, very thin Descemet's, anterior 1/3 of stroma is scarred and vascularized

Megalocornea

Horizontal diameter of cornea greater than 12 mm in newborn (>13 mm in adult)

Nonprogressive; most commonly X-linked (associated with anterior megalophthalmos), bilateral, 90% male

Associations: Marfan's syndrome, Alport's syndrome, Down's syndrome, dwarfism, craniosynostosis, facial hemiatrophy

Findings: large cornea; may have weak zonules, lens subluxation, hypoplastic iris, and ectopic pupil

Complications: ectopia lentis (enlarged limbal ring stretches the zonular fibers), glaucoma (due to angle abnormalities), cataract (PSC)

Microcornea

Corneal diameter less than 9 mm in newborn (<10 mm in adult)

Autosomal dominant or sporadic; unilateral or bilateral

Etiology: arrested corneal growth after 5th month of fetal development

Associations: dwarfism, Ehlers-Danlos syndrome

Findings: small cornea; often hyperopic (relatively flat corneas); may have cataract, coloboma, PHPV, microphakia; may develop angle-closure glaucoma or POAG

DDx: nanophthalmos (small but structurally normal eye), anterior microphthalmos (small anterior segment), microphthalmos (small malformed eye)

Posterior Keratoconus

Discrete posterior corneal indentation with stromal haze and thinning

Female > male

Nonprogressive, usually central and unilateral

Anterior corneal surface is normal

Vision usually good; causes irregular astigmatism

Pathology: loss of stromal substance; Descemet's may be thinned, but both Descemet's and endothelium are intact

Anterior Segment Dysgenesis (Mesodermal Dysgenesis Syndromes)

Bilateral, congenital, hereditary disorders affecting anterior segment structures

Axenfeld's anomaly: posterior embryotoxon (anteriorly displaced Schwalbe's line; found in 15% of normal individuals) with iris processes to scleral spur; 50% develop glaucoma; AD; mapped to chromosome 4q25 (RIEG1), 13q14 (RIEG2), 6p25 (FOXC1), 11p (PAX6)

Alagille's syndrome: Axenfeld's plus pigmentary retinopathy, corectopia, esotropia, and systemic abnormalities (absent deep tendon reflexes, abnormal facies, pulmonic valvular stenosis, peripheral arterial stenosis, biliary hypoplasia, and skeletal abnormalities); mapped to chromosome 20p12 (JAG1); ERG and EOG are abnormal

Rieger's anomaly: Axenfeld's plus iris hypoplasia with holes; 50% develop glaucoma; mapped to chromosome 4q25 (RIEG1), 13q14 (RIEG2), 6p25 (FOXC1), 11p (PAX6)

Rieger's syndrome: Rieger's anomaly plus mental retardation and systemic abnormalities (dental, craniofacial, genitourinary, and skeletal)

Peter's anomaly: central corneal leukoma (opacity due to defect in Descemet's membrane with absence of endothelium) with iris adhesions; lens involvement (cataract) may occur and 50% develop glaucoma; also associated with cardiac, craniofacial, and skeletal abnormalities; usually sporadic, bilateral (80%); mapped to chromosome 11p (PAX6)

BOX 5-1. DDx of Congenital Cloudy Cornea: STUMPED

Sclerocornea
Tears in Descemet's
Ulcers
Metabolic disease
Peter's anomaly
Edema (CHED)
Dermoids
Others: CHSD, rubella, posterior ulcer of von Hippel, posterior keratoconus, congenital corneal staphyloma

---

Sclerocornea

Scleralized (white vascularized opacification) cornea; peripheral or entire

Nonprogressive; sporadic (50%) or hereditary (50%); 90% bilateral

Corneoscleral limbus indistinct

Associations: persistent pupillary membrane, congenital glaucoma, cornea plana (80%)

Poor prognosis for corneal transplant

Descemet's Tear/Rupture

May be caused by forceps trauma (vertical or oblique) or glaucoma (horizontal or concentric to limbus; Haab's striae)

Acutely, edema occurs, scarring develops later

May cause astigmatism and amblyopia

Metabolic Disorders (Mucopolysaccharidoses, Mucolipidoses)

(see Table 5-4)

Congenital Hereditary Endothelial Dystrophy (CHED)

Rare, bilateral; mapped to chromosome 20p

Onset at or shortly after birth

Corneal clouding due to edema from defect of corneal endothelium and Descemet's membrane

2 forms:
  AR: more common, presents at birth, nystagmus, no pain or tearing, nonprogressive
  AD: later onset (2nd year of life), pain, tearing, photophobia, no nystagmus, progressive

No association with other systemic abnormalities

Findings: bilateral cloudy corneas, corneal edema

Pathology: thickened edematous stroma, massively thickened Descemet's, atrophic or nonfunctioning endothelium

Congenital Hereditary Stromal Dystrophy (CHSD) (AD)

Rare, nonprogressive, diffuse opacification of superficial cornea

Findings: flaky, feathery appearance of anterior stroma, clear peripherally; no corneal edema

May cause strabismus, nystagmus, and amblyopia

Dermoid

Smooth, solid, yellow-white choristoma that may extend into corneal stroma to cover visual axis or cause astigmatism

No hereditary pattern; 25% bilateral

2 types:
  Conjunctival (limbal) dermoid:
  Straddles limbus, most commonly in inferotemporal quadrant
  Isolated or associated with Goldenhar's syndrome (30%; includes accessory auricular appendages, aural fistulas, vertebral body abnormalities)
  May cause astigmatism and amblyopia
  Also associated with linear sebaceous nevus syndrome
  Dermolipoma of the conjunctiva:
  Usually located in superotemporal fornix; can extend deep into orbit
  Consists of adipose and connective tissue
  High surgical complication rate, with risk of marked ptosis, lateral rectus muscle paresis, and dry eye

Findings: dermoid, layer of lipid at leading edge in cornea; may cause proptosis, astigmatism-restricted motility, amblyopia

Pathology: thickened collagen fibers covered by skinlike epithelium; contains hair, sebaceous and sweat glands, and fat, and lined by squamous epithelium

Treatment: observation; excision for cosmesis or if visual axis is blocked (*caution*: may be full thickness; granulomatous reaction if ruptures)

Other Causes of Corneal Opacity

Interstitial keratitis: congenital syphilis causes keratitis with edema followed by stromal vascularization ("salmon patch"), blood flow stops and "ghost" vessels remain with corneal haze

Riley-day syndrome (AR): autonomic nervous system dysfunction due to block of NE production; Eastern European Jews
  Findings: decreased corneal sensation, lack of tearing, poorly reactive pupils, light-near dissociation; may develop neurotrophic keratitis with risk of perforation
  Other findings: poor pain, temperature, and taste sensation; spinal curvature; increased sweating; constipation; hypotension
  Crisis (lasts 1–10 days): emotional lability, profuse sweating, postural hypotension, vomiting; treat with diazepam (Valium) and hydration
  Increased risk with general anesthesia: exquisite sensitivity to thiopental sodium (Pentothal) (hypotension, cardiac arrest)
  Diagnosis: high urinary HVA and VMA, low HMPT

Infections

Syphilis

Congenital: maternal transmission after 4th month of gestation (50% for primary or secondary syphilis, 30% for untreated or late syphilis)

Findings: interstitial keratitis (33%), ectopia lentis, Argyll-Robertson pupil, optic atrophy, panuveitis with various retinal pigmentary changes (usually salt and pepper or pseudo-RP)

Other findings:
  Early: stillbirth, failure to thrive, rhinitis ("snuffles"), osteochondritis, pneumonia, hepatosplenomegaly
  Late: Hutchinson's teeth (peg-shaped), mulberry molars, saber shins, frontal bossing, saddle nose, deafness (5%), tabes dorsalis

Hutchinson's triad: interstitial keratitis, Hutchinson's teeth, deafness
  Interstitial keratitis (IK): immune response to treponemal antigens

Starts between age 5 and 20 years of age; triggered by minor corneal trauma

Bilateral with 2nd eye involvement at 1–2 months in 50%, 12 months in 75%

3 STAGES:

PROGRESSIVE: pain, photophobia, poor vision; blepharospasm, fine KP, perilimbal injection, diffuse or sectoral corneal haze (ground-glass appearance)

FLORID: acute inflammatory response; salmon patch of Hutchinson (cornea appears pink due to deep vascularization)

RETROGRESSIVE: vessels meet at center of cornea

LATE FINDINGS: ghost vessels, Descemet's folds, guttata, secondary glaucoma (iris/angle damage)

PATHOLOGY: stromal blood vessels just anterior to Descemet's

TREATMENT: steroids (do not prevent involvement of fellow eye); systemic penicillin

DDx: acquired syphilis (IK usually sectoral and less severe), leprosy (superficial avascular keratitis, usually superotemporal quadrant; later, leprous pannus of blood vessels, beading of corneal nerves)

Herpes Simplex (HSV)

Often asymptomatic primary infection before age 5; 3- to 5-day incubation period

Congenital: ocular involvement in 10% of disseminated cases

Findings: vesicular skin eruption, conjunctivitis, epithelial keratitis, stromal immune reaction, cataracts, necrotizing chorioretinitis

IRIS DISORDERS

Aniridia

Bilateral absence of iris, commonly a rudimentary iris stump exists

Incidence 1 in 100,000

Hereditary or sporadic; mapped to chromosome 11p13

3 types:

AN1 (85%): AD, only eye involvement

AN2 (13%): sporadic, associated with Wilms' tumor (Miller syndrome and WAGR [Wilms' tumor, aniridia, genitourinary abnormalities, and mental retardation])

AN3 (2%): AR, associated with mental retardation and ataxia (Gillespie's syndrome)

Findings: visual acuity usually 20/100 or worse, foveal and optic nerve hypoplasia, nystagmus, photophobia, amblyopia, strabismus

May have cataracts (50% to 85%), glaucoma (30% to 50%), and corneal pannus

Treatment: consider cosmetic/painted contact lenses for photophobia; peripherally painted IOLs and PMMA rings have been used with cataract surgery but are not FDA approved

Coloboma

Iris sector defect usually located in inferonasal quadrant

Due to incomplete closure of embryonic fissure

May have other colobomas (lid, ciliary body, choroid, retina, and optic nerve)

Associated with trisomy 13, 18, and 22; chromosome 18 deletion; Klinefelter's syndrome, Turner's syndrome, CHARGE, basal cell nevus syndrome, Goldenhar's syndrome, Meckel's syndrome, Rubinstein-Taybi syndrome, linear sebaceous nevus syndrome

Treatment: consider surgical repair in symptomatic cases

Congenital Iris Ectropion

Ectropion uveae: ectropion of posterior pigment epithelium onto anterior surface of iris

Associated with neurofibromatosis, Prader-Willi syndrome

Congenital iris ectropion syndrome: unilateral congenital iris ectropion, high iris insertion, smooth cryptless iris surface, dysgenesis of angle, and glaucoma

Congenital Iris Hypoplasia

Thin iris stroma with transillumination of entire iris

Associated with albinism

Congenital Miosis

May be associated with other anterior segment abnormalities

Etiology: absence or malformation of dilator pupillae muscle or contracture of fibrous material on pupil margin from tunica vasculosa lentis remnant or neural crest cell abnormalities

Congenital Mydriasis

Etiology: iris sphincter trauma, pharmacologic, neurologic disease

Corectopia

Displacement of pupil

Isolated or associated with ectopia lentis et pupillae, Axenfeld-Rieger syndrome, iridocorneal endothelial syndrome, uveitis, or trauma

Dyscoria

Abnormally shaped pupil

Isolated or associated with posterior synechiae, Axenfeld-Reiger syndrome, ectopia lentis et pupillae

Persistent Pupillary Membrane

Remnants of anterior tunica vasculosa lentis that appear as fine iris strands

Most common congenital ocular anomaly; occurs in 80% of dark-colored eyes and 35% of light-colored eyes

Rarely visually significant

Type I: iris to iris, bridging pupil

Type II: iris to lens; may have associated anterior polar cataract

Primary Iris Cysts

Due to spontaneous separation of pigmented and nonpigmented epithelium

Occur anywhere between pupil and ciliary body

Miotics can cause cysts at pupillary border

Congenital stromal cysts occur in infants and young children from sequestration of epithelium during fetal development

Brushfield's Spots

Focal areas of iris stromal hyperplasia surrounded by relative hypoplasia

Appear as ring of peripheral, elevated, white-grey spots (10–20/eye)

Occur in 85% of Down's syndrome patients

May be found in normal individuals (Kunkmann-Wolffian bodies)

Lisch Nodules

Neural crest hamartomas

Associated with neurofibromatosis type I

Number and frequency increase with age

Appear as tan nodules, usually in inferior iris

Juvenile Xanthogranuloma (JXG; Nevoxanthoendothelioma)

Histiocytic proliferation usually of skin

Yellow-orange nodules appear before 1 year of age

Orange because of vascularity (red) combined with high lipid content (yellow)

May involve iris (may cause spontaneous hyphema)

May involve muscles, salivary glands, stomach, and other internal organs

Rarely associated with an orbital granuloma (which causes proptosis)

Lesions often spontaneously regress by 5 years of age

Pathology: diffuse non-necrotizing proliferation of histiocytes with scattered touton giant cells (ring of nuclei separating a central eosinophilic cytoplasm from peripheral foamy [or clear] cytoplasm)

Treatment: iris lesions are treated with steroids, XRT, and excision

Medulloepithelioma (Diktyoma)

Primary neoplasm of ciliary body neuroectoderm (arises in nonpigmented epithelium); arises from primitive medullary epithelium that lines neural tube; can also arise in retina and ON

Occurs in both benign and malignant forms (locally invasive but limited metastatic potential)

May have heterotopic elements; no calcification

Unilateral, unifocal, usually arises before 6 years of age; no hereditary pattern

2 types:
  Nonteratoid or simple: pure proliferation of embryonic nonpigmented ciliary epithelium
  Teratoid: contains heterotopic elements such as cartilage, brain tissue, and rhabdomyoblasts

Findings: decreased vision, pain, strabismus, leukocoria, iris mass, fleshy pink to white peripheral fundus tumor; rubeosis, hyphema, glaucoma, lens coloboma occurs in some congenital cases

Pathology: undifferentiated round to oval cells containing little cytoplasm, organized into ribbon-like structures that have distinct cellular polarity; lined on one side by thin basement membrane; stratified sheets of cells are capable of forming mucinous cysts that are clinically characteristic; Flexner-Wintersteiner and Homer-Wright rosettes can be seen; called **teratoid medulloepithelioma** when composed of cells from 2 different embryonic germ layers; may contain cartilage, brain tissue, and rhabdomyoblasts

Treatment: resection (iridocyclectomy) or enucleation (not radiosensitive)

Prognosis: good if no extraocular extension; rarely metastasizes

LENS DISORDERS

Congenital Anomalies

Mittendorf's dot: small white opacity on posterior lens capsule that represents a remnant of the posterior vascular capsule (tunica vasculosa lentis) where hyaloid artery is inserted

Chicken tracks (epicapsular star): brown or golden flecks on anterior lens capsule; remnant of anterior tunica vasculosa lentis

Lenticonus: cone-shaped lens deformity due to central bulge in area of thin capsule; causes irregular myopic astigmatism; "oil-droplet" sign on retinoscopy; associated with cataract

Anterior: bilateral, male > female; associated with Alport's syndrome (anterior lenticonus, hereditary nephritis, and deafness)

Posterior: unilateral, sporadic, female > male, more common than anterior type, amblyopia common

Lens coloboma: focal flattening of lens edge due to absence of inferior zonules from ciliary body coloboma; not a true coloboma

Lentiglobus: generalized hemispherical deformity, very rare

Microphakia: small lens due to arrested development; associated with Lowe's syndrome

Microspherophakia: small, spherical lens, usually bilateral; zonules visible on pupillary dilation; iridodenesis; zonule rupture is common, pupillary block may occur especially with use of miotics (treat with cycloplegic to tighten zonules, flattening the lens and pulling it posteriorly)

Associated with Weill-Marchesani syndrome, hyperlysinemia, Lowe's syndrome, Alport's syndrome, congenital rubella, and Peter's anomaly

Treatment: cycloplegic (tightens zonules, flattening lens and pulling it posteriorly)

Congenital aphakia: rare, absence of lens

Ectopia Lentis (see Chapter 10, Anterior Segment)

Congenital Cataracts

Characteristics:

Bilateral: usually autosomal dominant (AD); consider diabetes, galactosemia, or Lowe's syndrome; require metabolic workup and treatment by age 3 months, or irreversible nystagmus with poor visual acuity (≤20/200) occurs. Opacities greater than 3 mm can be visually significant. Surgery often performed on the better-seeing eye first: lensectomy, anterior vitrectomy, and contact lens fitting for infants; posterior capsulotomy is necessary due to significant postoperative inflammation, which causes posterior capsular opacification

Unilateral: generally not metabolic or genetic; therefore, laboratory testing not needed. Usually local dysgenesis (PHPV, anterior polar, or posterior lenticonus). Often present with leukocoria and strabismus. Requires treatment by 6–8 weeks of life

Types: classified by location or etiology

Polar (subcapsular cortex and capsule): anterior or posterior, sporadic, or AD

ANTERIOR: usually small, bilateral, symmetric, nonprogressive; good visual prognosis; 90% are idiopathic. Remnant of the hyaloid system. Associated with microphthalmos and anterior lenticonus.

PATHOLOGY: fibrous plaque beneath folded anterior capsule secreted by irritated metaplastic epithelial cells.

POSTERIOR: larger, usually stable, but may progress; more visually significant; AD (bilateral) or sporadic (unilateral); often with associated defect of posterior capsule.

Associated with remnants of the tunica vasculosa lentis, posterior lenticonus, or lentiglobus

PATHOLOGY: posterior migration of lens epithelium.

Sutural (AD): bilateral opacities of Y sutures; rarely affects vision. Occurs during development of fetal lens nucleus

Nuclear (usually AD): bilateral, opacification of embryonic/fetal nucleus; typically axial, dense, bilateral, and larger than 3 mm; associated with small eye

Anterior pyramidal: congenital anterior subcapsular

Lamellar/zonular: bilateral, symmetric, appears like a sand dollar; circumscribed zone of opacity within lens, surrounding the nucleus. May be due to transient toxic exposure during embryogenesis (neonatal tetany); can be AD. Usually does not interfere with vision

Complete: no red reflex; unilateral or bilateral

Membranous: lens proteins resorb following trauma; anterior and posterior capsules fuse into a dense white membrane

Crystalline: rare, bilateral congenital cataract, with refractile, rhomboid crystals (containing tyrosine and cysteine) radiating outward from the center of the lens into the juvenile nucleus

Anterior axial embryonic: most common type of congenital/infantile cataract. White, clustered, punctate opacities near the Y-sutures; not visually significant

Coronary (cerulean): wart-like excrescences on capsule, eventually replaced by clumps of epithelium, resulting in granular debris in peripheral cortex

Pulverulent (AD): central, translucent, ovoid, and cluster of dot-like opacities in the fetal nucleus

Coronary (AD): associated with Down's syndrome; wreath of peripheral cortical opacities that encircle the nucleus in a radial fashion; smaller punctate bluish opacities within the nucleus

Etiology: 1/3 hereditary; 1/3 associated with systemic syndromes; 1/3 unknown origin

Etiology of bilateral cataracts:

Idiopathic (60%)

Intrauterine infection (3%): **TORCH** syndromes (**T**oxoplasmosis, **R**ubella, **C**MV, **H**erpes, syphilis)

Associated with ocular disorders: Leber's congenital amaurosis, retinitis pigmentosa (RP), persistent hyperplastic primary vitreous (PHPV), retinopathy of prematurity (ROP), aniridia, Peter's anomaly, ectopia lentis, posterior lenticonus, uveitis, tumors (retinoblastoma, medulloepithelioma)

Metabolic: galactosemia, hypocalcemia, Lowe's syndrome, congenital hemolytic jaundice, hypoglycemia, mannosidosis, Alport's syndrome, Fabry's disease

Hereditary (30%, usually AD):

WITHOUT SYSTEMIC ABNORMALITIES: AD, AR, X-linked

WITH CHROMOSOMAL ABNORMALITIES: trisomy 18, trisomy 21 (Down's syndrome), Turner's syndrome, trisomy 13 (Patau's syndrome), "cri-du-chat" syndrome

CRANIOFACIAL SYNDROMES: Crouzon's syndrome, Apert's syndrome, Hallermann-Streiff syndrome, Pierre Robin sequence

CNS ABNORMALITIES: Zellweger syndrome, Torsten-Sjögren syndrome, Marinesco-Sjögren syndrome, Lawrence-Moon-Biedl-Bardet syndrome, Norrie's disease, neurofibromatosis

SKIN ABNORMALITIES: Cockayne's syndrome, Rothmund-Thomson syndrome, Werner's syndrome, atopic dermatitis, ichthyosis, incontinentia pigmenti

Maternal drug ingestion/malnutrition
Trauma

Specific entities:

Galactosemia (AR): defect of 1 of 3 enzymes (galactose-1-P-uridyl transferase [most common], galactokinase, or UDP galactose-4-epimerase) causes inability to convert galactose into glucose; galactose converted into galactitol, which serves as osmotic agent for influx of fluid

FINDINGS: oil-droplet cataract (reversible early)

OTHER FINDINGS: mental retardation, hepatomegaly, jaundice, and malnutrition within 1st few weeks of life

TREATMENT: eliminate lactose from diet; fatal if untreated

Mannosidosis: α-mannosidase deficiency causes Hurler-like syndrome

FINDINGS: posterior spoke-like opacity; no corneal changes (unlike Hurler's)

OTHER FINDINGS: mental retardation, short stature, skeletal changes, hepatosplenomagaly

Fabry's disease: α-galactosidase A deficiency

FINDINGS: cornea verticillata; spoke-like cataract in 25%

OTHER FINDINGS: angiokeratomas, cardiovascular abnormalities, renal disorders, bouts of pain in digits

Hypocalcemia: either idiopathic or following surgery of parathyroid glands

Punctate iridescent opacities in anterior and posterior cortex

Lowe's (oculocerebrorenal) syndrome (X-linked): defect of amino acid metabolism; male > female

FINDINGS: congenital cataract (100%), usually bilateral; small, thin, discoid lens (microphakic) associated with retained lens nuclei; glaucoma (50%); congenital cataract and glaucoma are very rare

Female carriers have white, punctate cortical opacities and subcapsular plaque-like opacities

OTHER FINDINGS: renal tubular acidosis, aminoaciduria, renal rickets, mental retardation, muscular hypotonia, failure to thrive

Alport's syndrome (X-linked): triad of anterior lenticonus, deafness, and hemorrhagic nephropathy/renal failure

FINDINGS: conjunctival calcium crystals, corneal endothelial pigment, juvenile arcus, spherophakia, anterior polar cataract, retinal changes similar to retinitis pigmentosa or fundus albipunctatis, optic nerve drusen

Female carriers have lenticular changes

DIAGNOSIS: renal or skin biopsy (lack of α-5 type IV collagen in glomerular and epidermal basement membranes)

Hallermann-Streiff syndrome (mandibulo-oculofacial dysmorphia): hypoplasia of mandible with birdlike facies; one of the few syndromes with combined cataract and glaucoma

FINDINGS: microphakia, microcornea, glaucoma, and cataract (can develop within 1st few weeks of life); spontaneous rupture of lens capsule with absorption of lens proteins can occur; immune response to lens proteins resembles phacoanaphylactic uveitis

Intrauterine infections: usually occur early in first trimester because lens capsule is formed during week 5 of embryogenesis; rubella, HSV, mumps, toxoplasmosis, vaccinia, CMV

Hypoglycemia during pregnancy: congenital lenticular opacities; associated with optic atrophy, mental retardation

Down's syndrome: snowflake cataract, keratoconus

Diagnosis of bilateral cataracts: if AD pattern determined, no workup necessary

Urinalysis: amino acids (Lowe's syndrome), reducing substance after milk feeding (galactosemia)

Blood tests: calcium (hypocalcemia/hyperparathyroidism), glucose (hypoglycemia), red blood cell galactokinase, TORCH titers

Karyotyping: trisomy 13 (Patau's), 18, and 21 (Down's); Turner's syndrome, "cri-du-chat" syndrome

Bilateral audiograms: congenital rubella, Alport's syndrome

B-scan ultrasound: if no view of fundus

Etiology of unilateral cataracts:

Idiopathic (80%)

Ocular abnormalities (10%): PHPV, posterior lenticonus (90% unilateral), anterior segment dysgenesis, tumors (retinoblastoma, medulloepithelioma)

Trauma (9%)

Intrauterine infection: rubella; 33% unilateral

Diagnosis of unilateral cataracts: rule out trauma (child abuse), TORCH titers

DDx of leukocoria (white pupil): cataract, retinoblastoma, toxoplasmosis, toxocariasis, RD, ROP, PHPV, Coats' disease, coloboma, myelinated nerve fibers, retinal dysplasia, Norrie's disease, incontinentia pigmenti, retinoschisis, cyclitic membrane, medulloepithelioma

DDx of congenital cataracts and glaucoma: Lowe's syndrome, rubella, Hallermann-Streiff syndrome

> *Rubella*: due to maternal infection late in the first trimester of pregnancy
>
>> FINDINGS (in 50%): cataract (usually bilateral, pearly white nuclear opacification; retention of lens nuclei in embryonic nucleus. Virus remains viable in lens for years: viral shedding following cataract surgery can lead to intense and persistent AC inflammation), salt and pepper fundus (normal ERG), glaucoma (usually either cataract or glaucoma, rarely both), microphthalmos (15%), necrotizing iridocyclitis, corneal clouding
>>
>> OTHER FINDINGS (especially during 1st trimester): cardiac defects (patent ductus arteriosis), deafness (infection of the organ of Corti [90%]), and mental retardation

Complications of surgery: chronic aphakic glaucoma (15%). Usually discovered 5–6 years after surgery; increased risk with trauma, microcornea, PHPV, preexisting anterior segment abnormalities, and retained lens material

Prognosis:

> *Good*: lamellar cataracts (later onset and less risk of glaucoma)
>
> *Intermediate*: nuclear cataracts
>
> *Poor*: total cataracts (high incidence of microcornea, poor pupillary dilation, and increased risk of glaucoma). Microphthalmos, strabismus, nystagmus, and amblyopia. 90% of patients with visually significant congenital bilateral cataracts will develop nystagmus if not treated by 2 months of age. Nystagmus and amblyopia may not resolve even after cataract surgery

GLAUCOMA

Childhood Glaucoma

Several types of glaucoma typically categorized by age of onset

Congenital (occurs in infants <3 months old; may be primary, secondary, or associated with a syndrome)

Infantile (between 3 months and 3 years of age)

Juvenile (between 3 and 35 years of age)

Primary Congenital Glaucoma

Etiology: Mapped to chromosomes 1p36 (GLC3B), 2p21-p22 (GLC3A, CYP1B1). A mutation in the CYP1B1 gene accounts for ~85% of congenital glaucoma. AR in 10%; affected parent has 5% chance of having a child with infantile glaucoma

Epidemiology: occurs in 1 of 12,500 births; 40% present at birth; 86% present during first year of life; 70% bilateral; 70% males.

Symptoms: tearing, photophobia, blepharospasm, eye rubbing. If younger than age 3 months, usually present with corneal clouding or tearing; older than 3 years of age, usually asymptomatic with progressive myopia and insidious VF loss

Findings: IOP >21 mm Hg; C/D ratio >0.3 (present in only 2.6% of normal infants; cupping is reversible in childhood); buphthalmos ("bull's-eye"; horizontal corneal diameter >13 mm; limbal ectasia; stretching of zonules can lead to lens subluxation; irreversible); corneal clouding/edema/Haab's striae (circumferential or horizontal Descemet's ruptures [vs oblique or vertical with forceps injury]; may result in chronic corneal edema, scarring, and astigmatism); myopia.

Angle is of neural crest origin, as are facial bones, teeth, cartilage, and meninges; therefore, congenital glaucoma may be associated with malformation of these structures

Other ocular associations: microcornea, cornea plana, sclerocornea, Axenfeld's/Reiger's/Peter's anomaly (50%), aniridia (50% to 75% develop glaucoma by teens due to increased episcleral venous pressure, iris stump blocking TM, or angle malformation or agenesis), microspherophakia, nanophthalmos, PHPV, ROP, tumors (RB, JXG, medulloepithelioma), inflammation, trauma, steroid-induced

Associated syndromes: Lowe's syndrome (50%); Sturge-Weber syndrome (50%, especially if nevus flammeus involves upper lid, due to primary defect in angle and increased episcleral venous pressure); neurofibromatosis (25% if plexiform neurofibroma involves upper lid; may have hamartomatous infiltration of angle); congenital rubella (2% to 15%); also Marfan's syndrome, homocystinuria, Weill-Marchesani syndrome, Rubenstein-Taybi, Pierre Robin, nevus of Ota, trisomy 13 (Patau's), Hallermann-Streiff, Stickler's syndrome, mucopolysaccharidoses (Hurler's and Hunter's)

Diagnosis:

> *Examination under ansthesia* (EUA): usually required for complete evaluation. Remember, ketamine and succinylcholine raise IOP, general anesthesia (halothane, thiopental, tranquilizers, and barbituates) lowers IOP. Best time for IOP measurement is just as patient goes under and is not too deep

Gonioscopy: landmarks are often poorly recognized due to "Barkan's membrane" covering TM (but no histologic evidence of such a structure)
1. Open-angle with anterior iris insertion above scleral spur (usual configuration is flat iris insertion into trabecular meshwork; less commonly, concave insertion with plane of iris posterior to scleral spur and anterior iris sweeping upward and inserting into TM)
2. Thickening of TM
3. Peripheral iris stromal hypoplasia

Treatment: definitive treatment is surgical; medication is a temporizing measure
Goniotomy: perform in child <1½ years of age; TM incised under direct gonioscopic visualization; requires clear cornea. 77% success rate
Trabeculotomy (ab externo): if cornea hazy, if >1½ years old, or if goniotomy fails twice; Schlemm's canal is entered via an external incision, and the trabeculotome rotates into the AC and tears the TM; 77% success rate
If goniotomy and trabeculotomy fail, consider trabeculectomy with mitomycin C, drainage implant, cycloablation of CB

Primary infantile glaucoma (congenital glaucoma, trabeculodysgenesis)	
Secondary infantile glaucoma	
Associated with mesodermal neural crest dysgenesis	Iridocorneotrabeculodysgenesis
	• Rieger's anomaly or syndrome
	• Axenfeld's anomaly or syndrome
	• Peters' anomaly
	• systemic hypoplastic mesodermal dysgenesis (Marfan's syndrome)
	• systemic hyperplastic mesodermal dysgenesis (Weill–Marchesani syndrome)
	Iridotrabeculodysgenesis (aniridia)
Associated with phakomatoses and hamartomas	Neurofibromatosis (Von Recklinghausen's disease)
	Encephalotrigeminal angiomatosis (Sturge–Weber syndrome and variants, e.g. Klippel–Trénaunay–Weber syndrome)
	Angiomatosis retinae et cerebelli
	Oculodermal melanocytosis
Associated with metabolic disease	Oculocerebrorenal syndrome (Lowe's syndrome)
	Homocystinuria
Associated with inflammatory disease	Maternal rubella syndrome (congenital rubella)
	Herpes simplex iridocyclitis
Associated with mitotic disease	Juvenile xanthogranuloma (nevoxanthoendothelioma)
	Retinoblastoma
Associated with other congenital disease	Trisomy 13–15 syndrome (Patau's syndrome)
	Rubinstein–Taybi syndrome
	Persistent hyperplastic primary vitreous
	Congenital cataract
	• in phakic eyes
	• in aphakic eyes following surgery

Figure 5-6. Classification of the congenital and infantile glaucomas. (From Yanoff M, Duker JS [eds]: *Ophthalmology*, London, Mosby, 1999.)

UVEITIS

Anterior Uveitis

DDx: JRA, trauma, infection, tumor, sympathetic ophthalmia, sarcoidosis, phacoantigenic

Juvenile Rheumatoid Arthritis (JRA)

Most common cause of uveitis in children: seronegative (RF–), ANA-positive, pauciarticular (<5 joints) arthritis in children <16 years old; mostly girls

4 types (Table 5-2):
Pauciarticular (<5 joints), early onset: 80% female; 30% with chronic iridocyclitis; 25% of all JRA; RF–; 60% ANA+
Pauciarticular, late onset: 90% male; 15% of all JRA; RF–; ANA–; 75% HLA-B27; 15% acute iridocyclitis
Polyarticular (≥5 joints): 85% female; iridocyclitis rare; 40% of all JRA; 75% are RF–
Still's disease: throughout childhood; 60% male; small and large joints; iridocylitis rare; 20% of all JRA; RF–; ANA–; high fever, rash, organomegaly, polyserositis

Findings: chronic anterior uveitis (30%, usually bilateral; eyes are white and quiet even with active ocular inflammation [lots of flare]), glaucoma (20%), cataract (40%), band keratopathy (40%)

Other findings (30%): arthritis, fever, lymphadenopathy, maculopapular rash, myocarditis, hepatosplenomegaly

Treatment: topical steroids and cycloplegic; consider systemic steroids or sub-Tenon's steroid injection; treat complications. May require immunosuppressive agents, EDTA chelation for band keratopathy, treatment of secondary glaucoma, cataract surgery (eyes should be without AC reaction for at least 3 months; intraoperatively, anterior vitrectomy, synechialysis, removal of cyclitic membranes; no IOL; may be complicated by hypotony)

Intermediate Uveitis

Pars Planitis (see Chapter 8, Uveitis)

Posterior Uveitis

DDx: toxoplasmosis, toxocariasis, POHS, HSV, syphilis, Lyme disease, sympathetic ophthalmia, masquerade syndromes (RB, leukemia, lymphoma, melanoma, JXG, intraocular foreign body, RD, RP, MS)

Table 5-2. Classification of JRA

Type	Polyarticular RF-Negative	Polyarticular RF-Positive	Pauciarticular Type I	Pauciarticular Type II	Systemic (Still's Disease)
Age	Any	Late childhood	Early childhood	Late childhood	Any
Sex	90% girls	80% girls	80% girls	90% boys	60% boys
RF	Negative	Positive	Negative	Negative	Negative
ANA	25%	75%	60%	Negative	Negative
HLA-B27	N/A	N/A	N/A	75%	N/A
Joints	Any	Any	Large joints (knee, elbow, ankle)	Large joints (hip, SI joints)	Any
Uveitis	Rare	No	30% Chronic	15% Acute	Rare
Other findings	Low-grade fever, delayed growth, anemia, malaise	Low-grade fever, anemia, malaise, rheumatoid nodules	Few	Few	High fever, rash, organomegaly, polyserositis

Toxoplasmosis

Due to infection with *Toxoplasma gondii*, usually congenital (maternal infection during gestation)

70% of women are seronegative

Primary retinal infection with coagulative necrosis and secondary granulomatous choroiditis with vitritis; intraretinal cysts cause recurrent disease

Most common cause of posterior uveitis (25%); 98% congenital

Most common cause of pediatric uveitis (50% of posterior uveitis in children)

Tachyzoite form is responsible for inflammation

Congenital infection: transplacental transmission of *T. gondii*
  First-trimester infection: neonatal convulsions, intracerebral calcifications, retinitis
  Later infection: may have retinitis only

Findings: inactive chorioretinal scar in posterior pole, often in macula; active focal white fluffy lesion ("headlight in fog" appearance) occurs adjacent to old scar with granulomatous uveitis and vitritis; may have white spots along arterioles (Kyrieleis' plaques); may have microphthalmia, nystagmus, strabismus
  In AIDS: head CT may show ring-enhancing lesions; minimal AC reaction and vitritis because immunocompromised host is unable to mount normal immune response

Other findings:
  Congenital toxoplasmosis: stillbirth, mental retardation, seizures, hydrocephalus, microcephaly, intracranial calcifications, hepatosplenomegaly, vomiting, diarrhea
  Acquired toxoplasmosis: rash, meningoencephalitis, flu-like syndrome

Figure 5-7. Congenital toxoplasmic retinitis. Note inactive satellite scars at the macula, the inferior juxtapapillary scar, and the temporal pallor of the disc. (From Khanna A, Goldstein DA, Tessler HH: Protozoal posterior uveitis. In Yanoff M, Duker JS [eds]: *Ophthalmology*, London, Mosby, 1999.)

Figure 5-8. Viable and necrotic cysts of *Toxoplasma gondii* in the necrotic retina. (From Khanna A, Goldstein DA, Tessler HH: Protozoal posterior uveitis. In Yanoff M, Duker JS [eds]: *Ophthalmology*, London, Mosby, 1999.)

Pathology: round *Toxoplasma* cysts; chronic granulomatous choroiditis

Diagnosis: ELISA or IFA for *Toxoplasma* IgG or IgM

Treatment:

Indications: decreased vision; moderate to severe vitreous inflammation; lesions that threaten macula, papillomacular bundle, or optic nerve; small peripheral lesions may be observed (heal spontaneously)

Antibiotics: kill tachyzoites in retina during active retinitis, but do not affect cysts

CLINDAMYCIN: 300 mg qid (risk of pseudomembranous colitis)

SULFADIAZINE: 2 g loading, then 1 g qid

PYRIMETHAMINE (Daraprim): 75 mg loading, then 25 mg daily (bone marrow depression; prevent with use of folinic acid [leukovorin; 3–5 mg 2 times/week])

ALTERNATIVE: trimethoprim-sulfamethoxazole (Bactrim)

Steroids: systemic and periocular

Toxocariasis (Table 5-3)

Due to infection with 2nd-stage larval form of dog hookworm *Toxocara canis* (ocular larva migrans)

Acquired by ingestion of contaminated soil

Ocular larva migrans: usually unilateral, solitary lesion; does not complete life cycle (stool examination unnecessary), no other findings

Visceral larva migrans: fever, lymphadenopathy, hepatomegaly, pneumonitis, eosinophilia, no eye involvement

Findings: 3 clinical presentations depending on patient age (endophthalmitis, localized granuloma, or peripheral granuloma); vitreous abscess; dragging of macula temporally due to peripheral lesion results in apparent XT; often presents with leukocoria; traction RD can occur (Figure 5-9)

Other findings: may affect lungs and liver

DDx: as for leukocoria

Figure 5-9. Typical toxocara granuloma located over the optic nerve. In Yanoff M, Duker JS [eds]: *Ophthalmology*, London, Mosby, 1999.)

Diagnosis: AC tap for eosinophils; ELISA for Toxocara antibody titers; no ova/parasites in stool

Treatment: topical steroid and cycloplegic for active uveitis; vitrectomy, may require surgical repair of RD

METABOLIC DISORDERS

(Table 5-4)

RETINAL DISORDERS

Persistent Hyperplastic Primary Vitreous (PHPV)

Unilateral microphthalmia with spectrum of findings from prominent hyaloid vessel remnant with large Mittendorf's dot and Bergmeister's papillae to angle-closure from fibrovascular invasion of lens through posterior lens capsule

Due to incomplete regression of tunica vasculosa lentis and primary vitreous

Sporadic, 90% unilateral

Table 5-3. Clinical Presentations of Toxocariasis

	Chronic Endophthalmitis	Localized Granuloma	Peripheral Granuloma
Age range	2–9 years	6–14 years	6–40 years
Lesion	Exudation filling vitreous cavity, cyclitic membrane	Single localized granuloma in macula or peripapillary region	Peripheral granuloma with dense fibrotic strand, often to disc
Symptoms	Pain, photophobia, lacrimation, decreased vision, acute inflammation	Quite eye, decreased vision, strabismus	Decreased vision, strabismus
Course	Often leads to destruction of globe	Nonprogressive	Nonprogressive

Table 5-4. Metabolic Diseases with Eye Findings

Sphingolipidoses

Disease	Enzyme Deficiency	Inheritance	Findings	Other Findings
GM2 gangliosidoses				Normal at birth, motor deterioration starts at 3–5 months of age, rapid after 10 months of age
Type I (Tay-Sachs disease)	Hexosaminidase A	Autosomal recessive	Cherry red spot, optic atrophy, blindness, nystagmus, ophthalmoplegia	Death by 2–3 years of age
Type II (Sandhoff's disease)	Hexosaminidase B	Autosomal recessive	Cherry red spot, optic atrophy, blindness	Death by 2–12 years of age
Type III (Bernheimer-Seitelberger disease)	Hexosaminidase A (partial)	Autosomal recessive	Optic atrophy, pigmentary retinopathy	Death by 15 years of age
GM1 gangliosidoses				
Type I (Landing disease)	β-Galactosidase A, B, and C	Autosomal recessive	Cherry red spots in 50%, optic atrophy, high myopia, blindness, subtle corneal clouding, nystagmus	Psychomotor delay present at birth with rapid neurologic deterioration and death by 2 years of age
Type II (Derry disease)	β-Galactosidase B and C	Autosomal recessive	RPE degeneration, possible optic atrophy, nystagmus, esotropia	Neurologic deterioration in 1st or 2nd year of life, seizures, death between 3 and 10 years of age

Mucopolysaccharidoses

Disease	Enzyme Deficiency	Inheritance	Findings	Other Findings
MPS type 1-H (Hurler's)	α-Iduronidase	Autosomal recessive	Corneal clouding, RPE degeneration, optic atrophy, glaucoma	Onset between 6 and 24 months of age, gargoyls facies, mental retardation, dwarfism, skeletal dysplasia
MPS type 1-S (Scheie's)				Coarse facial features, claw-like hands, aortic valve disease
MPS type II (Hunter's)	Iduronate sulfatase	X-linked recessive	RPE degeneration, optic atrophy	Similar to 1-H, less skeletal deformity
MPS type III (Sanfilippo's)	4 types: A, B, C, D Heparan N-sulfatase; N-acetyl D-glucosaminidase; acetyl-CoA-glucosaminidase-N,N-acetyltransferase; N-acetylglucosamine-6-sulfate sulfatase	Autosomal recessive	RPE degeneration, optic atrophy	Mild dysmorphism, progressive dementia
MPS type IV (Morquio's)	2 types: A, B galactose-6-sulfatase; β-galactosidase	Autosomal recessive	Corneal clouding, optic atrophy	Short trunk, dwarfism, skeletal deformities, aortic valve disease, normal mental development
MPS type VI (Maroteaux-Lamy)	Arylsulfatase B	Autosomal recessive	Corneal clouding, RPE degeneration, optic atrophy	Normal mental development, similar to 1-H

Table 5-4.—cont'd

Mucopolysaccharidoses

Disease	Enzyme Deficiency	Inheritance	Findings	Other Findings
MPS type VII (Sly's)	β-Glucuronidase	Autosomal recessive	Corneal clouding	Onset after 4 years of age, similar to 1-H
MPS type VIII (Diferrante)	Glucosamine-S-sulfate sulfatase	Autosomal recessive	Clear cornea	

Lipidoses

Disease	Enzyme Deficiency	Inheritance	Findings	Other Findings
Fabry's disease	α-Galactosidase A	X-linked recessive	Whorl-like corneal changes, granular opacities of lens, tortuosity of retinal and conjunctival vessels	Systemic ischemia and infarction (cerebrovascular, cardiac, skin)
Metachromatic leukodystrophy	Arylsulfatase A	Autosomal recessive	Nystagmus, cherry red spot, optic atrophy	Weakness, mental deterioration, developmental delay, may be infantile, juvenile, or adult onset
Krabbe's disease	Galactocerebrosidase	Autosomal recessive	Optic atrophy, blindness	Rapidly progressive and fatal, usually with infantile onset
Gaucher's disease	β-Galactosidase	Autosomal recessive	RPE degeneration, EOM abnormalities	Hepatosplenomegaly, bone complications, neurologic deterioration
Niemann-Pick disease	Sphingomyelinase	Autosomal recessive	Corneal opacities, cherry red spot, lens opacities	Severity of disease varies depending on type, loss of motor and cognitive skills, splenomegaly

Others

Disease	Enzyme Deficiency	Inheritance	Findings	Other Findings
Cystinosis	Defective transport of cystine	Autosomal recessive	Corneal crystals, secondary photophobia and blepharospasm, RPE degeneration	Infantile and late-onset forms; renal failure (Fanconi's syndrome), CNS damage
Galactosemia	Gal-1-UDP transferase	Autosomal recessive	Cataract (oil-drop)	Failure to thrive, hepatomegaly and liver dysfunction, developmental delay
Mannosidosis	α-Mannosidase	Autosomal recessive	Corneal clouding, lens opacification	Coarse features, hepatosplenomegaly, mental deterioration, hearing loss
Mucolipidoses II and III	Multiple lysosomal enzymes	Autosomal recessive	Corneal clouding	Coarse features, psychomotor retardation, organomegaly, cardiorespiratory problems
Refsum's disease	Phytanic acid oxidase	Autosomal recessive	Retinal degeneration, optic disc pallor, cataracts	Peripheral neuropathy, cerebellar ataxia, elevated CSF protein
Adrenoleuko-dystrophy	Peroxisomal disorder	X-linked, autosomal recessive	Optic atrophy, RPE degeneration, strabismus	CNS demyelination, adrenal insufficiency, high long-chain fatty acid levels
Homocystinuria	Cystathionine synthase	Autosomal recessive	Dislocated lenses, optic atrophy, glaucoma	Osteoporosis, thromboembolic disease, seizures

Findings: microphthalmia, vascularized retrolental plaque (may contain cartilage), elongated ciliary processes, prominent radial vessels on iris surface, shallow AC, iris vascularization; may have cataract, angle-closure glaucoma, vitreous hemorrhage, retinal detachment

DDx of intraocular cartilage: PHPV, medulloepithelioma, teratoma, trisomy 13

Treatment: observation, lensectomy with or without vitrectomy

Prognosis: depends on degree of amblyopia; visual prognosis variable after surgery, often depends on status of posterior segment

Coloboma

Yellow-white lesion with pigmented margins due to incomplete closure of embryonic fissure

Usually inferonasal

Retina is reduced to glial tissue; no RPE; may have colobomas of other ocular structures

Retinopathy of Prematurity (ROP, Retrolental Fibroplasia)

Vasoproliferative retinopathy occurring almost exclusively in premature infants; occasionally in full-term infants

Risk factors: low birth weight (<1.5 kg; if <1.25 kg, 65% develop some degree of ROP), early gestational age (<33 weeks), supplemental oxygen (>50 days; controversial), coexisting illness

Risk increases exponentially the more premature and the smaller the infant: <2000 g (4 pounds, 7 ounces), earlier than 36 weeks (at 36 weeks, nasal retina completely vascularized; at 40 weeks, temporal retina fully vascularized)

2 phases:
   Acute: abnormal vessels develop in association with fibrous proliferation; >85% to 90% spontaneously regress
   Chronic: retinal detachment, temporal displacement of macula, severe vision loss; occurs in 15%

Classification: (International Classification of ROP [ICROP])
   Zone:
   1. Posterior pole, area enclosed by 60° diameter circle centered on optic nerve
   2. Area between edge of zone 1 and circle centered on optic disc and tangent to nasal ora serrata
   3. Remaining crescent of temporal peripheral retina anterior to zone 2

Extent: measured in clock hours of involvement
Stage:
1. Demarcation line between vascular and avascular retina (flat, white)
2. Ridge (elevated, pink/white)
3. Ridge with tufts of extraretinal blood vessels (popcorn)
4. Subtotal retinal detachment
   A. Extrafoveal
   B. Including fovea
5. Total RD with funnel (open or closed)

Figure 5-10. Stage 1 retinopathy of prematurity. The flat, white border between the avascular and vascular retina seen superiorly is called a demarcation line. (Reproduced from Earl A. Palmer, MD, and the Multicenter Trial of Cryotherapy for Retinopathy of Prematurity. From Yanoff M, Duker JS [eds]: *Ophthalmology*, London, Mosby, 1999.)

Figure 5-11. Stage 2 retinopathy of prematurity. The elevated mesenchymal ridge has height. Highly arborized blood vessels from the vascularized retina dive into the ridge. (Reproduced from Earl A. Palmer, MD, and the Multicenter Trial of Cryotherapy for Retinopathy of Prematurity. From Yanoff M, Duker JS [eds]: *Ophthalmology*, London, Mosby, 1999.)

Figure 5-12. Stage 3 retinopathy of prematurity. Vessels on top of the ridge project into the vitreous cavity. The extraretinal proliferation carries with it a fibrovascular membrane. Note the opalescent avascular retina anterior to the ridge. (From Sears J, Capone A; Retinopathy of primaturity. In Yanoff M, Duker JS [eds]: *Ophthalmology*, London, Mosby, 1999.)

Figure 5-13. Stage 3 retinopathy of prematurity. Note finger-like projections of extraretinal vessels into the vitreous cavity. Hemorrhage on the ridge is not uncommon. (From Sears J, Capone A: Retinopathy of prematurity. In Yanoff M, Duker JS [eds]: *Ophthalmology*, London, Mosby, 1999.)

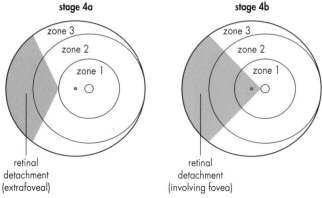

Figure 5-14. Stage 4a detachment spares the fovea. Stage 4b detachment involves the fovea. (From Sears J, Capone A: Retinopathy of prematurity. In Yanoff M, Duker JS [eds]: *Ophthalmology*, London, Mosby, 1999.)

Plus disease: engorged, tortuous vessels around disc, vitreous haze, and iris vascular congestion; progressive vascular incompetence throughout eye; poor prognostic sign

Threshold disease (level at which 50% go blind without treatment) = stage 3 in zone 1 or 2 with Plus disease and at least 5 contiguous or 8 cumulative clock hours of involvement; usually develops at 27 weeks postgestation

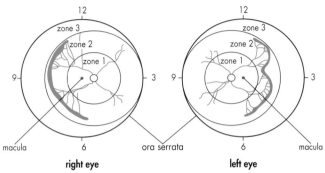

Figure 5-15. Definition of "threshold" retinopathy of prematurity. (From Sears J, Capone A: Retinopathy of prematurity. In Yanoff M, Duker JS [eds]: *Ophthalmology*, London, Mosby, 1999.)

Rush disease: plus disease in zone 1 or posterior zone 2; rapidly progressive

Prethreshold:
1. Zone 1, any stage
2. Zone 2, stage 2+ or 3
3. Zone 2, stage 3+ for >5 clock hours

DDx of peripheral vascular changes and retinal dragging: FEVR, incontinentia pigmenti (Bloch-Sulzberger syndrome), X-linked retinoschisis

DDx of temporally dragged disc: FEVR, *Toxocara*, congenital falciform fold

Diagnosis: screen infants <1250 g, on supplemental oxygen during first 7 days of life, or <27 weeks gestation

Treatment: observation, laser, cryo, surgery
   Cryotherapy for ROP Study (Cryo-ROP): determined whether treatment for ROP would prevent poor outcomes (see below)
   Treat with ablation of peripheral avascular retina: when patient reaches type 1 ROP, defined as:
   Zone 1, any stage with Plus disease
   Zone 1, stage 3
   Zone 2, stage 2 or 3 with Plus disease
   (Early Treatment of ROP Study [ETROP])
   Indirect argon green or diode laser photocoagulation: 500 μm spots to entire avascular retina in zone 1 and peripheral zone 2 (at least as effective as cryotherapy; Laser-ROP study)

Cryotherapy: to entire avascular retina in zone 2, but not ridge (cryo-ROP study)

Serial Exams: with type 2 ROP, defined as:
Zone 1, stage 1 or 2
Zone 2, stage 3

Surgery: vitrectomy with or without lensectomy, membrane peel, and possible scleral buckle for TRD or RRD (cicatricial ROP, stages 4 and 5)

Prognosis: depends on extent of disease; most cases resolve spontaneously without visible residua

Some develop cicatricial changes (retrolental fibroplasia):

GRADE I: myopia and peripheral glial scar (VA >20/40)

GRADE II: dragged retina, macular heterotopia (VA 20/50–20/200)

GRADE III: retinal fold (VA <20/200)

GRADE IV: partial retrolental membrane and RD (VA = HM or LP)

GRADE V: complete retrolental membrane and RD (VA = LP or NLP)

Complications:

Grade I–II: myopia (80%; due to forward displacement of lens-iris diaphragm), anisometropia, strabismus, amblyopia, macular heterotopia, pseudo-XT (change in angle κ due to macular dragging from peripheral cicatrization), increased risk of retinal tear or RD

Grade III–V: nystagmus, glaucoma, cataracts, heterochromia irides, rubeosis iridis, anterior uveitis, RD, band keratopathy, phthisis bulbi

MAJOR CLINICAL STUDY

Cryotherapy for ROP Study (Cryo-ROP)

Objective: to evaluate whether cryotherapy for ROP in preterm infants with birth weights <1251 g prevents unfavorable outcomes (posterior retinal fold, stage 4B or 5 retinal detachment, or visual acuity of 20/200 or worse)

Results:
The more posterior the zone and the greater the extent of stage 3+ ROP, the poorer the outcome

All unfavorable fundus structural outcomes and almost all unfavorable visual acuity outcomes occurred in eyes with zone 1 or 2 ROP and >6 sectors of stage 3+ disease

Fewer unfavorable outcomes occurred in treated vs control eyes (44.4% vs 62.1% for visual acuity; 27.2% vs 47.9% for fundus status)

Retinal detachments remained stable in treated eyes (22%) but continued to occur in control eyes (from 38.6% at 5.5 years to 41.4% at 10 years)

After 10 years, treated eyes were much less likely than control eyes to be blind

Conclusions:
Cryotherapy preserves visual acuity in eyes with threshold disease

Initial examination: 4–6 weeks after birth or at 30 weeks' gestational age (whichever is later), then every 2 weeks until vessels reach zone 3

Prethreshold disease: examine every week until regression or threshold disease develops

Threshold disease: perform cryotherapy within 72 hours of diagnosis

Laser photocoagulation or cryotherapy to avascular retina, 90% regression rate

After 1 week, plus disease is usually less if treatment will work, fibrovascular proliferation often takes 2 weeks to begin regressing; consider retreatment if ROP is worse after 1 week; retreat untreated areas

Stage 4 disease: 60% reattachment rate with scleral buckle; 5% obtain useful vision

Stage 5 disease: vitrectomy (very poor success rate)

Familial Exudative Vitreoretinopathy (FEVR) (AD or X-Linked Recessive)

Mapped to chromosome 11q13-q23 (EVR1), 11p13-p12 (EVR3)

Most are unaware that they have this disorder

Rare, progressive developmental abnormality of peripheral retinal vasculature (especially temporally)

Findings: similar to ROP (Figures 5-16 and 5-17)

Stage 1: avascular peripheral retina, white without pressure, vitreous bands, peripheral cystoid degeneration, microaneurysms, telangiectasia, straightened vessels, vascular engorgement; may have strabismus or nystagmus; most asymptomatic; may progress to stage 2

Stage 2: fibrovascular proliferation with neovascularization, exudates, dragging of disc and macula, retinal folds and detachments; visual loss after 2nd–3rd decade of life rare unless progress to stage 3

Figure 5-16. Fundus view of a patient who has familial exudative vitreoretinopathy. Note abnormally straightened retinal vasculature. (From Kimura AJ: Hereditary vitreoretinopathies. In Yanoff M, Duker JS [eds]: *Ophthalmology*, London, Mosby, 1999.)

Figure 5-17. Fluorescein angiogram of a patient who has familial exudative vitreoretinopathy. (From Kimura AJ: Hereditary vitreoretinopathies. In Yanoff M, Duker JS [eds]: *Ophthalmology*, London, Mosby, 1999.)

Stage 3: cicatrization with rhegmatogenous retinal detachments (10% to 20%; usually in 3rd–4th decade of life), may develop proliferative vitreoretinopathy; prognosis poor

Treatment: prophylactic laser treatment to avascular retina (controversial); may require RD repair

Coats' Disease
(Leber's Miliary Aneurysms)

Nonhereditary, proliferative exudative vascular disease

More common in males (10 : 1); bimodal distribution (peak in 1st decade and small peak in young adulthood [associated with hypercholesterolemia])

90% unilateral; 50% progressive

Findings: usually presents with leukocoria and strabismus; telangiectatic blood vessels leak (with large amount of subretinal lipid in outer plexiform layer), noncalcified yellow subretinal lesions, exudative RD in 66% (especially in patients <4 years old), microaneurysms, capillary nonperfusion

Pathology: triad of retinal vascular anomalies, subretinal and intraretinal cholesterol deposits, intraretinal PAS-positive deposits; loss of vascular endothelium and pericytes; gliotic retina over subretinal fluid with cholesterol clefts and hemosiderin-laden macrophages. Aspiration of subretinal exudates reveals cholesterol and pigment-laden macrophages

DDx: retinoblastoma, angiomatosis retinae (von Hippel–Lindau syndrome), PHPV

B-scan ultrasound: consider to rule out retinoblastoma

FA: blood-fluid levels; saccular aneurysms ("light bulb" dilatations) of retinal arterioles and venules (Figure 5-18)

Treatment: cryo or laser to stop leaking blood vessels

Norrie's Disease (X-Linked Recessive)

Defect of retinal development

Findings: bilateral leukocoria (white, often hemorrhagic retrolental mass), retinal dysplasia, peripheral NV, hemorrhagic RD, and retinal necrosis

Other findings: deafness, mental retardation

Shaken Baby Syndrome

30% to 40% of children subjected to child abuse will have ophthalmic sequelae

Most common in children <3 years old

Findings: diffuse retinal hemorrhages, papilledema, vitreous hemorrhage, retinal tissue disruption (retinoschisis, retinal breaks, folds); may resemble CRVO, Terson's syndrome, or Purtscher's retinopathy

Associated with other injuries: subdural hematoma, subarachnoid hemorrhage, bruises, fractures of long bones or ribs

Prognosis: poor due to macular scarring, vitreous hemorrhage, RD

A   B

Figure 5-18. A, The classic fundus picture of Coats' disease with massive lipid exudation that causes an exudative retinal detachment. **B**, Fluorescein angiogram from the same patient with large telangiectatic vessels and numerous leaking aneurysms. (From Mittra RA, Mieler WF, Pollack JS: Retinal arterial macroaneurysms. In Yanoff M, Duker JS [eds]: *Ophthalmology*, London, Mosby, 1999.)

Inherited Retinal Diseases

Fundus Flavimaculatus (AR)

Mapped to chromosome 1p21-p13 (ABCA4)

Findings: bilateral pisciform, yellow-white flecks at level of RPE

Predominantly involves peripheral retina with macula involved to a lesser degree; flecks, then macular degeneration

Central vision preserved until macula involved

Pathology: lipofuscin deposits within hypertrophied RPE cells

ERG: degree of abnormality correlates with amount of fundus involvement

Stargardt's Disease

Autosomal recessive or less often dominant; mapped to chromosome 1p21-p22 (STGD1), 4p (STGD4), 6q14 (STGD3)

Juvenile macular degeneration with flecks

Most common hereditary macular dystrophy

Onset in first 2 decades of life with decreased vision

Symptoms: decreased vision, nyctalopia

Findings: bilateral pisciform, yellow-white flecks at level of RPE; change with time (new ones appear, others disappear); beaten-metal appearance of fundus; foveal atrophy; bull's-eye maculopathy; may have salt and pepper pigmentary changes of peripheral retina

Pathology: RPE massively thickened by accumulation of lipofuscin

FA: dark choroid (85%) due to accumulation of lipofuscin in RPE; areas of hyperfluorescence do not directly correspond to flecks; pigmentary changes in macula appear as window defects

pisciform flecks   "bull's-eye" maculopathy

Figure 5-19. Stargardt's disease. (From Kaiser PK, Friedman NJ, Pineda II, R: *Massachusetts Eye and Ear Infirmary Illustrated Manual of Ophthalmology*, 2nd ed, Philadelphia, WB Saunders, 2004.)

"silent" choroid   pisciform flecks

Figure 5-20. Fluorescein angiogram of Stargardt's disease demonstrating dark choroid and hyperfluorescent pisciform flecks. (From Kaiser PK, Friedman NJ, Pineda II, R: *Massachusetts Eye and Ear Infirmary Illustrated Manual of Ophthalmology*, 2nd ed, Philadelphia, WB Saunders, 2004.)

ERG and EOG: normal or subnormal

Prognosis: 50% have at least 20/40 vision in one eye by age 19; only 22% have 20/40 vision by age 39; rapid progression to 20/200 – CF

Best's Disease (Vitelliform Dystrophy) (AD)

Variable penetrance; mapped to chromosome 11q13 (VMD2 [bestrophin])

Second most common hereditary macular dystrophy

Progressive with onset in 1st decade of life

Macular dystrophy in which RPE is primarily affected; form of exudative central macular detachment in which pigmentation can occur in end stages with atrophic scarring and/or CNV

Associated with strabismus and hyperopia

Symptoms: none or mild decreased vision initially; later decreases to 20/50–20/100; better vision than expected by clinical appearance

Findings: progressive macular changes; can get CNV
   Previtelliform stage: small round submacular yellow dot
   Vitelliform stage: yellow-orange egg yolk/fried egg appearance; can be multiple; usually between ages 3 and 15 (Figure 5-21)
   Scrambled egg stage: irregular subretinal spots; vision usually still good
   Cyst stage
   Pseudohypopyon stage: RPE atrophy
   Round chorioretinal atrophy stage: atrophic scar; vision usually stabilizes at 20/100

DDx: central serous chorioretinopathy, RPED, toxoplasmosis, macular coloboma, solar retinopathy, old foveal hemorrhage, adult vitelliform macular dystrophy, syphilis

FA: blockage by egg yolk lesion; window defect when cyst ruptures

Figure 5-21. Best's disease. Vitelliform stage. (Courtesy of Ola Sandgren, University Hospital of Umea, Sweden. From Parnell JR, Small KW: Macular dystropies. In Yanoff M, Duker JS [eds]: *Ophthalmology*, London, Mosby, 1999.)

Figure 5-22. North Carolina macular dystrophy. (From Parnell JR, Small KW: Macular dystrophies. In Yanoff M, Duker JS [eds]: *Ophthalmology*, London, Mosby, 1999.)

ERG: normal

EOG: abnormal (Arden ratio <1.6; also in carriers)

Dark adaptation: normal

Prognosis: good vision (20/30–20/100 range)

Familial Drusen (Doyne's Honeycomb Dystrophy) (AD)

Mapped to chromosome 2p16-p21 (EFEMP1)

Small yellow-white, round to oval deposits on Bruch's membrane; decreased vision after age 40

Complications: macular edema, hemorrhage, CNV

North Carolina Macular Dystrophy (AD)

Mapped to chromosome 6q14-q16 (MCDR1)

Onset in 1st decade with drusen progressing to chorioretinal atrophy with staphyloma of macula (Figure 5-22)

May develop CNV

ERG, EOG, and dark adaptation: normal

Pseudoinflammatory Macular Dystrophy (Sorsby's) (AD)

Mapped to chromosome 22q12-q13 (SFD [TIMP-3])

Atrophy, edema, hemorrhage, and exudate

Decreased acuity and color vision occurs between ages 40 and 50

ERG and EOG: subnormal late

Dark adaptation: delayed

Pattern Dystrophies (Usually AD)

Group of diseases with central pigmentary disturbance, good central vision, normal ERG, abnormal EOG

May develop CNV

Sjögren's reticular: fishnet configuration; fishnet is hypofluorescent on FA

Butterfly: gray-yellow butterfly lesion with surrounding depigmentation; onset between ages 20 and 50 with slightly reduced vision; mapped to chromosome 6p21 (RDS [peripherin])

Adult vitelliform: onset between ages 30 and 50; early ring-like area of RPE clumping that develops into symmetric, solitary yellow macula lesions (like Best's egg yolk lesions but smaller [1/2 DD in central fovea] and do not break up); often have central area of pigment; CNV is more common than in Best's disease; normal EOG

Progressive Cone Dystrophy

Autosomal dominant or less often X-linked; mapped to chromosome 6p21 (COD3), Xp21 (COD1) [RPGR]), Xq27 (COD2)

Progressive dysfunction of cones with normal rod function

Onset during first 3 decades of life with decreased vision, dyschromatopsia, photophobia

Symptoms: visual loss, photophobia (usually precede visible macular changes)

Findings: decreased vision (to 20/200), decreased color vision, central scotoma, nystagmus (25%), NFL loss, optic atrophy, macular degeneration (granular appearance early, then beaten-metal appearance); can have fine, golden subretinal deposits, bull's-eye maculopathy; can develop a pattern that mimics Stargardt's or fundus flavimaculatus (Figure 5-24)

VF: normal

FA: may show window defects early

ERG: absent photopic, normal scotopic

EOG: normal

Dark adaptation: rod phase only

Prognosis: poor vision (20/200 level) by 4th decade of life

Figure 5-24. The "bull's-eye" maculopathy in this 5-year-old male who has a cone-rod dystrophy is not found in all cases of this entity. (From Sieving PA: Retinis pigmentosa and related disorders. In Yanoff M, Duker JS [eds]: *Ophthalmology*, London, Mosby, 1999.)

Figure 5-23. Visual function test. (From Sieving PA: Retinis pigmentosa and related disorders. In Yanoff M, Duker JS [eds]: *Ophthalmology*, London, Mosby, 1999.)

Stationary Cone Disorders

Present at birth; nonprogressive

Complete rod monochromatism (congenital achromatopsia) (AR): mapped to chromosome 14 (ACHM1); absent or abnormal cones; nonprogressive
  Findings: severely reduced vision (20/200 level), complete color blindness, photophobia, nystagmus, normal retinal examination
  VF: central scotoma
  ERG: normal scotopic, abnormal photopic

Blue cone monochromatism (X-linked recessive):

Have only blue-sensitive cones
  Findings: decreased vision (20/40–20/200), photoaversion, nystagmus
  ERG: absent cone response, normal rod response

Tapetoretinal Degeneration

Processes that involve the outer half of the retina (photoreceptor/RPE); RPE = tapetum nigran (black carpet)

Retinitis Pigmentosa (RP)

Group of progressive dystrophies caused by abnormal photoreceptor protein production

Most common hereditary degeneration, incidence 1 : 5000

RP type I (rod-cone):
  Inheritance patterns:
    AR (37%): most common form; may be due to defects in 2 RPE genes (which provide instructions for vitamin A transport proteins): RPE 65, CRALBP
    X-LINKED RECESSIVE (4%): rarest and most severe form; poor prognosis; vision <20/100 by 3rd decade of life; carriers may have fundus changes
    AD (20%): least severe form, later onset; most likely to retain good vision
    SPORADIC (30% to 50%)
  Associations: keratoconus, macular cystoid degeneration, Coats' disease, optic disc drusen, astrocytic hamartoma of ON, myopia
  Symptoms: nyctalopia, "blue blindness," decreased vision late

Findings: pigmentary retinal changes (bone spicules), attenuated arteries, waxy pallor of optic nerve (due to glial membrane formation over disc), retinal atrophy with increased visibility of choroidal vessels, vitreous cells, cataract; some forms can have prominent subretinal exudation (Coats'-like disease) (Figure 5-25)

Pathology: photoreceptor atrophy including outer nuclear layer; inner retina well preserved; RPE cells invade retina and surround retinal vessels (bone spicules)

VF: inferotemporal scotoma, enlarges to form ring/annular scotoma; constricted

ERG: early, increased rod threshold with normal cone response and decreased scotopic b-wave; late, nonrecordable; abnormalities precede retinal changes and visual complaints

EOG: abnormal

Dark adaptation: prolonged

RP carriers:

  FUNDUS: bone spicules, salt and pepper changes, bronze sheen in macula

  ERG: decreased scotopic amplitude and delayed cone B-wave implicit time in X-linked carriers

  VITREOUS FLUOROPHOTOMETRY: abnormal in X-linked carriers

DDx of tunnel vision: glaucoma, functional, gyrate atrophy, vitamin A toxicity, occipital lobe stroke

DDx of nyctalopia: uncorrected myopia, vitamin A deficiency, zinc deficiency, choroideremia, gyrate atrophy, CSNB, Goldman-Favre disease

DDx of salt and pepper fundus: rubella retinopathy, Leber's congenital amaurosis, carrier states (albinism, RP, choroideremia), syphilis, cystinosis, phenothiazine toxicity, pattern dystrophy, following resolution of an exudative RD

Macular complications: CME (no leakage on FA), epiretinal membrane, atrophy

RP type II (cone-rod): AD, AR, or X-linked

  Findings: less pigment deposition; 50% are sine pigmento

  ERG: cones more affected than rods

Treatment: low vision aids, dark glasses; vitamin A slows reduction of ERG (controversial)

Prognosis: poor

RP Variants

Treatable RP: Bassen-Kornzweig (abetalipoproteinemia), Refsum's (elevated phytanic acid), gyrate atrophy (elevated ornithine)

Leber's congenital amaurosis (AR): mapped to chromosome 1p31 (LCA2), 14q11 (RPGRIP1), 17p13 (LCA1,LCA4), 19q13 (CRX)

  Infantile form of RP; blind or severe visual impairment in infancy or early childhood

Figure 5-25. "Typical" retinitis pigmentosa changes. (From Sieving PA: Retinis pigmentosa and related disorders. In Yanoff M, Duker JS [eds]: *Ophthalmology*, London, Mosby, 1999.)

Responsible for approximately 10% of blindness

Associations: keratoconus, hyperopia, cataract, macular coloboma, mental retardation, deafness, seizures, renal and musculoskeletal abnormalities

Findings: decreased vision (HM-CF), nystagmus, hyperopia, poorly reactive pupils, range of fundus appearance from normal (most common) to variety of pigmentary changes (granular, fleck, salt and pepper, sheen, or atrophic)

  OCULODIGITAL SIGN: child rubs eyes to elicit entopic stimulation of retina

Pathology: diffuse absence of photoreceptors

ERG: low or completely flat

Sector RP (AD or AR): retinal changes limited to focal area, usually inferonasal quadrant

  VF: abnormal

  ERG: abnormal; normal b-wave implicit time reflects nonprogression

  Prognosis: good

Unilateral RP: very rare

Inverse RP: posterior pole affected (rather than midperiphery): bone spicules in macula, normal periphery

  FA: dark choroid (probably variant of Stargardt's)

Retinitis punctata albescens (AR): small white spots in midperiphery of retina, no bone spicules

RP sine pigmento: no retinal pigmentary changes

Pseudoretinitis pigmentosa: migration of RPE melanin into sensory retina leading to bone spicule pattern

  Etiology: trauma, drug toxicity (chloroquine, chlorpromazine), infection/inflammation (syphilis, toxoplasmosis, measles, rubella), post-CVO, resolved exudative RD, ophthalmic artery occlusion

RP Syndromes

Usher's syndrome (AR): most common syndrome associated with RP; mapped to chromosome 1q41 (USH2A)

>*Findings*: RP and deafness; ataxia, MR, low phosphate (rickets), muscle wasting
>
>10% to 20% of RP patients are deaf; 5% of congenitally deaf individuals have Usher's type I
>
>>TYPE 1: night blindness (1st–2nd decade), profound deafness, unintelligible speech, ataxia
>>
>>TYPE 2: night blindness (2nd–4th decade), partial deafness, intelligible speech, no ataxia
>
>*DDx of deafness and RP*: Usher's, Hallgrenn's, Alstrom's, Laurence-Moon-Biedl-Bardet, and Cockayne's syndromes
>
>*Other eye syndromes associated with hearing loss*: Cogan's (IK + hearing loss), Stickler's (vitreous changes, joint and orofacial abnormalities, hearing loss), Waardenburg-Klein (iris heterochromia, white forelock), Duane's (15% have hearing loss)

Refsum's disease (AR): deficiency of phytanic acid oxidase interferes with fatty acid metabolism

>Phytanic acid accumulates in RPE cells, sensory retina deteriorates; onset in childhood
>
>Mapped to chromosome 7q21-q22 (PEX1), 10p15-p12 (PNYH)
>
>*Findings*: atypical RP (often sine pigmento or starts in macula), cataracts, prominent corneal nerves
>
>*Other findings*: ataxia, peripheral neuropathy, deafness, anosmia, ichthyosis, cardiac abnormalities, hypotonia, hepatomegaly, mental retardation
>
>*Diagnosis*: increased serum copper and ceruloplasmin; increased CSF protein without pleocytosis
>
>*Treatment*: dietary restriction of animal fats, milk products, leafy green vegetables

Bassen-Kornzweig syndrome (AR): hereditary abetalipoproteinemia; mapped to chromosome 4q24 (MTP)

>Inability to transport and absorb lipids because apolipoprotein B is a major protein of chylomicrons; deficiency in fat-soluble vitamins (A, D, E, and K)
>
>*Findings*: RP (usually without bone spicules); may have Bitot's spots on conjuctiva
>
>*Other findings*: ataxic neuropathy, growth retardation, coagulopathy
>
>*Diagnosis*: CBC, cholesterol (low), stool sample; elevated CSF protein; no apolipoprotein B-48 (low chylomicrons) or apolipoprotein B-100 (low LDL and VLDL)
>
>*Treatment*: vitamin A and E supplements
>
>*Other causes of treatable RP due to vitamin A deficiency*: chronic pancreatitis, cirrhosis, bowel resection

Lawrence-Moon-Biedl-Bardet syndrome (AR): mapped to chromosome 2q31 (BBS5), 3p13-p12 (BBS3), 11q13 (BBS1), 15q22-q23(BBS4), 6q21 (BBS2), 20p12 (BBS6)

>*L-M and B-B*: pigmentary retinopathy with flat ERG, mental retardation, hypogonadism, short stature
>
>*B-B*: polydactyly and obesity
>
>*L-M*: spastic paraplegia

Figure 5-26. Bardet-Biedl syndrome with extensive peripheral retinal pigment epithelium and parafoveal retinal pigment epithelium atrophy. (From Sieving PA: Retinis pigmentosa and related disorders. In Yanoff M, Duker JS [eds]: *Ophthalmology*, London, Mosby, 1999.)

Spielmeyer-Vogt-Batten-Mayou syndrome: neuronal ceroid lipofuscinosis

Onset between 2 and 4 years of age in Jewish females

>*Findings*: RP-like retinal degeneration with bull's-eye maculopathy
>
>*Other findings*: seizures, progressive dementia, ataxia
>
>*Pathology*: vacuolization of peripheral lymphocytes; metachromasia of skin fibroblasts in cell culture (carriers only)

Chronic progressive external ophthalmoplegia (CPEO): mitochondrial inheritance; 50% with positive family history

>*Findings*: retinal degeneration (salt and pepper changes with normal retinal function; progresses to RP-like disease), ptosis, ophthalmoplegia, strabismus
>
>*Other findings*: facial weakness, dysphagia, small stature, limb girdle myopathy, cardiac conduction defects (Kearn-Sayre syndrome)

Olivopontocerebellar atrophy: retinal degeneration; tremors, ataxia, dysarthria

Alstrom's disease: mapped to chromosome 2p13 (ALMS1)

RP with profound visual loss in 1st decade of life; diabetes, obesity, deafness, renal failure, baldness, acanthosis nigricans, hypogenitalism

Cockayne's syndrome: RP with profound visual loss by 2nd decade of life; dwarfism, deafness, mental retardation, premature aging, psychosis, intracranial calcifications

Neuronal ceroid lipofuscinosis (Batten's disease): juvenile or adult onset of seizures, dementia, ataxia, mental retardation

Central Areolar Choroidal Dystrophy (AD)

Mapped to chromosome 6p (RDS [peripherin]), 17p13 (CACD)

Decreased vision in 4th decade

Findings: RPE mottling in macula progressing to geographic atrophy (choroidal vessels visible)

central areolar choroidal dystrophy

Figure 5-27. Central geographic atrophy in a patient with central areolar choroidal dystrophy. (From Kaiser PK, Friedman NJ, Pineda II, R: *Massachusetts Eye and Ear Infirmary Illustrated Manual of Ophthalmology*, 2nd ed, Philadelphia, WB Saunders, 2004.)

central areolar choroidal dystrophy

Figure 5-28. Left eye of same patient as shown in Figure 5-27 demonstrating similar central geographic atrophy. (From Kaiser PK, Friedman NJ, Pineda II, R: *Massachusetts Eye and Ear Infirmary Illustrated Manual of Ophthalmology*, 2nd ed, Philadelphia, WB Saunders, 2004.)

FA: window defect of central lesion

ERG: normal or subnormal

EOG, dark adaptation: normal

Bietti's Crystalline Retinopathy (AR)

Decreased vision in 5th decade

Findings: yellow-white refractile spots throughout fundus, geographic atrophy; may have crystals in peripheral corneal stroma

Bietti's crystalline retinopathy

Figure 5-29. Bietti's crystalline retinopathy. (From Kaiser PK, Friedman NJ, Pineda II, R: *Massachusetts Eye and Ear Infirmary Illustrated Manual of Ophthalmology*, 2nd ed, Philadelphia, WB Saunders, 2004.)

FA: crystals hyperfluoresce, window defects and areas of blockage

ERG: reduced

Congenital Stationary Night Blindness (CSNB)

Poor night vision (nyctalopia)

Group of nonprogressive rod disorders classified by fundus appearance

Findings: normal vision, VF, and color vision; may show paradoxical pupillary dilation to light; no Purkinje shift (always most sensitive to 550 nm)

ERG: scotopic and photopic implicit times are identical; decreased scotopic ERG; photopic ERG almost normal

Normal fundus:
 Nougaret type (AD): no rod function; mapped to chromosome 3p21 (GNAT1)
 Riggs type (AR): some rod function

Schubert-Bornschein type (X-linked or AR): some or no rod function, myopia

Abnormal fundus:

Fundus albipunctatus (AR): mapped to chromosome 12q13-q14

FINDINGS: midperipheral deep yellow-white spots spare macula

ERG: normalization of scotopic after 4–8 hours of dark adaptation

ALPORT'S SYNDROME (AD): kidney failure, deafness, anterior lenticonus with anterior polar cataract; may have retinal appearance similar to fundus albipunctatus

A

B

Figure 5-31. Oguchi's disease. **A**, The yellowish metallic sheen is apparent nasal to the optic disc. **B**, After 3 hours of dark. (From Noble KG: Congenital stationary night blindness. In Yanoff M, Duker JS [eds]: *Ophthalmology*, London, Mosby, 1999.)

Figure 5-30. Fundus albipunctatus. This posterior pole and beyond show multiple small, discrete, round, white dots that spare the fovea. (From Noble KG: Congenital stationary night blindness. In Yanoff M, Duker JS [eds]: *Ophthalmology*, London, Mosby, 1999.)

Oguchi's disease: mapped to chromosome 2q37 (Oguchi 1, Arrestin, SAG), 13q34 (Oguchi 2 [RHOK])

MIZUO-NAKAMURA PHENOMENON: golden-brown fundus (yellow/gray sheen) in light-adapted state, normal-colored fundus in dark-adapted state (takes about 12 hours) (Figure 5-31)

ERG: absent b-wave; only scotopic a-wave

Kandori's flecked retina (AR): yellow-white spots scattered in equatorial region; spares macula

Choroideremia (X-Linked Recessive)

Mapped to Xq21

Progressive disorder of choriocapillaris; considered a form of rod cone degeneration

Onset during late childhood with nyctalopia, photophobia, constricted visual fields in affected males

Findings: early—degeneration of RPE and choriocapillaris in periphery (scalloped RPE atrophy); late—absence of RPE and choriocapillaris except in macula (Figure 5-32)

Female carriers have salt and pepper fundus

Pathology: defect in choroidal vasculature

ERG: markedly reduced; undetectable late

Gyrate Atrophy (AR)

Mapped to chromosome 10q26

Deficiency of ornithine aminotransferase; elevated ornithine levels (10–20× normal), low lysine levels; chorioretinal dystrophy itself is not due to high ornithine levels

Progressive retinal degeneration; starts peripherally and spreads toward posterior pole

Onset by 2nd decade of life with decreased vision, nyctalopia, and constricted visual fields

Figure 5-32. Fundus changes in the right eye from a patient with late-stage choroideremia. (From Grover S, Fishman GA: Choroidal dystrophies. In Yanoff M, Duker JS [eds]: *Ophthalmology*, London, Mosby, 1999.)

gyrate atrophy

Figure 5-33. Gyrate atrophy. (From Kaiser PK, Friedman NJ, Pineda II, R: *Massachusetts Eye and Ear Infirmary Illustrated Manual of Ophthalmology*, 2nd ed, Philadelphia, WB Saunders, 2004.)

Findings: scalloped areas of absent choriocapillaris and RPE in periphery with abrupt transition between normal and atrophic areas; eventually lose choriocapillaris and medium-sized choroidal vessels; myopia (90%), cataracts, vitreous degeneration, CME (Figure 5-33)

Other findings: seizures, structural changes in muscle and hair fibers

Diagnosis: blood tests (increased ornithine, decreased lysine), urinalysis (increased ornithine)
   Carrier: decreased levels of ornithine ketoacid transaminase

ERG and EOG: abnormal

Dark adaptation: prolonged

Treatment: restrict arginine and protein in diet; consider vitamin B_6 supplementation (pyridoxine; reduces ornithine)

Metabolic Diseases

Mucopolysaccharidoses (AR Except Hunter's [AD])

Accumulation of acid mucopolysaccharides due to lysosomal enzyme defects

Syndromes in which heparin sulfate accumulates are associated with pigmentary retinopathy

Findings: may have corneal clouding and/or pigmentary retinal changes
   Corneal clouding and retinopathy: Hurler's (type Ia), Scheie (type Ib)
   Retinopathy only: Hunter's (type II), Sanfilippo (type IV)
   Corneal changes only: Morquio (type V), Maroteaux-Lamy (type VI)
   No corneal clouding or retinopathy: Sly (type VII)

Sphingolipidoses (AR)

Accumulation of sphingolipids due to lysosomal enzyme defects

Sphingolipids accumulate in retinal ganglion cells; result in cherry red spot (macula has highest concentration of ganglion cells)

Cherry red spot: Tay-Sachs, Sandhoff's, Neimann-Pick, and Gaucher's disease
   Tay-Sachs: most common; hexosaminodase A deficiency; death by 3 years of age; cherry red spot and mental retardation
   Sandhoff's: similar to Tay-Sachs; extensive visceral involvement
   Niemann-Pick: cherry red spot, macular halo, optic atrophy; hepatosplenomegaly, infiltration of lungs, foam cells in bone marrow, no mental retardation

DDx of cherry red spot: CRAO, commotio retinae, macular hole, macular hemorrhage, ocular ischemic syndrome, subacute sclerosing panencephalitis, quinine toxicity, methanol toxicity

No cherry red spot: Fabry's and Krabbe's disease
   Fabry's (X-linked dominant): α-galactosidase A deficiency; accumulation of trihexosylceramide in smooth muscle of blood vessels; manifested in heterozygous females
     FINDINGS: cornea verticillata (corneal whorls), tortuous conjunctival and retinal vessels, posterior lenticular spoke–like changes
     OTHER FINDINGS: paresthesias in extremities, cutaneous telangiectases, poor temperature regulation, abdominal pain, anemia, renal failure, hypertension; vascular thromboses resulting in stroke and cardiac and renal disease; renal failure is leading cause of death
     DIAGNOSIS: failure to detect α-galactosidase in tears

Cystinosis

Amino acid disorder; lysosomes cannot excrete cystine

Findings: iridescent fusiform crystals in cornea, iris, lens, and retina; photophobia

> ***Infantile form*** (nephropathic form) (AR): Fanconi's syndrome: polyuria, growth retardation, rickets, progressive renal failure, salt and pepper fundus changes (but no visual disturbance)
>
> ***Adolescent form*** (AR): less severe nephropathy than in Fanconi's syndrome
>
> ***Adult form***: benign form; no renal problems

Treatment: cysteamine (systemically for renal disease, topically for corneal crystals)

Long-Chain 3-Hydroxyacyl-CoA Dehydrogenase Deficiency (LCHAD Deficiency)

Disorder of mitochondrial fatty acid beta-oxidation due to mutation of guanine to cytosine at position 1528

Findings: normal fundus at birth, followed by RPE pigment dispersion; eventually develop chorioretinal atrophy and occlusion of choroidal vessels; deterioration of central vision; may have posterior staphylomas, developmental cataracts, progressive myopia

Treatment: low-fat, high-carbohydrate diet with carnitine supplementation

Prognosis: usually fatal by 2 years of age (hepatic or cardiorespiratory failure) unless dietary treatment is started

Vitreoretinal Dystrophies

Vitreous abnormalities associated with schisis cavity at level of NFL and ganglion cell layer

Juvenile Retinoschisis
(X-Linked Recessive)

Mapped to Xp22 (XLRS1 [retinoschisin])

Males; bilateral; present at birth; progresses rapidly during first 5 years of life; stable by age 20

Cleavage of retina at NFL (in senile retinoschisis, cleavage is at outer plexiform layer)

Findings:

> ***Foveal retinoschisis*** (only abnormality in 50%): pathognomonic; earliest change is radial, spoke-like ILM folds centered on fovea because of dehiscence of NFL; appears like CME. Later, cystoid structure appears in fovea with round microcysts in perifoveal area and marked pigmentary degeneration; bullous schisis cavities

develop; retinal vessels are only remaining structure within inner layer and may bleed causing vitreous hemorrhage
> Marked sclerosis/sheathing of blood vessels with appearance of vitreous veils
> Vitreous cells (30%)
> True retinoschisis (NFL) in periphery in 50% (usually inferotemporal); does not extend to ora
> Vitreous syneresis
> Hyperopia
> Reduced vision (20/50–20/100 level)

Carriers have normal retinal appearance and function

VF: absolute scotoma

ERG: normal a-wave until late, reduced b-wave (especially scotopic) in proportion to amount of retinoschisis, markedly reduced oscillatory potentials

EOG: normal

FA: microcysts with no leakage

Complications: RD and VH (uncommon)

Goldmann-Favre Disease (AR)

Mapped to chromosome 15q23 (PNR)

Rare, vitreotapetoretinal degeneration with nyctalopia and constricted visual fields (like RP + juvenile retinoschisis)

Findings: decreased vision, nyctalopia, optically empty vitreous with strands and veils, bilateral central and peripheral retinoschisis, attenuated retinal vessels, peripheral bone–spicule retinal pigmentary changes, lattice degeneration, optic disc pallor, cataracts

ERG: markedly reduced

EOG: abnormal (distinguishes from juvenile retinoschisis)

Treatment: may require retinal surgery for retinal tears or detachments

Vitreoretinal Degenerations

Wagner Syndrome (AD)

Mapped to chromosome 5q13-q14 (WGN1), 12q13 (COL2A1)

Findings: vitreous liquefaction and veils, optically empty vitreous, no RD, equatorial and perivascular pigmented lattice-like changes, peripheral vessel sheathing, RPE atrophy, cataract (wedge and fleck opacities between ages 20 and 40), moderate myopia, optic atrophy

ERG: may be abnormal

Treatment: cataract extraction; genetic counseling

Jansen Syndrome (AD)

Wagner syndrome + RD

Stickler's Syndrome (AD)

Mapped to chromosome 1p21 (COL11A1), 6p21 (COL11A2), 12q13 (COL2A1)

Progressive arthro-ophthalmopathy; Wagner-like ocular changes with severe myopia and marfinoid habitus

Findings: optically empty vitreous with bands, lattice degeneration, RD (50%), optic atrophy, cataract, glaucoma, high myopia

Figure 5-34. Fundus view of the eye of a Stickler's syndrome patient. Note the radial perivascular pigmentary changes. (From Kimura AJ: Hereditary vitreoretinopathies. In Yanoff M, Duker JS [eds]: *Ophthalmology*, London, Mosby, 1999.)

Other findings: orofacial abnormalities (Pierre Robin anomaly: midfacial flattening and cleft palate), marfinoid habitus, hearing loss, mitral valve prolapse, joint abnormalities (hyperextensibility, enlargement, arthritis)

ERG: decreased b-wave

Hereditary Arthro-Ophthalmopathy (Weill-Marchesani–Like Variety)

Similar to Stickler's but short stature with stubby hands and feet; increased risk of ectopia lentis

Snowflake Degeneration (AD)

Very rare, progressive vitreoretinal degeneration

Manifests after 25 years of age

Findings: fibrillar condensation and liquefaction of vitreous; associated with peripheral NV, increased risk of RD, early cataracts

Stage 1: Extensive white without pressure
Stage 2: Snowflakes (white dots in superficial retina) within white without pressure
Stage 3: Sheathing of retinal vessels and early peripheral pigmentation
Stage 4: Disappearance of retinal vessels in periphery and increased retinal pigmentation

ERG: decreased scotopic B-wave amplitude

EOG: normal

Dark adaptation: elevated rod threshold later in disease

Albinism

Albinoidism: only minimal reduction in vision; no nystagmus

Albinism: AR or less frequently AD disorder characterized by decreased melanin and congenitally subnormal vision (foveal hypoplasia and nystagmus)

 Oculocutaneous: lack of pigmentation of skin, hair, and eyes

  TYROSINASE-NEGATIVE (no pigmentation): Defect in chromosome 11

   FINDINGS: decreased vision, iris transillumination, foveal hypoplasia, hypopigmented fundus, nystagmus, photophobia, high myopia, strabismus

   OTHER FINDINGS: hypopigmentation of skin and hair (white hair, pink skin)

  TYROSINASE-POSITIVE (some pigmentation): Defect in chromosome 15 (paternal = Prader-Willi syndrome; maternal = Angelman's syndrome)

  Ocular and systemic characteristics less severe

  2 POTENTIALLY LETHAL VARIANTS:

   CHÉDIAK-HIGASHI SYNDROME: large melanosomes on skin biopsy, reticuloendothelial dysfunction with pancytopenia, recurrent infections, and malignancies (leukemia, lymphoma)

   HERMANSKY-PUDLAK SYNDROME: clotting disorder due to abnormal platelets, commonly of Puerto Rican descent

 Ocular: abnormal melanogenesis limited to eye (decreased number of melanosomes)

  X-LINKED RECESSIVE: iris transillumination less prominent, female carriers with variable retinal pigmentation (mosaic pattern)

  Giant melanosomes in skin, normal pigmentation of skin

  Associated with deafness

  AUTOSOMAL RECESSIVE: both males and females affected

 ERG and EOG: supranormal

Aicardi's Syndrome (X-Linked Dominant)

Only females, lethal in males

Lacunar defects in RPE

Findings: widespread depigmented round chorioretinal lesions, ON head coloboma, microphthalmos

Other findings: infantile spasms, severe mental retardation, agenesis of corpus collosum

Colorblindness (Tables 5-5 and 5-6)

Incidence up to 13% of population

Red-green disorders are X-linked recessive (male preponderance); men and women can have tritan disorders (AD)

Congenital color vision defect typically redgreen; acquired color vision defect typically blueyellow

Color vision defects do not cause decreased vision, except for rod and blue cone monochromatism

Normal individuals are trichromats: 3 types of cones (red, green, blue); 92% of population

Prot = Red; Deuter = Green; Trit = Blue (Greek for 1st, 2nd, 3rd; order in which these deficits were described)

Anopia = absent; Anomaly = abnormal; An = unspecified

Anomalous trichromatism: all 3 cones present but in abnormal proportions; can distinguish fully saturated colors but have difficulty distinguishing colors of low saturation
    According to which pigment is abnormal, the disorders are called:
    Protanomaly: abnormal level of red pigment
    Deuteranomaly: abnormal level of green pigment
    Tritanomaly: abnormal level of blue pigment

Congenital dichromatism: substantial lack of one type of color cone
    Protanopia: red cones contain chlorolabe (green pigment)
    Deuteranopia: green cones contain erythrolabe (red pigment)
    Tritanopia: defect of blue cones

2 forms of congenital dyschromatopsia associated with low vision:
    Rod monochromatism (AR): cones are absent, therefore complete achromatopsia; poor vision and nystagmus in infants; ERG: normal under scotopic conditions; reduced during photopic conditions
    Blue cone monochromatism (X-linked recessive): nystagmus, decreased vision, photophobia, myopia

Tritan color defect and slightly subnormal vision: consider Kjer's dominant optic atrophy

Table 5-5. Incidences of Color Vision Abnormalities

Deuteranomaly	5% (XR)
Deuteranopia	1% (XR)
Protonanomaly	1% (XR)
Protonanopia	1% (XR)
Tritanomaly	0.0001% (AD)
Tritanopia	0.001% (AD)

Table 5-6. Comparison of Dyschromatopsias

Congenital Dyschromatopsia	Acquired Dyschromatopsia
Deuteranomalous trichromats are most common (5% of male population)	
Red-green axis	Blue-yellow axis
Males > females	Females = males
Nonprogressive	May be slowly progressive
Bilateral and symmetric	Unilateral or nonsymmetric
Normal eye examination	Associated with abnormality on eye examination
X-linked recessive	No heritability
Deep blue is perceived as purple	Deep blue is perceived as gray

Diagnosis: Farnsworth-Munsell 100 hue test: consists of 85 hue caps contained in 4 separate racks with 2 end caps fixed; patient arranges caps between fixed ends in order of hue; tests for both red-green and blue-yellow defects
    Farnsworth's panel D-15: derived from 100 hue test, but uses only 15 caps
    City university test: derived from 100 hue test, but 10 charts with a central color and 4 peripheral colors; select outer color that matches central color
    Pseudoisochromatic plates: Ishihara plates (for protanopes and deuteranopes; detect only redgreen defects), and Hardy-Rand-Ritter (HRR) polychromatic plates (test for both red-green and blue-yellow defects)
    Kollner's rule: errors made by persons with optic nerve disease tend to resemble those made by protans and deutans (red and green), whereas

errors made by individuals with retinal disease resemble those made by tritans (blue)

Congenital Hypertrophy of the RPE (CHRPE)

Usually unilateral, congenital, asymptomatic

Findings: flat, well-circumscribed black lesion with surrounding halo; larger lesions often contain depigmented lacunae (choroid visible through lacunae); multiple patches with sector distribution called "bear tracks" (Figures 5-35 and 5-38)

Figure 5-35. Typical congenital hypertrophy of retinal pigment epithelium. (From Augsburger JJ, Bolling JJ: Hypertrophy of retinal pigment epithelium. In Yanoff M, Duker JS [eds]: *Ophthalmology*, London, Mosby, 1999.)

Figure 5-36. Congenital hypertrophy of retinal pigment epithelium with prominent depigmented lacunae. (From Augsburger JJ, Bolling JJ: Hypertrophy of retinal pigment epithelium. In Yanoff M, Duker JS [eds]: *Ophthalmology*, London, Mosby, 1999.)

Pathology: melanosomes in RPE cells are larger and more spherical than normal; densely packed round melanocytes and increased thickness of RPE; focal areas of RPE loss (lacunae)

Atypical multifocal bilateral variant: occurs in 75% of patients with familial adenomatous polyposis (FAP: AD, high incidence of multiple adenomas of colon and rectum; eventually undergo malignant transformation; chromosome 5q. Gardner's syn-

Figure 5-37. Congenital hypertrophy of retinal pigment epithelium (grouped by pigmentation of retina). (From Augsburger JJ, Bolling JJ: Hypertrophy of retinal pigment epithelium. In Yanoff M, Duker JS [eds]: *Ophthalmology*, 2nd ed, St. Louis, Mosby, 2004.)

> Reactive hyperplasia of retinal pigment epithelium
>
> Massive gliosis of retina
>
> Combined hamartoma of retina
>
> Melanotic choroidal nevus or melanoma
>
> Bilateral diffuse uveal melanocytic proliferation associated with systemic carcinoma syndrome
>
> Adenoma or adenocarcinoma of retinal pigment epithelium
>
> Metastatic melanoma to retina

Figure 5-38. Differential diagnosis of congenital hypertrophy of the retinal pigment epithelium. (From Augsburger JJ, Bolling JJ: Hypertrophy of retinal pigment epithelium. In Yanoff M, Duker JS [eds]: *Ophthalmology*, London, Mosby, 1999.)

drome [variant of FAP]: combination of colonic polyps and extracolonic manifestations [osteomas, dermoid tumors])

Retinoblastoma

Most common intraocular malignancy in children

Incidence 1 in 20,000

No sex or race predilection

90% diagnosed by 5 years of age; fatal in 2–4 years if untreated

30% bilateral, 30% multifocal

Genetics: (Table 5-7)

Mapped to chromosome 13q14, must have gene defect on both chromosomes

Table 5-7. Chances of Having a Baby with Retinoblastoma

	Negative FH		Positive FH	
Offspring of	*Unilateral*	*Bilateral*	*Unilateral*	*Bilateral*
Parents with an affected child	1%	6%	40%	40%
Affected patient	8%	40%	40%	40%
Normal sibling of affected patient	1%	<1%	7%	7%

94% sporadic (75% somatic, 25% germinal mutation); 6% autosomal dominant

40% heritable, 80% penetrance

Most occur sporadically in infants with no family history; bilateral cases are usually familial (risk that additional offspring will have retinoblastoma is 40%)

75% are caused by mutation (inactivation of both RB genes) in a single retinal cell; these tumors are unilateral and unifocal; the chance of inactivation of both RB genes is very small

Parents with 1 affected child: 6% risk of producing more affected children

Parents with 2 or more affected children: 40% risk (because only 80% penetrance)

Retinoblastoma survivor with hereditary form: 50% chance of transferring to children (but children have only 40% chance of manifesting a tumor)

Presentation: leukocoria (60%), strabismus (22%), decreased vision (5%)

Findings: yellow-white retinal mass, rubeosis, pseudohypopyon, hyphema, angle-closure glaucoma, uveitis

2 forms:

Endophytic: arises from inner retina and grows toward vitreous; can simulate endophthalmitis; can have pseudohypopyon (Figure 5-39)

Exophytic: arises from outer retina and grows toward choroid causing solid RD; can extend through sclera; can simulate Coats' disease or traumatic RD

retinoblastoma

Figure 5-39. Retinoblastoma demonstrating discrete round tumor. (From Kaiser PK, Friedman NJ, Pineda II, R: *Massachusetts Eye and Ear Infirmary Illustrated Manual of Ophthalmology*, 2nd ed, Philadelphia, WB Saunders, 2004.)

Tumor necrosis when outgrows blood supply, then calcification (seen on CT and US); may develop NV glaucoma (17%); no macular tumors after 1.5 months of age

ON involvement: present in 29% of enucleated eyes

Risk for ON invasion: exophytic tumors >15 mm, and eyes that have secondary glaucoma

Second tumors: commonly present around age 17; osteogenic sarcoma of femur (most common), malignant melanoma of eye or orbit, leiomyosarcoma of eye or orbit, lymphoma, leukemia, rhabdomyosarcoma, medulloblastoma

Trilateral retinoblastoma: bilateral RB with a pinealoblastoma or parasellar neuroblastoma; occurs in 3% of chidren with unilateral RB and 8% with bilateral RB; 95% have a positive family history and/or other tumors; spontaneous regression occurs with subsequent necrosis and phthisis

Pathology: rosettes are histologic markers for tumor differentiation

In order of increasing differentiation:

Homer-Wright rosette: no lumen; nuclei surround tangle of neural filaments; reflects low-grade neuroblastic differentiation; can be found in other types of neuroblastic tumors (adrenal neuroblastoma, medulloblastoma)

Flexner-Wintersteiner rosette: ring of single row of columnar cells around central lumen; cells have eosinophilic cytoplasm and peripheral nuclei; photoreceptors contain cilia with a 9 + 0 pattern; represent early retinal differentiation; attempt of outer photoreceptor production; special stains show hyaluronidase-resistant acid mucopolysaccharides in lumen; also present in medulloepitheliomas (Figure 5-40)

Fleurettes: bouquet of pink bulbous neoplastic photoreceptor inner segments; highest degree of differentiation in retinoblastoma; found in relatively eosinophilic areas of tumor (photoreceptor differentiation) (Figure 5-41)

Pseudorosettes: circumferential arrangements of viable tumor cells surrounding a central vessel

Cells have round, spindle-shaped hyperchromatic nuclei and very little cytoplasm; high mitotic activity; as tumor grows, outgrows blood supply creating necrosis with areas of calcification (80%)

Figure 5-40. Flexner-Wintersteiner rosettes. (From Augsburger JJ, Bornfeld M, Giblin ME: Retinoblastoma. In Yanoff M, Duker JS [eds]: *Ophthalmology*, London, Mosby, 1999.)

Figure 5-42. RB demonstrating necrosis and optic nerve invasion. (From Yanoff M, Fine BS: *Ocular Pathology*, 5th ed, Philadelphia, Mosby, 2002.)

Figure 5-41. Homer-Wright rosettes. (From Augsburger JJ, Bornfeld M, Giblin ME: Retinoblastoma. In Yanoff M, Duker JS [eds]: *Ophthalmology*, London, Mosby, 1999.)

H&E stain:

BLUE AREAS: represent viable tumor; differentiated cells that have basophilic nuclei and little cytoplasm

PINK AREAS: represent necrotic tumor; lose basophilic nuclei and appear eosinophilic (pink)

PURPLE AREAS: represent calcified tumor; occur in necrotic areas; calcium stains purple (Figure 5-42)

DDx (DDx of leukocoria): cataract, retrolental mass (PHPV, ROP, Norrie's disease, RD), tumor (choroidal metastases, retinal astrocytoma), exudates (FEVR, Coats' disease, Eales' disease), change in retinal pigment (incontinentia pigmenti, high myopia, myelinated nerve fiber, retinal dysplasia, choroideremia, coloboma), infections (toxoplasmosis, toxocariasis, endophthalmitis)

Diagnosis:

LDH levels: ratio of aqueous:plasma LDH >1.0

Ultrasound: acoustic solidity and high internal reflectivity; calcium appears as dense echoes

FA: early hyperfluorescence with late leakage of lesions

CT scan: calcification; look for pineal tumor with CT or MRI, and for ON involvement

Metastatic workup: bone scan, bone marrow aspirate, LP (cytology)

Treatment:

Enucleation: all blind and painful eyes; affected eye in most unilateral cases; worse eye in most asymmetric cases; both eyes in many symmetric cases; excise at least 10 mm of ON to prevent spread

External beam radiation: salvageable eyes with vitreous seeding or large tumor; most eyes with multifocal tumors; eyes that have failed coagulation therapy; RB is very radiosensitive; used to treat most 2nd tumors

Episcleral plaque radiation: salvageable eyes with single medium-sized tumor that does not involve ON or macula, even with localized vitreous seeding

Photocoagulation/cryotherapy: occasional eyes with one or a few small tumors, not involving ON or macula

Prognosis: 90% to 95% of children with retinoblastoma survive (same with either growth pattern); 3% spontaneously regress

Metastases: most commonly to CNS along ON; 50% are to bone

Familial RB: location related to age, earliest in macula, later in periphery; 2nd eye tumor develops up to 44 months later; 45% mortality by age 35 (vs 19% long-term survival for all patients with RB by age 35); multiple primary tumors in an eye does not worsen prognosis

Increased risk of 2nd unrelated malignancy in 25% of children with heritable retinoblastoma

Poor prognostic signs: ON invasion, uveal invasion, extrascleral extension, multifocal tumors (represent seeding); delay in diagnosis, degree of differentiation

Bilateral involvement does not worsen prognosis; prognosis depends on status of tumor in worst eye; degree of necrosis and calcification does not influence prognosis

Reese-Ellsworth classification: predicts visual prognosis (not survival) in eyes treated by methods other than enucleation

Retinocytoma/Retinoma

Benign tumor with same appearance and genetics as RB

Pathology: numerous fleurettes among cells with varying degrees of photoreceptor differentiation

Differentiation from RB: more cytoplasm, more evenly dispersed nuclear chromatin, no mitoses, calcification may be present, and necrosis is usually absent in retinocytoma

13q Deletion Syndrome

Associated with retinoblastoma, microcephaly, hypertelorism, microphthalmos, ptosis, and epicanthus

Leukemia (Figures 5-43 and 5-44)

Most common malignancy of childhood

Usually affects choroid with retinal hemorrhages; usually unilateral

Symptoms: blurred vision, floaters

Findings: cellular infiltration of vitreous; infiltrative lesions of retina, optic nerve, or uvea; multiple hemorrhages, Roth spots; CWS, heterochomia irides, pseudohypopyon, spontaneous hyphema, uveitic glaucoma, cataract

Optic nerve infiltration causes loss of vision and papilledema

Figure 5-43. Leukemic infiltrate in optic nerve. (From Yanoff M, Fine BS: *Ocular Pathology*, 5th ed, Philadelphia, Mosby, 2002.)

Orbital infiltration (rare) causes proptosis, lid swelling, ecchymosis (1% to 2% of patients)

Treatment: emergent XRT for ON infiltration; patient is more susceptible to developing radiation optic neuropathy when chemotherapy is used concurrently

Prognosis: poor; high mortality; can be rapidly fatal if untreated

PHAKOMATOSES

Group of disorders (neurocutaneous syndromes) characterized by ocular and systemic hamartomas. Most are AD with variable penetrance except Sturge-Weber and Wyburn-Mason (no hereditary pattern) and ataxia-telangiectasia (AR)

Treatment: often requires CT scans and medical consultations; may require treatment of elevated IOP

Table 5-8. Genetics of the Phakomatoses

Disorder		Chromosome
Neurofibromatosis:	Type 1	17
	Type 2	22
Sturge-Weber		None
von Hippel–Lindau		3
Tuberous sclerosis		9
Ataxia-telangiectasia		11
Wyburn-Mason		None

Neurofibromatosis (AD)

Variable expressivity

Disorder of Schwann cells and melanocytes with hamartomas of nervous system, skin, and eye

2 types:

NF-1 (von Recklinghausen's syndrome): mapped to chromosome 17q11 (neurofibromin), 50% due to new mutation; 80% penetrance

More common form (prevalence 1 in 3000 to 5000)
Criteria (2 or more of the following):
6 or more café au lait spots >5 mm in diameter in prepubescent or >15 mm in postpubescent individuals
2 or more neurofibromas or 1 plexiform neurofibroma
Freckling of intertriginous areas
Optic nerve glioma
2 or more Lisch nodules
Osseous lesion (sphenoid bone dysplasia, thinning of long bone cortex)
First-degree relative with NF-1

A

B

C

D

Figure 5-44. Acute leukemia. **A**, A patient presented with a large infiltrate of leukemic cells positioned nasally within the conjunctiva of the right eye, giving this characteristic clinical picture. These lesions look similar to those caused by benign lymphoid hyperplasia, lymphoma, or amyloidosis. **B**, A biopsy of the lesion shows primitive blastic leukocytes. **C**, In another case, the iris is infiltrated by leukemic cell. A special stain (Lader stain) shows that some of the cells stain red, better seen when viewed under increased magnification in **D**. This red positivety is characteristic of myelogenous leukemic cells. (From Augsburger JJ, Tsiaras WG: Lymphoma and leukemia. In Yanoff M, Duker JS [eds]: *Ophthalmology*, London, Mosby, 1999.)

Findings: plexiform neurofibroma (plexus of abnormal markedly enlarged nerves; occur in 25%; 10% involve face, often upper eyelid or orbit; "bag of worms" appearance and S-shaped upper lid; congenital glaucoma in ipsilateral eye in up to 50%), fibroma molluscum, plexiform neurofibroma of conjunctiva, prominent corneal nerves, Lisch nodules (glial/melanocytic iris hamartomas), diffuse uveal thickening due to excess melanocytes and neurons (similar to ocular melanocytosis), ectropion uveae, retinal astrocytic hamartoma (less likely to be calcified than in tuberous sclerosis), increased incidence of myelinated nerve fibers and choroidal nevi (33%), ON glioma (juvenile pilocytic astrocytoma in >30%; may cause visual loss, hypothalamic dysfunction or hydrocephalus; neuroimaging shows fusiform enlargement of nerve with kinking; if have glioma, 25% have NF), meningioma, orbital plexiform neurofibroma, schwannoma, absence of sphenoid wing (pulsating exophthalmos)

Other findings: café au lait spots, intertriginous (axillary) freckling, cutaneous peripheral nerve sheath tumors

NF-2: mapped to chromosome 22q
Prevalence 1 in 50,000

Criteria:
Bilateral cerebellar-pontine angle tumors (acoustic neuromas; cause hearing loss, ataxia, headache)
First-degree relative with NF-2 and either a unilateral acoustic neuroma or 2 of the following: meningioma, schwannoma, neurofibroma, glioma, posterior subcapsular cataract
May have pheochromocytoma and other malignant tumors
No Lisch nodules

Encephalotrigeminal Angiomatosis (Sturge-Weber Syndrome)

Nonhereditary

No racial or sex predilection

Facial hemangioma: nevus flammeus (port wine stain) limited to first 2 divisions of CN 5; 5% to 10% bilateral

Findings: dilated tortuous vessels of the conjunctiva and episclera, congenital or juvenile glaucoma (25% risk, especially if upper lid involved), heterochromia irides (due to angiomas of iris), angiomas of episclera and CB, diffuse cavernous choroidal hemangioma ("tomato-ketchup" fundus [50%]), peripheral retinal AV malformations, may get RD or severe RPE alterations (pseudo-RP)

> *Mechanism of glaucoma*: neovascular, increased episcleral venous pressure, immature angle structures

Other findings: leptomeningeal vascular malformations (ipsilateral to port wine stain), central calcifications, mental retardation, seizures

Klippel-Trénaunay-Weber: variant of Sturge-Weber with cutaneous nevus flammeus, hemangiomas, varicosities, intracranial angiomas, and hemihypertrophy of limbs

> *Findings* (uncommon): congenital glaucoma, conjunctival telangiectasia; can have AV malformation similar to Wyburn-Mason

Angiomatosis Retinae (Von Hippel–Lindau Disease) (AD)

Incomplete penetrance; mapped to chromosome 3p26-p25 (VHL)

Prevalence 1 in 100,000

50% bilateral

Hamartomas of eye, brain (cerebellum), kidney/adrenal gland (3 names, 3 locations for tumors)

Findings: retinal angioma (hemangioma or hemangioblastoma; round orange-red mass fed by dilated tortuous retinal artery and drained by engorged vein; may be multifocal as well as bilateral; often in midperiphery, may be near disc; leaks heavily causing serous RD and/or macular edema; treat with yellow dye laser if enlarges)

Other findings: 25% of retinal capillary hemangiomas associated with CNS tumor (hemangioblastoma of cerebellum (60%); pons, medulla, and/or spinal cord is less common); visceral lesions (cysts and tumors of kidney, pancreas, liver, adrenal glands, including renal cell carcinoma [25%], pheochromocytoma [5%])

Von Hippel disease: only ocular involvement

Treatment: observation, cryotherapy, or laser photocoagulation

Tuberous Sclerosis (Bourneville's Disease) (AD or Sporadic)

Mapped to chromosome 9q34 (TSC1 [hamartin]), 16p13 (TSC2 [tuberin])

Prevalence 1 in 10,000 to 100,000

Triad of adenoma sebaceum, mental retardation, and epilepsy

Findings: astrocytic hamartoma of the retina (flat or mulberry-shaped with calcifications; usually in posterior pole; consists of nerve fibers and undifferentiated glial cells; occurs in 50%; bilateral in 15%), astrocytic hamartoma of the ON ("giant drusen"; benign)

Other findings:

> *Cutaneous*: facial angiofibroma (adenoma sebaceum; vascularized red papules in butterfly distribution, not present at birth, become visible between ages 2 and 5), ash leaf spots (hypopigmented spots that fluoresce under Wood's light, considered pathognomonic), shagreen patches (25%; areas of fibromatous infiltration, usually on trunk), periungual fibromas, may have café au lait spots
>
> *CNS*: subependymal hamartomas (calcify, forming "brain stones" with root-like appearance; concentrated in periventricular area), mental retardation (60%), seizures (80%), cerebral calcification
>
> *Other*: cardiac rhabdomyoma, spontaneous pneumothorax (from pleural cyst), renal angiomyolipomas

Early mortality

Ataxia-Telangiectasia (Louis-Bar's Syndrome) (AR)

Mapped to chromosome 11q22 (ATM)

Prevalence 1 in 40,000

Findings: prominent dilated conjunctival vessels, impaired convergence, nystagmus, oculomotor apraxia

Other findings: cutaneous telangiectasia in butterfly distribution during 1st decade of life, mental retardation, cerebellar ataxia (due to cerebellar atrophy), thymic hypoplasia with defective T-cell function and IgA deficiency with increased risk of infections, malignancy (leukemia/lymphoma)

Racemose Hemangiomatosis (Wyburn-Mason Syndrome)

Nonhereditary, usually unilateral

Findings: racemose hemangioma of retina (arteriovenous malformation with markedly dilated and tortuous shunt vessels); may have intraocular hemorrhage or glaucoma

Other findings: arteriovenous malformations in brain (may cause seizures, paresis, mental changes,

VF defects), orbit and facial bones; may have small facial hemangiomas

Others

Retinal Cavernous Hemangioma

Cluster of intraretinal aneurysms filled with venous blood

Appears as "cluster of grapes"

Vitreous hemorrhage is rare

May be associated with cutaneous and CNS hemangiomas

FA: fluid levels without leakage within lesions

Incontinentia Pigmenti (Bloch-Sulzberger Syndrome) (X-Linked Dominant)

Occurs exclusively in females (lethal in males)

Findings: proliferative retinal vasculopathy (resembles ROP); may have retinal detachment and retrolental membrane (Figure 5-45)

Other findings:
Skin lesions:
  STAGE 1 (at birth): erythematous macules, papules, and bullae on trunk and extremities (intraepithelial vesicles containing eosinophils)
  STAGE 2 (2 months of age): vesicles are replaced by verrucous lesions
  STAGE 3 (3–6 months of age): lesions take form of pigmented whorls on trunk
  STAGE 4: skin is atrophic with hypopigmented patches
Alopecia
CNS abnormalities: microcephaly, hydrocephalus, seizures, mental deficiency
Dental abnormalities: missing and cone-shaped teeth

Treatment: photocoagulation (variable results)

OPTIC NERVE DISORDERS

Aplasia

Complete absence of optic nerve; very rare; may occur with anencephaly or major cerebral maldevelopment

Hypoplasia

Variable visual compromise

Etiology unclear

Figure 5-45. Incontinentia pigmenti. The peripheral retina of a patient who has incontinentia pigmenti demonstrates somewhat elevated vessels with vessel walls. A majority of these vessels show nonperfusion. The more posterior retina was perfused, and the anterior retina was ischemic. (From Ebroom DA, Jampol JM: Proliferation retinopathies. In Yanoff M, Duker JS [eds]: *Ophthalmology*, London, Mosby, 1999.)

No sex predilection

Associations: aniridia, Goldenhar's syndrome, midline anomalies, endocrine abnormalities, congenital intracranial tumors (craniopharyngioma, optic glioma), maternal diabetes or drug ingestion during pregnancy (alcohol, LSD, quinine, dilantin)

Findings: double ring sign (thin ring of pigment surrounding nerve tissue; halo of retina and RPE partially covering lamina cribrosa), strabismus, amblyopia, nystagmus, RAPD, VF defects

Other findings: CNS abnormalities (45%), growth retardation, endocrine abnormalities

De Morsier's syndrome (septo-optic dysplasia): bilateral ON hypoplasia, septum pellucidum abnormality, pituitary and hypothalamus deficiency; associated with agenesis of the corpus callosum; may have chiasmal developmental anomalies with VF defects; at risk for sudden death

Treatment: brain MRI, endocrine workup

Coloboma

Due to incomplete closure of embryonic fissure; usually located inferonasal

Unilateral or bilateral

Variable visual acuity and visual field defects

Associated with other ocular colobomas

Findings: large anomalous discs, deep excavation with abnormal vascular pattern (ranges from complete chorioretinal coloboma to involvement of proximal portion of embryonic fissure causing only optic nerve deformity); may resemble physiologic cupping if mild

Morning Glory Disc

Probably represents a dysplastic coloboma

Generally unilateral

Female > male (2 : 1)

Often seen with high myopia

May be associated with cranial defects or other ocular anomalies

Findings: cup filled with glial tissue surrounded by pigment ring, adjacent retinal folds common; also described as funnel-shaped, enlarged, excavated disc with central white connective tissue; vessels radiate in spoke-like fashion; usually poor vision; may develop peripapillary RD

Optic Pit

Gray-white depression in optic disc usually in infero-temporal area

85% unilateral

Associated with peripapillary RPE disturbances

May develop serous retinal detachment extending from pit (40%)

Tilted Disc

Findings (any of the following may occur, alone or in combination): apparent tilting (usually inferiorly with superior pole of disc elevated), scleral crescent, situs inversus arteriosus (vessels emerge temporally from optic nerve [rather than nasally] and course nasally before sweeping temporally), myopia and/or astigmatism, reduced visual acuity, visual field defects (usually bitemporal and do not respect vertical midline)

Myelinated Nerve Fibers

Myelination begins at lateral geniculate body and usually ceases at lamina cribrosa; however, some retinal fibers may acquire myelin sheath during first month of life

More common in males

Unilateral or bilateral (20%)

Vision generally good unless macula involved

Findings: superficial white flame-shaped patches with feathery margins; usually peripapillary; can be extensive

Relative or absolute scotoma corresponds to area of myelination

Persistence of Hyaloid System

Common; ranges from tuft of glial tissue on disc (Bergmeister's papillae) to patent artery extending from disc to lens

Megalopapilla

Enlarged optic disc

Peripapillary Staphyloma

Posterior bulging of sclera in which optic disc occupies bottom of bulge

Optic Nerve Drusen

Superficial or buried hyaline bodies in prelaminar portion of optic nerve

Sporadic or AD; 75% bilateral

Incidence 0.3% to 1% clinically; 2% histopathologically

More common in Caucasians; no sex predilection

Associations: angioid streaks, retinitis pigmentosa, Alagille's syndrome (familial intrahepatic cholestasis, posterior embryotoxin, bilateral optic disc drusen [80%])

Findings: disc margins may show irregular outline, bumpy nodular chunky appearance to nerve head (pseudopapilledema); VF defects (especially with deep drusen; enlarged blind spot, arcuate scotoma, sectoral scotoma); may have transient visual obscurations, positive RAPD (unilateral ON drusen); often calcify with age

Pathology: hyaline bodies that become calcified; stain positively for amino acids, calcium, acid mucopolysaccharides, and hemosiderin; stain negatively for amyloid

Diagnosis: B-scan ultrasound, CT scan, autofluorescence

Complications: rarely visual loss due to axonal compression, AION, CNV, subretinal or vitreous hemorrhage, vascular occlusion

Melanocytoma (Magnocellular Nevus of the Optic Disc)

Deeply pigmented tumor with feathery border located over ON

Derived from uveal dendritic melanocytes

May have choroidal and NFL involvement

15% show minimal enlargement over 5 years

Findings: VF defect; may have positive RAPD (even with good vision)

Pathology: benign, plump, round polyhedral melanocytes

Malignant transformation very rare

Hereditary Optic Neuropathy

Kjer's syndrome (AD): dominant optic neuropathy; most common form of heritable optic atrophy; mapped to chromosome 3q28 (OPA1); insidious onset age of 4–8 years; bilateral and symmetric; mild decreased vision (20/40–20/200), blue-yellow dyschromatopsia, temporal wedge of disc pallor

Behr's syndrome (AR): infantile optic neuropathy; onset before age 10, male > female, nonprogressive; moderate to severe decreased vision, nystagmus, diffuse optic atrophy; ataxia, spasticity, hypotonia, mental retardation

Wolfram syndrome (AR): onset age 5–21 years; slowly progressive; decreased vision (<20/400), diffuse optic atrophy; DIDMOAD (Diabetes Insipidus, Diabetes Mellitus, Optic Atrophy, Deafness), ataxia, seizures, mental retardation

Leber's hereditary optic neuropathy (LHON): maternal mitochondrial DNA; point mutations in mitochondrial gene for NADH subunit 4 (position 11778 [31% to 90%], 3460 [8% to 15%], 14484 [10% to 15%]); male > female (9 : 1); maternal transmission to all sons (50% affected) and all daughters (15% of daughters affected, 85% are carriers); onset age 15–30; subacute sequential bilateral vision loss (20/200 or worse) over days; tobacco or alcohol can trigger decompensation

> *Findings*: disc hyperemia, peripapillary telangiectatic vessels (do not leak fluorescein, also found in 60% of asymptomatic family members), tortuous vessels, peripapillary NFL edema, late optic disc pallor; may have cardiac conduction abnormalities

DDx: acquired optic neuropathies: compressive (tumors [craniopharyngioma, optic nerve/chiasmal gliomas], hydrocephalus), toxic (anoxia at birth or in neonatal period), traumatic, infiltrative (leukemia, metabolic storage diseases)

Treatment: no treatment; genetic counseling

Mitochondrial Diseases

Maternal inheritance; children of both sexes affected; only female offspring can pass on

Findings: optic atrophy, CPEO, pigmentary retinopathy, retrochiasmal visual loss

Disorders:
> *Leber's hereditary optic neuropathy* (LHON): see earlier
> *Kearns-Sayre syndrome*: onset before age 20
> > FINDINGS: chronic progressive external ophthalmoplegia with ptosis, pigmentary retinopathy

(salt and pepper, bone spicules, and/or RPE atrophy), mild visual loss (50%)
> OTHER FINDINGS: neck and limb weakness, arrhythmias, cerebellar ataxia
> PATHOLOGY: "ragged-red" fibers (contain degenerated mitochondria) on muscle biopsy
> EKG: heart block
> CSF: elevated protein

MELAS: **M**itochondrial **E**ncephalopathy, **L**actic **A**cidosis, and **S**trokelike episodes

Onset before age 15; point mutations (3242, 3271) or deletions
> FINDINGS: retrochiasmal visual loss; recurrent attacks of headache, vomiting, seizures; transient focal neurologic deficits (hemiplegia, hemianopia/cortical blindness); psychiatric changes, hearing loss, short stature, muscle weakness
> DIAGNOSIS:
> Elevated serum and CSF lactate
> Ragged red fibers
> Abnormal mitochondria in blood vessels
> CT SCAN: basal ganglia calcification
> MRI: posterior cortex lesions, spare deep white matter; can resolve

Figure 5-46. MELAS syndrome demonstrating degenerated EOM with trichome stain shows "ragged red" fibers. (Case presented by Dr. R. Folberg to the meeting of the Verhoeff Society, 1993, and reported by Rummett V, et al: *Ophthalmology*, 100:1757, 1993.)

MERRF: **M**yoclonus, **E**pilepsy, and **R**agged **R**ed Fibers (Box 5-2)

BOX 5-2. Ocular Manifestations of Childhood Cerebral Degenerations

Conjunctival telangiectasia: ataxia telangiectasia, Fabry's disease
Glaucoma: MPS I—Scheie's, Zellweger's disease (rare)
Corneal opacity: MPS I, III, IV, VI; mucolipidoses III, IV; Fabry's disease, sialidosis with chondrodystrophy, Cockayne's disease, xeroderma pigmentosum, Zellweger's disease (occasionally), Wilson's disease (Kayser-Fleischer ring)

Lens opacity: Wilson's disease, galactosemia, Marinesco-Sjögren syndrome, Lowe's disease, cerebrocutaneous xanthomatosis, sialidosis, mannosidosis

Cherry red spot: Tay-Sachs disease, sialidosis, Niemann-Pick disease (50%), GM gangliosidosis (50%), Farber's disease, multiple sulfatase deficiency (metachromatic leukodystrophy variant)

Macular and pigmentary degeneration: ceroid lipofuscinosis, MPS 1-H, 1-S, II, III; mucolipidoses IV, Refsum's disease (phytanic acid lipidosis), Bassen-Kornzweig (abetalipoproteinemia), Kearns-Sayre syndrome

Optic atrophy: Krabbe's disease, metachromatic leukodystrophy, sphingolipidoses, adrenoleuko-dystrophy, Alexander's disease, spongy degeneration, Pelizaeus-Merzbacher disease, neuraxonal dystrophy, Alpers' disease, spinocerebellar degeneration, diseases with retinal pigmentary degeneration

Nystagmus: diseases with poor vision (searching nystagmus), Pelizaeus-Merzbacher disease, metachromatic leukodystrophy, Friedreich's ataxia, other spinocerebellar degenerations and cerebellar atrophies, neuraxonal dystrophy, ataxiatelangiectasia, Leigh's syndrome, Marinesco-Sjögren syndrome, opsoclonus-myoclonus syndrome, Chédiak-Higashi disease

Ophthalmoplegia: Leigh's syndrome, Kearns-Sayre syndrome, Niemann-Pick variant with vertical ophthalmoplegia, Gaucher's disease, Bassen-Kornzweig syndrome, ataxia-telangiectasia, Tangier's disease

Strabismus

ANATOMY AND PHYSIOLOGY

Subconjunctival Fascia (Figure 5-47)

Tenon's capsule
   Anterior: fuses with conjunctiva just behind limbus
   Posterior: separates orbital fat from muscles and globe

Intermuscular septum: extension of Tenon's, connects muscles

Check ligaments: connect muscles to overlying Tenon's and inserts on orbital walls to support globe

Lockwood's ligament: fusion of sheaths of inferior rectus and inferior oblique; attaches to medial and lateral retinaculi and supports globe

Extraocular Muscles (Figures 5-48 to 5-50) (Table 5-9)

All rectus muscles have 2 accompanying ciliary arteries, except lateral rectus, which has 1

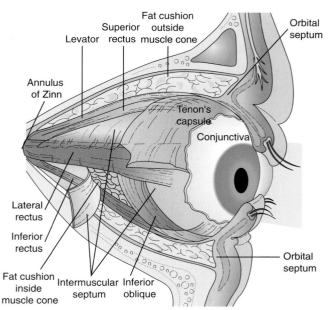

Figure 5-47. Muscle cone. (From Campolattaro BN, Wang FM: Anatomy and physiology of the extraocular muscles and surrounding tissues. In Yanoff M, Duker JS [eds]: *Ophthalmology*, 2nd ed, St. Louis, Mosby, 2004.)

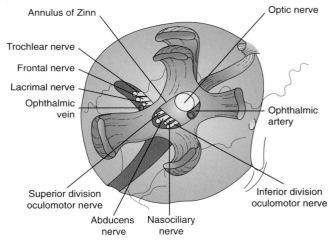

Figure 5-48. The annulus of Zinn and surrounding structures. (From Campolattaro BN, Wang FM: Anatomy and physiology of the extraocular muscles and surrounding tissues. In Yanoff M, Duker JS [eds]: *Ophthalmology*, 2nd ed, St. Louis, Mosby, 2004.)

Spiral of Tillaux: Continuous curve that passes through insertions of rectus muscles; the temporal aspect of vertical muscles lies farther from limbus than the nasal aspect (Figure 5-51)

Medial rectus (MR):

1. Pure adductor

2. Closest to limbus

3. Hardest to find if slipped because no fascial attachment to an oblique muscle

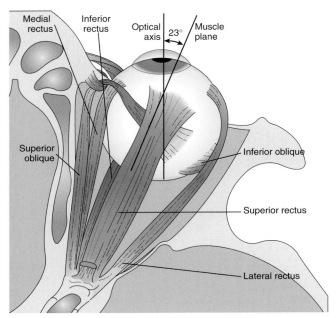

Figure 5-49. The extrinsic mucles of the right eyeball in the primary position, seen from above. The muscles are shown as partially transparent. (From Campolattaro BN, Wang FM: Anatomy and physiology of the extraocular muscles and surrounding tissues. In Yanoff M, Duker JS [eds]: *Ophthalmology*, 2nd ed, St. Louis, Mosby, 2004.)

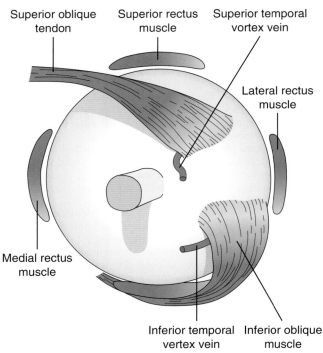

Figure 5-50. Posterior view of the eye with Tenon's capsule removed. (From Campolattaro BN, Wang FM: Anatomy and physiology of the extraocular muscles and surrounding tissues. In Yanoff M, Duker JS [eds]: *Ophthalmology*, 2nd ed, St. Louis, Mosby, 2004.)

Table 5-9. Extraocular Muscles

Muscle	Muscle Length (mm)	Tendon Length (mm)	Arc of Contact (mm)	Anatomic Insertion from Limbus	Action from Primary Position	Origin	Innervation
Medial rectus (MR)	40	4.5	7	5.5 mm	Adduction	Annulus of Zinn	CN 3, (inferior division)
Lateral rectus (LR)	40	7	12	6.9 mm	Abduction	Annulus of Zinn	CN 6
Superior rectus (SR)	40	6	6.5	7.7 mm	1. Elevation 2. Intorsion 3. Adduction	Annulus of Zinn	CN 3, (superior division)
Inferior rectus (IR)	40	7	6.5	6.5 mm	1. Depression 2. Extorsion 3. Adduction	Annulus of Zinn	CN 3, (inferior division)
Superior oblique (SO)	32	26	7–8	Posterior to equator in superotemporal quadrant	1. Intorsion 2. Depression 3. Abduction	Orbital apex above annulus of Zinn	CN 4
Inferior oblique (IO)	37	1	15	Posterior to equator in inferotemporal quadrant	1. Extorsion 2. Elevation 3. Abduction	Behind lacrimal fossa	CN 3, (inferior division)
Levator palpebrae	40	14–20	—	Septa of pretarsal orbicularis and anterior surface of tarsus	Lid elevation	Orbital apex above annulus of Zinn	CN 3, (superior division)

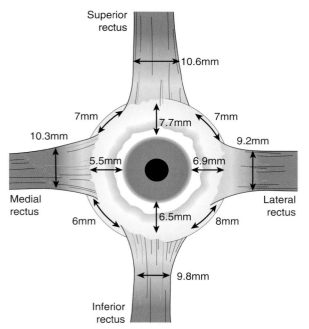

Figure 5-51. Spiral of Tillaux. The structure of the rectus muscle insertions. (From Campolattaro BN, Wang FM: Anatomy and physiology of the extraocular muscles and surrounding tissues. In Yanoff M, Duker JS [eds]: *Ophthalmology*, 2nd ed, St. Louis, Mosby, 2004.)

Lateral rectus (LR):

1. Pure abductor

2. Easiest exposure

3. Connected to inferior oblique

Superior rectus (SR):

1. Elevates, adducts, and incyclotorts

2. Inserts 23° temporal to visual axis in primary position; pure elevator only in 23° abduction

3. Fascial connections: SO, upper eyelid elevators (therefore, SR recession may cause lid retraction, and resection may cause fissure narrowing)

4. Passes over superior oblique

Inferior rectus (IR):

1. Depresses, abducts, and excyclotorts

2. Inserts 23° temporal to visual axis in primary position; pure depressor only in 23° abduction

3. Fascial connections: IO, lower eyelid retractors (Lockwood's ligament). Therefore, IR recession may cause lid retraction, and resection may cause fissure narrowing

Superior oblique (SO):

1. Incyclotorts, abducts, and depresses

2. Inserts 51° to visual axis; pure depressor only in 51° adduction

3. Passes inferior to SR

4. Arises from orbital apex above annulus of Zinn (lesser wing of sphenoid)

Inferior oblique (IO):

1. Excyclotorts, abducts, and elevates

2. Inserts 51° to visual axis

3. Passes inferior to IR

4. Originates from periosteum of maxillary bone

5. Inserts near macula

6. Avoid inferotemporal vortex vein during surgery

7. The inferior division of CN 3 up to the inferior oblique carries parasympathetic supply to iris constrictor; injury to these fibers results in mydriasis

Pediatric Eye Examination

Visual development:
> *At birth*: blinking response to bright lights
> *At 7 days*: vestibulo-ocular response
> *At 2 months*: fixation well developed
> *At 6 months*: VER acuity at adult level
> *At 2 years*: Snellen acuity at adult level
> *At 7 years*: stereoacuity at adult level

Hyperopia (average of 2 D) increases during first year of life; 50% have >1 D with-the-rule astigmatism; decreases after 7 years of age

Vision testing:
> *Infancy*: optokinetic response, forced preferential looking (Teller acuity cards), visual evoked response (VER)
> *Older children*: Allen pictures, HOTV or tumbling E, Snellen acuity

Sensory Testing

Binocular vision:
> *Horopter*: object points imaged on corresponding retinal points
> *Panum's fusional space*: region around horopter in which binocular vision exists (Figure 5-52)
> *Types of binocularity*:
>> SIMULTANEOUS PERCEPTION: ability to see 2 images, 1 on each retina (super-imposed, not blended)
>> FUSION: simultaneous perception of 2 similar images blended as 1

Table 5-10. Normal Fusional Amplitudes (prism diopters)

Testing Distance	Convergence	Divergence	Vertical
6 m	14△	6△	2.5△
25 cm	38△	16△	2.6△

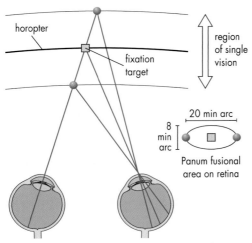

Figure 5-52. Panum's fusional area. The left eye fixates a square target, and a search object visible only to the right eye is moved before and behind this target. The ellipse of retinal area, for which typical dimensions are given for the parafoveal area, is the projection of Panum's fusional area. Diplopia is not perceived for 2 targets within this area. (From Diamond GR: Sensory status in strabismus. In Yanoff M, Duker JS [eds]: *Ophthalmology*, London, Mosby, 1999.)

STEREOPSIS: perception of 2 slightly dissimilar images blended as 1 with appreciation of depth

STEREOACUITY: occurs when retinal disparity is too small to cause diplopia, but too great to allow superimposition of fusion of the 2 visual directions. Normal is 20–50 seconds of arc

TITMUS STEREOTEST: readily available, monocular clues present. Determines NRC in binocular patient.

EXAMPLE: Fly = 3000 arc seconds; animals = 400, 200, 100 arc seconds; circles = 800 – 40 arc seconds

RANDOM DOT STEREOGRAMS: monocular clues absent but more difficult for children to understand

Sensory phenomena associated with strabismus:

Diplopia: simultaneous perception of similar images falling on noncorresponding retinal points

Visual confusion: simultaneous perception of dissimilar images falling on corresponding retinal points

Sensory adaptations to diplopia and visual confusion:

Suppression (scotoma): image from 1 eye is inhibited or does not reach consciousness (Figure 5-53)

CENTRAL: adaptation to avoid confusion

PERIPHERAL: adaptation to avoid diplopia

OBLIGATORY: present all the time

FACULTATIVE: present only when eyes are deviated

TESTS:

WORTH 4 DOT: with red lens over 1 eye and green lens over other eye, patient views red,

Figure 5-53. Suppression scotomas for esotropia (ET) and exotropia (XT).

green, and white lights. Green light is visible to eye under green lens, red light visible to eye under red lens, and white light visible to both eyes. Determines binocularity. May be used to define the size and location of a suppression scotoma in patients with strabismus (Figure 5-55)

Esotropic left eye with ARC and suppression or with monofixation syndrome, fixing with right eye

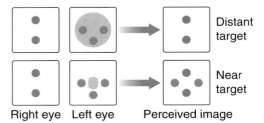

Esotropic right eye with ARC and suppression or with monofixation syndrome, fixing with left eye

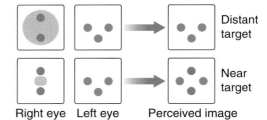

Figure 5-54. Possible Worth 4 Dot percepts in binocular patients. Note the similar distant responses in patients who have esotropia with abnormal retinal correspondence (ARC) and suppression and in those who have monofixation syndrome. Patients who have exotropia with ARC and suppression give the same responses, but the suppression scotoma is larger and shaped somewhat differently. The red lens is over the right eye, and the green lens is over the left eye. (From Diamond GR: Sensory status in strabismus. In Yanoff M, Duker JS [eds]: *Ophthalmology*, 2nd ed, St. Louis, Mosby, 2004.)

Performed at distance (central fusion) and at near (peripheral fusion)

Results:

Suppression: 2 red or 3 green lights seen

Fusion: 4 lights seen

Diplopia: 5 lights seen

Any strabismus in patient fixing right eye

Any strabismus in patient fixing left eye

Figure 5-55. Possible Worth 4 Dot responses in patients who do not have binocularity. The red lens is over the right eye, and the green lens is over the left eye. (From Diamond GR: Sensory status in strabismus. In Yanoff M, Duker JS [eds]: *Ophthalmology*, London, Mosby, 1999.)

4-PRISM DIOPTER TEST: for small suppression scotomas. 4-prism diopter prism placed base out over 1 eye; if suppression scotoma present, eye will not move

HORROR FUSIONIS: intractable diplopia with absence of central suppression

Abnormal retinal correspondence (ARC): (see following)

Monofixation syndrome: binocular sensory state in patients with small angle strabismus (<8 prism diopters; microtropia)

CHARACTERISTICS:

Central scotoma and peripheral fusion present with binocular viewing

Usually ET, may appear XT or orthophoric

Amblyopia common, usually mild

Stereoacuity reduced

Central or eccentric fixation

Typically occurs when preexisting strabismus is controlled nonoperatively or after surgery, but may occur in nonstrabismic patients, also from macular lesions and anisometropia

Decompensation occurs when the deviation changes from a latent to a manifest one

DIAGNOSIS: 4-prism diopter base-out prism test (used to shift image outside scotoma to cause eye movement). In normal patient, when prism is placed in front of 1 eye, eyes turn and then refixate

In monofixation syndrome, when prism is placed in front of normal eye, there is no refixation movement, and when prism is placed in front of eye with scotoma, there is no initial eye turn

Retinal correspondence: the ability of the sensory system to appreciate the perceived direction of the fovea and other retinal elements in each eye relative to each other

Corresponding retinal points: 2 retinal points (1 in each eye) that, when stimulated simultaneously, result in the subjective sensation that the stimulating target comes from the same direction in space. If diplopia occurs, then the 2 points are noncorresponding

Normal retinal correspondence (NRC): corresponding areas of the retina that have identical relationships to the fovea of each eye

CHARACTERISTICS:

Occurs in straight eyes under binocular conditions

Occurs in eyes in which the objective and subjective angles of strabismus are the same; measured with amblyoscope (patient superimposes dissimilar targets)

OBJECTIVE ANGLE: measured angle

SUBJECTIVE ANGLE: the amount of prism required to superimpose the images or promote fusion

Other dissimilar target tests: Lancaster red-green test and Hess screen; require NRC; used to measure paretic strabismus

Abnormal retinal correspondence (ARC): corresponding areas of the retina that have dissimilar relationships to their respective foveas. Sensory adaptation eliminates peripheral diplopia and confusion by permitting fusion of similar images projecting onto noncorresponding retinal areas

CHARACTERISTICS:

Change in visual direction of retinal points

Manifests only during binocular viewing

Objective and subjective angles are not equal

Sensory adaptation of immature visual system to strabismus

Prevents diplopia

Accompanied by scotoma

No fusional amplitudes and no stereopsis

Fovea in deviating eye and fovea in fixing eye do not have the same visual direction

Fovea of fixing eye shares common visual direction with peripheral area of the nonfixing eye

HARMONIOUS ARC: subjective angle is zero

UNHARMONIOUS ARC: subjective angle is greater than zero but less than objective angle

TESTS FOR ARC:

AFTERIMAGE TEST: label fovea of each eye with a linear light afterimage (vertical image for deviating eye and horizontal image for fixing eye). Each eye is stimulated individually (monocular), then patient draws perceived afterimages:

NRC: cross with central gap

ET with ARC: afterimages crossed

XT with ARC: afterimages uncrossed (Figure 5-56)

BAGOLINI LENSES: glasses have no dioptric power but have narrow striations running at 45° and 135°. With glasses on, patient fixes on a light and draws perceived image. Allows determination of strabismus as well as retinal correspondence. Break in line is proportional to size of suppression scotoma (Figure 5-57)

Test

Horizontal flash before fixing eye, vertical flash before nonfixing eye. Flash one eye at a time. After both eyes flashed, ask patient to close eyes; positive afterimage is seen. When eyes open, negative afterimage noted.

Results

Normal retinal correspondence | Abnormal retinal correspondence (assume right strabismus, vertical flash before right eye)

esotropia   exotropia

Figure 5-56. Afterimage test percepts, central fixation. Shown are those possible in patients who have central fixation and binocular vision. (From Diamond GR: Sensory status in strabismus. In Yanoff M, Duker JS [eds]: *Ophthalmology*, 2nd ed, St. Louis, Mosby, 2004.)

Figure 5-57. Possible Bagolini lens percepts, central fixation. (From Diamond GR: Sensory status in strabismus. In Yanoff M, Duker JS [eds]: *Ophthalmology*, London, Mosby, 1999.)

RED GLASS TEST: with red glass in front of deviating eye, patient fixes on light; angular deviation can be measured with a Maddox rod to determine retinal correspondence
ET: uncrossed images
XT: crossed images
Harmonious ARC: patient sees pink light
AMBLYOSCOPE: device with which patient views 2 dissimilar targets and attempts to superimpose them
NRC: objective and subjective angles of strabismus are equal
Harmonious ARC: subjective angle equals zero (arms of amblyoscope are parallel)

Unharmonious ARC: subjective angle is between zero and objective angle

Amblyopia

Unilateral or bilateral reduction of visual acuity that cannot be attributed directly to any structural abnormality of the eye or visual system. Due to disuse of fovea

Characteristics: prevalence 2% to 4%; may coexist with visual loss attributable to uncorrectable structural abnormality of the eye. Preventable or reversible with appropriately timed intervention

Types:
   Strabismic: crowding phenomenon (letters or symbols are more difficult to recognize if closely surrounded by similar forms; therefore, visual acuity may substantially improve with isolate letters); neutral density filters do not reduce acuity as much in the amblyopic eye as in the normal eye
   Refractive: high ametropia (hyperopia of +6 D, myopia of –10 to 12 D, astigmatism of 2.5 D) or anisometropia (1 to 1.5 D for hyperopia, 6 D for myopia, 2 to 3 D for astigmatism)
   Deprivation: media opacity, ptosis, occlusion
   Organic: optic nerve or retinal abnormality

Diagnosis: reduced visual acuity that cannot be entirely explained by physical abnormalities

Treatment: treat amblyopia before strabismus surgery (eliminate any obstacle to vision, remove significant congenital lens opacity by 2 months of age). Force use of poorer eye by limiting use of better eye (full-time occlusion, part-time occlusion, optical degradation of better eye, atropinization of better eye). Full-time occlusion for 1 week per year of age at most; continue until no further improvement. Reevaluate until 9 years of age

Prognosis: good for strabismic, poor for deprivation

Motor Testing

Ductions: monocular rotations of eye

Versions: conjugate binocular eye movements

Vergence: disconjugate binocular eye movement

Agonist: primary muscle moving eye in given direction

Synergist: secondary muscle that acts with agonist to move eye in given direction

Antagonist: muscle that acts to move eye in opposite direction as agonist

Yoke muscles: 2 muscles, 1 in each eye, that act to move respective eyes into a cardinal position

Cardinal positions: 6 positions of gaze in which 1 muscle of the eye is the prime mover

Midline positions: straight up and straight down from primary position

Table 5-11. Agonists, Synergists, and Antagonists

Agonist	Synergists	Antagonists
Medial rectus (MR)	SR, IR	LR, SO, IO
Lateral rectus (LR)	SO, IO	MR, SR, IR
Superior rectus (SR)	IO, MR	IR, SO
Inferior rectus (IR)	SO, MR	SR, IO
Superior oblique (SO)	IO, LR	IO, SR
Inferior oblique (IO)	SR, LR	SO, IR

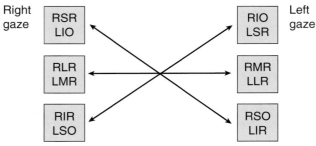

Figure 5-58. Cardinal positions and yoke muscles.

Hering's law (equal innervation): equal and simultaneous innervation to synergistic muscles; amount of innervation to eyes is determined by the fixating eye; therefore, the amount of deviation depends on which eye is fixating:

Primary deviation (paralytic strabismus): deviation measured with normal eye fixing

Secondary deviation (paralytic strabismus): deviation measured with paretic eye fixing; larger than primary deviation

Hering's law also explains the term "inhibitional paresis of the contralateral antagonist"

This is the incorrect impression that a muscle in the normal eye is responsible for the ocular misalignment and may occur in an SO palsy when the paretic eye fixes (e.g., in SO palsy, less innervation is required by the antagonist [IO], and therefore, less innervation is directed to the yoke [contralateral SR]). The contralateral antagonist is actually the antagonist of the yoke of the paretic muscle

Sherrington's law (reciprocal innervation): innervation to ipsilateral antagonist decreases as innervation to the agonist increases

Angle Kappa (κ): angle between visual axis and anatomic axis (pupillary axis) of eye

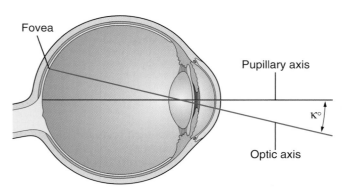

Figure 5-59. The angle κ. This is the displacement in degrees of the pupillary axis from the optic axis. The positive-angle κ provides the illusion of exotropia in the left eye. (From Diamond GR: Sensory status in strabismus. In Yanoff M, Duker JS [eds]: *Ophthalmology*, 2nd ed, St. Louis, Mosby, 2004.)

Positive-angle κ: temporal position of fovea relative to pupillary axis; causes slight temporal rotation of globe to keep image in focus; light reflex appears nasal. May cause a pseudoexotropia or increase the apparent degree of an XT, and lessen or mask an ET

EXAMPLES: ROP, *Toxocara*

Negative-angle κ: nasal position of fovea relative to pupillary axis; causes slight nasal rotation of globe to keep image in focus; light reflex appears temporal. May cause a pseudoesotropia or increase the apparent degree of an ET, and lessen or mask an XT

Eccentric fixation: consistent use of a nonfoveal region of retina for monocular viewing in an amblyopic eye; a monocular phenomenon

Detecting deviations:

Corneal light reflex: if equal, no manifest deviation (tropia) but may have latent deviation (phoria); if unequal, tropia is present

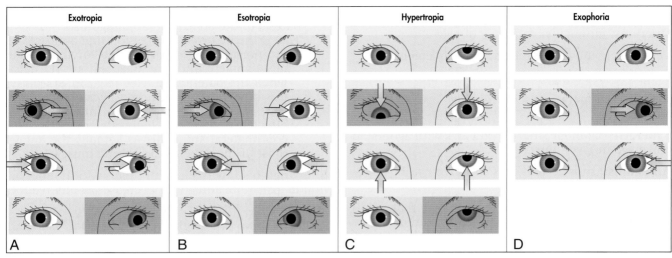

Figure 5-60. Cover test for tropias and phorias. **A**, For exotropia, covering the right eye drives inward movement of the left eye to take up fixation; uncovering the right eye shows recovery of fixation by the right eye and leftward movement of both eyes; covering the left eye discloses no shift of the preferred right eye. **B**, For esotropia, covering the right eye drives outward movement of the left eye to take up fixation; uncovering the right eye shows recovery of fixation by the right eye and rightward movement of both eyes; covering the left eye discloses no shift of the preferred right eye. **C**, For hypertropia, covering the right eye drives downward movement of the left eye to take up fixation; uncovering the right eye shows recovery of fixation by the right eye and upward movement of both eyes; covering the left eye shows no shift of the preferred right eye. **D**, For exophoria, the left eye deviates outward behind a cover and returns to primary position when the cover is removed. An immediate inward movement denotes a phoria, a delayed inward movement denotes an intermittent exotropia. (From Diamond G, Eggers H: *Strabismus and Pediatric Ophthalmology*, London, Mosby, 1993.)

Monocular cover-uncover test: tests for phoria or tropia by detecting movement of eyes when 1 eye is covered and then uncovered (Figure 5-60)

Measuring deviations:
Modified Krimsky's method: place prism over fixating eye to center the corneal light reflex over the pupil; place over deviating eye in incomitant or paralytic deviations (Figure 5-61)
Hirschberg's method: estimate each millimeter of decentration of corneal light reflex from the center of the pupil (1 mm equals 7° or 15 prism diopters of deviation) (Figure 5-62)
Simulataneous prism cover test or cover-uncover test: measures tropia
Alternate cover testing: measures tropia and phoria
Measurements are affected by corrective lenses: minus (concave lenses; myopia) measures more, and plus (convex lenses; hyperopia) measures less, due to the prismatic effect of the lenses. Difference = 2.5% × D

Other tests:
Double Maddox rod test: measures torsion
Parks-Bielschowsky 3-step test: identifies cyclovertical palsy
1. Which eye has hyperdeviation?
   Identify weak depressors in higher eye (IR, SO) and elevators in lower eye (IO, SR)
2. Is hyperdeviation greater in right or left gaze?
   Identify muscles that act in direction as hyperdeviation increases
      Right gaze: SR and IR of right eye, IO and SO of left eye

Left gaze: IO and SO of right eye, SR and IR of left eye
3. Is hyperdeviation greater with right or left head tilt?
   Identify torting muscles that act in direction as hyperdeviation increases
      Right head tilt:
         Intorsion of right eye (SR and SO)
         Extorsion of left eye (IO and IR)
      Left head tilt is reversed
      (Remember: **S**upinate—**s**uperiors **i**ntort)
   Circle involved muscles at each step described previously (see Figure 5-63). Muscle with 3 circles is the one with palsy

EXAMPLE: RSO palsy (Figure 5-63)

Forced duction test: determines deviation due to muscle restriction
Forced generation test: measures muscle strength

NYSTAGMUS

Oscillation of eyes

Childhood forms are most commonly congenital, latent, sensory, and spasmus nutans

Congenital

Benign disorder of eye movement calibration system (between sensory and motor systems)

Characteristics: long-standing, horizontal in all positions, may have rotary component, increases

A

B

C

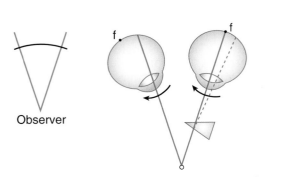

Observer

D

Figure 5-61. Modified Krimsky's method of estimating deviation. (From von Noorden GK: *Von Noorden-Maumenee's Atlas of Strabismus*, 3rd ed, St. Louis, Mosby, 1977.)

intensity with fixation, null point, no oscillopsia, may have head posture dampened by convergence (better near than distance vision), exponentially increasing velocity of slow phase, OKN reversal in 60%, strabismus in 33%, similar monocular and binocular vision (20/20–20/70), absent during sleeping, latent nystagmus can be present (cover 1 eye, nystagmus converts to jerk away from covered eye), may develop head oscillations at 3 months of age, wide-swinging eye movements; at 1 year, small pendular movements; at 2 years, jerk nystagmus with null zone, discover convergence dampens nystagmus and may develop nystagmus blockage syndrome

Waveform: exponentially increasing velocity of slow phase

A   Normal

B   15° ET

C   30° ET

D   45° ET

Figure 5-62. Hirschberg's method of estimating deviation. (From von Noorden GK: *Von Noorden-Maumenee's Atlas of Stabismus*, 3rd ed, St. Louis, Mosby, 1977.)

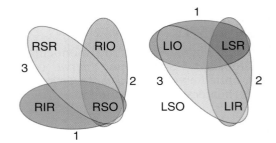

Figure 5-63. Parks-Bielschowsky 3-step test for RSO palsy.

Associations: albinism, aniridia, Leber's congenital amaurosis, ON hypoplasia, congenital cataracts, achromatopsia

Treatment: base-out prisms in glasses dampen nystagmus by forcing patient to converge (only fusional convergence [overcoming exophoria] diminishes the nystagmus; therefore, minus lenses that stimulate accommodative convergence do not dampen nystagmus); if head posture >50% of time, surgical correction (Kestenbaum procedure)

Distinguish congenital nystagmus from latent nystagmus:

Cover 1 eye: latent nystagmus worsens

Reversal of normal OKN response: congenital nystagmus

Dampens with convergence: congenital nystagmus

Examine slow-phase velocity: increases (congenital), decreases (latent)

Latent

Jerk nystagmus during monocular viewing away from covered eye

Associated with congenital esotropia and DVD

Pure form is rare

Etiology: abnormal cortical binocularity, proprioceptive imbalance, defective egocentric localization

Characteristics: cover 1 eye and uncovered eye develops nystagmus, fast phase to side of fixing eye; long-standing; normal OKN response; nulls with adduction; normal vision when both eyes open, vision decreases when each eye is tested separately; may have strabismus, especially infantile esotropia, DVD (50%)

Waveform: exponentially decreasing velocity of slow phase

Alexander's rule: intensity increases when looking toward fast phase and decreases when looking toward slow phase (i.e., adduction nulls; therefore, no head posture)

Treatment: surgery for strabismus or head turn

Sensory

Pendular nystagmus due to visual loss; more common than congenital nystagmus

Etiology: aniridia, albinism, rod monochromatism (achromatopsia), CSNB, optic nerve coloboma, cataracts, optic nerve hypoplasia, Leber's congenital amaurosis, bilateral macular coloboma

Spasmus Nutans

Benign form of nystagmus consisting of fine, rapid, often monocular or markedly asymmetric eye movements

Diagnosis of exclusion

Onset during first year of life with spontaneous resolution by age 3 years

Triad of findings: eye movements, head nodding/bobbing, torticollis (diagnosis can be made in absence of head nodding)

Waveform: high frequency, low amplitude, pendular, asymmetric (dissociated form of nystagmus)

DDx: chiasmal glioma, subacute necrotizing encephalomyopathy

Neuroimaging: rule out tumor

Acquired Nystagmus (see Chapter 4, Neuro-ophthalmology)

OCULAR ALIGNMENT

Horizontal Deviations

At birth, 40% of infants are orthophoric, 33% are XT, 3% to 5% are ET

Sensory deprivation, in a child (< age 6) usually causes ET; in an adult, usually causes XT

Orthophoria: normal alignment; no latent or manifest deviation exists. Eyes are straight

Comitant: deviation is equal in all positions of gaze

Incomitant: deviation varies in different positions of gaze (paralytic or restrictive etiologies)

Esodeviations: latent or manifest convergence of the visual axes

Most common deviation (50% to 75%)

Types:

PSEUDOESOTROPIA: patient is orthophoric but has appearance of esotropia. Due to broad nasal bridge, prominent medial epicanthal folds, or negative-angle κ

ESOPHORIA (E): latent deviation controlled by fusional mechanisms; may manifest under certain conditions (fatigue, illness, stress, or tests that dissociate eyes [alternate cover test])

INTERMITTENT ESOTROPIA (E(T)): deviation that is sometimes latent and sometimes manifest; partially controlled by fusional mechanisms

ESOTROPIA (ET): manifest deviation (Box 5-3)

Exodeviations: latent or manifest divergence of the visual axes

Less common than ET

Account for 25% of strabismus in children

In neonates, up to 60% have a constant, transient exodeviation

Most common form is intermittent exotropia

Types:

PSEUDOEXOTROPIA: patient is orthophoric but has appearance of exotropia. Due to positive-angle κ without other abnormalities, macular heterotopia (temporally dragged macula [PHPV, ROP, toxocariasis] with large angle κ), wide interpupillary distance

EXOPHORIA (X): latent deviation. Detected by alternate cover testing. May be related to asthenopia

INTERMITTENT EXOTROPIA (X(T)): deviation that is sometimes latent and sometimes manifest; partially controlled by fusional mechanisms

BOX 5-3. **Classification of Esotropia**

Infantile
    Classic congenital
    Early-onset accommodative
    Duane's type I
    Abducens paralysis from birth trauma
    Nystagmus blockage syndrome
    Möbius' syndrome
Acquired
    Accommodative
        Refractive
        Nonrefractive
        Mixed (partially accommodative and partially
            basic)
        Decompensated
    Nonaccommodative
        Stress-induced acquired
        Cyclic
        Acute comitant
        Sensory deprivation
        Divergence insufficiency
        Divergence paralysis
        Spasm of near synkinetic reflex
        Restrictive (thyroid-related, medial orbital wall
            fracture, over-resected MR)
        Lateral rectus weakness (CN 6 palsy,
            iatrogenic/surgical [slipped, detached, over-
            recessed LR])

EXOTROPIA (XT): manifest deviation
    BASIC: exodeviation equal at distance and near
    DIVERGENCE EXCESS: exodeviation greater at distance than near by at least 10 prism diopters
    Types:
        Simulated (pseudodivergence excess): enhanced fusional convergence at near related to accommodation 30-minute patch test: binocular fusional impulses suspended and exodeviation becomes equal at distance and near. If near deviation increases to close to distance deviation with +3.00 lenses, then high AC/A ratio exists
        True: after 30-minute patch test, still has divergence excess at distance
    CONVERGENCE INSUFFICIENCY: near exotropia is greater than distance exotropia

Congenital Esotropia

1% to 2% of all strabismus

Equal sex distribution

Present by 6 months of age

Family history of strabismus is common

Increased frequency in cerebral palsy or hydrocephalus

Findings: deviation usually ≥30 prism diopters, low amounts of hyperopia, often cross fixation with equal visual acuity in each eye, rarely develop normal binocular vision (even with surgery)

Associations:
    Dissociated vertical deviation (DVD) in 70%
    Overaction of inferior obliques in 70%
        Involved eye elevates with adduction
        Onset usually in second year of life; greatest occurrence between ages 3 and 7
        Treat with IO weakening procedure
    Latent nystagmus
        Congenital, conjugate, horizontal jerk nystagmus that occurs under monocular conditions
        When 1 eye is occluded, nystagmus develops in both eyes with fast phase toward the fixing eye and slow phase toward the occluded eye
        MANIFEST LATENT NYSTAGMUS: nystagmus present when both eyes are open
            Because of induced nystagmus in the uncovered eye with latent nystagmus, binocular visual acuity is better than when each eye is tested individually
        NYSTAGMUS BLOCKAGE SYNDROME: overaccommodation to dampen nystagmus results in ET at near (usually large). Can differentiate from essential infantile esotropia (EIE) with manifest latent nystagmus because nystagmus does not increase with occlusion of 1 eye. Nystagmus dampens in convergence or adduction and increases in primary or lateral gaze. Adduction continues even when 1 eye is occluded, and head turn occurs toward the uncovered eye when the fellow eye is occluded. With adduction effort, the pupil constricts, demonstrating that accommodative mechanisms are present. May treat with large (6 mm+) bimedial resections using a Faden suture
    Asymmetry of the monocular, optokinetic motion–processing response
        Nasal to temporal smooth pursuit less well developed than temporal to nasal pursuit
        Can establish congenital nature of ET in an older patient
        Asymmetry also seen in healthy newborns and disappears by 6 months of age

Diagnosis:
    Demonstrate potential for full abduction with vestibular ocular reflex and doll's head maneuver to rule out congenital CN 6 palsy
    Look for synkinetic lid or eye movements with attempted horizontal gaze to rule out Duane's syndrome
    Rule out accommodative component with glasses if older than age 1 or phospholine iodide 0.06% or 0.12%

Treatment:
    Nonsurgical:
        Correct amblyopia before surgery

Cross fixation suggests equal visual acuity of both eyes

Early surgery (as early as 6 months):

Potential for sensory binocular fusion

Aim for alignment within 10 PD of orthophoria

PROCEDURES:

Bilateral medial rectus recession

Recess medial rectus muscle and resect lateral rectus muscle of 1 eye

Associated surgery of inferior obliques if overaction present

3 or 4 muscle surgeries for large deviation

Accommodative Esotropia

Onset 6 months to 7 years

May be intermittent at onset

Often, positive family history

Associated with amblyopia (generally from anisometropia)

May be precipitated by trauma or illness

Types: (Table 5-12)

Accommodative convergence to accommodation (AC/A) ratio:

Normally between 3 : 1 and 5 : 1 prism diopters per diopter of accommodation

High AC/A ratio: usually present when near deviation exceeds distance deviation by >10 to 15 PD

Calculation (2 methods):

HETEROPHORIA METHOD: AC/A = IPD + [(N − D)/Diopt]

IPD = interpupillary distance (cm)

N = near deviation

D = distance deviation

Diopt = accommodative demand at fixation distance

EXAMPLE: near deviation = 35; distance deviation = 10; accommodative demand = 20 cm (5D); IPD = 60 mm (6 cm). Therefore, AC/A = 6 + [(35 − 10)/5] = 11 : 1

LENS GRADIENT METHOD: AC/A = (WL − NL)/D

WL = deviation with lens in front of eye

NL = deviation without lens in front of eye

D = dioptric power of lens used

EXAMPLE: near deviation with a +1.00 lens is 50 PD and without a lens is 35 PD. Therefore, AC/A = (50 − 35)/ 1.00 = 15 : 1

Natural history:

Hyperopia may decrease with age

AC/A ratio may normalize, and fusional divergence can improve

May begin to reduce strength of glasses and bifocals slowly as child gets older

Treatment: correct refractive error and treat amblyopia; consider surgery for residual component

Satisfactory: residual esotropia less than 10 prism diopters. Peripheral fusion and expansion of fusional amplitudes possible

Unsatisfactory: try atropine with glasses or long-acting cholinesterase inhibitors; recheck refraction for increased or latent hyperopia

Echothiophate (phospholine iodide) causes accommodation that removes convergence with accommodative effort

Table 5-12. Types of Accommodative Esotropia

Type	Characteristics	Treatment
Refractive accommodative (normal AC/A ratio)	• Esotropia at distance and near within 10 prism diopters • High hyperopia (range +3.00 to +10.00, average = +4.00)	• Full cycloplegic refraction • Treat amblyopia
Nonrefractive accommodative (high AC/A ratio)	• Lower amount of hyperopia (average = +2.25) • Esotropia greater at near than at distance (may resolve with age) • Esotropia reduced at near with plus lens	• Consider bifocal when esotropia at near exceeds distance by 10 prism diopters (executive type) • Consider miotics (phospholine iodide 0.125% or 0.025%) • Surgery if needed for residual esotropia
Mixed mechanism	• Partially accommodative • Angle of deviation reduced but not eliminated with spectacles	• Full cycloplegic refraction • Surgery for nonaccommodative component
Decompensated accommodative	• Residual esotropia after correction with full cycloplegic refraction • Occurs more commonly with high AC/A ratio	• Full cycloplegic refraction • Surgery

Nonaccommodative, Acquired ET

Stress-induced acquired ET: breakdown of fusional divergence that occurs after illness, emotional trauma, or injury. Requires surgery

Cyclic ET: intermittent, usually present every other day (48-hour cycle) and becomes constant with time
  V-pattern ET is common; amblyopia can develop
  On days when ET is not present, normal binocular visual acuity with good stereovision
  Treat with full hyperopic correction
  May also require surgery if glasses do not fully correct deviation
  Phenobarbital and amphetamines can alter the frequency of the cycles

Sensory deprivation ET: due to loss of vision in 1 or both eyes; identify and treat obstruction to vision

Divergence insufficiency: ET greater at distance than near
  Fusional divergence is reduced
  Treat with base-out prisms (to correct diplopia) or surgery
  Rule out divergence paralysis
    Associated with pontine tumors, head trauma, or other neurologic abnormalities
    May mimic bilateral CN 6 paralysis

Spasm of near synkinetic reflex (ciliary spasm):
  Intermittent episodes of sustained convergence with accommodative spasm and miosis
  Findings: headache, blurred distance visual acuity, abnormally close near point, and fluctuating visual acuity
    Recent onset of myopia is present in history (pseudomyopia)
    Variable angle of deviation
    Monocular abduction is normal
    Large difference between manifest and cycloplegic refraction
  Treatment: cycloplegia may break spasm; on post-cycloplegic refraction push plus

Incomitant ET:
  Etiology:
    MR restriction: thyroid, orbital wall fractures, or excessively resected MR muscle
    Slipped muscle following strabismus surgery
    Neurogenic: CN 6 palsy (spontaneous or due to intracranial lesions [33%], infections, or birth trauma)
    Myasthenia gravis

Consecutive esotropia: follows surgery for exotropia; rule out slipped muscle

Prism Adaptation Test: prisms are used to help patients obtain binocular fusion while awaiting surgical alignment of the eyes. Used to preoperatively predict which patients will develop residual esotropia after surgery. Patients who respond with increasing deviation are given stronger prism until orthophoria is obtained. The largest angle is the target for surgical correction

Intermittent Exotropia

Most common form of XT

Onset varies from infancy to age 4

May be progressive

Often have reflex closure of 1 eye in bright light

Suppression only when eyes are deviated (facultative suppression)

Amblyopia uncommon

Natural history:
  Phase 1: X(T) at distance and straight at near
    Present when fatigued
    May see double
    Most maintain excellent stereovision
  Phase 2: X(T) becomes more constant at distance with X(T) at near
    Suppression increases
  Phase 3: XT at far and near
    Often no diplopia because of suppression
    Most common cause of a constant XT

Treatment:
  Treat amblyopia
  Alternate occlusion therapy
  Induce accommodative convergence by prescribing overminus spectacles (also for consecutive exotropia)
  Prism therapy with base-in prisms
  Fusional convergence training (progressive base-out prism to induce convergence)
  Surgery for increased tropic phase, poor recovery of fusion once tropic, increasing ease of dissociation, XT greater than 50% of time at home
    PROCEDURES:
      Bilateral lateral rectus recession
      Recess lateral rectus and resect medial rectus of 1 eye
      3 of 4 muscle surgeries for large deviation

Congenital Exotropia

Rare

May be primary (otherwise healthy patients) or secondary (from ocular or systemic abnormalities)

Usually large angle of deviation (average >35 prism diopters)

Amblyopia is uncommon; similar refractive error to general population

Most resolve by age 6 months; if not, consider surgery

Associations: DVD and oblique muscle overaction; orbital or skull defects, neurologic disease, or other ocular, genetic, or systemic conditions

Convergence Insufficiency

Exophoria greater at near than at distance (not exotropic at near)

Reduced near point of convergence and amplitudes of convergence

Female > male

Common in teenagers and young adults

Associations: can be exacerbated by fatigue, drugs, uveitis, or Adie's tonic pupil; may also follow head trauma

Associated with systemic illnesses, or as a conversion reaction

Findings: asthenopia, diplopia; may have reduced amplitude of accommodation and remote near point of accommodation

Treatment:
Observation
Orthoptic exercises to improve fusional amplitudes
Base-out prisms
Rarely surgery (medial rectus resection)

Convergence Paralysis Secondary to Intracranial Lesion

Normal adduction and accommodation

XT and diplopia on attempted near fixation

Associations: Parinaud's syndrome

Treatment: base-in prisms or occlusion of 1 eye to relieve diplopia

Sensory Exotropia

Due to loss of vision or long-standing poor vision in 1 eye

Children younger than age 5 with unilateral vision loss may develop ET or XT; adults usually develop XT

Angle of deviation may be variable and usually increases with time

Consecutive Exotropia

Follows previous strabismus surgery for esotropia

Vertical Deviations

Dissociated Vertical Deviation (DVD; DHD [Dissociated Horizontal Deviation]; DTD [Dissociated Torsional Deviation])

Intermittent deviation of nonfixing eye consisting of upward excursion, extorsion, excyclotorsion, abduction, or lateral deviation

Exact etiology unknown but associated with early disruption of binocular development

Usually asymptomatic because of poor fusion and suppression

Often asymmetric

Does not obey Hering's law (fellow eye does not exhibit refixation movement in opposite direction)

Occurs with eye occlusion or visual inattention

May be latent or manifest

Usually presents before 12 months of age

Usually more marked when patient is fatigued, daydreaming, under stress, or sick

Associations: nystagmus (latent or manifest latent), inferior oblique overaction, often occurs in patients with history of congenital ET; isolated in 40% of patients

Findings: slow movement of eye in the characteristic direction

Amount of deviation variable; therefore, accurate measurements difficult to obtain

Dissociated deviation occurs in all directions of gaze

Diagnosis:
Bielschowsky's phenomenon:
50% of patients with DVD
Elevated eye will drift downward when light in fixing eye is reduced
Conversely, increased illumination in an eye with DVD will cause it to drift up
Red lens phenomenon:
Place red lens over either eye while patient fixates on light source
Red image is always seen below the white image
In patients with a true hypertropia, the red image is seen above or below the primary image, depending on whether the red filter is placed in front of the hyperdeviated or hypodeviated eye

Treatment:
Increase fusional mechanisms: give optimal spectacle correction; switch fixation to nonpreferred eye
Surgery:
INDICATIONS:
Increasing size or frequency of manifest DVD
Abnormal head position
PROCEDURES:
SR recession
IR resection
IO weakening or anterior transposition (in patients with IOOA and DVD)
CAUTIONS: perform bilateral surgery (unilateral surgery often reveals occult contralateral DVD); often recurs or persists after surgery

Inferior Oblique Overaction (IOOA)

Occurs in 2/3 of patients with congenital ET

Usually bilateral and asymmetric

Early surgery for ET is important for development of binocular vision but does not reduce incidence of IO dysfunction

May be primary (due to paralysis of the antagonist [SO]) or secondary

Findings: when fixing eye is abducted, adducting eye is elevated

> When fixing eye is adducted, abducted eye is depressed
> V-pattern deviation
> Primary position extorsion of fundus on indirect ophthalmoscopy

Treatment:

> ***Surgery***: IO weakening procedure (recession, myectomy, anteriorization)

Inferior Oblique Palsy

Rare

Usually idiopathic but may follow orbital trauma, viral illness, or other neurologic problems

May be bilateral

Findings: eye is hypotropic when fixing with normal eye

> Hypertropia of normal eye when fixing with involved eye
> Deviation worsens with gaze into field of action of involved inferior oblique
> Deviation is worse with head tilt opposite of paretic eye
> Poor elevation in adduction
> Normal forced duction (distinguishes from Brown's syndrome)
> A pattern

Treatment:

> ***With associated SO overaction***: SO weakening procedure. If hyperdeviation develops in downgaze, then weaken contralateral IR
> ***IO palsy with hypotropia in primary gaze and no SO overaction***: IR recession (2.5 prism diopters per mm of recession)

Superior Oblique Overaction

Less common than IO overaction or DVD

Findings: A pattern

> Associated with depression on attempted adduction if fixing with uninvolved eye
> May have associated horizontal deviation

Treatment: weaken overacting SO, with tenotomy (uncontrolled) or silicone spacer (controlled)

Superior Oblique Palsy

Most common isolated cyclovertical muscle palsy

Congenital (75%):

> Large fusional amplitudes (as much as 15 prism diopters or more)
> SO tendon often long or floppy; sometimes absent
> Long-standing CN 4 palsy results in ocular torticollis, which can lead to facial asymmetry
> Examine old photographs to determine duration of head tilt
> Can mimic a double elevator palsy (if fixation preference is for the affected eye, the contralateral SR muscle can appear to underact (inhibitional palsy of the contralateral antagonist) and the contralateral IR can undergo contracture, leading to double elevator palsy)

Acquired: often due to trauma (long course of 4th nerve makes it especially vulnerable)

> ***Findings***: diplopia (vertical, horizontal, or torsional)
> In long-standing cases of SO palsy, comitance develops and the deviation becomes more difficult to localize (hypertropia can be present in all fields of gaze)

Bilateral: objective torsion is often >10° of excyclotorsion (measure with double Maddox rod)

> Often have inferior oblique overaction with V-pattern ET and chin-down head posture
> Alternate hypertropia with head tilt

Diagnosis: Parks-Bielschowsky 3-step test (i.e., right superior oblique palsy produces right hypertropia in primary gaze, worsens in left gaze and in right head tilt)

Treatment: surgery

> ***Indications***: significant head tilt, large hypertropia in primary gaze, diplopia
> ***Procedures***:
> > If deviation in primary gaze is less than 15 prism diopters, operate on 1 muscle; if deviation greater than 15 prism diopters, operate on 2 or more muscles
> > With IO overaction, weaken ipsilateral IO (corrects approximately 15 prism diopters of vertical deviation)
> > If hyperdeviation is greater than 15 prism diopters in primary gaze, strengthen ipsilateral IR or weaken contralateral SR
> > With no inferior oblique overaction, consider weakening ipsilateral SR or recessing contralateral IR; SO tuck may also be considered if there is laxity of the tendon
> > Knapp classification for treatment of superior oblique palsy offers guidance
> > > General principle is to match the fields of greatest deviation to the muscles that work

most in those field to guide surgical approach

Check traction test in operating room to assess laxity of superior oblique tendon

Torsional symptoms:

Most people can tolerate 7° of torsion

Consider Harada-Ito procedure: lateral transposition of anterior portion of SO tendon; corrects excyclotorsion only; no effect on vertical deviation or fusion

Inferior Rectus Palsy

Due to trauma to CN 3 or IR

May occur at time of injury or repair of an orbital fracture

May resolve with time

Double Elevator Palsy (Monocular Elevation Deficiency)

Sporadic, unilateral defect of upgaze associated with ipsilateral ptosis

There are 2 elevators of eye—the SR (provides most of elevation) and the IO

May be supranuclear (may not involve both elevators)

May be congenital or acquired (cerebrovascular disease, tumor, or infection)

Types:

IR restriction:

Positive forced ductions to elevation

Positive force generation (no muscle paralysis)

Normal saccades of SR

Elevator weakness:

Free forced ductions to elevation

Reduced force generation (muscle paralysis)

Reduced velocities of upgaze movements

Combination: IR restriction plus weak elevators

Positive forced ductions to elevation

Reduced force generation (muscle paralysis)

Reduced velocities of upgaze movements

Findings: unilateral limitation of upgaze above midline with accompanying ptosis in both adduction and abduction

Variable head position (normal or chin-up)

Hypotropia increases on upgaze

Fixing with involved eye causes large secondary hypotropia in nonparetic eye

Treatment: surgery

Indications: chin-up head position, large vertical deviation in primary position, poor fusion in primary position

Procedures:

DOUBLE ELEVATOR PALSY WITH TIGHT IR: IR recession

DOUBLE ELEVATOR PALSY WITH SR WEAKNESS: Knapp procedure (elevation and transposition of MR and LR to the side of SR)

DOUBLE ELEVATOR PALSY WITH PTOSIS: correct strabismus then residual ptosis

Brown's Syndrome (SO Tendon Sheath Syndrome)

Inability to elevate the eye in adduction, both actively and passively on forced duction testing

May be congenital or acquired (traumatic, inflammatory, iatrogenic [following SO tuck, glaucoma drainage implant, scleral buckle])

Findings: limitation of elevation in adduction

Less elevation deficiency in midline

Minimal or no elevation deficiency in abduction

V-pattern divergence in upgaze

Restricted forced ductions

Minimal or no superior oblique overaction

"Clicking" may occur and suggests a trochlear problem

Anomalous head posture or hypotropia in primary position may be present

Treatment:

Observation: spontaneous improvement may occur

Surgery:

INDICATIONS: abnormal head position, large hypotropia in primary position, constant deviation causing amblyopia and threatening binocularity

PROCEDURE: superior weakening procedure (SO tenectomy, tenotomy, or silicone spacer)

COMPLICATION: SO palsy

A and V Patterns

Change in horizontal deviation as eyes move between upgaze and downgaze

Up to 50% of all strabismus has an associated A or V pattern

May present as compensatory head posture (chin-up or chin-down) in child with binocular function

A pattern:

Increasing convergence or decreasing divergence in upgaze

Increasing divergence in downgaze

Clinically significant when eyes diverge >10 prism diopters from upgaze to downgaze

V pattern:

Increasing convergence or decreasing divergence in downgaze

Increasing divergence in upgaze

Clinically significant when eyes converge >15 prism diopters from upgaze to downgaze

Etiology:

Oblique muscle dysfunction (obliques are abductors, IO overaction creates a V pattern)

Horizontal rectus muscle dysfunction

Vertical rectus muscle dysfunction

Structural factors (e.g., craniosynostosis is associated with a V pattern, abnormal insertions of rectus muscles, absence of SO tendon)

Diagnosis: measure deviation in primary position, then with eyes directed 25° in upgaze and downgaze

Treatment: surgery

Indications: abnormal head position; to improve motor alignment

Procedures:

If no oblique muscle overaction present, vertical transposition of horizontal muscles

Corrects about 15 prism diopters of the A and V patterns

Muscles are transposed 1/2 to 1 tendon width up or down

Transposition is in the direction of the desired weakening

Mnemonic: MALE (**M**edial rectus to **A**pex of pattern; **L**ateral rectus to the **E**mpty space)

Figure 5-64. Direction of muscle transposition for A and V patterns.

If oblique muscle overaction present, oblique muscle weakening

IO WEAKENING: corrects 15 prism diopters or more of eso shift in upgaze, with no effect on horizontal alignment in primary gaze

BILATERAL SO TENOTOMIES: corrects up to 30–40 prism diopters of eso shift in downgaze; torsional symptoms may occur in patients with good fusion

SPECIAL FORMS OF STRABISMUS

Duane's Retraction Syndrome

Usually sporadic, may be inherited

Co-contraction of medial and lateral rectus muscles causes retraction of the globe with secondary narrowing of the palpebral fissure

Vertical deviations may be present with characteristic upshoot or downshoot (leash phenomenon)

Bilateral in 15% to 20%

Head turn common (for fusion)

Etiology: abnormal innervation of lateral rectus by a branch of CN 3; electromyography shows decreased firing of lateral rectus during abduction and paradoxical innervation of the lateral rectus during adduction

Exact etiology unclear, proposed mechanisms include hypoplasia of 6th nerve nucleus, midbrain pathology, fibrosis of lateral rectus

Types:

Type 1 (most common): limitation of abduction

Retraction and narrowing of palpebral fissures in adduction

Appears esotropic

Type 2: limitation of adduction

Appears exotropic

Type 3: limitation of abduction and adduction

Associations: deafness, crocodile tears, syndromes (Goldenhar's syndrome, Klippel-Feil syndrome, Wildervanck's syndrome [Duane's syndrome associated with Klippel-Feil], Thalidomide toxicity, Fetal alcohol syndrome, Cat-Eye syndrome)

Treatment:

Correct any refractive error

Treat amblyopia

Surgery

INDICATIONS: abnormal head position or deviation in primary gaze

PROCEDURES:

For esotropia, recession of medial rectus muscle

For globe retraction, simultaneous lateral rectus recession

For upshoot or downshoot, splitting of lateral rectus or Faden procedure

Avoid muscle resection (increases globe retraction, upshoots and downshoots)

Möbius' Syndrome

CN 6 and 7 palsies

Due to aplasia of involved brain stem nuclei

Associations: congenital facial diplegia (mask facies); combined CN 6, 7, 9, and 12 palsies; gaze palsy (PPRF involvement); chest, limb, tongue defects

Findings: esotropia with limitation of abduction, exposure keratitis from poor lid closure

Congenital Fibrosis Syndrome

Group of congenital anomalies characterized by variable amounts of restriction of extraocular muscles and replacement of the muscles with fibrous tissue

Nonprogressive

1 or more muscles may be involved

Positive forced duction testing

Types:
    Congenital fibrosis syndrome:
        Most severe
        Usually autosomal dominant, may be recessive
        All extraocular muscles involved, including levator (with ptosis)
    Congenital fibrosis of inferior rectus:
        Sporadic or familial
        Levator may be involved
    Strabismus fixus:
        Severe esotropia
        Horizontal rectus muscles involved (usually MR, occasionally LR)
    Vertical retraction syndrome:
        SR fibrosis (inability to depress eye)
    Congenital unilateral fibrosis:
        Enophthalmos and ptosis
        Fibrosis of all muscles, including levator

Chronic Progressive External Ophthalmoplegia (CPEO)

Sporadic or familial (mitochondrial DNA)

May present at any age

Associations:
    Kearns-Sayre: triad of CPEO, retinal pigmentary changes, and cardiomyopathy
    Bassen-Kornzweig syndrome (abetalipoproteinemia): retinal pigmentary changes similar to RP, diarrhea, ataxia, and other neurologic signs
    Refsum's disease: RP-like syndrome with elevated phytanic acid levels
    Oculopharyngeal dystrophy (AD): difficulty swallowing
    Cardiac conduction defects

Findings: severe ptosis with complete ophthalmoplegia, absent Bell's phenomenon, no restrictions on forced ductions, large-angle strabismus (often exotropia)

Orbital Floor Fracture

Findings: ecchymosis, diplopia in some or all positions of gaze immediately after injury, paresthesia or hypesthesia in distribution of infraorbital nerve, entrapment of inferior rectus muscle or inferior oblique muscle; may have associated ocular damage, may have associated wall fractures (e.g., medial wall with medial rectus entrapment)

Diagnosis:
    Forced duction testing
    Orbital imaging
Treatment:
    Observation: usually 5 to 10 days until edema and hematoma resolve, then reevaluate
    Surgery

Following Surgery

Commonly after cataract, scleral buckle, and glaucoma drainage implant procedures

May be transient and resolve spontaneously

Horizontal, vertical, or torsional

Etiology:
    Mechanical: adhesions, mass effect (implant or buckle)
    Motor: trauma, ischemia, slipped or disinserted muscle, toxicity (local anesthetic; most commonly IR fibrosis with hypotropia in primary gaze that worsens in abduction; positive forced ductions)
    Sensory: fusion breakdown, anisometropia, anisokonia, image distortion

Treatment: observation, prism spectacles, surgery

Other Forms of Strabismus

Myasthenia gravis, thyroid-related ophthalmopathy, CN 3 palsy, skew deviation

STRABISMUS SURGERY

Indications:
    Establish binocularity
    Improve fusion
    Improve symptoms or appearance
Anesthesia:
    Topical: may consider for recession procedures
    Retrobulbar: use shorter-acting anesthetic for adjustable sutures
    General: for children; consider in adults undergoing bilateral surgery
Incisions:
    Fornix: in superior or inferior cul-de-sac on bulbar conjunctiva
    Limbal: conjunctival/Tenon's flap at limbus
    Swan: over the muscle (causes more scarring)

Weakening Procedures

Recession: most common technique used to weaken rectus muscles by moving muscle posteriorly; also used to weaken inferior oblique

Myotomy (cutting across muscle) **or myectomy** (excising a portion of muscle): used to weaken inferior oblique

Denervation and extirpation: used to weaken inferior oblique by ablating all muscle within Tenon's capsule

Tenotomy (cutting across tendon) **or tenectomy** (excising a portion of tendon): most commonly used to weaken superior oblique

Posterior fixation suture (Faden procedure): suture placed 11–18 mm from insertion through belly of muscle and sclera to weaken muscle only in its field of action; decreases mechanical advantage of muscle acting on globe; often combined with recession

Strengthening Procedures

Resection: used to strengthen rectus muscles by excising portion of muscle and reattaching muscle at its insertion site

Advancement (moving muscle forward): often used for muscles previously recessed, also in Harada-Ito procedure

Tuck: technique used to strengthen superior oblique by shortening the tendon (may produce iatrogenic Brown's syndrome)

Other Techniques

Adjustable suture: slipknot or noose suture to enable muscle adjustment postoperatively under topical anesthesia

Transposition: moving muscle out of original plane of action; used in cases of paralysis, double elevator palsy, or A and V patterns

Harada-Ito procedure: anterior temporal displacement of anterior half of superior oblique tendon; used to correct excyclotorsion

Kestenbaum procedure: bilateral resection/recession to dampen nystagmus in patients with nystagmus and head turn; eyes are surgically moved toward direction of head turn

Botulinum toxin (Botox): interferes with release of acetylcholine to paralyze muscle into which it is injected. When an extraocular muscle is paralyzed by Botox, the antagonist contracts to change the alignment of the eyes

Used in cases of paralytic strabismus to prevent contracture of muscles or postoperative residual strabismus, and when surgery is inappropriate

General Principles

Needles: use spatulated needles (cutting surface on the side) to decrease risk of perforation (sclera is thinnest just posterior to insertion of rectus muscles [0.3 mm])

Vertical deviations: in general, surgery should be performed on muscles whose field of action is in same field as the vertical deviation (e.g., left hypertropia that is greatest down and to patient's right might be addressed by either weakening right inferior rectus or strengthening left superior oblique)

Horizontal incomitancy: can be treated by adjusting amount of surgery performed on each muscle (i.e., if exotropia increases from right gaze to primary gaze to left gaze, consider larger recession on left lateral rectus to have a greater effect on exotropia to left [in field of action of that muscle])

Distance-near disparity: perform surgery on lateral rectus muscles if exodeviation is greater at distance than at near. Perform surgery on medial rectus muscles if esodeviation is greater at near than at distance

Complications of Strabismus Surgery

Residual strabismus (most common): alignment in postoperative period can change due to poor fusion, poor vision, altered accommodation, and contracture of scar tissue

Scleral perforation: usually only creates a chorioretinal scar but can also lead to vitreous hemorrhage, retinal tear, retinal detachment, or endophthalmitis. If suspected during surgery, perform indirect ophthalmoscopy to determine whether a perforation is present; consider retinal laser treatment, cryotherapy, or observation

Infection: uncommon; includes endophthalmitis, cellulitis, and subconjunctival abscess

Foreign body granuloma: may develop weeks after surgery, often at suture site. Localized, elevated, slightly hyperemic, tender mass, usually <1 cm; may require surgical excision

Conjunctival inclusion cyst: may occur when conjunctiva is buried during closure of incision. Appears days to weeks later as noninflamed, transluscent mass under conjunctiva. May resolve spontaneously or require excision if symptomatic

Conjunctival scarring: can occur with orbital fat encroaching under bulbar conjunctiva because of inadvertent openings through Tenon's capsule

Fat adherence syndrome: violation of Tenon's capsule with prolapsed orbital fat into sub-Tenon's space can lead to fibrofatty scar. May have positive traction test and restricted motility

Delle: thin, dehydrated area of cornea caused by elevated limbal conjunctiva that prevents adequate corneal lubrication during blinking

Anterior segment ischemia: most blood to anterior segment supplied by anterior ciliary arteries that travel in rectus muscles. Usually occurs with surgery on 3 or more muscles. Corneal edema and anterior uveitis are present. Treat with topical steroids

Diplopia

Change in eyelid position: most commonly with surgery of vertical rectus muscles

Lost or slipped muscle: when only the capsule is sutured to insertion site, muscle can slip back; prevented with locking bites during suturing

Oculocardiac reflex: slowing of heart rate with traction on extraocular muscles

Malignant hyperthermia: acute metabolic disorder that may be fatal if diagnosis or treatment is delayed. Triggered by inhalation agents and succinylcholine. Signs include tachycardia, unstable BP, arrhythmias, increased temperature, muscle rigidity, cyanosis, dark urine

Review Questions *(Answers start on page 360)*

1. The approximate age of onset for accommodative ET is closest to
   a. 1 year old
   b. 3 years old
   c. 5 years old
   d. 7 years old

2. A 15-year-old girl with strabismus is examined, and the following measurements are recorded: distance deviation of 10 prism diopters, near deviation of 35 prism diopters at 20 cm, and interpupillary distance of 60 mm. Her AC/A ratio is
   a. 11 : 1
   b. 10 : 1
   c. 5 : 1
   d. 3 : 1

3. Duane's syndrome is thought to be due to a developmental abnormality of the
   a. trochlear nucleus
   b. motor endplate
   c. oculomotor nucleus
   d. abducens nucleus

4. The most helpful test in a patient with aniridia is
   a. EKG
   b. abdominal ultrasound
   c. chest X-ray
   d. CBC

5. The best test for an infant with a normal fundus and searching eye movements is
   a. VER
   b. ERG
   c. EOG
   d. OKN

6. The most common congenital infection is
   a. toxoplasmosis
   b. HSV
   c. CMV
   d. rubella

7. ARC is most likely to develop in a child with
   a. congenital esotropia
   b. amblyopia and suppression
   c. alternating exotropia
   d. small-angle esotropia

8. Which of the following most accurately reflects what a patient with harmonious ARC reports when the angle of anomaly is equal to the objective angle?
   a. fusion
   b. crossed diplopia
   c. simultaneous macular perception
   d. uncrossed diplopia

9. The inferior oblique muscle is weakened most by which procedure?
   a. disinsertion
   b. recession
   c. myotomy
   d. anteriorization

10. The test that gives the best dissociation is
    a. Maddox rod
    b. Worth 4 Dot
    c. Bagolini glasses
    d. Red glass

11. The 3-step test shows a left hypertropia in primary position that worsens on right gaze and with left head tilt. The best surgical procedure is
    a. RIR resection
    b. RSO tuck
    c. LIR recession
    d. LIO weakening

12. In the treatment of a superior oblique palsy, Knapp recommended all of the following except
    a. SO plication
    b. recession of the contralateral IR
    c. IO weakening
    d. resection of the contralateral SR

13. The best results of cryotherapy for ROP occur for treatment of disease in which location?
    a. zone 1
    b. anterior zone 2
    c. posterior zone 2
    d. zone 3

14. Characteristics of congenital ET include all of the following except
    a. dissociated vertical deviation
    b. cross fixation
    c. amblyopia
    d. inferior oblique overaction

15. The contalateral antagonist of the right superior rectus
    a. passes under another muscle
    b. causes incyclotorsion when paretic
    c. adducts the eye
    d. is innervated by the inferior division of CN 3

16. With respect to Panum's area, physiologic diplopia occurs at what point?
    a. on the horopter
    b. within Panum's area
    c. in front of Panum's area
    d. none of the above

17. The best treatment of an A pattern ET with muscle transposition is
    a. MR resection with upward transposition
    b. LR resection with upward transposition
    c. MR recession with downward transposition
    d. LR resection with downward transposition

18. A superior rectus Faden suture is used for the treatment of which condition?
    a. Duane's syndrome
    b. dissociated vertical deviation
    c. Brown's syndrome
    d. double elevator palsy

19. Which medication should be administered to a child who develops trismus under general anesthesia?
    a. atropine
    b. Tensilon
    c. lidocaine
    d. dantrolene

20. Congenital superior oblique palsy is characterized by all of the following except
    a. excyclotorsion <10°
    b. head tilt
    c. facial asymmetry
    d. <10 D of vertical vergence amplitudes

21. Which of the following statements regarding monofixation syndrome is false?
    a. There is no diplopia with the 4 prism diopter base-out prism test.
    b. Fusion with the Worth 4 Dot test is absent at distance.
    c. Fusional vergence amplitudes are absent.
    d. Titmus test for fly is normal.

22. Iridocyclitis is most commonly associated with which form of JRA?
    a. Still's disease
    b. polyarticular
    c. spondyloarthropathy
    d. pauciarticular

23. Congenital rubella is most commonly associated with
    a. retinal pigment epitheliopathy
    b. cataracts
    c. glaucoma
    d. strabismus

24. The most common cause of proptosis in a child is
    a. idiopathic orbital inflammation
    b. orbital cellulitis
    c. cavernous hemangioma
    d. Graves' disease

25. Which form of rhabdomyosarcoma has the worst prognosis?
    a. botryoid
    b. pleomorphic
    c. alveolar
    d. embryonal

26. Which of the following conditions is the least common cause of childhood proptosis?
    a. cavernous hemangioma
    b. rhabdomyosarcoma
    c. lymphangioma
    d. mucocele

27. A child with retinoblastoma is born to healthy parents with no family history of RB. The chance of RB occurring in a second child is approximately
    a. 5%
    b. 25%
    c. 40%
    d. 50%

28. The best chronologic age to examine a baby for ROP is
    a. 28 weeks
    b. 32 weeks
    c. 36 weeks
    d. 40 weeks

29. All of the following are associated with trisomy 13 except
    a. anophthalmos
    b. retinal dysplasia
    c. epiblepharon
    d. intraocular cartilage

30. Paradoxical pupillary response does not occur in
    a. achromatopsia
    b. CSNB
    c. Leber's congenital amaurosis
    d. albinism

SUGGESTED READINGS

American Academy of Ophthalmology: Pediatric Ophthalmology and Strabismus, vol 6. San Francisco, AAO, 2004.

Burian HM, von Noorden GK: Binocular Vision and Ocular Motility: Theory and Treatment of Strabismus. St. Louis, Mosby, 1974.

Del Monte MA, Archer SM: Atlas of Pediatric Ophthalmology and Strabismus Surgery. Philadelphia, Butterworth-Heinemann, 1991.

Nelson LB, Harley RB: Harley's Pediatric Ophthalmology, 4th edition. Philadelphia, WB Saunders, 1998.

Nelson LB, Catalano RA: Atlas of Ocular Motility. Philadelphia, WB Saunders, 1997.

Von Noorden GK: Atlas of Strabismus, 4th edition. St. Louis, Mosby, 1983.

Von Noorden GK, Campos EC: Binocular Vision and Ocular Motility: Theory and Treatment of Strabismus, 6th edition. St. Louis, Mosby, 2002.

CHAPTER 6

Orbit/Lids/Adnexa

ANATOMY

IMAGING

ORBITAL DISORDERS

EYELID DISORDERS

NASOLACRIMAL SYSTEM DISORDERS

ORBITAL SURGERY

ANATOMY

Table 6-1

Dimensions

Orbit: pear-shaped (widest diameter is 1 cm posterior to orbital rim); 40 mm wide, 35 mm high, 45 mm deep, volume = 30 cc

Optic nerve: orbital length = 25 mm; length from globe to optic foramen = 18 mm; width = 1.5 mm in globe, 3.5 mm posterior to lamina cribrosa (due to myelin), 5.0 mm with the addition of the optic nerve sheath (see Figure 4-2)

Proptosis: measure with Hertel exophthalmometer (Table 6-2)

Apertures

Figures 6-1 to 6-3

Superior orbital fissure:
Separates greater and lesser sphenoid wings
Between roof and lateral wall
Transmits: CN 3, 4, V_1, and 6, superior orbital vein, and sympathetic fibers to iris dilator

Optic canal (orbital foramen):
Within lesser wing of sphenoid: 10 mm long
Enlarged with ON glioma
Transmits: Optic nerve (CN 2), ophthalmic artery, and sympathetic nerves to ocular and orbital blood vessels

Inferior orbital fissure:
Bordered medially by maxillary bone, anteriorly by zygomatic bone, and laterally by greater wing of sphenoid
Transmits: CN V_2, zygomatic nerve, inferior ophthalmic artery, venous communication between ophthalmic vein and pterygoid plexus, sphenopalatine ganglion branches

Nasolacrimal canal:
Runs from lacrimal sac fossa to inferior meatus under the inferior turbinate
Contains the nasolacrimal duct
Lateral wall = maxillary bone
Medial wall = lacrimal bone and inferior turbinate

Zygomaticofacial and zygomaticotemporal canals:
Transmit: vessels and branches of the zygomatic nerve through the lateral wall to cheek and temporal fossa

Ethmoidal foramina:
Transmit: anterior and posterior ethmoid arteries
Potential route for spread of infectious sinusitis

Frontosphenoidal foramina:
Transmit: anastomosis between the middle meningeal and lacrimal arteries, which provides collateral blood supply to the orbit (Figure 6-3)

Foramen ovale:
Transmits: CN V_3

Foramen rotundum:
Transmits: CN V_2

Foramen lacerum:
Transmits: internal carotid artery

Vascular Supply to Eye

(Figures 6-4 to 6-6)

Ophthalmic artery: 1st branch of internal carotid within skull
Central retinal artery:
Enters optic nerve 13 mm posterior to globe
Supplies blood to inner 2/3 of retina
Posterior ciliary arteries:

Table 6-1. **Osteology**

Orbit	Bones	Related Structures/Miscellaneous
Roof	Sphenoid (lesser wing) Frontal	Lacrimal gland fossa Trochlea Supraorbital notch (medial)
Lateral wall	Sphenoid (greater wing) Zygomatic	Lateral orbital tubercle of Whitnall Strongest orbital wall Lateral orbital rim at equator of globe
Floor	Maxilla Palatine Zygomatic	Contains infraorbital nerve and canal Forms roof of maxillary sinus
Medial wall	Sphenoid Maxilla Ethmoid Lacrimal	Lacrimal sac fossa Adjacent to ethmoid and sphenoid sinuses Posterior ethmoidal foramen Weakest orbital wall

Table 6-2. **Hertel Exophthalmometry Measurements**

	Mean (mm)	Upper Limit of Normal (mm)
Caucasian male	16.5	21.7
Caucasian female	15.4	20
African American male	18.5	24.7
African American female	17.8	23.0

Figure 6-1. Bony anatomy of the orbit in frontal view. (From Dutton JJ: *Atlas of Clinical and Surgical Orbital Anatomy*, Philadelphia, WB Saunders, 1994.)

Long posterior ciliary arteries supply anterior segment

Short posterior ciliary arteries supply choroid

Optic nerve head is primarily supplied by blood from the vascular circle of Zinn-Haller

Collection of anastomotic arteries arising from the short posterior ciliary arteries

Venous system:

Orbital veins do not have valves

Superior ophthalmic vein:

Exits via superior orbital fissure into the cavernous sinus

2 superior vortex veins

Inferior ophthalmic vein:

Also exits via superior orbital fissure

2 inferior vortex veins

Central retinal vein:

Joins superior or inferior ophthalmic vein

Leaves nerve 10 mm behind globe

Innervation of Eye

Sensory innervation provided by ophthalmic and maxillary division of trigeminal nerve (CN 5) (Figure 6-7)

Ophthalmic division (V_1):

Nasociliary nerve:

Enters orbit within the annulus of Zinn

Short ciliary nerves pass through ciliary ganglion without synapsing

Long ciliary nerves supply iris, cornea, and ciliary muscle

Frontal nerve:

Enters orbit above annulus of Zinn

Divides into supraorbital nerve and supratrochlear nerve

Innervates medial canthus, upper lid, and forehead

Lacrimal nerve:

Figure 6-2. Orbital apex, superior and inferior orbital fissure. MR, medial rectus; IR, inferior rectus; LR, lateral rectus; SR, superior rectus; L, levator; SO, superior oblique. Note that the trochlear nerve lies outside the muscle cone.

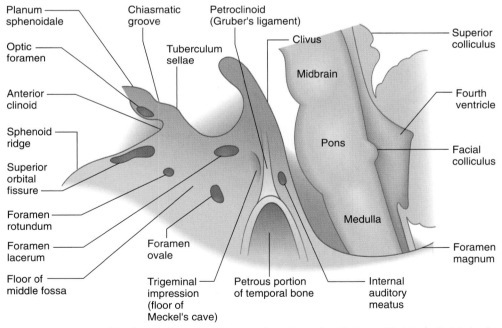

Figure 6-3. Schematic representation of the landmarks, temporal view. (From Bajandas FJ, Kline BK: *Neuro-Ophthalmology Review Manual,* Thorofare, NJ, Slack, 1988.)

supraorbital artery

dorsal nasal artery

anterior ethmoidal artery

ophthalmic artery

medial posterior ciliary artery

lateral posterior ciliary artery

zygomaticotemporal artery

zygomaticofacial artery

central retinal artery

Figure 6-4. Arterial supply to the orbit, in coronal view. (From Dutton JJ: *Atlas of Clinical and Surgical Orbital Anatomy*, Philadelphia, WB Saunders, 1994.)

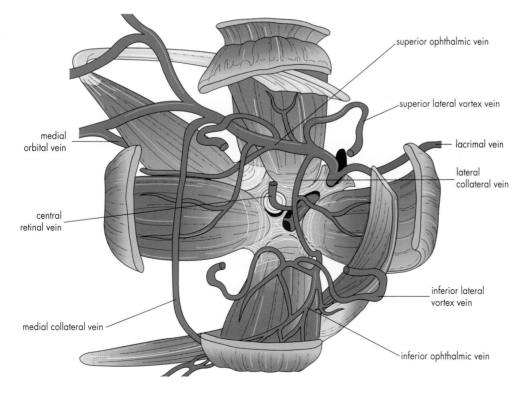

medial orbital vein

central retinal vein

medial collateral vein

superior ophthalmic vein

superior lateral vortex vein

lacrimal vein

lateral collateral vein

inferior lateral vortex vein

inferior ophthalmic vein

Figure 6-5. Orbital veins. Venous drainage from the orbit, in coronal view. (From Dutton JJ: *Atlas of Clinical and Surgical Orbital Anatomy*, Philadelphia, WB Saunders, 1994.)

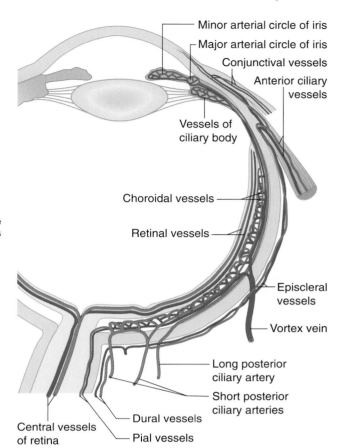

Minor arterial circle of iris
Major arterial circle of iris
Conjunctival vessels
Anterior ciliary vessels
Vessels of ciliary body
Choroidal vessels
Retinal vessels
Episcleral vessels
Vortex vein
Long posterior ciliary artery
Short posterior ciliary arteries
Dural vessels
Central vessels of retina
Pial vessels

Figure 6-6. Vascular supply to the eye. All arterial branches originate with the ophthalmic artery. Venous drainage is through the cavernous sinus and the pterygoid plexus.

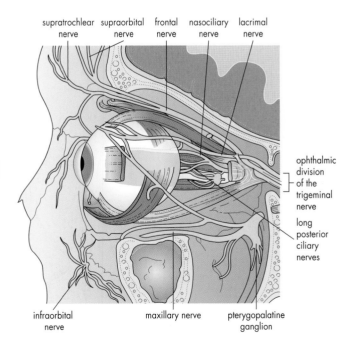

supratrochlear nerve
supraorbital nerve
frontal nerve
nasociliary nerve
lacrimal nerve
ophthalmic division of the trigeminal nerve
long posterior ciliary nerves
infraorbital nerve
maxillary nerve
pterygopalatine ganglion

Figure 6-7. Sensory nerves of the orbit, in lateral view. (From Dutton JJ: *Atlas of Clinical and Surgical Orbital Anatomy*, Philadelphia, WB Saunders, 1994.)

Enters orbit above annulus of Zinn

Innervates upper eyelid and lacrimal gland

Maxillary nerve (V₂):

Passes through foramen rotundum, then passes through inferior orbital fissure

Divides into infraorbital nerve, zygomatic nerve, and superior alveolar nerve

Parasympathetic innervation:

Controls accommodation, pupillary constriction, and lacrimal gland stimulation

Enters eye as short posterior ciliary nerves after synapsing in the ciliary ganglion

Sympathetic innervation:

Controls pupillary dilation, vasoconstriction, smooth muscle function of eyelids and orbit, and hidrosis

Dysfunction: Horner's syndrome (ptosis, miosis, anhidrosis, and vasodilation)

Nerve fibers follow arterial supply as well as long ciliary nerves

Sinuses

Figure 6-8

Frontal:

Not radiographically visible before age 6

Drains into anterior portion of the middle meatus

Ethmoid:

Multiple thin-walled cavities

First sinus to aerate

Anterior and middle air cells drain into the middle meatus

Posterior air cells drain into the superior meatus

Ethmoidal sinusitis is the most common source of infection that leads to orbital cellulitis

Sphenoid:

Rudimentary at birth

Reaches full size after puberty

Optic canal is superior and lateral to sphenoid sinus

Drains into sphenoethmoid recess of each nasal fossa

Maxillary:

Largest sinus

Roof contains the infraorbital nerve

Drains into middle meatus

Soft Tissues

Periorbita:

Periosteum is attached firmly at the orbital rim and suture lines

Arcus marginalis: fusion of periosteum and orbital septum at orbital rim

Fuses with the dura covering the optic nerve

Annulus of Zinn:

Fibrous tissue ring arising from periorbita that surrounds the optic canal

Origin of the 4 recti muscles

Fuses with dura covering ON at apex

Adipose tissue:

Surrounds most of orbital contents; divided by fine fibrous septa

Preaponeurotic fat pads: lie immediately posterior to orbital septum

2 FAT PADS IN UPPER LID: anterior to levator aponeurosis; nasal pad smaller and paler than

Figure 6-8. Relationship of the orbits to the paranasal sinuses: FS, frontal sinus, ES, ethmoid sinus; MS, maxillary sinus; SS, sphenoid sinus. (Reprinted with permission from Slamovits TL: Basic and Clinical Science Course, Section 7: Orbit, Eyelids and Lacrimal System, San Francisco, American Academy of Ophthalmology, 1993.)

central pad; with aging, nasal pad moves anteriorly and may cause bulging of upper nasal orbit

3 FAT PADS IN LOWER LID: anterior to capsulopalpebral fascia; inferior oblique muscle separates the nasal and middle pads; lateral pad is small and more inferior

Lacrimal gland:

2 lobes: orbital (larger) and palpebral, separated by levator aponeurosis

Ducts from both lobes pass though the palpebral lobe and empty into the superior fornix

Innervation: secretomotor from superior salivatory nucleus via CN 7; sensory from CN 5; sympathetic from superior cervical ganglion via deep petrosal nerve, pterygopalatine ganglion, and zygomatic nerve

Blood supply: lacrimal artery

Accessory lacrimal glands: glands of Wolfring located in tarsus and glands of Krause located in the conjunctival fornices

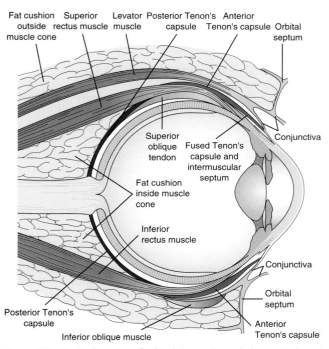

Figure 6-9. Sagittal section of orbital tissues through the vertical recti. (Adapted from Parks MM: Extraocular muscles. In Duane TD: *Clinical Ophthalmology*, Philadelphia, Harper and Row, 1982.)

Eyelid

Lamellae of upper eyelid:

Anterior: skin, orbicularis

Posterior: tarsus, levator aponeurosis, Müller's muscle, palpebral conjunctiva (Figure 6-10)

Skin:

Thinnest skin of the body, no subcutaneous fat layer

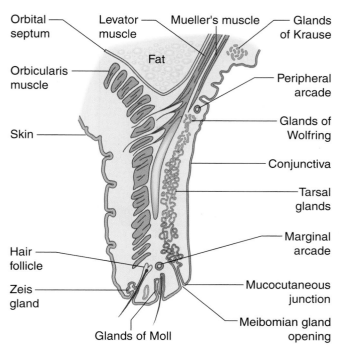

Figure 6-10. Cross section of upper eyelid. Note position of cilia, tarsal gland orifices, and mucocutaneous junction. (Reprinted with permission from Grand MG: Basic and Clinical Science Course, Section 2: Fundamentals and Principles of Ophthalmology. San Francisco, American Academy of Ophthalmology, 1993.)

Upper eyelid crease approximates attachments of the levator aponeurosis to the pretarsal orbicularis and skin

Histology of epidermis:

BASILAR LAYER (stratum basalis): cuboidal cells with scant cytoplasm; responsible for generating superficial layers

PRICKLE CELL LAYER: multiple layers of cells with abundant cytoplasm attached to each other by desmosomes

GRANULAR CELL LAYER (stratum granulosum): cells contain granular material that stains blue with H&E

KERATIN LAYER: superficial, acellular keratin devoid of nuclei; stains pink with H&E

Orbicularis oculi:

Main protractor of the eyelid; acts as lacrimal pump; innervated by CN 7

3 anatomic parts: palpebral portion (pretarsal and preseptal) involved with involuntary blinking; orbital portion involved with voluntary, forced lid closure (Figure 6-11)

PRETARSAL: overlies tarsus, originates from lateral orbital tubercle, forms muscle of Riolan (seen as gray line at lid margin)

SUPERFICIAL HEAD: medially inserts into anterior lacrimal crest, contributes to medial canthal tendon, laterally inserts into zygomatic bone

Figure 6-11. The orbicularis and frontalis muscles. (From Dutton JJ: *Atlas of Clinical and Surgical Orbital Anatomy*, Philadelphia, WB Saunders, 1994.)

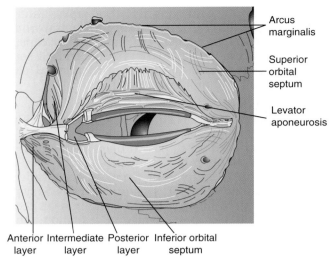

Figure 6-12. The orbital septum. (From Dutton JJ: *Atlas of Clinical and Surgical Orbital Anatomy*, Philadelphia, WB Saunders, 1994.)

DEEP HEAD: medially inserts into posterior lacrimal crest, called Horner's muscle, surrounds canaliculi facilitating tear drainage, laterally inserts into lateral orbital tubercle, contributes to lateral canthal tendon

PRESEPTAL: overlies orbital septum

Originates from anterior limb of the medial canthal tendon, and from posterior lacrimal crest and lacrimal sac fascia

Forms lateral palpebral raphe overlying the lateral orbital rim

ORBITAL: lies beneath skin

Thickest portion of orbicularis

Inserts at medial canthal tendon

Interdigitates with the frontalis muscle superiorly at eyebrow

Other muscles of forehead and eyebrow:
Occipitofrontalis: moves scalp anteriorly and posteriorly; raises eyebrows; innervated by CN 7
Corrugator: pulls medial eyebrow inferiorly and medially producing vertical glabellar wrinkle; originates from nasal process of frontal bone; inserts laterally into subcutaneous tissue; innervated by CN 7
Procerus: pulls forehead and medial eyebrow inferiorly producing horizontal lines in nose; interdigitates with inferior edge of frontalis; innervated by CN 7

Orbital septum: (Figure 6-12)
Dense fibrous sheath that acts as barrier between the orbit and eyelid; stops spread of infection
Originates from periosteum of the superior and inferior orbital rims
Inserts into levator aponeurosis superiorly (2–5 mm above superior tarsal border in non-Asians) and into lower eyelid retractors inferiorly (capsulopalpebral fascia just below inferior tarsal border)

Medially inserts into lacrimal crest
Structures posterior to the septum: palpebral lobe of lacrimal gland, lateral canthal tendon, trochlea of superior oblique muscle

Upper eyelid retractors: (Figure 6-13)
Levator palpebrae:
Originates from lesser wing of sphenoid above annulus of Zinn
Innervated by CN 3
MUSCULAR PORTION: 40 mm
APONEUROTIC PORTION: 14–20 mm and has lateral and medial extensions (horns) (Figure 6-14)
LATERAL HORN:
Inserts onto lateral orbital tubercle
Divides lacrimal gland into orbital and palpebral portions
MEDIAL HORN:
Inserts onto posterior lacrimal crest
More delicate and weaker than lateral horn
Anterior portion inserts into septa between pretarsal orbicularis muscle bundles
Posterior portion inserts onto anterior surface of lower half of tarsus; forms eyelid crease
Disinsertion of aponeurosis results in loss of eyelid crease
Whitnall's ligament (superior transverse ligament): condensation of levator muscle sheath
Visible as horizontal white line 10 mm above superior edge of tarsus
Arises from the sheath of anterior portion of levator muscle
Medially attaches to trochlea
Laterally forms septa through stroma of lacrimal gland and attaches to inner aspect of lateral orbital wall 10 mm above orbital tubercle
Acts to change direction of pull of levator and serves as check ligament to prevent excessive lid elevation

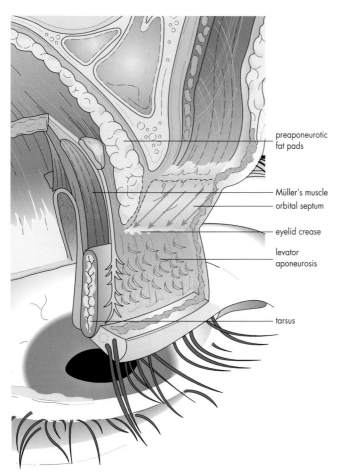

Figure 6-13. The orbital septum inserts into the levator aponeurosis *(arrows)*. The preaponeurotic fat pads are located posterior to the septum. In downgaze, the lid crease becomes attenuated (weakened), and in a normal young eyelid, the fold is absent. (From Zide BW, Jelks BW: *Surgical Anatomy of the Orbit*, New York, Raven Press, 1985.)

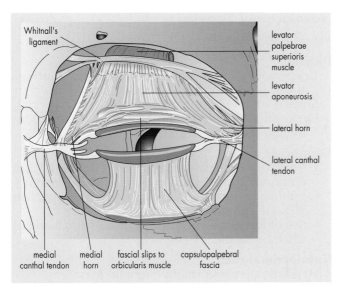

Figure 6-14. The levator aponeurosis, and the medial and lateral canthal tendons. (Adapted from Dutton JJ: *Atlas of Clinical and Surgical Orbital Anatomy*, Philadelphia, WB Saunders, 1994.)

Müller's muscle (superior tarsal muscle):
Posterior to levator aponeurosis
Sympathetic innervation
Originates from undersurface of levator approximately at level of Whitnall's ligament
Inserts into upper border of tarsus
12–15 mm long; raises eyelid 2 mm
Peripheral arterial arcade found between aponeurosis and Müller's muscle

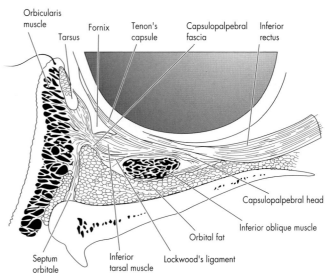

Figure 6-15. Anatomy of the lower eyelid retractors. (Adapted from Hawes MJ, Dortzbach RK: The microscopic anatomy of the lower eyelid retractors, *Arch Ophthalmol* 100:1313–1318, 1982.)

Lower eyelid retractors:
Capsulopalpebral fascia: analogous to levator aponeurosis
Originates from inferior rectus muscle sheath, divides as it encircles inferior oblique muscle, and then joins to form Lockwood's ligament
Fuses with septum and inserts into inferior tarsus
Lockwood's suspensory ligament: analogous to Whitnall's ligament
Arises posteriorly from fibrous attachments to inferior side of the IR muscle and continues anteriorly as capsulopalpebral fascia
Medial and lateral horns attach to retinacula forming a suspensory hammock for the globe
Inferior tarsal muscle: analogous to Müller's muscle
Sympathetic innervation
Arises from capsulopalpebral fascia

Tarsus:
Dense connective tissue plate in each eyelid
Contains meibomian glands
29 mm long and 1 mm thick; tapered at ends
Rigid attachments to periosteum medially and laterally

Superior tarsal plate: 10 mm in height
Inferior tarsal plate: 4 mm in height

Medial canthal tendon:
Fusion of tendinous insertions of pretarsal and preseptal orbicularis muscles
Attaches to tarsal plates
Anterior limb: attaches to frontal process of maxillary bone and serves as origin of superficial head of pretarsal orbicularis; passes in front of lacrimal sac and attaches to anterior lacrimal crest
Posterior limb: attaches to posterior lacrimal crest; passes behind lacrimal sac. More important than anterior limb for normal medial canthal appearance and function (maintaining apposition of lids to globe)

Lateral canthal tendon:
Broad band of connective tissue from lateral borders of upper and lower tarsal plates
Inserts onto lateral orbital tubercle of Whitnall; 3 mm superior to medial canthal tendon insertion

Eyelid margin: 3 distinguishing landmarks
Lash line: 2–3 rows of lashes; 100 in upper lid, 50 in lower lid; 10-week growth, 5-month resting phase
Gray line: border of pretarsal orbicularis (muscle of Riolan); junction of anterior and posterior lamellae; vascular watershed
Meibomian gland orifices: 30 in upper lid, 20 in lower lid

Vascular supply: (Figure 6-16)
Upper lid: internal carotid artery → ophthalmic artery → superior marginal arcade (deep to orbicularis and anterior surface of tarsus)
Lower lid: external carotid artery → facial artery → angular artery → inferior marginal arcade
Angular artery is 6–8 mm medial to medial canthus, posterior to orbicularis, 5 mm anterior to lacrimal sac
Peripheral and marginal arcades allow for anastomosis between the ICA and ECA
Venous drainage:
    PRETARSAL: angular vein medially, superficial temporal vein temporally
    POST-TARSAL: orbital vein, anterior facial vein, and pterygoid plexus

Innervation:
Sensory: CN V_1 (upper lid), CN V_2 (lower lid)
Motor: CN 3, CN 7, sympathetics

Lymphatic drainage:
Submandibular nodes: drain medial 1/3 of upper lid, medial 2/3 of lower lid
Preauricular nodes: drain medial 2/3 of upper lid, medial 1/3 of lower lid
No lymphatic vessels or nodes are found within the orbit
Lymphatic vessels are found in the conjunctiva

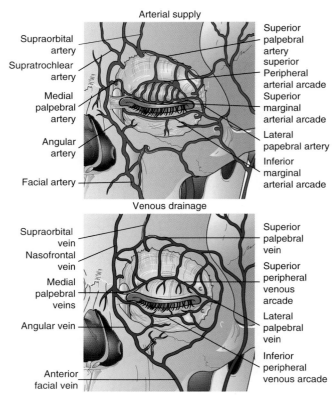

Figure 6-16. Arterial supply to, and venous drainage from, the eyelids. (From Dutton JJ: *Atlas of Clinical and Surgical Orbital Anatomy*, Philadelphia, WB Saunders, 1994.)

Glands of the eyelids: (Table 6-3)
Eccrine: secretion by simple exocytosis
Holocrine: secretion by release of entire cellular contents (disruption of cell)
Apocrine: secretion by pinching or budding off of a portion of cellular cytoplasm

Nasolacrimal System

Figure 6-17

Puncta:
Upper and lower; 6 mm from medial canthus, lower is slightly more temporal
Slightly inverted against globe
Open into ampulla (2 mm long) oriented perpendicular to eyelid margin

Canaliculi:
10 mm long (2 mm vertical segment [ampulla] and 8 mm horizontal portion parallel to lid margin)
Combine to form single common canaliculus in 90% of individuals
Valve of Rosenmüller prevents reflux from lacrimal sac into canaliculi

Nasolacrimal sac:
10 mm long, occupies the lacrimal fossa
Lies between anterior and posterior crura of the medial canthal tendon, anterior to orbital septum
Middle meatus of nose, medial to sac

Table 6-3. **Glands of the Eyelids**

Gland	Location	Type	Function	Pathology
Lacrimal	Superotemporal orbit	Eccrine	Reflex tear (aqueous) secretion	Dacryoadenitis Tumors
Accessory lacrimal: Krause Wolfring	Fornix Just above tarsus	Eccrine	Basal tear (aqueous) secretion	Sjögren's syndrome GVH disease Rare tumors (BMT)
Meibomian	Within tarsus	Holocrine	Lipid secretion Retards tear evaporation	Chalazion Sebaceous carcinoma
Zeis	Near lid margin Caruncle Associated with cilia	Holocrine	Lipid secretion Lubricates cilia	External hordeolum Sebaceous carcinoma
Moll	Near lid margin	Apocrine	Modified sweat glands Lubricates cilia	Ductal cyst Apocrine carcinoma
Sweat		Eccrine	Electrolyte balance	Ductal cyst Syringoma Sweat gland carcinoma
Goblet cells	Conjunctiva Plica Caruncle	Holocrine	Mucin secretion Enhances corneal wetting	Dry eye

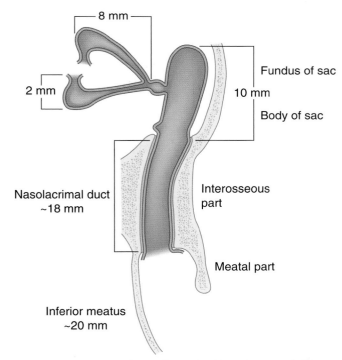

Figure 6-17. Excretory lacrimal system. (From Basic and Clinical Science Course, Section 2, Fundamentals and Principles of Ophthalmology. San Francisco, American Academy of Ophthalmology, 1993.)

Nasolacrimal duct:
15 mm long
Passes inferiorly, posteriorly, and laterally within canal formed by maxillary and lacrimal bones
Extends into inferior meatus, which opens under inferior turbinate (2.5 cm posterior to naris)
Partially covered by valve of Hasner

Lacrimal pump:
Lids close: pretarsal orbicularis contracts, compresses ampulla, shortens canaliculus; punctum moves medially; lacrimal sac expands, creates negative pressure, draws fluid from canaliculus into sac
Lids open: muscles relax, lacrimal sac collapses, tears forced into nose, punctum moves laterally, tears enter canaliculus

IMAGING

Ultrasound

Optimal sound wave frequency is 10 MHz

Higher frequencies give better resolution, lower frequencies provide better penetration (Table 6-4)

MRI

Strong magnetic field results in alignment of nuclei of atoms with odd numbers of protons or neutrons

Radiofrequency pulse disturbs the alignment by energizing protons or neutrons

Table 6-4. **Ultrasound Characteristics of Lesions**

Good Sound Transmission	Poor Sound Transmission
Cavernous hemangioma	Metastatic cancer
Lymphangioma	Orbital pseudotumor
Mucocele	Glioma
Dermoid	Neurofibroma
High Reflectivity	**Low Reflectivity**
Neurofibroma	Metastatic cancer
Fresh hemorrhage	Orbital pseudotumor
Hemangioma	Cyst
Thyroid eye disease	Mucocele Varix Dermoid Lymphoma

When pulse terminates, protons return to previous alignment and emit absorbed energy as radiofrequency signal, generating an image

Can provide axial, coronal, and sagittal views

Relaxation times:

Longitudinal relaxation time (T1): time required for net bulk magnetization to realign itself along original axis

Blood, orbital fat, melanin, and mucus appear bright

Acute hemorrhage, vitreous, optic nerve sheath, and extraocular muscles appear dark

Most orbital tumors are hypointense to fat on T1-weighted images

EXCEPTIONS: mucinous lesions (orbital dermoid cyst, mucocele), lipoma, liposarcoma, melanoma, subacute hemorrhage

Gadolinium: bright white on T1-weighted images

Must perform fat suppression on T1-weighted images when gadolinium is used

Fat suppression renders orbital fat hypointense and permits better visualization of optic nerve and extraocular muscles

Transverse relaxation time (T2): mean relaxation time

Based on interaction of hydrogen nuclei within a given tissue

Provides more information about pathologic processes

Helps differentiate melanotic lesions from hemorrhagic process

Vitreous is bright on T2-weighted images

Blood and fat appear dark

Demyelinating plaques of MS are best seen with T2-weighted images (hyperintense foci, usually in periventricular white matter)

Advantages: better for soft tissues and posterior fossa, sagittal sections, no artifacts from bone or teeth, no ionizing radiation

Disadvantages: poor bony detail, longer imaging time, more expensive, certain contraindications

Contraindications: patients with retained metallic foreign body, pacemaker, aneurysm clip

CT Scan

Use with orbital trauma to detect foreign body or calcification, or for evaluation of orbital soft tissue lesion with suspicion of bony erosion

Bone and metal appear bright

Advantages: better bony detail and for acute hemorrhage, sinuses, and trauma; shorter imaging time; less expensive

Disadvantages: poor posterior fossa detail; no sagittal sections, ionizing radiation

Table 6-5. **CT and MRI Characteristics of Lesions**

Most Common Orbital Lesions with Well-Circumscribed Appearance on CT and MRI	Most Common Orbital Lesions with Ill-Defined Appearance on CT and MRI
Children: Dermoid cyst Lymphangioma Rhabdomyosarcoma ON glioma	Children: Capillary hemangioma Orbital pseudotumor Plexiform neurofibroma Leukemic infiltrate Eosinophilic granuloma
Adults: Cavernous hemangioma Neurofibroma Neurilemmoma Fibrous histiocytoma Lymphoproliferative disorders	Adults: Orbital pseudotumor Metastasis Leukemic infiltrate Primary malignant tumor Lymphoproliferative disorders

Radiographs

Specific views can be helpful, especially when CT is unavailable or to quickly rule out a metallic foreign body

Plain film radiography also detects sinus pathology, calcification, hyperostosis, and lytic lesions

Canthomeatal line: radiographic baseline of skull (line between lateral canthal angle and tragus of ear)

Waters view: occipitomental; head extended until canthomeatal line lies at 37° to the central beam; best view of orbital roof and floor

Caldwell view: posteroanterior view with central beam tilted 25° toward feet; best view of superior and lateral orbital rim, medial wall, and ethmoid and frontal sinuses

Lateral view: best for evaluation of sella turcica

Submental vertex view: basal or Hirtz view with head tilted back until canthomeatal line is perpendicular to central beam; best view of sphenoid and ethmoid sinuses, nasal cavities, and zygomatic arch

Oblique (×2) views: PA view with central beam tilted 32° toward feet and 37° from perpendicular; best views of optic foramina

ORBITAL DISORDERS

Congenital and Developmental Anomalies

(see Chapter 5, Pediatrics/Strabismus)

Trauma

Orbital Contusion

Bruising from blunt trauma

Pain, decreased vision

Often have associated lid, orbit, and ocular injuries

Treatment: ice compresses, systemic NSAIDs

Orbital Fractures

Fractures of orbital bones, often associated with ocular or intracranial injuries

Orbital floor (blow-out):
  Maxillary bone
  Posterior medial floor is weakest area
  May have enophthalmos, diplopia, infraorbital hypesthesia, orbit or lid emphysema, and medial wall fracture
  Orbital contents may become entrapped in maxillary sinus with resultant restriction of ocular motility, diplopia, and globe ptosis

Medial wall:
  Maxillary, lacrimal, and ethmoid bones
  Associated with depressed nasal bridge, telecanthus, floor fracture
  Complications: epistaxis from injury of anterior ethmoidal artery, CSF rhinorrhea, lacrimal drainage injury, orbit or lid emphysema

Orbital apex:
  Can involve optic canal and superior orbital fissure
  Complications: CSF rhinorrhea, carotid-cavernous fistula

Orbital roof:
  Uncommon
  May affect frontal sinus, cribriform plate, and brain
  Complications: CSF rhinorrhea, pneumocephalus

Zygomatic (tripod):
  Fracture of zygoma at 3 sites (zygomaticomaxillary suture, zygomaticofrontal suture, and zygomatic arch) and orbital floor
  Findings: discontinuity of orbital rim, flattening of malar eminence, enophthalmos, infraorbital hypesthesia, trismus, orbit or lid emphysema, downward displacement of lateral canthus

LeFort (I, II, III):
  I: low transverse fracture of maxillary bone above teeth; no orbital involvement
  II: pyramidal fracture of nasal, lacrimal, and maxillary bones; involves medial orbital floors
  III: craniofacial dysjunction; involves orbital floor, lateral and medial walls; may involve optic canal
  CT scan: identify and localize fracture and coexisting injuries

Treatment:
  Systemic steroids and antibiotics
  Surgical repair depends on type, location, and severity of fracture and associated findings

Intraorbital Foreign Bodies

Commonly associated with intraocular and/or optic nerve injury

Inert material can be well tolerated and may be observed

Copper and organic material are poorly tolerated and must be removed

Often asymptomatic, but may have pain or decreased vision

CT scan (MRI is contraindicated for metallic foreign bodies)

Treatment: systemic antibiotics, tetanus booster, consider surgical removal

Orbital (Retrobulbar) Hemorrhage

Compartment syndrome due to bleeding in orbit with globe and nerve compression

Ocular emergency

Findings: pain, decreased vision, subconjunctival hemorrhage, proptosis, restriction of ocular motility, increased IOP, tense orbit

Treatment: lateral canthotomy and cantholysis

Degeneration

Atrophia Bulbi

Progressive degeneration and decompensation of globe following severe injury

3 stages: atrophia bulbi without shrinkage, atrophia bulbi with shrinkage, atrophia bulbi with disorganization (phthisis bulbi)

Increased risk of intraocular malignancy

Annual B-scan to rule out malignancy

Findings: cataract, retinal detachment, hypotony, corneal edema, globe shrinkage, intraocular hemorrhage, inflammation, calcification, and disorganization

Treatment: topical steroid and cycloplegic for pain; consider retrobulbar alcohol injection or enucleation for severe pain

Infections

Bacterial

Preseptal cellulitis, orbital cellulitis (see Chapter 5, Pediatrics/Strabismus)

Fungal

Most commonly *Phycomycetes*

Mucormycosis:
  Most common and virulent fungal orbital disease
  Black eschar may be visible in nose or palate
  Nonseptated large branching hyphae, with invasion of blood vessels, thrombosis, and necrosis
  Intracranial spread is hematogenous via ophthalmic artery
  Risk factors: diabetes mellitus (70%), immunosuppression (18%), renal disease (5%), leukemia (3%)
  Findings: painful orbital apex syndrome, proptosis, ptosis, ophthalmoplegia, decreased vision, corneal anesthesia; may develop retinal vascular occlusions
  Treatment: requires immediate and emergent management
  Surgical débridement, IV amphotericin B; control underlying illness

Aspergillosis:
  Septated branching hyphae
  Disseminated form: occurs in immunosuppressed hosts; widespread necrotizing angiitis, thrombosis, endophthalmitis
  Local form: sclerosing granulomatous infiltrative mass that originates in the sinus; proptosis, periorbital pain, visual loss
  Treatment: surgical débridement, amphotericin B, flucytosine, rifampin (IV and oral)

Viral

Dengue fever:
  Flavivirus

75% with ocular soreness and pain on eye movement

Parasitic

Trichinosis:
  Trichinella spiralis
  Larvae from ingestion of raw meat migrate to muscle and brain and become encysted
  Associated with fever, myalgia, diarrhea, eosinophilia, and periorbital edema

Cysticercosis:
  Taenia solium
  Larvae penetrate intestinal wall, enter bloodstream, and migrate to eyes, lungs, brain, muscle, and connective tissue

Inflammation

Idiopathic Orbital Inflammation (Orbital Pseudotumor)

Idiopathic inflammatory disease of orbital tissues

Patchy infiltrate of lymphocytes, plasma cells, and eosinophils

Findings: acute orbital pain, lid erythema and edema, lacrimal gland enlargement, restricted eye movements, proptosis, diplopia, increased IOP; may have impaired vision from optic nerve involvement

Adults: usually unilateral; bilateral cases need workup for vasculitis and lymphoproliferative disorders

Children: bilateral in 33%; commonly have headache, fever, vomiting, and lethargy; may have associated papillitis or iritis

DDx: thyroid-related ophthalmopathy, orbital cellulitis, tumor, vasculitis, trauma, AV fistula, cavernous sinus thrombosis, CN palsy

Diagnosis:
  Lab tests: eosinophilia, elevated ESR, positive ANA, CSF pleocytosis
  CT scan: enlargement of extraocular muscles and tendons, ring sign (contrast enhanced sclera), enlarged lacrimal gland
  B-scan ultrasound: may show acoustically hollow area corresponding to edematous Tenon's capsule

Treatment: systemic NSAIDs, systemic steroids (60–120 mg oral prednisone, taper slowly over months); consider radiation if unresponsive to steroids, perform biopsy first; chemotherapy (cyclophosphamide)

Orbital myositis: localized to extraocular muscles

MR and LR most commonly involved (33% each), IR 10%

Findings: diplopia, pain, proptosis, ptosis, conjunctival injection, and chemosis
Complications: fibrosis with strabismus

Tolosa-Hunt syndrome: localized to superior orbital fissure, optic canal, and cavernous sinus
Findings: painful ophthalmoplegia, decreased vision

Sclerosing orbital pseudotumor: fibrosis of orbit and lacrimal gland
Insidious onset
More steroid resistant
Pain is less common, and eye is often white and quiet
Associated with retroperitoneal fibrosis
A-scan ultrasound: low reflectivity (seen with both orbital pseudotumor and lymphoma)

Thyroid-Related Ophthalmopathy

Autoimmune disease with spectrum of ocular manifestations

Most common cause of unilateral or bilateral proptosis in adults

Most common cause of acquired diplopia in adults

Women affected 8–10× more often than men

Patient can be hyperthyroid, euthyroid, or hypothyroid; most commonly associated with Graves' disease

Associated with myasthenia gravis (in 5% of patients with Graves' disease)

Usually asymptomatic

Findings: eyelid retraction (90%), proptosis (63%), restrictive myopathy with diplopia; overaction of levator (secondary to restrictive myopathy of inferior rectus muscle); pseudoretraction (secondary to proptosis); lagophthalmos; lid lag on downgaze (von Graefe's sign); dry eye (due to corneal exposure and infiltration of lacrimal glands); conjunctival injection and chemosis; corneal exposure (from combination of eyelid retraction, proptosis, and lagophthalmos); increased IOP on upgaze; choroidal folds or disc hyperemia; compressive optic neuropathy (<5%) with decreased acuity and color vision, RAPD, and VF defect

Werner Classification of Eye Findings in Graves' Disease (**NO SPECS**):
No signs or symptoms
Only signs
Soft tissue involvement (signs and symptoms)
Proptosis
Extraocular muscle involvement
Corneal involvement
Sight loss (optic nerve compression)

Pathology: enlargement of extraocular muscles; patchy infiltrates of lymphocytes, monocytes, mast cells, and fibroblasts; fibroblasts produce mucopolysaccharides, which leads to increased water content of muscles; inflammation spares tendons

Figure 6-18. Thyroid-related ophthalmopathy demonstrating thickened extraocular muscles with inflammatory cell infiltrate and fluid. (Courtesy of Dr. RC Eagle, Jr. Reported in Hufnagel TJ et al: *Ophthalmology* 91:1411, 1984.)

CT scan: enlargement of extraocular muscles sparing tendons; inferior rectus > medial rectus > superior rectus > obliques > lateral rectus

Treatment: control underlying thyroid abnormality; ocular lubrication; consider lid taping or tarsorrhaphy; systemic steroids; radiation (effects take 2–4 weeks)
Surgery:
ORBITAL DECOMPRESSION: perform before strabismus surgery; 2, 3, or 4 walls; 80% will experience postoperative diplopia
STRABISMUS SURGERY: perform before lid surgery is undertaken
INDICATIONS: diplopia, abnormal head position, large-angle strabismus
Strabismus must be stable for at least 6 months
Avoid if anterior inflammatory signs present
Recession of affected muscles is mainstay of treatment, avoid resections (can exacerbate restrictions already present)
Vertical muscle surgery can affect eyelid position (recession of inferior rectus can cause increased lid retraction due to connection of IR to lower lid retractors; recession of IR can decrease upper lid retraction in that the SR now has to work less against the tight IR [thus, the associated levator muscle is less stimulated, causing less eyelid retraction])
Beware late slippage of inferior rectus
Consider adjustable sutures
LID SURGERY: eyelid retraction repair; perform after orbital decompression and strabismus surgery

Sarcoidosis

(see Chapter 8, Uveitis)

Chronic, idiopathic, multisystem, granulomatous disease primarily affecting lung, skin, eye

More common among young African Americans

Findings: panuveitis, keratitis, pars planitis, chorioretinitis, optic nerve involvement, orbital apex syndrome, ptosis, conjunctival nodules, dacryoadenitis

Pathology: noncaseating granulomas and Langhans' giant cells

Diagnosis: CXR, PPD and controls, angiotensin-converting enzyme (ACE), serum lysozyme, gallium scan, pulmonary function tests

Treatment: systemic steroids, chemotherapy; treat ocular complications

Wegener's Granulomatosis

Systemic disease of necrotizing vasculitis and granulomatous inflammation involving sinuses, respiratory system, kidneys, and orbit

Findings: painful proptosis, reduced ocular motility, chemosis, scleritis, keratitis, optic nerve edema, nasolacrimal duct obstruction

Diagnosis: ANCA (positive in 67%)

Treatment: systemic steroids, immunosuppressive therapy

Vascular Abnormalities

Varix

(see Chapter 5, Pediatrics/Strabismus)

AV Fistula

Direct or indirect communication between carotid artery and venous structures of the cavernous sinus

Direct carotid-cavernous sinus fistula: high flow; associated with head trauma, especially basal skull fracture; due to spontaneous rupture of aneurysm

> *Findings*: dilated corkscrew scleral/episcleral vessels, conjunctival injection and chemosis, elevated IOP on involved side, proptosis (may be pulsatile), orbital bruit that may be abolished by ipsilateral carotid compression, dilated tortuous retinal veins, may develop ischemic maculopathy or retinal artery occlusion, enlarged cup-to-disc ratio, ophthalmoplegia (often CN 6), anterior segment ischemia
>
> *CT/MRI scan*: dilated superior ophthalmic vein
>
> *Treatment* (for severely affected patients): embolization, surgical ligation

Dural-sinus fistula: low-flow communication between meningeal branches of carotid artery and dural walls of cavernous sinus; often asymptomatic; associated with hypertension, atherosclerosis, and connective tissue diseases; may close spontaneously

Tumors

(Table 6-6)

Hamartomas: growth arising from tissue normally found at that site (e.g., nevus, neurofibroma, neurilemmoma, schwannoma, glioma, hemangioma, hemangiopericytoma, lymphangioma, trichoepithelioma)

Choristomas: growth arising from tissue not normally found at that site (e.g., dermoid cyst, dermatolipoma)

Cystic Tumors

(see Chapter 5, Pediatrics/Strabismus)

Table 6-6. **Common Orbital Tumors**

In Children (see Chapter 5, Pediatrics/Strabismus)	In Adults
90% are benign; 10% are malignant	Mucocele
Rhabdomyosarcoma (most common primary orbital malignancy)	Cavernous hemangioma
Capillary hemangioma (most common benign primary orbital tumor)	Meningioma
Lymphangioma	Fibrous histiocytoma
Neuroblastoma (most common metastasis to orbit)	Neurilemmoma
Dermoid (most common noninflammatory orbital mass)	Pleomorphic adenoma (BMT)
Teratoma	Lymphoid tumors
ON glioma	Metastatic tumors
Granulocytic sarcoma ("chloroma")	
Burkitt's lymphoma	
Histiocytic tumors	

Vascular Tumors

Lymphangioma

(see Chapter 5, Pediatrics/Strabismus)

Capillary Hemangioma

(see Chapter 5, Pediatrics/Strabismus)

Cavernous Hemangioma

Most common benign orbital tumor in adults (usually middle-aged women)

Findings: slowly progressive proptosis; may induce hyperopia, may also have retinal striae, IOP elevation, strabismus, or optic nerve compression

Growth may accelerate during pregnancy

Pathology: encapsulated lesion composed of blood-filled cavernous spaces, lined by endothelial cells

Figure 6-19. Cavernous hemangioma demonstrating large, blood-filled spaces and fibrous septa. (Case presented by Dr. WC Frayer to the meeting of the Verhoeff Society, 1989. From Yanoff M, Fine BS: *Ocular Pathology*, 5th ed, St. Louis, Mosby, 2002.)

CT scan: well-demarcated, encapsulated, intraconal mass

MRI: hypointense to fat on T1-weighted images, hyperintense to fat and equivalent to vitreous on T2-weighted images

A-scan ultrasound: high internal reflectivity

Treatment: observation, surgical excision

Hemangiopericytoma

Rare tumor of abnormal pericytes surrounding blood vessels

Occurs in middle-aged adults

More common in women

Often located in superior orbit

Can metastasize to lung, bone, liver

Findings: slowly progressive proptosis

CT scan: well-circumscribed, encapsulated mass

A-scan ultrasound: low to medium internal reflectivity

Treatment: complete surgical excision

Neural Tumors

Optic Nerve Glioma

(see Chapter 5, Pediatrics/Strabismus)

Neurofibroma

(see Chapter 5, Pediatrics/Strabismus)

Neurilemmoma (Schwannoma)

Encapsulated tumor consisting of benign proliferation of Schwann cells

No malignant potential

Occurs in middle-aged individuals

Lesion can be painful due to perineural spread and compression of nerve

Usually located in the superior orbit causing gradual proptosis and globe dystopia

Schwannomas can grow along any peripheral or cranial nerve, most commonly CN 8 (acoustic neuroma)

Rarely associated with neurofibromatosis

Pathology: stains with S-100
>   ***Antoni A***: spindle cells arranged in interlacing cords, whorls, or palisades; contains Verocay bodies (collections of cells resembling sensory corpuscles)

Figure 6-20. Antoni A pattern demonstrating palisading spindle cells with Verocray bodies (areas that appear acellular). (From Yanoff M, Fine BS: *Ocular Pathology*, 5th ed, St. Louis, Mosby, 2002.)

Antoni B: loose, myxoid; stellate cells with a mucoid stroma

Figure 6-21. Antoni B pattern demonstrating necrosis with inflammatory cells. (From Yanoff M, Fine BS: *Ocular Pathology*, 5th ed, St. Louis, Mosby, 2002.)

CT scan: well-circumscribed, fusiform mass

Treatment: complete surgical excision

Meningioma

Optic nerve sheath meningioma:
  More common in women
  Accounts for 33% of all primary optic nerve tumors
  Increased incidence in neurofibromatosis
  Arises from arachnoid cells in the meninges
  Pathology: sheets of cells or whorls; psammoma bodies (calcified) in the center of whorls
  Findings: decreased visual acuity and color vision, visual field loss, proptosis, disc edema or pallor, optociliary shunt vessels
  Spencer's triad: optociliary shunts, optic atrophy, optic nerve meningioma
  CT scan: tubular enlargement of optic nerve that enhances with gadolinium; optic foramen enlargement
  Treatment: observation, surgical excision

Sphenoid wing meningioma:
  Most common tumor to spread to orbit from intracranial space
  Findings: temporal fullness, proptosis, lid edema
  CT scan: hyperostosis and calcifications
  Treatment: observation, surgical excision

Rhabdomyosarcoma

(see Chapter 5, Pediatrics/Strabismus)

Lymphoid Tumors

Spectrum of disorders characterized by abnormal proliferation of lymphoid tissue

Usually occur in adults 50–70 years old; rare in children

Cause painless proptosis

Conjunctival or lacrimal gland lesions

Tissue biopsy with immunohistochemical studies required for diagnosis

All lymphoid lesions of orbit must have a workup for systemic lymphoma, including CBC with differential, serum protein electrophoresis (SPEP), physical examination for lymphadenopathy, CT of thoracic and abdominal viscera, and bone scan

Perform every 6 months for 2 years

Bone marrow biopsy (better than bone marrow aspirate)

Monoclonal proliferations do not all progress to systemic disease; some polyclonal proliferations do progress

Benign Reactive Lymphoid Hyperplasia

Findings: bilateral painless lacrimal gland enlargement, limitation of ocular motility, visual disturbances

Pathology: mature lymphocytes with reactive germinal centers; T cells, 60%–80% with scattered polyclonal B cells; high degree of endothelial cell proliferation

Atypical Lymphoid Hyperplasia

Low-grade lymphoma, no mitotic activity

Pathology: follicles and polymorphous response consistent with benign process

40% develop systemic disease within 5 years

Orbital Lymphoma

Orbital lymphoma occurs primarily in adults and usually involves superior orbit (only Burkitt's occurs in children)

Findings: limitation of ocular motility, painless lacrimal gland swelling, conjunctival salmon patches, visual changes

Pathology: atypical immature lymphocytes with mitoses; diffuse or follicular growth; monoclonal B-cell proliferations 60%–90% with scattered or reactive T cells; involves reticuloendothelial system, including retroperitoneal lymph nodes (Figure 6-22)

CT scan: putty-like molding of tumor; orbital tissues not displaced

Treatment: radiotherapy for localized orbital disease, chemotherapy for systemic involvement

Prognosis: location appears more important than histopathology for determining systemic involvement: lymphoma of eyelids (67% have systemic involvement) > orbit (35%) > conjunctiva (20%)

Figure 6-22. A, Nodular lymphoid infiltrate. **B,** Higher magnification shows uniform lymphocyte infiltrate with mitotic figures. (From Yanoff M, Scheie HG: Malignant lymphoma of the orbit—difficulties in diagnosis, *Surv Ophthalmol* 12:133–140, 1967.)

Malignant lymphoma: 60% risk of systemic lymphoma

Plasmacytoma

Tumor composed of plasma cells

Pathology: plasmacytoid lymphocytes, immunoblasts, mature plasma cells

DDx: Waldenström's macroglobulinemia, multiple myeloma, lymphoma with immunoglobulin production

Granulocytic Sarcoma ("Chloroma")

(see Chapter 5, Pediatrics/Strabismus)

Burkitt's Lymphoma

(see Chapter 5, Pediatrics/Strabismus)

Systemic Lymphoma and Waldenström's Macroglobulinemia

Solid infiltrating tumor with putty-like molding of tumor to preexisting structures

Pathology: Dutcher bodies (intranuclear PAS-positive inclusions of immunoglobulin)

Fibro-osseous Tumors

Fibrous Dysplasia

(see Chapter 5, Pediatrics/Strabismus)

Ossifying Fibroma

Variant of fibrous dysplasia

Occurs in second and third decades of life

More common in women

Well-circumscribed, slow-growing, monostotic lesion

Pathology: vascular stroma containing lamellar bone with a rim of osteoid and osteoblasts

Osteoma

Dense bony lesions originating in the frontal and ethmoid sinus

Well-circumscribed, slow-growing mass

Symptoms secondary to sinus obstruction and intracranial or intraorbital extension

Pathology: lamellar bone with variable amounts of fibrous stroma

Fibrous Histiocytoma

Firm orbital mass composed of fibroblasts and histiocytes

Usually benign (malignant in 10%)

Distinguished from hemangiopericytoma only on biopsy

Most common mesenchymal orbital lesion of adults

Pathology: storiform (cartwheel or spiral), nebular pattern of tumor cells (fibroblasts); both fibrous histiocytoma and hemangiopericytoma are spindle cell tumors, and they can be difficult to differentiate

Figure 6-23. Histiocytes *(on left)* and fibrous *(on right,* with storiform [matted] appearance) components. (From Jones WD 3rd, Yanoff M, Katowitz JA: Recurrent facial fibrous histiocytoma. *Br J Plast Surg* 32:46–51, 1979.)

CT scan: well-circumscribed mass anywhere in the orbit (upper nasal most common)

Treatment: surgical excision; moderate risk of recurrence

Histiocytosis X

(Langerhans' cell histiocytosis) (see Chapter 5, Pediatrics/Strabismus)

Juvenile Xanthogranuloma

(JXG; nevoxanthoendothelioma) (see Chapter 5, Pediatrics/Strabismus)

Epithelial Lacrimal Gland Tumors

50% of lacrimal gland lesions are inflammatory and lymphoproliferative

50% of lacrimal gland tumors are of epithelial origin

50% of epithelial tumors are benign pleomorphic adenomas

50% of malignant tumors are adenoid cystic carcinomas

Pleomorphic Adenoma (Benign Mixed Tumor)

Most common epithelial tumor of the lacrimal gland

Occurs in 4th–5th decade of life

More common in men

Slow onset (6–12 months)

Firm mass in lacrimal fossa with painless proptosis; globe often displaced medially and downward

Progressive expansile growth may indent bone of lacrimal fossa

Tumor growth stimulates periosteum to deposit a thin layer of new bone (cortication)

Pathology: proliferation of epithelial cells into a double layer, forming lumina with ductal and secretory elements; ductal inner cells secrete mucus; outer stromal cells give rise to fibrous stroma and osteoid and cartilaginous metaplasia, pseudoencapsulated with surface bosselations (Figure 6-24)

CT scan: well-circumscribed but may have nodular configuration

Treatment: complete en bloc excision without biopsy; biopsy or incomplete excision may result in recurrence and malignant transformation into pleomorphic adenocarcinoma

Pleomorphic Adenocarcinoma (Malignant Mixed Tumor)

Rapid, progressive, painful proptosis

Figure 6-24. BMT demonstrating ductal structures in a myxoid stroma. (From Yanoff M, Fine BS: *Ocular Pathology*, 5th ed, St. Louis, Mosby, 2002.)

Long history of mass in lacrimal fossa

Occurs in elderly individuals

Pathology: similar to benign mixed tumor but with foci of malignant change

Treatment: radical orbitectomy and bone removal

Adenoid Cystic Carcinoma

Most common malignant tumor of the lacrimal gland

Highly malignant

Presents in 4th decade of life

Rapidly progressive proptosis, pain and paresthesia due to perineural invasion and bony destruction

Pathology: small, benign-appearing cells arranged in nests, tubules, or in a "Swiss-cheese" (cribriform) pattern

Figure 6-25. Adenoid cystic carcinoma demonstrating characteristic "Swiss-cheese" appearance. (From Yanoff M, Fine BS: *Ocular Pathology*, 5th ed, St. Louis, Mosby, 2002.)

CT scan: poorly circumscribed mass, bony destruction, calcifications

Treatment: removal of any bone that is involved, exenteration, adjunctive radiation and chemotherapy

Prognosis: poor; survival rate of 20%–70%

Sinus Tumors

Sinus Mucocele

Cystic, slowly expanding sinus lesion

Entrapment of mucus in aerated space due to obstruction of sinus ostia

Exerts pressure on surrounding bony structures

May become infected (mucopyocele)

Causes of ostial obstruction: inflammation with scarring, congenital narrowing of ostia, trauma, osteomas, polyps, septal deviation, mucus retention cysts

Associated with cystic fibrosis

Must rule out encephalocele and meningocele

Findings:
  Frontoethmoid sinus (most common location): outward and downward displacement of globe, fullness in superonasal and medial canthal regions, above the medial canthal tendon
  Sphenoid and posterior ethmoid sinus: visual symptoms, retrobulbar pain; may have cranial nerve palsies; 50% have nasal symptoms
  Maxillary sinus (rare): upward displacement of globe, erosion of orbital floor may cause enophthalmos

CT scan: homogeneous opacified cyst with bowing of sinus wall and attenuation/erosion of bone MRI scan; highly variable signal intensities

Treatment: surgical excision with IV antibiotics; reestablish normal drainage; obliteration of sinus (only if frontal)

Sinus Carcinoma

Usually squamous cell

Most commonly from maxillary sinus

No early signs except for sinusitis

Late findings: nonaxial proptosis, epiphora, epistaxis, infraorbital anesthesia

Metastatic Tumors

In contrast to adults, pediatric tumors metastasize to the orbit more frequently than to the uvea

Orbital metastases produce rapid painful proptosis with restricted ocular motility

Neuroblastoma

(see Chapter 5, Pediatrics/Strabismus)

Leukemia

(see Chapter 5, Pediatrics/Strabismus)

Ewing's Sarcoma

(see Chapter 5, Pediatrics/Strabismus)

Breast Carcinoma

Most common primary source of orbital metastasis in women

May occur many years after primary diagnosis

May elicit a fibrous response and cause enophthalmos and ophthalmoplegia

May respond to hormonal manipulation

Lung Carcinoma

Most common primary source of orbital metastasis in men

Very aggressive

Prostate Carcinoma

May present similarly to acute pseudotumor

Less aggressive than lung carcinoma

EYELID DISORDERS

Congenital Anomalies

(see Chapter 5, Pediatrics/Strabismus)

Trauma

Lid Laceration

Partial- or full-thickness cut in eyelid that may involve the lid margin, canthus, or canaliculus

Treatment: antibiotics, tetanus booster; surgical repair; technique depends on severity and location of injury

Lid Avulsion

Complete or partial tearing of eyelid with or without tissue loss

Treatment: technique of repair depends on severity and location of injury
  Small defect (<25%): direct closure
  Moderate defect (25%–50%): Tenzel's flap

Large defect (>50%): bridge flap reconstruction (Cutler-Beard [for upper lid] or Hughes' [for lower lid] procedure with flap advancement)

Inflammation

Hordeolum

Obstruction and infection of Zeiss (external hordeolum, stye) or meibomian (internal hordeolum, chalazion) glands

Painful erythematous eyelid swelling

Accumulation of secretions causes acute inflammatory response

Lipogranuloma formation (chalazion) often evolves from internal hordeolum

Pathology: epithelioid and giant cells surrounding empty lipid vacuoles, zonal granulomatous inflammation (zonal lipogranuloma)

Figure 6-26. Chalazion demonstrating epithelioid and giant cells surrounding clear areas that contained lipid. (From Yanoff M, Fine BS: *Ocular Pathology*, 5th ed, St. Louis, Mosby, 2002.)

Treatment: warm compresses, topical antibiotic ointment, lid scrubs (for associated blepharitis); if no response, consider local steroid injection, or incision and curettage

Blepharitis

Inflammation of lid margin

Anterior lid margin disease: seborrheic or staph blepharitis

Posterior lid margin disease: meibomitis

Angular blepharitis: associated with *Moraxella*

Associated with dry eyes, acne rosacea, and chalazia

Symptoms: burning, itching, redness, tearing

Findings: lid thickening, crusting, scurf, collarettes, inspissated meibomian glands

Treatment: lid scrubs, topical antibiotic ointment, lubrication (for associated dry eye); consider oral tetracycline/doxycycline

Acne Rosacea

Idiopathic, chronic skin disorder with erythema, pustules, papules, and telangiectasia of facial skin

Rhinophyma occurs late

Ocular involvement in >50% (blepharitis, chalazia, keratoconjunctivitis sicca, keratitis)

Treatment: lid scrubs, oral tetracycline/doxycycline, oral flaxseed oil and omega-3 fatty acids, lubrication (for associated dry eye), topical metronidazole to facial skin

Contact Dermatitis

Inflammation of lid skin due to exogenous irritant or allergic hypersensitivity reaction

Red, swollen, itchy periorbital skin

Erythematous, scaling lesions; may have vesicles or weeping areas

Treatment: eliminate inciting agent; use mild steroid cream

Infections

Molluscum Contagiosum

Shiny, white-yellow papule with central umbilication

Infection by poxvirus

Spread by direct contact

Usually asymptomatic

Pathology: lobular acanthosis, large basophilic poxviral intracytoplasmic inclusions composed of nucleic acids from DNA virus (Figure 6-27)

Can cause follicular conjunctivitis and punctate keratitis

Treatment: surgical excision, cryo, incision and curettage

Phthiriasis Palpebrum/Pediculosis

Lice infection of lashes

Spread by direct contact, usually sexually transmitted

Produces blepharoconjunctivitis

Findings: follicles, injection, small white eggs (nits) and lice attached to lashes

Figure 6-27. Intracytoplasmic, eosinophilic molluscum bodies in epidermis; they become larger and more basophilic near the surface. (Courtesy of Dr. WC Frayer. From Skin and lacrimal drainage system. In Yanoff M, Fine BS: *Ocular Pathology*, 5th ed, St. Louis, Mosby, 2002.)

Treatment: remove nits and lice, topical ointment to suffocate lice, delousing creams and shampoo

Verruca Vulgaris (Papilloma)

Pink, pedunculated or sessile mass

Associated with papillomavirus (HPV)

Usually asymptomatic

Often multiple and resolve spontaneously

Herpes Infection

Herpes simplex virus (HSV):
  Primary infection causes vesicular dermatitis
  May be associated with follicular conjunctivitis and keratitis
  Treatment: antibiotic ointment to skin lesions, topical antiviral if eye involved

Varicella zoster virus (VZV):
  Vesicular dermatitis with ulceration, crusting, and scarring
  Reactivation of latent infection along distribution of trigeminal nerve (most often V_1)
  Dermatomal distribution, does not cross midline
  May have constitutional symptoms and ocular involvement
  Treatment: antibiotic ointment to skin lesions, (see Chapter 7, Cornea/External Disease for ocular involvement)

Leprosy

Organism is acid-fast bacillus *Mycobacterium leprae*

Tuberculoid and lepromatous leprosy can affect lids

Findings: loss of lashes, trichiasis, ectropion, and exposure keratitis

Treatment: systemic antibiotics (dapsone, rifampin)

Malposition and Other Disorders

Blepharospasm

Bilateral, intermittent, involuntary contractions of orbicularis and facial muscles causing uncontrolled blinking; may cause functional blindness

Etiology unknown but may be due to abnormality of basal ganglia

Usually occurs in 5th–7th decade of life; female > male (3 : 1)

Absent during sleep

Meige's syndrome: essential blepharospasm with facial grimacing

DDx: secondary blepharospasm (due to ocular irritation), hemifacial spasm (usually unilateral, due to compression of CN 7, can be caused by CPA tumor, present during sleep), myokymia, Tourette's syndrome, trigeminal neuralgia, basal ganglia disease, tardive dyskinesia

Consider CT/MRI scan to rule out posterior fossa lesion

Treatment: Botox (botulinum toxin type A) injections, surgery (excision of lid protractors or differential section of CN 7), medications (tetrabenazine, lithium, carbidopa, clonazepam)
  Botox: derived from *C. botulinum*, freeze-dried solution 5.0 units/1.0 mL; subcutaneous injection, no more than 200 units/month
    MECHANISM: blocks neuromuscular conduction by binding to receptors on nerve terminals and stops release of ACh by disrupting calcium metabolism; does not cross blood-brain barrier
    INDICATIONS: blepharospasm (effective in 90%, lasts 3 months), hemifacial spasm (lasts 4 months), strabismus (lasts 1–8 weeks)
    ADVERSE EFFECTS (no systemic toxicity): exposure keratopathy, ptosis, diplopia, flaccid lower lid ectropion

Blepharochalasis

Idiopathic inflammatory edema of the eyelids

Familial, most often in young women

Recurrent attacks of transient, painless eyelid edema resulting in atrophy, wrinkling, and redundancy of eyelid skin

May develop ptosis and herniation of orbital lacrimal gland

Dermatochalasis

Redundancy of eyelid skin with orbital fat prolapse due to involutional changes

Blepharoptosis (Acquired)

Eyelid malposition characterized by drooping upper eyelid

Myogenic:
Uncommon
From local or systemic muscular disease (e.g., myotonic dystrophy, chronic progressive external ophthalmoplegia, myasthenia gravis)
Treat underlying condition; usually requires frontalis sling

Involutional (aponeurotic):
Most common form of ptosis
Disinsertion of levator aponeurosis
Caused by aging or chronic inflammation
May be exacerbated by eye surgery or trauma
High eyelid crease with good levator function
Ptotic lid in all positions of gaze (no lid lag on downgaze as in congenital cases)
May have thinning of eyelid above tarsal plate

Neurogenic:
Etiology: CN 3 palsy, aberrant regeneration of CN 3 (Marcus Gunn jaw-winking ptosis), Horner's syndrome, multiple sclerosis, ophthalmoplegic migraine
Treatment for Horner's: shorten Müller's muscle (Putterman [conjunctival-Müller's muscle resection]) or Fasanella-Servat (tarsoconjunctival resection) procedure

Mechanical:
Etiology: mass effect of orbital or eyelid tumors, dermatochalasis, blepharochalasis, cicatrix

Traumatic:
Due to trauma to levator aponeurosis
May have lagophthalmos from cicatricial changes
May improve spontaneously, therefore observe for 6 months

Examination:
Palpebral fissure height (PF): normally 10–11 mm in primary gaze
Marginal reflex distance (MRD): distance between corneal light reflex and upper lid margin in primary gaze; normally 4 mm
Levator function (LF): distance of upper lid excursion while frontalis is immobilized; normal >12 mm, fair if 6–11 mm, poor if <5 mm
2.5% phenylephrine test: activates sympathetic fibers of Müller's muscle; resulting lid elevation simulates position after Müller's muscle resection

DDx: pseudoptosis (nanophthalmos, microphthalmos, phthisis bulbi, hypertropia, dermatochalasis, enophthalmos, contralateral eyelid retraction or proptosis)

Treatment: eyelid crutches, levator aponeurosis advancement, levator muscle resection, Müller's muscle resection, frontalis suspension with autogenous fascia lata, banked fascia lata, or synthetic materials

Surgical complications: overcorrection or undercorrection, lid lag, lagophthalmos, exposure keratopathy

Eyelid Retraction

Upper eyelid at or above superior limbus

Lower eyelid exposing sclera

DDx: thyroid-related ophthalmopathy (most common, lateral upper eyelid more retracted than medial eyelid, fibrous contraction of eyelid retractors), orbital pseudotumor (IOI), pharmacologic (phenylephrine, α-agonists, cocaine), resection of superior rectus, overcorrection of ptosis, contralateral ptosis (Hering's law)

Treatment: lubrication; surgical repair (levator aponeurosis recession, levator myotomy, spacer insertion, full-thickness skin graft for lower eyelid, hard palate grafts for lower eyelid)

Ectropion

Eversion of eyelid margin; may cause keratinization and hypertrophy of conjunctiva

Involutional:
Most common cause of ectropion
Often in lower eyelid
Etiology: horizontal laxity, disinsertion of lower eyelid retractors
Diagnosis: snap-back test
Treatment: horizontal eyelid shortening, lateral canthoplasty, repair of lower eyelid retractors

Paralytic:
Occurs after CN 7 palsy
Frequent complaints of tearing from chronic reflex secretion
Treatment: lubrication, taping of temporal lower eyelid, moisture chamber goggles, lateral tarsorrhaphy, horizontal tightening procedure, hard palate mucosal graft for lower eyelid elevation, gold weight implantation to aid in closure of upper eyelid

Cicatricial:
Etiology: burns, trauma, tumor, infection, chronic inflammation causing secondary anterior lamellar contraction (acne rosacea, atopic dermatitis, eczema, herpes zoster dermatitis, scleroderma, epidermolysis bullosa, porphyria, xeroderma pigmentosum)
Treatment: revision and relaxation of cicatrix, horizontal tightening procedure, may require vertical lengthening with full-thickness graft

Mechanical:
 Etiology: tumors of eyelid, herniated orbital fat, poorly fitted spectacles, chronic edema
 Treat underlying condition

Entropion

Inversion of eyelid margin

Lower eyelid entropion usually involutional

Upper eyelid entropion usually cicatricial

Symptoms: tearing, foreign body sensation, redness

Congenital:
 Very rare; due to epiblepharon or tarsal kink (see Chapter 5, Pediatrics/Strabismus)
 Usually does not require treatment

Spastic:
 Associated with ocular inflammation, trauma, and prolonged patching
 Squeezing of eyelids causes inward rolling of eyelid margin
 Ocular surface irritation perpetuates cycle
 Treatment: taping of eyelid, cautery, Botox injection, Quickert suture

Involutional:
 Etiology: canthal tendon laxity (horizontal lid laxity, diagnose with snap-back test), eyelid retractor dehiscence (vertical lid laxity), overriding preseptal orbicularis muscle, involutional enophthalmos
 Treatment: Quickert suture, horizontal lid-shortening procedure (Bick, lateral tarsal strip, marginal wedge resection), vertical lid-shortening procedure (Jones, Hotz, Wies marginal rotation), retractor advancement, excision of preseptal orbicularis

Cicatricial:
 Shortening of posterior lamella
 Etiology: ocular cicatricial pemphigoid, Stevens-Johnson syndrome, trachoma, herpes zoster dermatitis, surgery, trauma, chemical burns
 Digital pressure on inferior border of tarsus corrects eyelid position in involutional entropion but not cicatricial entropion
 Treatment: lubrication, avoid surgery during acute phase of autoimmune disease, remove lashes in contact with cornea, use tarsal fracture operation, apply tarsoconjunctival grafts or hard palate mucosal grafts to replace scarred tarsus; may require symblepharon ring and amniotic membrane graft to prevent recurrent scarring

Trichiasis

Misdirection of eyelashes with contact with ocular surface

May be associated with posterior lamellar scarring

Associated with distichiasis, entropion, OCP, Stevens-Johnson syndrome, entropion, chronic blepharitis, chemical burns

Symptoms: tearing, foreign body sensation, redness

Treatment: lubrication, epilation, electrolysis, cryo-destruction with double-freeze/thaw technique, argon laser, full-thickness wedge resection

Symblepharon

Adhesion between conjunctival surfaces (palpebral and bulbar)

Due to inflammation, trauma, or surgery

Bilateral in ocular cicatricial pemphigoid and Stevens-Johnson syndrome

Floppy Eyelid Syndrome

Easily everted upper eyelids

Chronic papillary conjunctivitis due to lid autoeversion during sleep with resultant mechanical irritation from bed sheets

Associated with obesity, keratoconus, eyelid rubbing, and sleep apnea

Treatment: lubrication, tape/patch/shield lids during sleep; consider horizontal eyelid tightening

Madarosis

Loss of eyelashes and/or eyebrows due to local or systemic disorders

DDx: eyelid neoplasms, chronic blepharitis, trauma, burns, trichotillomania, alopecia, seborrheic dermatitis, chemotherapy agents, malnutrition, lupus, leprosy

Poliosis/Vitiligo

Premature whitening of the eyelashes/eyebrows (poliosis) or skin (vitiligo) due to local systemic disorders

Associated with Vogt-Koyanagi-Harada syndrome, sympathetic ophthalmia, Waardenburg syndrome, tuberous sclerosis, radiation, and dermatitis

Eyelid Tumors

Benign Tumors

Squamous Papilloma

Keratinized epidermal fronds with fibrovascular cores

Most common benign lesion of eyelid

Associated with papovavirus (HPV) infection

May be sessile or pedunculated

Pathology: papillary configuration, proliferating fibrovascular tissue covered by hyperplastic prickle cell layer of the epidermis, hyperkeratosis and parakeratosis may be present, vacuolated cells containing virus particles may be seen in the upper squamous layer

Figure 6-28. Squamous papilloma demonstrating acanthosis and hyperkeratosis. (From Yanoff M, Fine BS: *Ocular Pathology*, 5th edition. St. Louis, Mosby, 2002.)

Treatment: surgical excision, cryo or laser ablation

Seborrheic Keratosis

Papillomatous proliferation of suprabasalar (prickle) cells

Pigmented keratin crust with greasy "stuck-on" appearance

Occurs in elderly

Pathology: acanthosis, hyperkaratosis, parakeratosis, and squamous eddies may be present

Figure 6-29. Seborrheic keratosis appears as blue lesion above skin surface with blue basaloid cells and keratin cysts. (From Yanoff M, Fine BS: *Ocular Pathology*, 5th ed, St. Louis, Mosby, 2002.)

Inverted Follicular Keratosis

Nodular or verrucous lesion

Looks like a cutaneous horn

Inflamed seborrheic keratosis

Pathology: acanthosis, squamous and basal cell proliferation

Cysts

Epithelial lined chambers filled with debris

Epidermal Inclusion Cyst (Epidermoid Cyst)

Single-lumen, round or oval lesion lined by keratinized, stratified squamous epithelium (epidermis) and filled with cheesy keratin debris

Occurs after a fragment of epidermis is carried into the subepithelium by trauma

Trapped but viable epithelium proliferates and produces keratin

Rupture can cause a foreign body granulomatous reaction

Dermoid Cyst

Lined by keratinized squamous epithelium and dermal appendages such as hair shafts and sebaceous glands

Contains keratin, cilia, and sebum

Often congenital

Can be found in eyelid or orbit

Hydrocystoma (Sudiforous Cyst)

Multilocular, branching lumen that appears empty or contains serous fluid

Lined by a double row of cuboidal epithelium (resembling sweat duct)

Most are eccrine hydrocystomas (can be apocrine if arising from the glands of Moll)

Occur most commonly at eyelid margin or lateral canthus

Sebaceous Gland Tumors

Congenital Sebaceous Gland Hyperplasia

Proliferation of normal sebaceous glands

20% degenerate into basal cell carcinoma

Acquired Sebaceous Gland Hyperplasia

Multiple well-circumscribed yellow nodules

Lobules of mature sebaceous glands around a dilated duct

Muir-Torre syndrome: multiple sebaceous neoplasms, keratoacanthomas, and visceral tumors (especially GI)

Sweat Gland Tumors

Syringoma

Waxy, yellow nodules on lower lid

Usually occur in young women

Benign proliferation of eccrine ductal structures

Hydrocystoma

Translucent, bluish cyst

Arises from eccrine or apocrine glands

Tumors of Hair Follicle Origin

Trichoepithelioma

Firm, skin-colored nodule

More common in women

Usually occurs on forehead, eyelids, nasolabial fold, and upper lip

Pathology: basaloid cells surrounding a keratin center

Multiple lesions: Brooke's tumor (AD)

Trichofolliculoma

A keratin-filled dilated cystic hair follicle, surrounded by immature hair follicles

Appears as a small umbilicated nodule usually with central white hairs

Tricholemmoma

Small crusty lesion with rough ulcerated surface

Usually occurs on face

Arises from glycogen-rich clear cells of the outer hair sheath

May resemble basal, squamous, or sebaceous cell carcinoma

Cowden's disease (AD): multiple facial tricholemmomas; marker for breast (40%) or thyroid cancer

Pilomatrixoma ("Calcifying Epithelioma of Malherbe")

Solitary, firm, deep nodule with overlying normal, pink, or bluish skin

Freely movable subcutaneous pink-purple nodule

Most common cystic lesion of childhood

In young adult, arises from hair matrix of upper lid or brow

Occurs on the eyelid, face, neck, or arms

Can range from 5–30 mm in diameter

May resemble an epidermal cyst

Associated with myotonic dystrophy and Gardner's syndrome

Precancerous Lesions

Actinic Keratosis

Most common precancerous lesion

Related to sun exposure

Occurs in middle-aged individuals

Scaly, white, flat-topped lesion with surrounding erythema

Common on face, eyelid, and scalp

May be single or multiple

12% evolve into squamous cell carcinoma

May also evolve into basal cell carcinoma

Pathology: elastotic degeneration in the dermis, overlying hyperkeratosis, focal parakeratosis, clefts in dyskeratotic areas (Figure 6-30)

Treatment: surgical excision, cryo or freezing with liquid nitrogen

Nevus

Congenital or acquired hamartoma

Can be flat, but is usually elevated and pigmented

Arises from neural crest cells

Pigmentation and size tend to increase during puberty

With time, nevi tend to move deeper, migrating into the dermis

Contains benign-appearing dermal melanocytes

Malignant transformation is rare

Classified by location

Junctional nevus:
    Flat, occurs at epidermal/dermal junction
    Greatest malignant potential

Figure 6-30. Actinic keratosis appears as pink papillomatous lesion with marked hyperkeratosis and acanthosis about skin surface. (From Yanoff M, Fine BS: *Ocular Pathology*, 5th ed, St. Louis, Mosby, 2002.)

Figure 6-31. Compound nevus with cells at junction and in dermis. (From Yanoff M, Fine BS: *Ocular Pathology*, 5th ed, St. Louis, Mosby, 2002.)

Compound nevus:
    Both intradermal and junctional components (Figure 6-31)
    Slightly elevated or papillomatous
    Often pigmented
    Junctional component gives malignant potential

Intradermal nevus:
    Most common
    Most benign
    Can be papillomatous, dome-shaped, or pedunculated
    Slightly pigmented or amelanotic
    Hair shafts indicate intradermal variety

Kissing nevus:
    Congenital
    Involves both upper and lower lids
    Secondary to fusion of lids during embryonic development

Spindle cell nevus:
    Compound nevus of childhood
    Bizarre cellular components
    No malignant potential

Giant hairy nevus of the face and scalp:
    Congenital
    Thickened eyelids can cause amblyopia

Nevus of Ota (Oculodermal Melanocytosis)

(see Chapter 5, Pediatrics/Strabismus)

Lentigo Maligna (Melanotic Freckle of Hutchinson)

Acquired cutaneous pigmentation

Often periocular

Occurs in middle-aged or older individuals

Conjunctival pigmentation may be noted

No episcleral pigmentation

Melanoma arises in approximately 30%

Cutaneous counterpart of primary acquired melanosis (PAM) of the conjunctiva

Xeroderma Pigmentosa (AR)

Defect in DNA repair (UV light endonuclease)

Freckles and scaling at early age

Susceptible to a variety of malignant tumors (basal cell carcinoma, squamous cell carcinoma, malignant melanoma, sarcoma)

3% incidence of skin malignant melanoma

Malignant Epithelial Tumors

Risk factors: increased age, sun exposure, fair skin, previous history of skin cancer, positive family history

Basal Cell Carcinoma (BCC)

Most common malignancy of the eyelid (90%)

40 times more common than squamous cell carcinoma

Develops on sun-exposed skin in elderly patients

Location (in order of frequency): lower lid, medial canthus, upper lid, outer canthus

Poorest prognosis when found in medial canthus in that tumor often extends deeper and can involve lacrimal drainage system

Morbidity and mortality occur from local invasion of skull and CNS

Rarely metastasizes

Pathology: blue basaloid tumor cells arranged in nests and cords (H&E stain), peripheral palisading commonly seen

A

B

Figure 6-32. A, BCC appears as blue nests of basal cells proliferating over pale pink desmoplasia (dermal fibroblast proliferation). **B,** Basal cell nests with peripheral palisading and mitotic figures. (Courtesy of HG Scheie. From Yanoff M, Fine BS: *Ocular Pathology*, 5th ed, St. Louis, Mosby, 2002.)

Nodular basal cell carcinoma:
  Most common form
  Firm, raised, pearly, discrete mass
  Often with telangiectases over tumor margin
  If center is ulcerated, called a rodent ulcer

Morpheaform basal cell carcinoma: (Figure 6-33)
  Less common, but much more aggressive
  Firm, flat lesion with indistinct borders
  Penetrates into dermis
  Pagetoid spread can occur

Figure 6-33. Morpheaform type demonstrating thin cords of basal cells. (From Yanoff M, Fine BS: *Ocular Pathology*, 5th ed, St. Louis, Mosby, 2002.)

Tumor cells may line up in single cell layer ("Indian-file" pattern)

Treatment: excisional biopsy, wide excision with frozen section, Mohs' micrographic surgery, may require supplemental cryotherapy or radiation therapy, exenteration for orbital extension

Squamous Cell Carcinoma (SCC)

Flat, keratinized, ulcerated, erythematous plaque

Can arise de novo or from preexisting actinic keratosis

May spread by direct extension or may metastasize via local lymphatics or hematogenously

May be associated with HIV and HPV infection

More aggressive than basal cell carcinoma

Usually occurs on lower eyelid

Pathology: pink dyskeratotic cells forming keratin pearls (H&E stain), cord-like infiltrating strands into the dermis containing atypical anaplastic cells (Figure 6-34)

Treatment: excisional biopsy, wide excision with frozen section, Mohs' micrographic surgery, may require supplemental cryotherapy or radiation therapy, exenteration for orbital extension

Keratoacanthoma

Dome-shaped squamous lesion

Central keratin-filled crater and elevated rolled edges

Occurs in elderly; clinically resembles basal cell carcinoma

Previously considered a form of pseudoepitheliomatous hyperplasia, now classified as a squamous carcinoma

Rapid onset (4–8 weeks)

A

B

Figure 6-34. SCC demonstrating **A**, pink epithelial cells invading dermis with overlying ulceration. **B**, squamous cells in dermis making keratin. (From Yanoff M, Fine BS: *Ocular Pathology*, 5th ed, St. Louis, Mosby, 2002.)

Spontaneous involution

May cause permanent damage to lid margin

May cause madarosis (loss of lashes)

Pathology: acanthotic, hyperkeratotic, dyskeratotic epithelium and inflammatory cells

Figure 6-35. Keratoacanthoma appears as cup-shaped lesion with central keratin core above skin surface. (From Yanoff M, Fine BS: *Ocular Pathology*, 5th ed, St. Louis, Mosby, 2002.)

Treatment: observation, surgical excision, local steroid injection

Sebaceous Adenocarcinoma (Figure 6-36)

Orange-yellow nodule

Highly malignant and lethal tumor

Second most common malignancy of the eyelid (after BCC)

Occurs in the elderly (6th–7th decade of life)

5 year mortality rate = 30%

Arises from meibomian glands, glands of Zeis, and glands of caruncle

Regional lymph node and hematogenous metastasis

Upper lid more commonly involved (greater number of meibomian glands)

Can masquerade and be misdiagnosed as a recurrent chalazion or chronic blepharitis

Often associated with madarosis

Pathology: lobules of anaplastic cells with foamy, lipid-laden, vacuolated cytoplasm, large hyperchromic nuclei, skip areas and pagetoid invasion (spread of tumor into conjunctival epithelium), positive lipid stains (Oil-red-O stain) (Figure 6-36)

Treatment: wide excision with frozen section and conjunctival map biopsy, exenteration for orbital extension or pagetoid spread, radiotherapy for palliation

Muir-Torre syndrome: multiple sebaceous neoplasms, keratoacanthomas, and visceral tumors (especially GI)

Malignant Melanoma (MM) (Figure 6-37)

<1% of all eyelid cancers

Lentigo maligna melanoma (Hutchinson's malignant freckle) (10%):
Flat, pigmented macule with irregular borders
Arises from lentigo maligna (see Precancerous lesions)
Occurs in sun-exposed areas of elderly patients
Fascicles of spindle-shaped cells
10% metastasize; 5 year survival = 90%

Superficial spreading melanoma (80%):
Occurs in younger individuals
Sun exposed and non-exposed skin (this form is not directly related to sun exposure)
5 year survival = 69%
Initial horizontal growth phase before invading deeper
Findings: spreading macule with irregular outline, variable pigmentation, invasive phase marked by papules and nodules
Pathology: pagetoid nests in all levels of epidermis

Figure 6-36. Sebaceous adenocarcinoma **A,** Large, foamy tumor cells in epidermis demonstrating pagetoid spread. **B,** Oil-red-O stains fat in cells. (From Yanoff M, Fine BS: *Ocular Pathology*, 5th ed, St. Louis, Mosby, 2002.)

Figure 6-37. Malignant melanoma. (From Yanoff M, Fine BS: *Ocular Pathology*, 5th ed, St. Louis, Mosby, 2002.)

Nodular melanoma (10%):
   Most common type of melanoma in the eyelid
   Usually occurs in 5th decade of life
   More common in men (2 : 1)
   Always palpable
   More aggressive, with early vertical invasion
   5 year survival = 44%

20% of nodular and 50% of superficial spreading arises from nevi

Signs of transformation: change in color, change in shape or size, crusting, bleeding

Treatment: wide surgical excision, lymph node dissection if microscopic evidence of lymphatic or vascular involvement

Prognosis: depends on depth of vertical invasion; <0.75 mm indicates favorable prognosis

Neurogenic Tumors

Neurofibroma

(see Chapter 5, Pediatrics/Strabismus)

Nodular form (fibroma molluscum):
   Usually not associated with neurofibromatosis (NF)

Plexiform form:
   Associated with NF
   Produces S-shaped lid deformity

Pathology: combined proliferation of axons, Schwann cells, and endoneural fibroblasts

Treatment: observation or resection

Neurilemmoma (Schwannoma)

(see Orbit section)

Solitary eyelid nodule composed of Schwann cells

Usually located near medial canthus

Usually not associated with NF

Pathology: proliferation of Schwann cells

Treatment: local excision

Merkel Cell Tumor

Rare, vascular, red-blue, sausage-shaped lesion

Rapid growth from Merkel cells (mechanical receptors for touch; APUD system)

Usually occurs in upper lid

Occurs in older individuals

Metastasis and death in 30% of patients

Treatment: wide excision with immunohistochemical stains, lymph node dissection, radiation therapy

Vascular Tumors

Lymphangioma

(see Chapter 5, Pediatrics/Strabismus)

Capillary Hemangioma

(see Chapter 5, Pediatrics/Strabismus)

Cavernous Hemangioma

Appears as a port wine stain (nevus flammeus)

Associated with Sturge-Weber syndrome

Grows with the patient; does not involute

Pathology: dilated capillaries without endothelial cell proliferation

Kaposi's Sarcoma

Malignant soft tissue sarcoma (solitary or multiple)

More common in immunocompromised patients and those of Mediterranean descent

May involve orbit

Nontender, violaceous nodules and plaques

May cause lid distortion with edema and entropion

Treatment: complete surgical excision, also responsive to radiotherapy and chemotherapy

Other Lesions

Xanthelasma

Soft, flat or slightly elevated yellow plaques

More common on the medial aspect of the eyelids

2/3 of patients have normal serum lipids

Can occur in hyperlipid syndromes such as familial hypercholesterolemia, juvenile xanthogranuloma, histiocytosis X

Associated with Erdheim-Chester disease (lipoid granulomatosis):
   Multisystem disease with lipogranuloma formation in the liver, heart, kidneys, lungs, and bones
      Findings: proptosis and xanthelasma-like lesions
      Pathology: histiocytes and Touton giant cells

Pathology: aggregates of lipid-containing macrophages (foam cells) with surrounding inflammation

Treatment: observation; may recur after excision

Sarcoidosis

Slightly elevated, umbilicated papules

Noncaseating granulomas

Amyloidosis

Confluent, yellow, waxy papules

May hemorrhage with minor trauma

Pathology: heterogeneous group of substances that stains with Congo red

Necrobiotic Xanthogranuloma

Zonal granuloma with necrobiotic center

Associated with JXG, monoclonal gammopathies, and plasma cell dyscrasias

Pathology: Touton giant cells and xanthoma cells

Mycosis Fungoides

Cutaneous T-cell lymphoma

Pathology: Lutzner cells and Pautrier abscesses

NASOLACRIMAL SYSTEM DISORDERS

Obstructions

Congenital tearing: (see Chapter 5, Pediatrics/Strabismus)
   Must rule out congenital glaucoma; also consider corneal trauma, trichiasis, and superficial foreign body

Acquired tearing:
   Etiology: primary idiopathic hypersecretion, ocular surface irritation with reflex tearing, outflow obstruction
   Diagnosis:
      DYE DISAPPEARANCE TEST:
         Instill fluorescein in inferior fornix of both eyes, wait 5 minutes, then evaluate for asymmetric clearance of dye from tear meniscus
      JONES I TEST:
         Perform dye disappearance test
         Attempt to recover fluorescein in inferior nasal meatus with cotton-tipped applicator
         Abnormal result (no fluorescein) occurs in 33% of normal individuals
      JONES II TEST:
         Perform Jones I test
         Irrigate saline into nasolacrimal system
         Dye recovery from nose indicates functional occlusion of nasolacrimal duct
         Clear saline recovery indicates canalicular occlusion or nonfunctioning lacrimal pump
      DACRYOSCINTOGRAM: instillation of technetium 99, physiologic test
      DACRYOCYSTOGRAM: injection of Lipiodol (radiopaque) outlines drainage system
      PROBING AND IRRIGATION

Punctal Obstruction

Etiology: senile, cicatrizing (ocular cicatrical pemphigoid, Stevens-Johnson syndrome), trauma, tumor, drug-induced

Treatment: dilation, punctoplasty, reapposition of puncta

Canalicular Obstruction

Etiology: trauma, toxic medications (antivirals, strong miotics, epinephrine), infections (HSV, EBV, trachoma), dacryolith, inflammation (ocular cicatrical pemphigoid, Stevens-Johnson syndrome), allergy, radiation, tumor, canaliculitis

Treatment:
Repair of canalicular system (in trauma)
Partial obstruction: Crawford tubes or Viers rods
Obstruction within 8 mm of punctum: Jones tubes
Obstruction >8 mm from punctum: DCR with O'Donoghue tubes

Nasolacrimal Duct Obstruction

Etiology: involutional stenosis (most common cause, more common in women [2 : 1], inflammatory infiltrates compress nasolacrimal duct), trauma, chronic sinus disease, nasal polyps, dacryocystitis, granulomatous disease (e.g., sarcoidosis, Wegener's granulomatosis)

Treatment: silicone intubation, dacryocystorhinostomy (DCR)

Lacrimal Sac Obstruction

Etiology: trauma, acute or chronic dacryocystitis

Treatment: DCR

Infections

Canaliculitis

Infection of canaliculus, usually chronic

Organisms: *Actinomyces israelii* is most common (filamentous Gram-positive rod). Also, *Candida albicans, Aspergillus, Nocardia asteroides*, HSV, and VZV

More commonly occurs in middle-aged women

Symptoms: tearing, redness, pain, discharge

Findings: erythematous, dilated, tender, pouting punctum; expressible discharge, recurrent conjunctivitis; may have bloody tears

Grating sensation with probing

Often find sulfur granules

Treatment: warm compresses, probing and irrigation with penicillin, canalicular curettage, incision and débridement

Dacryocystitis

Infection of nasolacrimal sac

Organisms: *Staphylococcus, Streptococcus, Pseudomonas, Haemophilus influenzae* (young children; less common now that children are vaccinated against *H. flu*), *Klebsiella, Actinomyces, Candida*

Findings:
Acute: edema, erythema, and distention below the medial canthal tendon; may result in mucocele formation, chronic conjunctivitis, or orbital cellulitis
Chronic: distended lacrimal sac, minimal inflammation

Treatment: warm compresses, topical and systemic antibiotics, incision and drainage if abscess present, avoid irrigation and probing during acute infection, DCR after acute inflammation subsides

Dacryoadenitis

Acute or chronic inflammation of lacrimal gland

Etiology:
Acute: infection (*Staphylococcus, N. gonorrheae*, mumps, EBV, VZV)
Chronic: inflammation or infection (IOI, sarcoidosis, Mikulicz's syndrome, lymphoid lesions, syphilis, TB)

Symptoms: swelling, redness; may have pain, tearing, discharge with acute infection

Findings: enlarged lacrimal gland; may have tenderness, fever, preauricular lymphadenopathy, globe dystopia, restricted ocular motility

Diagnosis: CT scan; consider culture, laboratory tests (serologies), and biopsy

Treatment: may require systemic antibiotics, incision and drainage, or excision

Tumors of the Lacrimal Sac

Rare; secondary to dacryocystitis

Findings: painless mass located above medial canthal tendon, tearing, may have bloody tears; bleeding with probing

Must be differentiated from dacryocystitis

Dacryocystogram outlines tumor

Squamous papilloma: most common primary lacrimal sac tumor

Squamous cell carcinoma: most common primary malignant lacrimal sac tumor

Lymphoma: second most common primary malignant lacrimal sac tumor

Lacrimal sac can be invaded by other malignant tumors of eyelids and conjunctiva

ORBITAL SURGERY

Evisceration

Removal of intraocular contents leaving the sclera intact

Table 6-7. **DDx of Common Disorders**

Epithelial Eyelid Lesions

Slow-growing:
  Squamous cell papilloma
  Actinic keratosis
  Seborrheic keratosis
  Basal cell carcinoma
  Squamous cell carcinoma

Fast-growing:
  Molluscum contagiosum
  Keratoacanthoma

Subepithelial Eyelid Lesions

Cystic
  Cyst of Moll
  Cyst of Zeiss
  Sebaceous cyst
Solid
  Meibomian cyst
  Hordeolum
  Chalazion
  Xanthelasma
  Sebaceous adenocarcinoma

Pseudoproptosis

High myopia (axial myopia)
Contralateral enophthalmos
Shallow orbits (Crouzon's, Apert's syndrome)
Buphthalmos
Contralateral ptosis
Upper lid retraction

Infantile Proptosis

Capillary hemangioma (most common)
Orbital cellulitis
Dermoid
Encephalocele
Histiocytosis X
Leukemia
Retinoblastoma
Craniofacial disorders

Childhood Proptosis

Orbital cellulitis (most common)
Capillary hemangioma
Dermoid cyst
Inflammatory pseudotumor
Lymphangioma
Metastatic neuroblastoma
Granulocytic sarcoma
Orbital extension of retinoblastoma
Optic nerve glioma
Rhabdomyosarcoma
Lymphoma/leukemia
Meningioma
Neurofibromatosis
Spheno-orbital encephalocele
Optic nerve glioma
Plexiform neurofibroma in the orbit

Adult Proptosis

Thyroid-related ophthalmopathy (50%)
Hemangioma
Orbital pseudotumor

Pigmented Eyelid Lesions

Nevus
Pigmented basal cell carcinoma
Lentigo maligna (Hutchinson's freckle)
Malignant melanoma
Oculodermal melanocytosis (nevus of Ota)

Enlarged Extraocular Muscles on CT Scan

Thyroid-related ophthalmopathy (muscle tendons spared)
Orbital pseudotumor (muscle tendons involved)
Metastatic cancer
Lymphoma
Infection
Carotid-cavernous sinus fistula
Acromegaly
Amyloid
Nodular fasciitis
Fibrous histiocytoma
Tenon's cyst
Wegener's granulomatosis

Enhancing Lesions with Contrast

Cavernous hemangioma
Neurilemmoma
Fibrous histiocytoma
Hemangiopericytoma

Lacrimal Gland Inflammation/Swelling

Mumps
Glandular fever
Suppurative adenitis
Extension of conjunctivitis
Tuberculosis
Sarcoidosis
Malignant lymphoma
Lacrimal gland tumor
Thyroid-related ophthalmopathy
Orbital pseudotumor

Unilateral Periorbital Inflammation

Ruptured dermoid cyst
Rhabdomyosarcoma
Orbital pseudotumor
Leukemia
Eosinophilic granuloma
Infantile cortical hyperostosis

Enophthalmos

Orbital floor fracture
Metastatic tumors with sclerosis (breast carcinoma)

Painless Proptosis

Cavernous hemangioma
Optic nerve tumor
Neurofibroma
Neurilemmoma
Benign lacrimal gland tumors
Rhabdomyosarcoma
Fibrous histiocytoma
Lymphoma
Osteoma

Table 6-7. **DDx of Common Disorders—cont'd**

Bilateral Proptosis	*Painful Proptosis*
Thyroid-related ophthalmopathy (most common)	Orbital pseudotumor
Orbital pseudotumor	Posterior scleritis
Wegener's granulomatosis	Dacryoadenitis
Orbital lymphoma	Orbital hemorrhage
Metastatic tumor	Malignant lacrimal gland tumor
Chloroma	Nasopharyngeal carcinoma
Metastatic neuroblastoma	Lymphangioma
Crouzon's disease	Orbital abscess
Cavernous sinus thrombosis	Wegener's granulomatosis
Acromegaly	Primary orbital tumors
Histiocytosis X	Hemangioma
Multiple myeloma	Lacrimal gland tumors
	Optic nerve meningioma or glioma
	Rhabdomyosarcoma

Indications: blind painful eye, process not involving sclera

Complications: implant extrusion due to epithelial downgrowth and poor closure

Enucleation

Removal of entire globe and portion of optic nerve

Implant material: PMMA, silicone, hydroxyapatite

Integrated implant: painted prosthesis fits into implant

Indications: blind painful eye, intraocular malignancy, after severe trauma to avoid sympathetic ophthalmia

Exenteration

Removal of all orbital contents

Indications: adenoid cystic carcinoma, mucormycosis, orbital extension of sebaceous cell, basal cell, and squamous cell carcinomas

Dacryocystorhinostomy (DCR)

Creation of passage between lacrimal sac and nasal cavity

Osteotomy is made by removing the lacrimal sac fossa and superior nasal wall of NLD at level of middle turbinate; bony window should measure 15 mm × 15 mm

Indications: focal distal canalicular obstuctions and NLDOs

Complications: failure due to obstruction at common canaliculus or at bony ostomy site

Review Questions *(Answers start on page 361)*

1. The most common causitive organism of canaliculitis is
   a. *Candida albicans*
   b. HSV
   c. *Actinomyces israelii*
   d. *Nocardia asteroides*

2. Sequelae of a CN 7 palsy may include all of the following except
   a. filaments
   b. ptosis
   c. decreased vision
   d. dry eye

3. Which procedure is the best treatment option for the repair of a large upper eyelid defect?
   a. Cutler-Beard
   b. Bick
   c. Hughes
   d. Fasanella-Servat

4. The extraocular muscle with the largest arc of contact is the
   a. LR
   b. IO
   c. MR
   d. SO

5. The risk of systemic involvement is highest for an ocular lymphoid tumor in which location?
   a. orbit
   b. eyelid
   c. conjunctiva
   d. bilateral orbit

6. The rectus muscle with the shortest tendon of insertion is the
   a. IR
   b. SR
   c. MR
   d. LR

7. Which of the following bones does not make up the medial orbital wall?
   a. lacrimal
   b. maxilla
   c. sphenoid
   d. palatine

8. Which of the following clinical features is least commonly associated with a tripod fracture?
   a. restriction of the inferior rectus
   b. flattening of the malar eminence
   c. hypesthesia
   d. displacement of the lateral canthus

9. A carotid-cavernous fistula can be differentiated from a dural-sinus fistula by all of the following characteristics except
   a. proptosis
   b. afferent pupillary defect
   c. bruit
   d. CN 6 palsy

10. Basal cell carcinoma is least likely to occur at which site?
    a. upper eyelid
    b. medial canthus
    c. lower eyelid
    d. lateral canthus

11. All of the following are sites of attachment of the limbs of the medial canthal tendon except
    a. frontal process of the maxillary bone
    b. anterior lacrimal crest
    c. orbital process of the frontal bone
    d. posterior lacrimal crest

12. Which muscle is most commonly responsible for vertical diplopia after 4-lid blepharoplasty?
    a. superior oblique
    b. inferior oblique
    c. superior rectus
    d. inferior rectus

13. Congenital and involutional ptosis can be distinguished by all of the following except
    a. degree of levator function
    b. presence of lid crease
    c. width of palprebal fissure
    d. presence of jaw wink

14. Congenital obstruction of the lacrimal drainage system usually occurs at the
    a. valve of Rosenmüller
    b. common canaliculus
    c. lacrimal sac
    d. valve of Hasner

15. What is the correct order of structures that would be encountered when the upper eyelid is penetrated 14 mm above the lid margin?
    a. preseptal orbicularis muscle, orbital septum, levator aponeurosis, Müller's muscle
    b. preseptal orbicularis muscle, orbital septum, levator muscle
    c. pretarsal orbicularis muscle, levator muscle, conjunctiva
    d. pretarsal orbicularis muscle, levator aponeurosis, orbital septum, fat

16. What is the best treatment option for a child who develops recurrent proptosis after upper respiratory infections?

   a. observation
   b. XRT
   c. chemotherapy
   d. surgery

17. All of the following are features of mucormycosis except
    a. internal ophthalmoplegia
    b. ipsilateral CN 7 palsy
    c. diplopia
    d. involvement of the first branch of the trigeminal nerve

18. All of the following are associated with blepharophimosis except
    a. trisomy 18
    b. ectropion
    c. AR inheritance
    d. wide intercanthal distance

19. Which of the following is the most important test to perform in a patient with a capillary hemangioma?
    a. ECHO
    b. hearing test
    c. EKG
    d. bleeding time

20. For entropion repair, the lateral tarsal strip is sutured
    a. below and anterior to the rim
    b. below and posterior to the rim
    c. above and anterior to the rim
    d. above and posterior to the rim

21. Staged surgery for a patient with severe thyroid-related ophthalmopathy is best done in what order?
    a. decompression, strabismus, lid repair
    b. strabismus, decompression, lid repair
    c. lid repair, decompression, strabismus
    d. decompression, lid repair, strabismus

22. Which of the following best explains why when a ptotic lid is lifted, the contralateral lid falls?
    a. inhibition of Müller's muscle
    b. Sherrington's law
    c. relaxation of the frontalis muscle
    d. Hering's law

23. Which study is most helpful in the evaluation of a patient with opsoclonus?
    a. EKG
    b. MRI
    c. ERG
    d. angiogram

24. What is the most appropriate treatment for a benign mixed tumor of the lacrimal gland?
    a. radiation
    b. excision
    c. observation
    d. biopsy

25. What is the most appropriate treatment for a biopsy-positive basal cell carcinoma of the lower eyelid?
   a. cryotherapy to the cancer and margins
   b. local antimetabolite treatment
   c. radiation with 2500 rads to the lesion and margins
   d. excision with frozen section control of the margins

26. CT enhancement is most associated with which lesion?
   a. rhabdomyosarcoma
   b. glioma
   c. lymphangioma
   d. meningioma

27. Which of the following factors is least likely to contribute to the development of entropion?
   a. preseptal orbicularis override
   b. horizontal lid laxity
   c. posterior lamella foreshortening
   d. capsulopalpebral fascia disinsertion

28. A 24-year-old woman presents after blunt trauma to the left orbit with enophthalmos and restriction of upgaze. Which plain film radiographic view would be most helpful?
   a. Caldwell view
   b. lateral view
   c. Waters view
   d. axial view

29. All of the following may cause enophthalmos except
   a. breast carcinoma
   b. lymphoma
   c. orbital floor fracture
   d. phthisis bulbi

30. All of the following nerves pass through the superior orbital fissure except
   a. CN 3
   b. CN 4
   c. CN V_2
   d. CN 6

SUGGESTED READINGS

American Academy of Ophthalmology: Orbit, Eyelids and Lacrimal System, vol 7. San Francisco, AAO, 2004.

Bosniak SL: Principles and Practice of Ophthalmic Plastic and Reconstructive Surgery. Philadelphia, WB Saunders, 1996.

Collin JRO: Manual of Systematic Eyelid Surgery, 3rd edition. Philadelphia, Butterworth-Heinemann, 2002.

Dutton JS: Atlas of Clinical and Surgical Orbital Anatomy. Philadelphia, WB Saunders, 1994.

Levine MR: Manual of Oculoplastic Surgery, 3rd edition. Philadelphia, Butterworth-Heinemann, 2003.

McCord C, Chen W, Khan JA: Color Atlas of Cosmetic Blepharoplasty. Philadelphia, Elsevier (in press).

Putterman AM: Cosmetic Oculoplastic Surgery Eyelid Forehead and Facial Techniques, 3rd edition. Philadelphia, WB Saunders, 1999.

Rootman J: Diseases of the Orbit, 2nd edition. Philadelphia, Lippincott Williams and Wilkins, 2002.

Smith BC, Nesi FA, Cantarella VH, Bittman M: Smith's Ophthalmic Plastic and Reconstructive Surgery, 2nd edition. St. Louis, Mosby, 1998.

CHAPTER 7

Cornea/External Disease

ANATOMY/PHYSIOLOGY

CONJUNCTIVAL DISORDERS

CORNEAL DISORDERS

SCLERAL DISORDERS

SURGERY

ANATOMY/PHYSIOLOGY

Conjunctiva

Nonkeratinized stratified columnar epithelium with goblet cells (most numerous in fornices) underlying loose stromal tissue (substantia propria)

Palpebral conjunctiva: firmly adherent to tarsus

Bulbar conjunctiva: loosely adherent to globe except at limbus where it fuses with Tenon's capsule

Plica semilunaris: narrow fold of medial bulbar conjunctiva near caruncle; rudimentary structure analogous to nictitating membrane in certain animals

Caruncle: tissue at medial canthus intermediate between conjunctiva and skin; contains accessory dermal appendages

Precorneal Tear Film

3 layers:
  Lipid: outer layer; reduces evaporation; cholesterol and lipids; produced by meibomian, Zeis', and Moll's glands
  Aqueous: middle layer; provides oxygen to epithelium; 98% water, 2% protein, pH = 7.35; produced by lacrimal and accessory lacrimal glands (Krause's and Wolfring's), basal secretion rate =

2 μL/min; lysozyme (antibacterial enzyme) constitutes 30% of total protein in tear film; also, lactoferrin, IgA, electrolytes, oxygen
  Mucin: inner layer; reduces surface tension and allows aqueous tear film to be spread evenly; glycoproteins; produced by conjunctival goblet cells (glands of Manz and crypts of Henle, primarily in fornix)

Cornea (Figure 7-1)

Average measurements:
  Diameter: vertical = 11.5 mm, horizontal = 12.5 mm; at birth, horizontal diameter = 9.5 to 10.5, reaches adult size by age 2
  Thickness: central = 550 microns (μm), peripheral = 1.0 mm; typically, inferotemporal paracentral cornea is thinnest, superior paracentral cornea is thickest
  Radius of curvature: 7.8 mm anteriorly; 6.2 to 6.8 mm posteriorly (peripheral cornea is flatter)
  Power: anterior surface = +49 D, posterior surface = –6D, total = 43 D
  Refractive index: 1.36

Epithelium: 50 μm thick; hydrophobic (hydrophilic molecules penetrate poorly)
  Smooth refractive surface; protects against infection
  Aerobic metabolism (accounts for 70% of ATP production)
  Oxygen is obtained via diffusion from the tear film when the eye is open and from the lid vasculature when the eye is closed; also, small amount from the aqueous
  Regenerates from limbal stem cells (turnover = 6–7 days)
  Approximately 4 to 6 cells thick centrally and 7 to 10 cells thick at limbus
  Layers:
    TOP: 3 to 4 layers of squamous cells (uppermost are apical cells)

Figure 7-1. Normal cornea. (From Yanoff M, Fine BS: *Ocular Pathology*, 5th ed, St. Louis, Mosby, 2002.)

MIDDLE: 1 to 3 layers of wing cells (flattened polygonal shape)

DEEP: 1 layer of basal cells

Cells:

    APICAL CELLS: secrete proteins that form the glycocalyx extending from epithelial surface into mucin layer of tear film

    WING CELLS: tightly packed, linked by desmosomes; form protective barrier

    BASAL CELLS: anchor epithelium to stroma by hemidesmosomes; secrete basement membrane

    NERVE CELLS: epithelium contains sensory nerve endings

Pathology:

    CORNEAL EPITHELIAL EDEMA:

        INTRACELLULAR: due to epithelial hypoxia and nutritional compromise; associated with contact lens use; fine, frosted-glass appearance (Sattler's veil)

        INTERCELLULAR: due to elevated IOP; causes microcystic edema and epithelial bullae

    CORNEAL FILAMENTS: composed of mucus and desquamated epithelial cells; due to increased mucus production and abnormal epithelial turnover

Basal lamina: scaffold for epithelium; adjacent to Bowman's membrane; secreted by basal epithelium

    Composed of type IV collagen

    2 layers: lamina lucida and lamina densa

    Basal epithelium is secured by hemidesmosomes; adheres to stroma by anchoring fibrils

Bowman's membrane: 10 μm thick; type I collagen enmeshed in GAG matrix, rich in fibronectin, acellular

    Formed from secretion from both basal epithelial cells and stromal keratocytes

    Not a true basement membrane

    Heals with scarring; does not regenerate

Stroma: 480 μm thick centrally, 900 μm peripherally; 78% water by weight

    Type I collagen in mucopolysaccharide matrix

    Collagen lamellae: 250 sheets composed of parallel small-diameter (20–30 nm) fibrils

    Glycosaminoglycans: maintain lamellar spacing, contain water

    Keratan sulfate

    Cells: keratocytes (produce tropocollagen; in wound repair, tropocollagen is different, resulting in nonparallel collagen fibrils and opacity), Langerhans' cells, pigmented melanocytes, lymphocytes, macrophages, histiocytes

    Matrix metalloproteinases (MMP): family of enzymes that break down components of the extracellular matrix; help maintain the normal corneal structure; play a critical role in restructuring the cornea after injury

        MMP-1 (collagenase-1): breaks down collagen types I, II, and III

        MMP-2 (gelatinase A): breaks down collagen types IV, V, and VII, as well as gelatins and fibronectin

        MMP-3 (stomalysin): breaks down proteoglycans and fibronectins

        MMP-9 (gelatinase B): breaks down collagen types IV, V, and VII, as well as gelatins and fibronectin

        MMP-1, 2, and 3 are made by the stroma; MMP-9 is made by the epithelium; only MMP-2 is found in healthy cornea, the others are found only after injury

    Pathology: during processing, stromal lamellae separate forming clefts (artifact); if these are absent, suggests corneal edema (lamellae are same thickness, but space between fills with fluid)

Descemet's membrane: 3 to 12 μm thick; PAS-positive basement membrane

    Anchors endothelium to stroma

    Type IV collagen secreted by endothelial cells

    2 layers:

        FETAL BANDED LAYER: anterior layer (closer to stroma), striated pattern; organized collagen lamellae (like stroma); no change with age (3 μm)

        ADULT NONBANDED LAYER: posterior layer (closer to endothelium), no striations; nonorganized; thickens with age (2–10 μm)

    Regenerates after damage as long as endothelium is intact

    Pathology:

        BREAKS: edges tend to coil or roll into a scroll shape (Haab's striae, forceps injury, hydrops) (Figure 7-2)

        FOCAL THICKENING: Fuchs' dystrophy, iridocorneal touch, vitreocorneal touch, guttata (Figure 7-3)

Endothelium: 4 to 6 μm thick

    Monolayer of interdigitating hexagonal cells joined by tight junctions

Figure 7-2. Hydrops demonstrating corneal edema (thickening) with breaks in Descemet's membrane. (From Yanoff M, Fine BS: *Ocular Pathology*, 5th ed, St. Louis, Mosby, 2002.)

Figure 7-3. PAS stain demonstrating guttata as wartlike excrescences of Descemet's membrane. (From Yanoff M, Fine BS: *Ocular Pathology*, 5th ed, St. Louis, Mosby, 2002.)

Transports nutrients into cornea, pumps fluid out of cornea

Rich in mitochondria; metabolizes carbohydrates at 5 to 6 times the rate of epithelium

2 functions:
1. Barrier between stroma and anterior chamber
2. Keeps cornea dehydrated and clear

1 million cells at birth (~3800 endothelial cells/mm^2); loss of approximately 50% with aging; adjacent cells stretch to fill gaps (no regeneration)

Morphology: at least 60% of cells should be hexagonal; less than this represents unhealthy cornea

Pathology:
  PLEOMORPHISM: variation in cell shape
  POLYMEGATHISM: variation in cell size
  Responses to stress (large, unusually shaped cells); surgery, contact lens wear, certain drugs may cause an osmotic challenge or inhibition of the Na$^+$/K$^+$ pump causing stromal edema

EXAMPLE: diabetes (buildup of sorbitol in endothelial cells with hyperglycemia); contact lens (inhibits Na$^+$/K$^+$ pump and cells swell); earliest endothelial change (endothelial bleb response) occurs within minutes of insertion of a thick, soft or rigid contact lens (resolves rapidly after lens removal or slowly after 30 minutes of lens wear)

SCHWALBE'S LINE: termination of corneal endothelium (junction between endothelium and trabecular meshwork)

POSTERIOR EMBRYOTOXIN: thickening and anterior displacement of Schwalbe's line

Innervation:
Innervation to cornea occurs via CN V$_1$

Approximately 70 to 80 branches of long posterior ciliary nerves enter peripheral cornea after myelin sheath is lost 1 to 2 mm before limbus

Stains:
  Fluorescein: stains epithelial defects; negative staining occurs in areas of epithelial irregularity
    PATTERN GIVES CLUE TO ETIOLOGY:
      INTERPALPEBRAL: KCS
      HORIZONTAL BAND ACROSS INFERIOR 1/3 OF CORNEA: lagophthalmos/exposure
      SUPERIOR PUNCTATE: SLK, floppy eyelid syndrome
      CENTRAL PUNCTATE: focal epithelial keratitis (Thygeson's SPK, EKC, molluscum)
      INFERIOR PUNCTATE: blepharitis
      PERILIMBAL (360°): soft contact lens wear
  Rose bengal: stains tissue deficient of albumin and mucin, including devitalized cells
  Lissamine green: devitalized cells, CIN; more comfortable than rose bengal

Special techniques:
  Pachymetry: measures corneal thickness
  Keratometry: measures corneal curvature (only 2 points 3 mm apart in paracentral region)
  Topography: measures curvature of entire cornea

Limbus:
Area 1 to 2 mm wide at which cornea and sclera meet; contains corneal epithelial stem cells, goblet cells, lymphoid cells, Langerhans' cells, mast cells (see Chapter 10, Anterior Segment)

Sclera:
White fibrous layer composed of collagen and elastin

0.66 mm thick at muscle insertion; 0.33 mm beneath recti; 1.0 mm posteriorly

3 layers (ill defined): episclera, sclera proper, and lamina fusca

CONJUNCTIVAL DISORDERS

Inflammation

Follicles

Gray-white round elevations with avascular center and vessels at periphery

Well-circumscribed focus of lymphoid hypertrophy (lymphocytes with a germinal center) due to reactive hyperplasia

Generally most prominent in inferior fornix (except in trachoma)

Papillae

Small to large elevations with central vascular tuft and pale avascular valleys

Epithelial proliferation, hypertrophy, and infoldings; hyperplasia of vascular stroma with chronic inflammatory cells

Usually upper eyelid

Nonspecific reaction to conjunctival inflammation (edema and leakage of fluid from vessels)

Subepithelial substantia propria of tarsal and limbal conjunctivae contains fibrous tissue septa that interconnect to form polygonal lobules with a central vascular bundle

Giant papillae: >1 mm in diameter

Chemosis

Conjunctival edema; may be caused by allergy or infection, or may be idiopathic

Phlyctenule

Usually unilateral; more common in children

Etiology: type IV hypersensitivity reaction to *Staphylococoi*, coccidioidomycosis, *Candida*, HSV, LGV, TB

Findings: round, elevated, focal, sterile infiltrate on bulbar conjunctiva, limbus, or cornea; overlying epithelium breaks down (stains with fluorescein); may have corneal vascularization

Pathology: infiltration of lymphocytes; atypical ulceration; fibrosis

Treatment: topical steroids and antibiotic

Degenerations

Amyloidosis

Yellow-salmon, subepithelial, interpalpebral plaque in primary localized disease

Systemic amyloidosis is not associated with conjunctival amyloid but is associated with amyloid of lid

Pathology: acellular eosinophilic material that stains with Congo red, thioflavin T, metachromatic with crystal violet, apple-green birefringence and dichroism with polarization microscopy

Concretions (Lithiasis)

Small, round, yellow-white deposits in palpebral conjunctiva

May contain calcium

May erode through conjunctiva and abrade ocular surface causing foreign body sensation

Treatment: remove with needle if erodes through conjunctiva

Conjunctivochalasis

Redundant, loose, nonedematous inferior bulbar conjunctiva interposed between globe and lower eyelid

Due to elastoid degeneration, possible mechanical factor from dry eye (lid rubbing, dry conjunctiva)

Symptoms: tearing (interference with tear meniscus and inferior punctal occlusion), irritation

Pingueculum

Small nodule composed of abnormal subepithelial collagen; may calcify

Located at limbus, nasal more common than temporal; does not involve cornea

Caused by actinic (UV light) exposure

Pathology: elastoid degeneration (basophilic degeneration of collagen)

Pingueculitis: inflamed pingueculum due to dryness and irritation
   Treatment: lubrication, short course of topical steroids

Pterygium

Interpalpebral, wing-shaped, fibrovascular tissue that invades cornea

Associated with actinic exposure

Findings: Stocker's line (corneal iron line at head of pterygium); may induce astigmatism with flattening in meridian of pterygium; may decrease vision if crosses visual axis

Pathology: elastoid degeneration with destruction of Bowman's membrane; may have epithelial dysplasia

Treatment: observation or surgical excision
   Up to 50% recurrence rate with primary excision (50% within 4 months, 95% within 1 year)
   Decreased risk of recurrence with amniotic membrane (15%), conjunctival autograft (5%), or mitomycin application at surgery

Deposits

Exogenous

Argyrosis, mascara, adenochrome (topical epinephrine is metabolized to melanin)

Endogenous

Addison's disease, Nelson's syndrome, alkaptonuria (AR, absence of homogentisic acid oxidase)

Biopsy: for cystinosis or oxalosis, fix in 50% alcohol so crystals do not dissolve; if urate suspected, use absolute alcohol

Conjunctival Telangiectasia

Associated with Louis-Barr syndrome (ataxia-telangiectasia), Osler-Weber-Rendu (hereditary telangiectasia), Sturge-Weber syndrome, diabetes, sickle cell disease, Fabry's disease, increased orbital pressure (C-C fistula), blood-filled lymphatic tissue, irradiation

Allergy

Type I hypersensitivity reaction: airborne allergens (pollen, mold, dander) cross-link IgE receptors on mast cells causing degranulation with release of histamine, eosinophil chemotactic factors, platelet-activating factor, major basic protein, and prostaglandin D_2

Symptoms: itching (H_1 receptors), hyperemia (H_2 receptors)

Conjunctival scraping: abundant eosinophils (normally, there are very few)

Treatment: topical antihistamine (Emadine, Livostin), mast cell stabilizer (Alamast, Alocril, Alomide, Crolom), antihistamine/mast cell stabilizer combination (Optivar, Patanol, Zaditor, Elestat), NSAID (Acular), steroid, artificial tears, cold compresses

Allergic Conjunctivitis

20% of the US population have allergies

90% of patients with systemic allergies will have ocular symptoms

Most commonly seasonal or perennial allergic conjunctivitis

Associated with allergic rhinitis

Symptoms: itching, tearing, redness

Findings: lid swelling, chemosis, injection

Giant Papillary Conjunctivitis

Etiology: allergic reaction to material coating a foreign body (e.g., contact lens [CL], exposed suture, ocular prosthesis); true giant papillae also occur in vernal and atopic keratoconjunctivitis

Atopic individuals are at higher risk

Symptoms: itching, tearing, mucus discharge, CL discomfort, then intolerance

Findings: giant papillae (>1.0 mm) on upper palpebral conjunctiva

Treatment: removal of inciting factor (e.g., CL, suture), topical allergy medication; symptoms resolve months before the giant papillae resolve; avoid thimerosal

Atopic Keratoconjunctivitis (AKC)

Atopy: hereditary allergic hypersensitivity (10%–20% of population)

Types I and IV hypersensitivity reactions

Onset usually between ages 30 and 50 years

Clinical diagnosis (atopic skin disease [eczema], hay fever, asthma)

Eczema (atopic dermatitis): 3% of population; AKC in 15% to 40% of those with atopic dermatitis

Symptoms: itching, burning, photophobia, tearing, blurred vision

Findings: atopic dermatitis of eyelids (may have blepharitis, madarosis [loss of lashes], punctal ectropion), papillary conjunctivitis (small or medium-sized papillae in inferior fornix); may develop symblepharon, corneal vascularization, and scarring

Associated with keratoconus (10%), subcapsular cataracts (Maltese cross-pattern), HSV keratitis

Pathology: mast cell infiltration of conjunctival epithelium

Treatment: topical allergy medication; consider systemic antihistamine, cyclosporine (up to 5 mg/kg/day)

Vernal Keratoconjunctivitis (VKC)

(see Chapter 5, Pediatrics/Strabismus)

Toxic Keratoconjunctivitis

Etiology: direct contact of medication or chemical substance with ocular surface

Findings: redness, follicles, papillae, keratitis (SPK, occasionally pseudodendrite)

Superior Limbic Keratoconjunctivitis (SLK)

Recurrent inflammation of superior bulbar and palpebral conjunctiva; unknown etiology

Associated with CL wear and thyroid dysfunction (50%)

Female preponderance (70%), onset usually between ages 30 and 55 years

Recurrent episodes; lasts 1 to 10 years, eventually resolves permanently

70% bilateral; symptoms worse than signs

Symptoms: foreign body sensation, burning, photophobia, blurred vision

Findings: hyperemia, thickening, redundancy of superior bulbar conjunctiva with fine punctate staining (rose bengal), velvety papillary hypertrophy of upper palpebral conjunctiva, micropannus, filamentary keratitis (50%), decreased Schirmer's test (25%)

Pathology: thickening and keratinization of superior bulbar conjunctiva with loss of goblet cells

Conjunctival scraping: neutrophils, lymphocytes, plasma cells

Treatment: variety of options, usually requires scarring of superior bulbar conjunctiva
  Steroids of little use
  Pressure patch
  Large-diameter bandage contact lens
  Mechanical scraping of affected area may provide temporary relief
  Topical silver nitrate solution 0.5% to 1.0% to produce chemical burn, can retreat for recurrence (never use silver nitrate stick)
  Thermocauterization of upper bulbar conjunctiva
  Recession or resection of upper bulbar conjunctiva

Conjunctivitis Associated with Systemic Diseases

Mucocutaneous disorders: Stevens-Johnson syndrome, ocular cicatricial pemphigoid (OCP), bullous pemphigoid, pemphigus, epidermolysis bullosa, dermatitis herpetiformis, arthropathies (Reiter's syndrome, psoriatic arthritis), infections (Parinaud's oculoglandular syndrome, Kawasaki's disease), Wegener's granulomatosis

Infectious Conjunctivitis

May be hyperacute, acute, or chronic

Findings: papillae, follicles, conjunctival injection, chemosis, discharge; may have preauricular lymphadenopathy, lid swelling, membranes, keratitis, corneal infiltrates, AC reaction
  Subepithelial infiltrates (SEI): collections of inflammatory cells (mostly lymphocytes) at level of Bowman's membrane and anterior stroma
    Typically occur 2 weeks after onset of EKC, can last months
    Thought to be immunologic response to viral antigens trapped in stroma

May cause decreased vision, glare, and photophobia
  DDx: hypoxia (contact lens overwear), infectious keratitis, EKC, Thygeson's SPK, hypersensitivity (staph marginal keratitis), medication (postsurgical topical NSAID without concomitant topical steroid), corneal graft rejection, Reis-Bucklers' dystrophy, Cogan's dystrophy
  TREATMENT: topical steroids (SEIs fade but may return if steroids abruptly discontinued)
Subconjunctival hemorrhages: hemorrhagic conjunctivitis
  ETIOLOGY: coxsackie A24, Picorna (enterovirus 70), EKC (adenovirus types 8 and 19)
True membrane: fibrin exudation, inflammatory cells, and invasion by vessels; firmly adherent to epithelium, bleeding occurs when peeled (diphtheria, *gonococcus*, β-hemolytic *streptococcus*, Stevens-Johnson syndrome)
Pseudomembrane: less adherent fibrin exudate (HSV, EKC, PCF, bacterial, chlamydial, VKC, chemical burn, OCP, foreign body, ligneous, Kawasaki's disease, GVHD)

DDx of conjunctivitis with preauricular lymphadenopathy: EKC, HSV, *Gonococcus*, *Chlamydia*, Parinaud's oculoglandular syndrome, Newcastle's disease

DDx of acute follicular conjunctivitis: EKC, PCF, chlamydial, primary HSV, medicamentosa (antivirals, atropine, Propine, Iopidine, Alphagan, neomycin), viral lid infections (verruca, molluscum), Newcastle's disease, acute hemorrhagic (enteroviral) conjunctivitis

DDx of chronic follicular conjunctivitis (>4 weeks): chlamydial, medicamentosa, viral lid lesion, HSV, psittacosis, Lyme disease, Parinaud's oculoglandular syndrome, chronic fiber granuloma (nylon in fornix), type I hypersensitivity (atopic)

Viral

Adenovirus

Most common; double-stranded DNA; primary infection provides lifelong immunity

Findings: initially diffuse epithelial keratitis with normal vision; later, focal epithelial keratitis, coalescence of fine spots that become subepithelial infiltrates

Epidemic keratoconjunctivitis (EKC): adenovirus types 8 and 19; bilateral in 75% to 90%
  Findings: preauricular lymphadenopathy, follicular conjunctivitis, lid swelling, watery discharge, pseudomembrane, subconjunctival hemorrhage, conjunctival scarring (symblepharon), SEIs; rarely, corneal edema, AC reaction, hypopyon; pharyngitis and rhinitis in 50%

Treatment: steroids are useful primarily with a true membrane or vision worse than 20/40 from SEIs

Pharyngoconjunctival fever (PCF): adenovirus types 3 and 7; young children; spread by respiratory secretions
  Findings: fever, pharyngitis, folliclular conjunctivitis; may have punctate keratitis, rarely SEIs

Newcastle's Disease

Unilateral follicular conjunctivitis, pneumonitis, preauricular lymphadenopathy

Occurs in poultry handlers; self-limited, lasts 1 week

Etiology: RNA virus; causes fatal disease in turkeys and other birds

Measles

Conjunctivitis, epithelial keratitis

Molluscum Contagiosum

Chronic follicular conjunctivitis associated with elevated umbilicated lid lesions

Due to release of toxic viral products

Treatment: excision of lesions or cryosurgery

Bacterial

Hyperacute

Copious purulent discharge, marked conjunctival injection and chemosis

Neisseria gonorrheae: preauricular lymphadenopathy, corneal infiltrates; can penetrate intact corneal epithelium; can perforate within 48 hours

Diagnosis: Gram's stain (Gram-negative intracellular diplococci)

Treatment: systemic ceftriaxone (1 g IM if no corneal involvement; 1 g IV or IM qd × 5 days with corneal involvement); topical antibiotic (fluoroquinolone or bacitracin); erythromycin or doxycycline × 1 week (to cover concurrent *Chlamydia* infection)

Acute

Purulent discharge, not as severe as hyperacute

Streptococcus pneumoniae, Staphylococcus, Haemophilus (less common now that children are vaccinated against *H. flu*), *Pseudomonas*

Treatment: topical antibiotic (Polytrim or fluoroquinolone); add systemic antibiotic for *H. flu*

Chronic

Staphylococcus, Moraxella, occasionally Gram-negative rods

Diagnosis: culture

Treatment: topical antibiotic (Polytrim)

Chlamydial

Inclusion Conjunctivitis (TRIC)

Chlamydia trachomatis serovars D to K

Chronic, follicular conjunctivitis

Associated with urethritis (5%)

Findings: bulbar follicles, subepithelial infiltrates, no membranes

Trachoma

Bilateral keratoconjunctivitis

Chlamydia trachomatis serovars A to C

Findings (progressive): bilateral infection of upper tarsal and superior bulbar conjunctiva, papillary reaction, follicles, repeated infections, conjunctival scarring, tarsal shortening, entropion, trichiasis, corneal abrasion, corneal pannus, corneal scarring, cicatrized limbal follicles (Herbert's pits)

Classification:
  MacCallan (old):
    STAGE **1** = simple conjunctivitis with immature follicles
    STAGE **2A** = mostly follicles
    STAGE **2B** = mostly papillae
    STAGE **3** = cicatrizing with trichiasis, entropion, horizontal palpebral conjunctival scar (Arlt's line)
    STAGE **4** = inactive with varying degrees of scarring, ptosis, xerosis
  World Heath Organization (new):
    TF = TRACHOMATOUS INFLAMMATION (follicular): >5 follicles larger than 0.5 mm on upper tarsus
    TI = TRACHOMATOUS INFLAMMATION (intense): inflammatory thickening obscuring >50% of large, deep tarsal vessels
    TS = TRACHOMATOUS CICATRIZATION (scarring): visible white lines or sheets of fibrosis (Arlt's line)
    TT = TRACHOMATOUS TRICHIASIS: at least one misdirected eyelash
    CO = CORNEAL OPACITY: obscuring at least part of pupil margin, causing vision worse than 20/60

Pathology: epithelial cells contain initial bodies (basophilic intracytoplasmic inclusions of Halberstaedter and Prowazek); Leber's cells (macrophages in conjunctival stroma with phagocytosed debris)

Treatment: systemic and topical antibiotics (tetracycline) during active disease; management of dry eyes; removal of misdirected lashes

Other Conjunctivitis

Ligneous

(see Chapter 5, Pediatrics/Strabismus)

Parinaud's Oculoglandular Syndrome

Monocular granulomatous conjunctivitis, with necrosis and ulceration of follicles; fever, malaise, lymphadenopathy; may have rash

Pathology: follicles and granulomas

DDx: cat-scratch disease (*Bartonella henselae*), tularemia, sporotrichosis, TB, syphilis, LGV, *Actinomyces*, mononucleosis, *Rickettsia*, coccidioidomycosis

Diagnosis: PCR assay

Reiter's Syndrome

Triad of urethritis, uveitis, and arthritis; conjunctivitis in 30%; may have keratoderma blenorrhagicum

Etiology: nongonococcal urethritis, *Chlamydia*, bowel infection; 85% HLA-B27 positive

Staphylococcal Disease

Blepharitis, conjunctivitis, keratitis (SPK, marginal infiltrates), phlyctenule

Floppy Eyelid Syndrome

Autoeversion of eyelids during sleep with mechanical irritation on bedsheets causes papillary reaction on tarsal conjunctiva

Associated with obesity, keratoconus, eyelid rubbing, and sleep apnea

Treatment: lubrication, tape/patch/shield lids during sleep; consider horizontal eyelid tightening

Cystic Lesions

Simple Cyst

Serous

Inclusion Cyst

Clear cyst lined by normal epithelium

Congenital or acquired (post surgery or trauma)

Dislodged epithelium undergoes cavitation within stroma

Lined by nonkeratinized stratified squamous epithelium; contains mucin (goblet cells)

Treatment: complete excision; recurs if not completely excised

Tumors

Hamartoma: growth arising from tissue normally found at that site

> EXAMPLE: hemangioma, nevus

Choristoma: growth arising from tissue not normally found at that site

> EXAMPLE: dermoid, ectopic lacrimal gland

Congenital

(see Chapter 5, Pediatrics/Strabismus)

Squamous

Squamous Papilloma

Benign proliferation of conjunctival epithelium, appears as sessile or pedunculated fleshy mass with prominent vascular tufts

Sessile: broad base, usually older patients, often located at limbus

Pedunculated: usually caused by HPV, occurs in children, often located near caruncle; frequently recurs after excision; can regress spontaneously

Pathology: vascular cores covered by acanthotic, nonkeratinized, stratified squamous epithelium

Figure 7-4. Squamous papilloma demonstrating acanthotic epithelium with blood vessels. (From Yanoff M, Fine BS: *Ocular Pathology*, 5th ed, St. Louis, Mosby, 2002.)

Treatment:
   Adults: excisional biopsy with cryotherapy to rule out dysplastic or carcinomatous lesion; incomplete excision may result in multiple recurrences

Rare risk of malignant transformation

Conjunctival Intraepithelial Neoplasia (CIN)

Premalignant lesion

Replacement of conjunctival epithelium by atypical dysplastic squamous cells

Usually transluscent or gelatinous appearance; <10% exhibit leukoplakia (keratinization)

Carcinoma in situ: total replacement of epithelium by malignant cells; BM intact; no invasion into substantia propria; characterized by leukoplakia, thickened epithelium, and abnormal vascularization

Usually begins at limbus and spreads onto cornea

Associated with HPV 16 and 18, and actinic exposure

Men > women; occurs in older, fair-skinned individuals

Pathology: dysplastic epithelium spreads anterior to Bowman's membrane, fine vascularity with hairpin configuration (similar to papilloma), anaplastic cells, dyspolarity

Figure 7-6. Squamous cell carcinoma demonstrating cells in substantia propria forming keratin pearls. (From Yanoff M, Fine BS: *Ocular Pathology*, 5th ed, St. Louis, Mosby, 2002.)

Figure 7-5. CIN demonstrating full-thickness atypia and loss of polarity. (From Yanoff M, Fine BS: *Ocular Pathology*, 5th ed, St. Louis, Mosby, 2002.)

Treatment: wide local excision with cryotherapy; remove involved corneal epithelium (use fluorescein or rose bengal to delimit); consider mitomycin; excise until margins are clear

Squamous Cell Carcinoma

Malignant cells have broken through epithelial basement membrane

Most common malignant epithelial tumor of conjunctiva; rarely metastasizes

Most common in Africa and Middle East

Appearance similar to carcinoma in situ

Pathology: invasive malignant squamous cells with penetration through basement membrane

Treatment: wide excision with removal of surrounding conjunctiva and some scleral lamellae

Cryotherapy reduces recurrence rate from 40% to <10%

Enucleation for intraocular involvement

Exenteration for intraorbital spread

Mucoepidermoid Carcinoma

Rare variant of squamous cell carcinoma with malignant goblet cells

Typically occurs in individuals >60 years old

Very aggressive, can invade globe through sclera

Suspect in cases of recurrent squamous cell carcinoma

Pathology: epidermoid and mucinous components; stains with mucicarmine, Alcian blue, and colloidal iron

Treatment: wide local excision with cryotherapy; high recurrence rate

Melanocytic

Racial Melanosis

Light brown, flat, perilimbal pigmentation; increased melanin in basal epithelium

Most common in pigmented individuals

No malignant potential

Freckle

Congenital; increased melanin in basal epithelium; normal number of melanocytes

Nevus

Congenital nests of benign nevus cells along basal epithelial and/or substantia propria

20% to 30% amelanotic

Freely movable over globe

May have epithelial inclusion cysts

Often enlarges or becomes more pigmented during puberty or pregnancy

3 types:

Junctional: nevus cell confined to epithelial/subepithelial junction (anterior to basement membrane); often seen during 1st and 2nd decades of life; appearance similar to PAM with atypia

Compound (most common): nevus cells in epithelial and subepithelial locations; cystic or solid epithelial rests are very common; epithelial inclusion cysts common

Subepithelial: nevus cells confined to substantia propria; malignant transformation possible

Figure 7-7. Nevus with subepithelial rests of nevus cells. (From Yanoff M, Fine BS: *Ocular Pathology*, 5th ed, St. Louis, Mosby, 2002.)

Primary Acquired Melanosis (PAM, Acquired Melanosis Oculi)

Unilateral, flat, diffuse, patchy, brown pigmentation; waxes and wanes

Proliferation of intraepithelial melanocytes; no cysts

Most frequently on bulbar conjunctiva or in fornices, but can occur on palpebral or tarsal conjunctiva

Analogous to lentigo maligna of skin

Occurs in middle-aged to elderly whites

20% to 30% risk of malignant transformation, nodular thickening is indication for excisional biopsy

PAM without atypia: very low risk for melanoma

Figure 7-8. PAM with pigmentation throughout the epithelium. (From Yanoff M, Fine BS: *Ocular Pathology*, 5th ed, St. Louis, Mosby, 2002.)

PAM with atypia: high risk for melanoma (46%)

20% if atypical melanocytes confined to basal epithelium

75% if epithelioid cells present

90% if intraepithelioid pagetoid spread present

Treatment: observe with photographs; biopsy-thickened areas (does not increase risk of metastasis); complete excision if malignant

Congenital Ocular Melanosis

(see Chapter 5, Pediatrics/Strabismus)

Secondary Acquired Conjunctival Melanosis

Addison's disease, radiation, pregnancy, topical epinephrine

Malignant Melanoma

Rare, variably pigmented, elevated mass most commonly on bulbar conjunctiva

May see feeder vessel

Arises from PAM (55%) or preexisting nevi (25%), or de novo

Pathology: intraepithelial pagetoid spread; need to bleach specimen to determine amount of atypia (Figure 7-9)

Treatment: document with photos; complete excision (no touch technique) with clear margins, partial lamellar sclerectomy, and cryotherapy

Recurrence is usually amelanotic

Prognosis: 20% mortality; 25% risk of metastases (regional lymph nodes and brain)

If more than 2 mm thick, increased risk of metastasis and mortality

Involvement of caruncle, fornices, palpebral conjunctiva has worst prognosis

Figure 7-9. Malignant melanoma appears as pigmented tumor with loss of polarity. (From Yanoff M, Fine BS: *Ocular Pathology*, 5th ed, St. Louis, Mosby, 2002.)

Better prognosis than cutaneous melanoma

Exenteration does not improve survival

Vascular

Pyogenic Granuloma

Exuberant proliferation of granulation tissue

Vascular mass with smooth convex surface occurring at site of previous surgery (usually strabismus or chalazion excision)

Pathology: loose fibrous stroma containing multiple capillaries and inflammatory cells

Treatment: topical steroids; excision with conjunctival graft or cryotherapy

Kaposi's Sarcoma

Red mass, often multifocal

Stages 1 and 2: patchy and flat, <3 mm in height, <4 months in duration

Stage 3: more nodular, >3 mm in height, longer duration

Associated with AIDS (20%)

Pathology: proliferation of capillaries, endothelial cells, and fibroblast-like cells (Figure 7-10)

Treatment: excision, XRT, paclitaxel (Taxol) (inhibits mitosis)

Cavernous Hemangioma

Red patch; may bleed

Associated with other ocular hemangiomas or systemic disease

Pathology: endothelial lined canals with RBCs

Figure 7-10. Kaposi's sarcoma demonstrating neoplastic cells and vascular spaces. (From Yanoff M, Fine BS: *Ocular Pathology*, 5th ed, St. Louis, Mosby, 2002.)

Lymphangioma

Cluster of clear cysts; may have areas of hemorrhage

Pathology: dilated lymphatic vessels

Treatment: excision if small

Lymphoid

(see Chapter 6, Orbit/Lids/Adnexa)

Smooth, flat, fleshy, salmon-colored mass; single or multiple

Occurs in substantia propria; overlying epithelium is smooth; can be bilateral

Most commonly in fornix

20% associated with systemic disease (but systemic lymphoma rarely presents in conjunctiva)

Spectrum of disease from benign to malignant; cannot distinguish clinically; requires immunohistochemical studies

Requires systemic workup, including CT scan, bone scan, SPEP, medical consultation

DDx: leukemia, metastases

Treatment: low-dose XRT, surgery, local chemotherapy

Metastatic

Very rare to conjunctiva

Fleshy yellow-pink mass

Breast, lung, cutaneous melanoma (usually pigmented)

Other Tumors

Fibrous Histiocytoma

Yellow-white mass composed of fibroblasts and histiocytes

Extends from limbus to peripheral cornea

Pathology: storiform pattern

Treatment: local excision

Benign Hereditary Intraepithelial Dyskeratosis (BHID)

AD with high penetrance

Originally seen in triracial families in Halifax County, North Carolina (Haliwa Indians)

Usually presents in 1st decade of life

Symptoms: itching, burning, photophobia

Findings: bilateral dyskeratotic lesions (plaques with gelatinous base and keratinized surface) involving bulbar conjunctiva near limbus; may have similar plaques on buccal mucosa or oropharynx

Pathology: acanthosis, dyskeratosis, prominent rete pegs; no malignant potential

DDx: Bitot's spot, pingueculum, squamous papilloma, squamous cell carcinoma

Treatment: observe; topical steroids (severe symptoms); excision (diagnostic; lesions recur)

Pseudoepitheliomatous Hyperplasia

Benign proliferation of conjunctiva onto corneal epithelium

Usually occurs away from limbus (in contrast to squamous hyperplasia or carcinoma)

Develops over weeks to months

Findings: raised, whitened hyperkeratotic surface (cannot differentiate clinically from dysplasia)

Pathology: thickened squamous epithelium; occasional mitotic figures; no atypia; no clear demarcation between normal and abnormal cells

Treatment: excision

Caruncle Tumors

Benign

Papilloma (30%), nevus (25%), inclusion cyst, sebaceous hyperplasia, sebaceous adenoma, pyogenic granuloma

Oncocytoma (oxyphilic adenoma): arises from metaplasia of ductal and acinar cells of accessory lacrimal glands; composed of polyhedral cells arranged in nests, cords, or sheets; eosinophilic cytoplasm correlates with abundance of mitochondria; more common in women

Malignant (5%)

Squamous cell carcinoma, malignant melanoma, sebaceous adenocarcinoma

CORNEAL DISORDERS

Congenital

(see Chapter 5, Pediatrics/Strabismus)

Trauma

Abrasion

Epithelial defect, most commonly traumatic (e.g., fingernail, plant branch)

Increased risk of infection, especially in contact lens wearer

Symptoms: foreign body sensation, pain, tearing, redness, photophobia

Findings: epithelial defect stains with fluorescein, conjunctival injection, ciliary flush; may have mild AC reaction

Treatment: topical antibiotic, consider topical NSAID, cycloplegic, bandage contact lens, or patching for pain control (never patch CL wearer because of increased risk of microbial keratitis)

Foreign Body

May be superficial or deep

Often metal (usually associated with adjacent rust ring), glass, or organic material

Treatment: removal of FB, topical antibiotic; old deep inert material may be observed

Laceration

Partial- or full-thickness cut in cornea

Requires surgical repair and topical antibiotic and steroid; complications include scarring and irregular astigmatism, which if affect vision, may be treated with rigid contact lens or keratoplasty

Recurrent Erosion

Spontaneous epithelial defect

Associated with anterior basement membrane dystrophy (ABMD) in 50% or previous corneal abrasion; also occurs in other corneal dystrophies

Abnormal adhesion of epithelium to Bowman's membrane allows spontaneous sloughing

Symptoms usually occur in morning upon awakening (epithelium swells 4% overnight, and mechanical force of lids rubbing across corneal surface when open eyes or blink can dislodge epithelium)

Duration of symptoms depends on size of erosion

Findings: epithelial defect (may be partially healed), ABMD (irregular epithelium, areas of negative stain)

Treatment: lubrication, hypertonic saline (Muro 128 5% ointment qhs × 3 months); if recurs, consider bandage contact lens, epithelial débridement, anterior stromal puncture/reinforcement (avoid visual axis because of scarring), laser (PTK with excimer laser, or Nd:YAG with stain); also, consider treatment with matrix metalloproteinase-9 inhibitors (doxycycline 50 mg PO bid × 2 months and topical steroids tid × 2–3 weeks); débridement for subepithelial scarring

Burns

Acid: denatures and precipitates tissue proteins
  Sulfuric (batteries): most common
  Sulfurous (bleach): penetrates more easily than other acids
  Hydrofluoric (glass polishing): increased penetration
  Hydrochloric: severe burn only with high concentration
  Acetic: mild burn if concentration <10%
  Pathology: superficial coagulative necrosis of conjunctiva and corneal epithelium

Alkali: denatures but does not precipitate proteins, also saponifies fat; therefore penetrates deeply
  Ammonia (fertilizers), *lye* (drain cleaners): produce most serious injury
  Lime (plaster, cement): most common; toxicity increased by retained particulate matter; less penetration
  Also, *MgOH* (fireworks), *KOH*
  Pathology: conjunctival and corneal epithelial loss with corneal clouding and edema; conjunctival and corneal necrosis; ischemia from thrombosis of conjunctival and episcleral vessels

Radiation: thermal burn (similar to acid burn)
  UV light (snow blindness, arc-welding): punctate epithelial keratitis 8 to 12 hours after exposure; completely resolves
  Ionizing radiation: superficial keratitis; then stromal disruption from keratocyte damage; corneal drying secondary to keratinization of conjunctiva

Grading systems:
  Grade I: corneal epithelial damage, no ischemia; full recovery
  Grade II: stromal haze but iris details seen, ischemia <1/3 of limbus; good prognosis, some scarring
  Grade III: total corneal epithelial loss, stromal haze, obscuration of iris; ischemia from 1/3 to 1/2 of limbus; guarded prognosis

Grade IV: cornea opaque; ischemia >1/2 of limbus; poor prognosis, risk of perforation
McCulley Classification:
  1. **IMMEDIATE PHASE**: extent of ocular surface involvement
  2. **ACUTE PHASE**: 0–7 days
  3. **EARLY REPARATIVE PHASE**: 7–21 days
  4. **LATE REPARATIVE PHASE**: 3 weeks to several months

Treatment:
  Copious irrigation; débridement of necrotic conjunctiva and particulate matter; check pH level
  Topical (10%) and oral sodium ascorbate (aids collagen synthesis and scavenges superoxide radicals)
  Collagenase inhibitors (acetyl cysteine or EDTA)
  Steroids for first 5 to 10 days only (reduce corneal and intraocular inflammation, help prevent symblepharon but can enhance collagenase-induced corneal melting, which often begins 1–2 weeks after injury)
  Topical antibiotic
  Ocular hypotensive medication for elevated IOP
  Cycloplegic
  Citrate (chelates calcium)
  During first 1 to 3 weeks:
    PROMOTE EPITHELIAL HEALING: artificial tears, tarsorrhaphy, bandage CL
    LIMIT ULCERATION AND SUPPORT REPAIR: ascorbate × 21 days, steroids × 1 week; if epithelium does not heal, consider conjunctival flap, tissue glue, or keratoplasty to prevent perforation
    TREAT SYMBLEPHARON: lyse with glass rod; consider vitamin A to improve goblet cell function
    TREAT GLAUCOMA: topical medication; may eventually require surgery
    SURGERY: limbal autograft or keratoepithelioplasty (if epithelium not healed after 3 weeks); penetrating keratoplasty (poor results; better if performed 1–2 years after injury; may need limbal stem cell transplant)

Complications: cataract, glaucoma, uveitis, symblepharon, entropion, xerosis, retrocorneal membrane, neurotrophic keratitis, corneal ulceration, anterior segment ischemia, and neovascularization

Ocular Surface Disease

Causes tear film disturbance and dry eye

Due to deficiency in tear film component(s)

Aqueous Deficiency

Lacrimal gland dysfunction (aplasia, surgical removal), infiltration (sarcoidosis, thyroid disease, lymphoma, amyloidosis, TB), inflammation (mumps, Sjögren's syndrome), denervation (Riley-Day [familial dysautonomia], Shy-Drager [adult dysautonomia, idiopathic autonomic dysfunction], Möbius' syndrome), drugs that decrease lacrimal secretion (antihistamines, diuretics, anticholinergics, psychotropics)

Keratoconjunctivitis Sicca

Adult women (95%), often associated with Sjögren's syndrome

Diagnostic criteria for Sjögren's syndrome:
Keratoconjunctivitis sicca
Xerostomia (decreased parotid flow rate)
Lymphocytic infiltration on labial salivary gland biopsy
Laboratory evidence of systemic autoimmune disease (positive ANA titer, rheumatoid factor, or SS-A or SS-B antibody; associated with HLA-B8 [90%])

Symptoms: burning, dryness, foreign body sensation, tearing; worse later in day, with prolonged use of eye, and in dry or windy environments

Findings: decreased tear meniscus height (normal = 0.5 mm), decreased tear breakup time (<10 seconds), increased mucus, filaments in severe cases, interpalpebral corneal and conjunctival staining with rose bengal/lissamine green or fluorescein, Schirmer's test (<10 mm/5 min), increased tear osmolarity (>302 mOsm)

Pathology: lymphocytic infiltration of lacrimal gland

Treatment: lubrication with artificial tears and ointments, punctal occlusion, humidifier, moisture chamber goggles; consider acetylcysteine (Mucomyst) or bandage contact lens for filaments; topical cyclosporine

Mikulicz's syndrome: lacrimal and parotid gland swelling and keratoconjunctivitis sicca due to sarcoidosis, TB, lymphoma, leukemia

Mucin Deficiency

Goblet cell dysfunction due to conjunctival scarring and keratinization (vitamin A deficiency, OCP, Stevens-Johnson syndrome, alkali burns, trachoma, graft-versus-host disease); impression cytology measures number of goblet cells

Xerophthalmia

Epithelial keratinization due to vitamin A deficiency

Vitamin A required for conjunctival goblet cell mucin production, corneal stromal metabolism, retinal photoreceptor metabolism, normal iron metabolism, normal growth, resistance to measles

Incidence 5 million new cases/year; affects 20 to 40 million children worldwide

Usually in developing countries (50% in India); in developed countries, due to lipid malabsorption (short bowel syndrome, chronic liver dysfunction, cystic fibrosis) and poor diet (chronic alcoholism)

Findings: night blindness (nyctalopia), conjunctival xerosis (leathery appearance) and Bitot's spots (gray foamy plaques), corneal xerosis with keratomalacia, ulceration, and scarring, xerophthalmic fundus (fine white mottling)

Treatment: 200,000 IU vitamin A (IM or PO)

Stevens-Johnson Syndrome

Young people; 25% recurrence, 10% to 33% mortality

Etiology: drugs (sulfa, antibiotics, barbituates, phenytoin [Dilantin]), infection (herpes, *Mycoplasma*), idiopathic

Findings: acute pseudomembranous conjunctivitis, symblepharon, persistent epithelial defects, dry eye, trichiasis, corneal scarring, vascularization, erosions, and ulcers

Other findings:
Erythema multiforme: cutaneous bullous eruptions (target lesions), crusting, rash involves face, mucosal ulceration and strictures, sore throat, fever, arthralgias
ERYTHEMA MULTIFORME MINOR: no mucous membrane involvement
ERYTHEMA MULTIFORME MAJOR: mucous membrane ulceration; 20% mortality from secondary infection

Pathology: occurs at mucocutaneous junction
Early: epithelial thinning with fibrinous exudate and stromal lymphocytic infiltration
Late: patchy epidermalization with keratinization and subepithelial fibrosis

Treatment: topical antibiotic, steroid, lubrication, symblepharon lysis

Ocular Cicatricial Pemphigoid

Bullous disease of mucous membranes resulting in scarring

Usually women age >60 years old

Etiology: probably autoimmune (immune complexes present in basement membrane zone)

Associated with HLA-B12 and with medications (pilocarpine, phospholine iodide, timolol, epinephrine, idoxuridine)

Findings: symblepharon, ankyloblepharon, trichiasis, entropion, subconjunctival fibrosis, severe dry eye, corneal ulcers, vascularization, and scarring

Other findings:

Skin: recurrent vesiculobullous lesions of inguinal region and extremities, scarring lesions on scalp and face

Mucous membranes (nose, pharynx, larynx, esophagus): strictures, dysphagia

Pathology: occurs at level of basement membrane (subepithelial bullae); epithelial thinning, loss of goblet cells, keratinization, subepithelial inflammation and fibrosis; IgA in conjunctival basement membrane zone; mostly polys; antigen-antibodies are deposited below epidermis

Pemphigus vulgaris: antigen-antibodies located within epithelium (intraepithelial acantholysis with epithelial bullae)

Conjunctival scraping: lymphocytes, plasma cells, eosinophils

Treatment: lubrication, immunosuppressive therapy, dapsone, cyclophosphamide, surgery

PK: poor success rate

Keratoprosthesis: limited success for end-stage disease

Prognosis: remissions and excacerbations

Lipid Deficiency

Meibomian gland disease (blepharitis, meibomitis, acne rosacea)

Acne Rosacea

Chronic oculodermal disorder affecting sebaceous glands of face (including meibomian glands)

Type IV hypersensitivity may play a role

Common between ages 40 and 60 years

Findings: chronic blepharitis, meibomitis, lid margin telangiectasia, conjunctival hyperemia, abnormal tear film (foam, mucin particles, excess oil), decreased tear film breakup time, meibomian gland plugging, recurrent chalazions; may develop peripheral corneal infiltrates, vascularization, scarring, thinning, ulceration, and rarely perforation

Other findings: acne-like skin changes, telangiectatic vessels, papules, and rhinophyma

Pathology: granulomatous inflammation

Treatment: warm compresses, lid scrubs, antibiotic ointment, systemic doxycycline or erythromycin, oral flaxseed oil and omega-3 fatty acids, lubrication (for associated dry eye); metronidazole to facial skin

Other Factors

Lid abnormalities: increased evaporative loss (lagophthalmos, Bell's palsy, ectropion, entropion, thyroid disease); treat with lid taping, tarsorrhaphy, surgical repair of underlying abnormality

Aging: reduced basal tear secretion

Environment: wind, low humidity

Medications: antihistamines, phenothiazines, anticholinergics, β-adrenergic blocking agents, diuretics, retinoids, estrogens, preservatives (benzalkonium chloride, thimerosal, polyquad)

Inflammation

Interstitial Keratitis

Etiology:

Bacteria: syphilis (congenital [90%; most common cause of bilateral IK] or acquired), relapsing fever (Borrelia), TB (unilateral, sectoral), leprosy, LGV

Virus: HSV, EBV, measles, mumps, rubella, influenza, smallpox, vaccinia

Protozoa: leishmaniasis, African sleeping sickness (Taenia cruzi), malaria, onchocerciasis, cysticercosis (Taenia solium)

Other causes: sarcoidosis, Hodgkin's disease, Kaposi's sarcoma, mycosis fungoides, incontinentia pigmenti, hidradenitis suppurativa, Cogan's syndrome (vertigo, tinnitus, hearing loss, IK)

Can be initiated by minor corneal trauma in patient with congenital syphilis

Findings: neovascularization appears as salmon patch, results in hazy corneal scarring, regression of vessels leaves ghost vessels (clear branching pattern within the scar); may develop secondary glaucoma from iris/angle damage

Pathology: diffuse lymphocytic infiltrate with thickened corneal stroma

Treatment: topical steroids

Cogan's Syndrome

Ocular inflammation (usually IK) with Meniere's-like vestibular dysfunction

Most likely autoimmune

Affects young adults, average age of onset is 29 years

Associated with antecedent upper respiratory illness (50%) and vascular inflammatory disease (10%; aortic insufficiency, aortitis, necrotizing large vessel [Takayasu's-like], and polyarteritis nodosa)

Symptoms: pain, redness, photophobia

Findings: SEIs, IK, conjunctivitis, iritis, scleritis, episcleritis

Other findings: sudden onset of Meniere's-like symptoms (nausea, emesis, tinnitus, decreased hearing, severe vertigo; may have nystagmus); 80% progress to deafness without systemic steroids

DDx of keratitis with vestibuloauditory symptoms: syphilis, polyarteritis nodosa, Wegener's granulomatosis, sarcoidosis, VKH, sympathetic ophthalmia, cerebellopontine angle tumor

Audiogram: most pronounced loss at extreme frequencies, relative sparing of midrange

Treatment: systemic steroids to prevent permanent hearing loss

Thygeson's Superficial Punctate Keratopathy

Associated with HLA-DR3; 90% bilateral; spontaneous remissions and exacerbations for years

Symptoms: photophobia, foreign body sensation, burning, tearing

Findings: coarse, punctate, gray-white snowflake opacities in corneal epithelium with faint subepithelial haze; raised center breaks through epithelial surface and stains with fluorescein during acute attack; during remissions, inactive lesions appear flat and do not stain; no associated conjunctivitis or iritis

Treatment: topical steroids (symptomatic relief and rapid resolution of lesions, but may prolong course of disease), therapeutic contact lens, trifluoridine (Viroptic; may help, but idoxuridine does not work and can cause subepithelial scarring), topical cyclosporine (may also be beneficial)

Without treatment symptoms last for 1 to 2 months, then remission; recurrences can begin 6 to 8 weeks later

Filamentary Keratitis

Strands composed of mucus and desquamated epithelial cells adherent to cornea at one end

Due to increased mucous production and abnormal epithelial turnover

Etiology: keratoconjunctivitis sicca, SLK, recurrent erosions, bullous keratopathy, prolonged patching, HSV keratitis, neurotrophic keratitis, neuroparalytic keratopathy, ectodermal dysplasia, trauma, atopic dermatitis, adenoviral keratoconjunctivitis, topical medication toxicity (medicamentosa), ptosis

No filaments in OCP because mucus production is diminished in this disorder

Treatment: acetylcysteine (Mucomyst), lubrication, remove filaments, bandage contact lens, treat underlying disorder

Degenerations

Pannus

Peripheral ingrowth of subepithelial fibrovascular tissue, usually superiorly

Inflammatory: destruction of Bowman's membrane (i.e., trachoma)

Degenerative: Bowman's membrane remains intact; may contain fatty plaque deposits (i.e., chronic edema)

Most commonly due to contact lens wear

White Limbal Girdle of Vogt

Small, white, fleck and needle-like deposits at temporal and nasal limbus

Pathology: subepithelial elastotic degeneration of collagen (sometimes with calcium particles)

Corneal Arcus

Arcus senilis: hazy white peripheral corneal ring with intervening clear zone between limbus

Arcus juvenilis: arcus in person <40 years old; associated with hyperlipoproteinemia types 2, 3, and 4

Pathology: lipid deposition in stroma

DDx: LCAT deficiency, fish eye disease, Tangier's disease

Carotid ultrasound: for unilateral arcus senilis (may have stenosis on uninvolved side)

Furrow Degeneration

Thin area peripheral to arcus senilis, more apparent than real; nonprogressive; asymptomatic

Crocodile Shagreen

Mosaic, polygonal, hazy, gray opacities separated by clear zones; "cracked-ice" appearance

Extends to periphery

Anterior crocodile shagreen: occurs at level of Bowman's membrane

Posterior crocodile shagreen: occurs at level of Descemet's membrane

Salzmann's Nodular Degeneration

Blue-white elevated nodules; more common in older females

Etiology: chronic inflammation (e.g., old phlyctenulosis, trachoma, IK, staph hypersensitivity)

Pathology: replacement of Bowman's membrane by hyaline and fibrillar material

Treatment: superficial keratectomy, PTK

Polymorphic Amyloid Degeneration

Bilateral, symmetric, small stellate flecks or filaments in deep stroma

Slowly progressive; usually seen in patients >50 years old; asymptomatic

Not associated with systemic amyloid

Spheroidal Degeneration (Labrador Keratopathy, Actinic Keratopathy, Lipid Droplet Degeneration, Bietti's Hyaline Degeneration, Keratinoid Degeneration)

Bilateral; male > female

Etiology: combination of genetic predisposition, actinic exposure, and age

3 types:
Type 1 (most common): involves peripheral cornea in horizontal meridian; occurs after age 30
Type 2: associated with other corneal pathology; may involve central cornea; occurs earlier in life
Type 3: involves conjunctiva

Usually asymptomatic

Findings: translucent, golden brown, spherical, superficial, stromal and conjunctival proteinaceous deposits

Pathology: extracellular basophilic material

Cornea Farinata (AD)

Involutional change

Tiny, dot- and comma-shaped, deep stromal opacities; may contain lipofuscin (degenerative pigment)

Hassall-Henle Bodies

Small, peripheral, wart-like excrescences (gutatta) of Descemet's membrane (protrude toward AC)

Normal senescent change; rare before age 20 years

Depositions

Band Keratopathy

Interpalpebral band of subepithelial hazy white opacities with ground-glass, Swiss-cheese appearance; begins at limbus

Etiology: uveitis, interstitial keratitis (IK), superficial keratitis, phthisis, sarcoidosis, trauma, intraocular silicone oil, systemic disease (hypercalcemia, vitamin D intoxication, Fanconi's syndrome, hypophosphatemia, gout, "milk-alkali" syndrome, myotonic dystrophy, chronic mercury exposure)

Pathology: calcification of epithelial basement membrane, Bowman's membrane, and anterior stroma, with destruction of Bowman's membrane; calcium salts are extracellular when process is due to local ocular disease, calcium salts are intracellular when process is due to alteration of systemic calcium metabolism

Treatment: chelation with topical disodium EDTA

Gout and hyperuricemia cause brown band from deposition of urate

Lipid Keratopathy

Diffuse or crystalline yellow stromal deposits

Due to lipid exudation from corneal vascularization

Coat's White Ring

Small, discrete, grey-white dots

Follows metallic foreign body

Mucopolysaccharidoses

AR, except Hunter's (X-linked recessive)

Most have corneal clouding (stromal; progressive), retinopathy (RPE degeneration), and optic atrophy

Corneal clouding: Hurler's, Scheie's, Morquio's, and Maroteaux-Lamy
Corneal clouding and retinopathy: Hurler's, Scheie's
Corneal clouding only: Morquio's, Moroteaux-Lamy

Retinopathy only: Hunter's, Sanfilippo's

No corneal clouding or retinopathy: Sly's

Sphingolipidoses

AR, except Fabry's (X-linked recessive)

Most affect retina (except Fabry's)

Fabry's disease (α-galactosidase deficiency):
Occurs in female carriers and 90% of affected males
Findings: cornea verticillata (whorl-like opacities in basal epithelium), cataracts (spoke-like lens opacities)
Other findings: angiokeratomas; vascular anomalies of heart, kidney, and brain; burning pain in hands and feet
DDx of cornea verticillata: amiodarone, chloroquine, hydroxychloroquine, indomethacin, phenothiazine

Dyslipoproteinemias

Fish eye disease: diffuse clouding, denser in periphery

Hyperlipoproteinemia types 2, 3, and 4: arcus

LCAT deficiency: dense arcus and diffuse, fine, gray stromal dots

Tangier's disease (AR): HDL deficiency, relapsing polyneuropathy, small deep stromal opacities

Hypergammaglobulinemia

Crystals

Cystinosis

Amino acid metabolic disorder; lysosomes cannot excrete cystine

3 forms:
  Infantile (Fanconi's syndrome) (AR): polyuria, growth retardation, rickets, progressive renal failure; salt and pepper–like fundus (no visual disturbance), only form with retinopathy; most die before puberty
  Adolescent (AR): less severe
  Adult (uncertain inheritance): benign; no renal problems; deposits limited to anterior segment

Symptoms: photophobia

Findings: iridescent, fusiform, cystine crystals in conjunctiva, cornea, iris, lens, and retina

Treatment: cysteamine (systemic for renal disease; topical for corneal crystals)

Ochronosis (Alkaptonuria)

Melanin-like pigment (alkapton; peripheral epithelium and superficial stroma)

Tyrosinemia Type II (Richner-Hanhart Syndrome) (AR)

Deposits in epithelium and subepithelial space due to tyrosine aminotransferase deficiency

Refractile branching linear opacities, may have dendritic pattern

Triad of painful hyperkeratotic skin lesions (on palms and soles), keratitis, and mental retardation

Wilson's Disease (Hepatolenticular Degeneration) (AR)

Increased copper levels due to deficiency in ceruloplasmin

Copper deposition in
  Basal ganglia: spasticity, dysarthria, tremor, ataxia
  Liver: cirrhosis
  Eye: Kayser-Fleischer ring (copper deposition in peripheral Descemet's; starts superiorly, then inferiorly, medially, and temporally); sunflower cataract

DDx of Kayser-Fleischer ring: primary biliary cirrhosis, chronic active hepatitis, multiple myeloma, chronic cholestatic jaundice

Treatment: oral tetrathiomolybdate (penicillamine), followed by oral zinc maintenance; Kayser-Fleischer rings resolve with adequate treatment

Chalcosis

Copper (Descemet's), due to intraocular foreign body composed of <85% copper

Siderosis

Iron (stroma)

Iron Lines

Due to stagnation of tears (basal epithelium)

Fleischer ring: base of cone in keratoconus

Stocker's line: head of pterygium

Ferry's line: adjacent to filtering bleb

Hudson-Stähli line: horizontal at lower 1/3 of cornea; normal aging, nocturnal exposure

Argyrosis

Silver (deep stroma/Descemet's)

Chrysiasis

Gold (peripheral deep stroma)

Krukenberg's Spindle

Melanin (on endothelium)

Plant Sap

From *Dieffenbachia*

Ulcers

Corneal Melt (Noninfectious Ulcer)

Nonimmune mediated: traumatic, eyelid abnormalities (entropion, ectropion, trichiasis, exposure, lagophthalmos), neurotrophic cornea, acne rosacea, keratomalacia, gold toxicity

Systemic immune mediated: primary keratoconjunctivitis sicca, Sjögren's syndrome, ocular cicatricial pemphigoid, Stevens-Johnson syndrome, rheumatoid arthritis, SLE, Wegener's granulomatosis, polyarteritis nodosa

Localized immune mediated: Mooren's ulcer, Staph marginal ulcer, vernal keratoconjunctivitis

Peripheral Corneal Ulcers

Mooren's Ulcer

Chronic, painful, progressive ulceration

Typically begins nasally or temporally and spreads circumferentially (up to 360°)

Type II hypersensitivity reaction

Associated with hepatitis C, Crohn's disease, and hydradenitis

Symptoms: photophobia, decreased vision (irregular astigmatism)

Findings: undermined leading edge with overhanging margin, absent epithelium in active areas; may have conjunctival injection

2 variants:
  USA: unilateral disease of elderly (males = females), usually less aggressive; perforation rare
  Africa: severe bilateral disease in young patients; rapidly progressive with risk of perforation

Diagnosis of exclusion (rule out rheumatologic and autoimmune diseases)

Pathology: adjacent conjunctiva contains increased plasma cells, immunoglobulin, and complement

Treatment: steroids, immunosuppressive agents (methotrexate, cyclosporine), NSAIDs, bandage contact lens, conjunctival recession or resection; may require corneal glue or penetrating or lamellar keratoplasty for perforation

Terrien's Marginal Degeneration

Painless, progressive, bilateral, troughlike stromal thinning; starts superiorly

Young to middle-aged men (75%)

Findings: leading edge of lipid, steep central edge, sloping peripheral edge, intact epithelium, superficial vascularization; can progress circumferentially or centrally; induces "against-the-rule" astigmatism; may perforate with mild trauma, rarely spontaneously

Staph Marginal Ulcer

Hypersensitivity reaction

Findings: initial subepithelial infiltrate with peripheral clear zone, progresses to shallow ulcer; adjacent conjunctival injection; blepharitis

Treatment: resolves spontaneously, topical steroids may help; treat blepharitis

Marginal Keratolysis/Peripheral Ulcerative Keratitis (PUK)

Ulceration is typically peripheral and unilateral, can be central and bilateral

Due to elevated collagenase; melting stops when epithelium heals

Associated with dry eyes (Sjögren's) and sytemic disease:
  Rheumatoid arthritis: painless guttering or acute painful ulceration; also may have scleritis

Wegener's granulomatosis: 60% have ocular involvement, most commonly PUK; also, may have scleritis, conjunctivitis, orbital involvement with proptosis, retinal vasculitis, and AION
Polyarteritis nodosa: may be presenting feature; also may have pale yellow, waxy, raised, friable conjunctival vessels, scleritis, conjunctivitis, and retinal vasculitis
SLE: rare manifestation
Scleroderma: also may have keratoconjunctivitis sicca and trichiasis
Others: relapsing polychondritis, inflammatory bowel disease, Behçet's disease

Diagnosis: blood tests as for scleritis (CBC, ESR, ANA, RF, ANCA)

Treatment: lubrication, punctal occlusion, tarsorrhaphy; consider immunosuppressive agents (topical cyclosporine), conjunctival recession or resection; treat underlying disease

Fuchs' Superficial Marginal Keratitis

Marginal infiltrates initially, then pseudopterygium with severe corneal thinning underneath

Risk of perforation with surgery or trauma

Microbial Keratitis (Infectious Ulcer)

Bacterial

Most common

Penetration of intact epithelium: *Neisseria, Corynebacterium diphtheriae, Shigella, H. aegyptus, Listeria monocytogenes*

Through epithelial defect: any organism; most commonly *Staphylococcus, Streptococcus,* and *Pseudomonas*

Risk factors: corneal trauma or surgery, contact lens wear, epithelial ulceration, dry eye, lid abnormalities

Signs of improvement: decrease in infiltrate (density/size), stromal edema, endothelial plaque, AC reaction, hypopyon; and reepithelialization

Treatment:
  Empiric: topical fortified antibiotics (vancomycin or cefazolin, plus tobramycin alternating q1h) or fluoroquinolone (Ocuflox, Ciloxin, Quixin, Zymar, or Vigamox q15min for 2–3 hours, then q1h); consider subconjunctival antibiotic injection (if noncompliant)
  If no response to empiric therapy: antibiotic resistance (change regimen based on culture results); fungal, protozoal, or viral process; poor compliance (admit to hospital); anesthetic abuse
  Topical cycloplegic
  Topical steroid (should be avoided until improvement is noted [usually after 48–72 hours], then dosed at lower frequency than topical antibiotic)

Complications:

Spread to adjacent structures: sclera (*Pseudomonas*), intraocular (rare in absence of corneal perforation; filamentous fungi may penetrate intact Descemet's membrane)

Corneal damage: scarring, neovascularization, endothelial dysfunction (corneal edema), descemetocele, perforation

Synechiae and secondary glaucoma

Cataract

Syphilis

(see Chapter 5, Pediatrics/Strabismus)

Crystalline Keratopathy

Often caused by *Streptoccus viridans*, also *Candida*

Associated with chronic topical steroid use (post corneal graft)

Branching, cracked-glass appearance without epithelial defect

Herpes Simplex (HSV)

Second most common cause of corneal blindness in United States (trauma is first)

Often asymptomatic primary infection before age 5 years, 3- to 5-day incubation period

Generally unilateral but can be bilateral

Congenital: see Chapter 5, Pediatrics/Strabismus

Vesicular blepharitis: primary or secondary HSV

Lymphadenopathy does not occur in recurrent HSV

Perilimbal involvement is atypical, dendrite uncommon

Acute follicular conjunctivitis: primary or recurrent HSV; usually unilateral punctate epithelial keratitis near limbus, preauricular lymphadenopathy; may develop dendrite and pseudomembrane, may have vesicular skin eruption; bulbar conjuntival ulceration is rare but specific

Primary HSV epithelial keratitis:
Multiple small dendrites, stromal infiltrates; no conjunctivitis
Heals in 1 to 2 weeks with corneal scarring
Lid lesions occur (uncommon in recurrences except in children) but without scarring
Associated with decreased corneal sensation and patchy iris atrophy near pupillary margin
Cultures: positive in 75%
Pathology: intranuclear viral inclusions and multinucleated giant cells with Giemsa stain
Prognosis: risk of recurrence is 30% within 2 years; can be induced by many stimuli (stress, sun exposure, fever, corneal trauma or surgery)

Recurrent HSV: due to latent virus in Gasserian ganglion

Epithelial keratitis: infectious dendritic ulcer caused by live virus in basal epithelium
Usually single dendrite with central trough (stains with fluorescein), heaped-up vesicular cells on either side (stain with rose bengal or lissamine green), and terminal bulbs (accumulations of vesicular cells)
May have stromal edema or infiltrate, iritis (few KP)
TREATMENT: topical antiviral (trifluridine [Viroptic] 9×/day, or vidarabine [Vira A] or idoxuridine 5×/day; use for 1–2 weeks, then taper for 1 week; beware of toxicity from overuse), cycloplegia, consider débridement
Dendrite usually resolves in 1 week; if still present after 10 days, possible resistance, so switch medication
Antiviral toxicity (idoxuridine > vidarabine > trifluridine > acyclovir): punctate epithelial keratopathy, follicular conjunctivitis, indolent corneal ulceration, preauricular ly phadenopathy with idoxuridine, punctal stenosis
Steroids reduce scarring; taper very slowly, critical dose variable (may need steroids for years); potentiate but do not activate live virus

Necrotizing keratitis: antigen-antibody complement mediated
Ulceration with infiltrate and thinning, stromal inflammation, AC reaction
TREATMENT: steroid and antiviral

Metaherpetic/trophic ulcer: chronic sterile macroulceration
Oval-shaped with smooth edges, no staining with rose bengal at edge; no stromal inflammation
Associated with overuse of topical antivirals
TREATMENT: lubrication; may take months to heal owing to damaged basement membrane, impaired corneal innervation, and abnormal tear film; may require tarsorrhaphy, bandage contact lens

Immune ring (Wessely's ring): type III hypersensitivity reaction
Ring of HSV antigen precipitates and neutrophils around area of stromal edema

Disciform keratitis: focal nummular stromal edema due to delayed hypersensitivity reaction
Localized fine KP, no necrosis; may have iritis, increased IOP (trabeculitis)
If severe: diffuse stromal edema, Descemet's folds; may have hypopyon, rarely corneal vascularization
Culture negative
PATHOLOGY: granulomatous reaction, sometimes with retrocorneal membrane
TREATMENT: topical steroid (cover with antiviral to prevent epithelial recurrence and antibiotic ointment to prevent secondary bacterial infection)

Keratouveitis: marked corneal edema (limbus to limbus) and AC reaction with KP
Significant bulbar injection; may have hypopyon, rubeosis, spontaneous hyphema, elevated IOP

Live virus present
TREATMENT: topical steroids plus oral or topical antiviral; consider antibiotic ointment

Diagnosis:

Papanicolaou smear: intranuclear inclusion bodies (Lipschütz bodies), Cowdry type A (eosinophilic) intranuclear inclusions

Tzanck's prep: multinucleated giant cells with Giemsa stain

Culture: only 60% positive if swab active dendrite

Immunofluorescence: detects HSV antigen

Treatment: depends on lesion (see earlier); corneal tranplant (PK) for visually significant scarring

Herpetic Eye Disease Study (HEDS):

STROMAL DISEASE: treatment with topical steroids and trifluridine (Viroptic) is better than Viroptic alone (prednisolone acetate 8×/day and viroptic qid for 1 week, then 10-week taper; supports immune mediated mechanism for stromal disease); no benefit to concomitant oral acyclovir

IRITIS: acyclovir (400 mg 5×/day), in addition to topical Viroptic and steroid, is better than topicals alone

PROPHYLAXIS: acyclovir (400 mg bid for 1 year) decreases by 50% risk of recurrent HSV keratitis

Complications: uveitis, glaucoma, episcleritis, scleritis, secondary bacterial keratitis, corneal scarring and ghost vessels, corneal perforation, punctal stenosis

MAJOR CLINICAL STUDY

Herpetic Eye Disease Study (HEDS)

Objective: Five trials to evaluate the role of steroids and antiviral medication in the treatment and prevention of ocular HSV disease:

1. **Efficacy of oral acyclovir in treating stromal keratitis (non-necrotizing [disciform] and necrotizing)**: 10-week course of ACV 400 mg 5×/day or placebo, in addition to topical steroids and trifluridine:

2. **Efficacy of topical corticosteroids in treating stromal keratitis**: 10-week tapering course of prednisolone phosphate or placebo in addition to topical trifluridine (prednisolone acetate 8×/day and trifluridine [Viroptic] qid × 1 week, then gradual taper over 10 weeks)

3. **Efficacy of oral acyclovir in treating iridocyclitis**: 10-week course of ACV 400 mg 5×/day or placebo, in addition to topical steroids and trifluridine

4. **Efficacy of oral acyclovir in preventing stromal keratitis or iritis in patients with epithelial keratitis**: 3-week course of ACV 400 mg 5×/day or placebo, in addition to topical trifluridine

5. **Efficacy of oral acyclovir in preventing recurrent ocular HSV disease**: 12-month course of ACV 400 mg bid or placebo and 6-month observation period for patients with a history of ocular HSV within the preceding year

6. **Determinants of recurrent HSV keratitis**: analyzed the placebo group from the acyclovir prevention trial

Results:

1. Oral acyclovir, in addition to topical steroids and trifluridine (Viroptic), for the treatment of stromal keratitis did not improve the number of treatment failures, time to resolution of keratitis, or 6-month best-corrected visual acuity

2. Topical corticosteroids reduced the risk of persistent or progressive stromal keratitis by 68% and shortened the duration of keratitis

3. Trial was stopped due to slow recruitment. Treatment failure occurred in 50% of the ACV group vs 68% of the placebo group

4. Oral acyclovir did not reduce the risk of stromal keratitis or iritis development in patients with epithelial keratitis. Stromal keratitis or iritis developed in 11% of patients in the ACV group vs 10% in the placebo group, and such an occurrence was more common in those with a previous history of stromal keratitis or iritis (23% vs 9% without previous history)

5. Oral acyclovir reduced the risk of recurrent ocular disease during the treatment period (19% vs 32%), especially in the stromal keratitis subset (14% vs 28%). Recurrence of nonocular HSV disease was also lower in the treated group (19% vs 36%). No rebound in the rate of disease was seen during the 6-month observation period after treatment

6. In the placebo group of the previous trial, 18% developed epithelial keratitis and 18% developed stromal keratitis. Previous epithelial keratitis did not significantly affect the subsequent risk of epithelial keratitis, and previous stromal keratitis significantly increased the subsequent risk of stromal keratitis (10×)

Conclusions:

1. Oral acyclovir is not useful for the treatment of stromal keratitis

2. Topical corticosteroids are beneficial for the treatment of stromal keratitis

3. Results were not statistically significant but suggest a possible benefit of oral acyclovir for the treatment of iridocyclitis

4. In patients with epithelial keratitis, a 3-week course of oral acyclovir has no apparent benefit in preventing stromal disease or iritis

5. Oral acyclovir prophylaxis significantly reduces the risk of recurrent ocular and orofacial HSV disease, especially in patients with previous stromal keratitis

6. In patients with ocular HSV disease in the previous year, a history of epithelial keratitis is not a risk factor for recurrent epithelial keratitis, but a history of stromal keratitis increases the risk of subsequent stromal keratitis, and this risk is strongly associated with the number of previous episodes

Herpes Zoster Ophthalmicus (HZO)

Herpes zoster involvement of first branch of trigeminal nerve CN 5 (V_1)

Unilateral dermatomal vesicular eruption (obeys midline)

After chickenpox, 20% risk of developing herpes zoster (shingles)

Most common single dermatome is CN 5: ophthalmic (V_1) > maxillary (V_2) > mandibular (V_3)

3 branches of ophthalmic division: frontal nerve > nasociliary nerve > lacrimal nerve

Hutchinson's sign: involvement of skin on tip of nose (nasociliary nerve) increases risk of ocular involvement

Symptoms: 2- to 3-day prodrome (fever, headache, paresthesia)

Findings:

Lid: vesicles, cicatricial changes (ectropion, entropion, madarosis, ptosis), blepharitis

Conjunctiva: follicular conjunctivitis, pseudomembranes

Cornea: keratitis

PUNCTATE EPITHELIAL: precursor to dendrite; viral replication with epithelial destruction

DENDRITIC: blunt ends, no terminal bulbs, no ulceration, minimal staining; self-limited (appears within a few days of rash, resolves in 4–6 days)

INFLAMMATORY ULCERATION: immune response; often peripheral; may lead to perforation

DENDRITIFORM EPITHELIAL PLAQUES (delayed mucous plaques): can occur at any time even weeks later; linear or branching, sharply demarcated gray-white lesion on epithelial surface; mild fluorescein staining, vivid rose bengal staining; interference with normal mucous-epithelial interaction, no active virus replication

STROMAL: occurs in 50% with epithelial disease within first 1 to 3 weeks; nummular subepithelial infiltrates and disciform keratitis beneath initial keratitis; immune response (may develop ring)

ENDOTHELIITIS: occurs in 10% with epithelial disease; bullous keratopathy (corneal edema out of proportion to stromal infiltrate), few KP, iritis

NEUROTROPHIC KERATOPATHY: occurs in 20%; due to decreased corneal sensation; leads to ulceration

Also, STROMAL SCARRING, PANNUS, EXPOSURE KERATOPATHY (due to lid abnormalities)

Iris: segmental atrophy due to vasculitis with necrosis; Argyll-Robertson pupil (ciliary ganglion involvement)

Uveitis: can occur months later; may have elevated IOP, 45% develop glaucoma

Retina: central retinal artery occlusion, acute retinal necrosis (ARN); progressive outer retinal necrosis (PORN) in patients with AIDS

Optic nerve: ischemic optic neuropathy

CN palsy (3, 4, or 6): occurs in 25%; self-limited; may involve pupil

Syndromes:

RAMSAY HUNT SYNDROME: CN 5 and 7 involvement with facial paralysis

ZOSTER SINE HERPETAE: zoster-type dermatomal pain without rash

Diagnosis: characteristic skin lesions, Tzanck's prep, serology, culture, ELISA

Treatment:

Oral antiviral within 5 days of onset: acyclovir (800 mg 5×/day), famciclovir (Famvir, 500 mg tid), or valacyclovir (Valtrex, 1000 mg tid) × 7 days; IV acyclovir × 10 to 14 days if immunocompromised

Reduces time course (formation of new lesions, healing of lesions, period of viral shedding)

Reduces risk and severity of ocular involvement if started within 2 to 3 days

Oral steroid: prednisone 60 mg qd × 1 week, then 30 mg qd × 1 week, then 15 mg qd × 1 week

Reduces time course

Reduces duration and severity of acute pain

Reduces incidence of postherpetic neuralgia

For intraocular and ocular surface involvement: topical steroid, cycloplegic, and antibiotic

For postherpetic neuralgia: capsaicin cream (Zostrix; depletes substance P), cimetidine, tricyclic antidepressants (amitriptyline, desipramine), carbamazepine (Tegretol), gabapentin (Neurontin), lidocaine (Lidoderm patch)

Complications:

Postherpetic neuralgia: pain persisting after resolution of rash; occurs in 10% of all zoster patients, 10% to 20% with HZO, and >50% of those age >60 years; 50% resolve within 1 month, 80% within 1 year

Meningoencephalitis and myelitis: rare; occurs 7 to 10 days after rash with fever, headache, cranial nerve palsies, hallucinations, altered sensorium; most common in patients with cranial zoster, dissemination, or immunocompromised (may be fatal in AIDS)

Granulomatous arteritis: contralateral hemiplegia weeks to months after acute disease; involves middle cerebral artery; 65% are >60 years old; 25% mortality

Orbital apex syndrome: optic neuropathy, ophthalmoplegia, and anesthesia

Chickenpox

Findings: papillary conjunctivitis, "pock" lesions on bulbar conjunctiva and at limbus, keratitis (dendritic, disciform, interstitial)

Fungi

Types:

Molds (filamentous): form hyphae

Table 7-1. **Comparison of Herpetic Epithelial Keratitis**

Lesion	HSV Dendrite	HZV Pseudodendrite
Appearance	Delicate, fine, lacy ulcer	Coarse, ropy, elevated, "painted-on" lesion Smaller, less branching than HSV dendrite
	Terminal bulbs	Blunt ends (no terminal bulbs)
	Epithelial cells slough	Epithelial cells are swollen and heaped-up
Staining	Base with fluorescein Edges with rose bengal	Poor with fluorescein and rose bengal
Treatment	Do not use steroids	Good response to steroids

Note: Active viral replication in epithelial lesions occurs in both HSV and HZV

Other causes of pseudodendrite: *Acanthamoeba*, tyrosinemia II, epithelial healing ridge

SEPTATE: most common cause of fungal keratitis; most common in southern/southwestern United States—*Fusarium* (*F. solani* is most virulent), *Aspergillus*, *Cuvularia*, *Paecilomyces*, *Penicillium*, *Phialophora*

NONSEPTATE: *Mucor* (rare cause of keratitis)

Yeast: *Candida* (most common cause of mycotic ocular infections in northern United States), *Cryptococcus* (associated with endogenous endophthalmitis; rarely keratitis)

Dimorphic fungi: grow as yeast or mold—*Histoplasma, Blastomyces, Coccidioides*

Risk factors:

Molds: corneal injury especially from tree branch or vegetable material, soft contact lens wear

Yeast: therapeutic soft contact lens wear, topical steroid use, nonhealing epithelial defect, decreased host resistance

Findings: satellite infiltrates, feathery edges, endothelial plaque; can penetrate Descemet's membrane

Treatment: topical antifungal (natamycin 5% [filamentous], clotrimazole [*Aspergillus*], amphotericin B 0.15% [yeast], flucytosine 1%, ketoconazole 2%, miconazole 1%, itraconazole 1%, fluconazole 0.5%); cycloplegic

Corneal epithelium is significant barrier to natamycin penetration

Acanthamoeba

22 species; exists as trophozoite or cyst

90% initially misdiagnosed as HSV

Risk factors: cleaning soft contact lenses with homemade saline solution; swimming or hot tubbing while wearing contact lenses

Prevention: heat disinfectant (75°C)

Findings: epithelial cysts (can look like EKC with subepithelial infiltrates and punctate keratopathy), perineural infiltrate (enlarged corneal nerves, decreased corneal sensation, pain [perineuritis]), ring-shaped infiltrate, corneal edema, pseudodendrite, iritis, hypopyon (30%–40%), scleritis; may perforate

Diagnosis: calcofluor white, Giemsa stain, culture (non-nutrient agar with *E. coli* overlay; can grow on blood or chocolate agar but not as well), confocal microscopy

Pathology: oval amoebic double-walled cysts in stroma

Treatment: débridement if infection limited to epithelium (may be curative), topical agents

  Antibacterial: neomycin, paromomycin (Humatin) 1% 6 to 8×/day

  Antifungal: miconazole 1%, clotrimazole 1%; ketoconazole or itraconazole (oral)

  Antiparasitic: propamidine isethionate (Brolene) 0.1% 6×/day, hexamidine (Desomedine) 0.1%, pentamidine (Biocide), polyhexamethylene biguanide (PHMB, Baquacil; swimming pool cleaner) 0.02%, chlorhexidine 0.02%

  Steroid: controversial

30% recurrence after penetrating keratoplasty

Microsporidia

Obligate intracellular spore-forming parasite (*Encephalitozoon hellem, E. cuniculi*)

Keratitis in HIV-positive patients

Symptoms: blurred vision, photophobia, foreign body sensation

Findings: diffuse punctate epithelial erosions and intraepithelial opacities; may have sinusitis

Diagnosis: epithelial cells with cytoplasmic inclusions on Giemsa stain

Treatment: fumagillin (10 mg/ml), itraconazole, albendazole

Onchocerciasis

(see Chapter 8, Uveitis)

Leprosy

(see Chapter 8, Uveitis)

Epstein-Barr Virus (EBV)

Findings: multifocal stromal keratitis; may rarely have episcleritis, follicular conjunctivitis, uveitis, optic neuritis

Diagnosis:

Antibodies: viral capsid antigen IgM and IgG and early antigen-diffuse (EA-D) peak at 6 to 12 weeks; VCA-IgM and Epstein-Barr nuclear antigen (EBNA) are detectable for life; heterophile antibodies (IgM that reacts to horse and sheep blood cells) peak at 2 to 3 weeks and last 1 year (Monospot test)

Lymphocytosis: occurs in 70%; peaks at 2 to 3 weeks

Liver enzymes: elevated

Ectasias

Keratoconus

90% bilateral; onset typically around puberty

Associations:

Systemic conditions: atopy (eye rubbing), Down's syndrome, connective tissue disease (Ehlers-Danlos syndrome, Marfan's syndrome, osteogenesis imperfecta)

Ocular conditions: aniridia, retinitis pigmentosa, VKC, Leber's congenital amaurosis, ectopia lentis, floppy eyelid syndrome, CHED, PPMD

Findings: inferior corneal protrusion, stromal thinning at cone apex (apical thinning), apical scarring, Fleischer ring (epithelial iron deposition at base of cone), Vogt's striae (fine deep striae anterior to Descemet's membrane; disappear with external pressure), prominent corneal nerves, scissors reflex on retinoscopy, Munson's sign (angulation of lower lid on downgaze due to corneal protrusion), Rizzutti's sign (conical reflection of light from temporal light source on nasal iris); may develop hydrops

Hydrops: acute corneal edema and clouding due to break in Descemet's membrane; painful or painless; decreased IOP; heals over 6 to 10 weeks; scarring can occur occasionally with stromal neovascularization

Pathology: breaks in Bowman's membrane, stromal folds, superficial scarring, stromal thinning; Descemet's is normal unless hydrops has occurred (breaks with curled edges covered by adjacent endothelial cells and new Descemet's)

DDx: contact lens-induced corneal warpage, pellucid marginal degeneration, keratoglobus

Diagnosis: corneal topography (irregular astigmatism, central or inferior steepening), keratometry (steep readings, irregular mires)

Treatment: contact lens (rigid, piggyback), penetrating keratoplasty; supportive for hydrops (topical steroids, cycloplegic, bandage contact lens)

Posterior Keratoconus

(see Chapter 5, Pediatrics/Strabismus)

Keratoglobus

Rare, sporadic, globular corneal deformity

Associated with connective tissue disorders, Leber's congenital amaurosis

Findings: bilateral corneal thinning, maximal in midperiphery at base of protrusion

Treatment: CL (rigid), penetrating keratoplasty

Pellucid Marginal Degeneration

Onset age 20 to 40 years old; no sex predilection; more common in Europeans and Japanese

Findings: bilateral, inferior corneal thinning with protrusion above thinnest area; no vascularization; acute hydrops rare

Pathology: resembles keratoconus

Diagnosis: corneal topography (irregular, against-the-rule astigmatism with inferior annular pattern of steepening)

Treatment: large penetrating keratoplasty

Dystrophies

Inherited genetic disorders (usually defective enzyme or structural protein)

AD, except macular, type 3 lattice, gelatinous, and nystagmus-associated form of CHED that are AR

Genetics: many dystrophies have a mutation of the BIGH-3 (TGFBI) gene on chromosome 5. These dystrophies tend to be AD and include granular, Avellino's, lattice types 1 and 3, Reis-Bucklers', and Thiel-Benke's

Onset by age 20 years, except anterior basement membrane dystrophy (ages 30–40), pre-Descemet's (ages 30–40), and Fuchs' (ages 40–50)

Not associated with systemic diseases, except central crystalline dystrophy (associated with hypercholesterolemia with or without hyperlipidemia), and type 2 lattice (Meretoja's syndrome associated with systemic amyloidosis)

Affect central cornea, except Meesmann's, macular, fleck, CHED, and CHSD, which extend to limbus

Anterior

Anterior Basement Membrane (Cogan's Microcystic; Map, Dot, Fingerprint) (AD)

Most common anterior corneal dystrophy

Usually bilateral, can be asymmetric; primarily affects middle-aged women

Symptoms more common in those >30 years old

Symptoms: usually asymptomatic; may have pain, redness, tearing, irritation (recurrent erosions), or decreased vision (subepithelial scarring)

Findings: irregular and often loose epithelium with characteristic appearance (map, dot, fingerprint):
  Map lines: subepithelial connective tissue
  Microcysts: white, putty-like dots (degenerated epithelial cells trapped in abnormal epithelium)
  Fingerprints: parallel lines of basement membrane separating tongues of reduplicated epithelium

May develop recurrent erosions (10% with dystrophy get erosions, 50% with erosions have dystrophy) or decreased vision or monocular diplopia from subepithelial scarring (irregular astigmatism)

Pathology: epithelial reduplication with excess subepithelial and intraepithelial production of basement membrane material and collagen (due to poor epithelial adhesion to basement membrane)

Figure 7-11. ABMD demonstrating cysts and aberrant production of basement membrane material in the epithelium. (From Yanoff M, Fine BS: *Ocular Pathology*, 5th ed, St. Louis, Mosby, 2002.)

Treatment: none unless symptomatic. For erosions, treat with lubrication, hypertonic saline (Muro 128 5% ointment qhs × 3 months); if recurs, consider bandage contact lens, epithelial débridement, anterior stromal puncture/reinforcement (avoid visual axis because of scarring), laser (PTK with excimer laser, or Nd:YAG with stain); also consider treatment with matrix metalloproteinase-9 inhibitors (doxycycline 50 mg PO bid × 2 months and topical steroids tid × 2–3 weeks); débridement for subepithelial scarring

Meesmann's (AD)

Appears early in life

Minimal symptoms, good vision

Findings: tiny epithelial vesicles, most numerous interpalpebrally, extend to limbus

Pathology: epithelial cells contain PAS-positive material (peculiar substance); thickened epithelial basement membrane

Figure 7-12. Meesmann's dystrophy with Periodic Acid-Schiff stain. (From Yanoff M, Fine BS: *Ocular Pathology*, 5th ed, St. Louis, Mosby, 2002.)

No treatment

Gelatinous Drop–Like (AR)

Rare; occurs in 1st decade

Symptoms: decreased vision, photophobia, tearing

Findings: central, mulberry-like, subepithelial opacity

Pathology: absence of Bowman's layer; amyloid

Reis-Bucklers' (Corneal Dystrophy of Bowman's Membrane Type I) (AD)

Mapped to chromosome 5q (BIGH3)

Appears early in life

Findings: subepithelial, irregularly shaped rings with scalloped edges and geographic gray-white reticular opacification, greatest centrally; epithelial erosions, corneal scarring

Pathology: absence of Bowman's layer and replacement by connective tissue; irregular saw-toothed epithelium; curly filaments (electron microscopy); stain with Masson's trichrome

Treatment: penetrating keratoplasty (recurrence is common)

Thiel-Behke's Dystrophy (Corneal Dystrophy of Bowman's Membrane Type II)

Honeycomb pattern; BIGH-3 gene defect

Stromal

Mnemonic: **M**arilyn **M**onroe **A**lways **G**ets **H**er **M**en in **LA** **C**ounty

Refers to name of dystrophy, substance deposited in cornea, special stain (for the 3 classic dystrophies)

Macular, Mucopolysaccharide, Alcian blue
Granular, Hyaline, Masson's trichrome
Lattice, Amyloid, Congo red

Macular (AR)

Mapped to chromosome 16q; error in synthesis of keratan sulfate

Most severe but least common of the 3 classic stromal dystrophies

Deposits present in 1st decade of life

Symptoms: decreased vision in 1st to 2nd decade of life

Findings: gray-white stromal opacities at all levels extending to periphery with diffuse clouding (no intervening clear spaces), central thinning; may have guttata

Pathology: mucopolysaccharide deposits, stain with Alcian blue and colloidal iron

Figure 7-13. Deposits in macular dystrophy stain with Alcian blue. (From Yanoff M, Fine BS: *Ocular Pathology*, 5th ed, St. Louis, Mosby, 2002.)

Treatment: penetrating keratoplasty; PTK (less useful, lesions extend though entire stroma and erosions rare)

Granular (AD)

Most common stromal dystrophy

Mapped to chromosome 5q (BIGH3)

Deposits present in 1st decade of life, can remain asymptomatic for decades

Symptoms: mild irritation, decreased vision

Findings: discrete focal, white, granular deposits in central anterior stroma with intervening clear areas; recurrent erosions rare

Superficial variant: looks like Reis-Bucklers'

Pathology: hyaline deposits, stain with Masson's trichrome

Figure 7-14. Deposits in granular dystrophy stain red with trichrome. (From Yanoff M, Fine BS: *Ocular Pathology*, 5th ed, St. Louis, Mosby, 2002.)

Treatment: penetrating keratoplasty, PTK

Lattice

Mapped to chromosome 5q (BIGH3)

Deposits present in 1st decade

Symptoms: pain, decreased vision in 2nd to 3rd decade of life

Findings: branching refractile lines in anterior stroma (best seen in retroillumination), central subepithelial white dots, stromal haze with ground-glass appearance, peripheral cornea typically clear (depends on type); eventually recurrent erosions with scarring

Types:

Type I (Biber-Haab-Dimmer) (AD): classic lattice dystrophy; starts centrally, spares periphery, no systemic amyloid; BIGH-3 gene defect

Type II (Meretoja's syndrome) (AD): Finnish descent; systemic amyloidosis (facial mask; dry, lax skin; blepharochalasis, dermatochalasis; pendulous ears; cranial and peripheral nerve palsies); corneal involvement more peripheral and moves centrally

Type III (AR): Japanese descent, adult onset, thicker lattice lines, limbus to limbus, no recurrent erosions; BIGH-3 gene defect

Pathology: amyloid deposits, stain with Congo red, thioflavin T, metachromatic with crystal violet, apple-green birefringence and dichroism with polarization microscopy (Figure 7-15)

Treatment: penetrating keratoplasty (recurrence more likely than in macular or granular, but less likely than in Reis-Bucklers')

Figure 7-15. Deposits in lattice dystrophy. (From Yanoff M, Fine BS: *Ocular Pathology*, 5th ed, St. Louis, Mosby, 2002.)

Avellino's

Mapped to chromosome 5q (BIGH3)

First identified in family from Avellino, Italy

Findings: appears like granular dystrophy with interspersed lattice lines; granular deposits occur early in anterior stroma, lattice findings occur later in deeper stroma; stromal haze; may get erosions

Pathology: hyaline and amyloid deposits; stain with Masson's trichrome and Congo red

Central Crystalline (Schnyder's) (AD)

Mapped to chromosome 1p

Slowly progressive, rarely reduces vision enough to require corneal transplantation

Findings: minute yellow-white crystals just beneath Bowman's membrane in central doughnut-like pattern, diffuse stromal haze, dense arcus with age, limbal girdle of Vogt; no recurrent erosions; hyperlipidemia or hypercholesterolemia (33%); may have short forearms and genu valgum

Pathology: cholesterol and neutral fat deposits, stain with Oil-red-O

Can recur in graft

Fleck (Francois-Neetans') (AD)

Congenital, nonprogressive, asymmetric or unilateral

Usually not present before age 15

Vision usually not affected

Findings: discrete, flat, gray-white, dandruff-like speck and ring-shaped opacities, extending to periphery; decreased corneal sensation

Associated with limbal dermoid, keratoconus, central cloudy corneal dystrophy (Francois'), punctate cortical lens changes, pseudoxanthoma elasticum, atopy

Pathology: glycosaminoglycan and lipid deposits, stain with Alcian blue and colloidal iron (GAGs), Sudan black and Oil-red-O (lipid)

Central Cloudy (Francois')

Nonprogressive

Vision usually not affected

Findings: multiple, nebulous, polygonal gray areas separated by cracklike intervening clear zones (looks similar to crocodile shagreen); most dense centrally and posteriorly, fade anteriorly and peripherally

Posterior Amorphous Stromal (AD)

Early in life, minimally progressive or nonprogressive

Findings: diffuse gray-white stromal opacities concentrated in posterior stroma, mostly centrally but extends to periphery

Associated with hyperopia, central thinning, flat corneal topography, anterior iris abnormalities, fine iris processes extending to Schwalbe's line

Congenital Hereditary Stromal (CHSD)

(see Chapter 5, Pediatrics/Strabismus)

Endothelial

Cornea Guttata

Beaten metal appearance

Pathology: thickened Descemet's with localized excrescences of collagen; variable endothelial size and shape and reduced number on specular microscopy

Most never develop corneal edema

Fuchs'

Most common in postmenopausal women

Symptoms: blurred vision (initially, only in morning; later, all day); may have pain (ruptured bullae)

Findings: guttata, stromal edema, Descemet's folds, endothelial pigment dusting, epithelial bullae, subepithelial fibrosis; may develop degenerative pannus

Pathology: guttata, thickened BM, atrophic endothelium with areas of cell dropout, endothelial cell polymegathism and pleomorphism

Treatment: hypertonic ointment, PK, contact lens or conjunctival flap (Gunderson) for comfort

Posterior Polymorphous (PPMD)
(AD, Occasionally AR)

Minimally or nonprogressive; occurs early in life

Vision usually normal

Endothelium behaves like epithelium, forming multiple layers with occasional migration of cells into angle causing glaucoma (15%)

Findings: isolated grouped vesicles, geographically shaped discrete gray lesions, broad bands with scalloped edges; variable amounts of stromal edema, corectopia, and broad iridocorneal adhesions

Pathology: irregular blebs or vacuoles at level of Descemet's surrounded by gray opacification, thickened Descemet's, abnormal endothelial cells (resemble epithelial cells; contain keratin, microvilli, desmosomes)

DDx: Haab's striae in congenital glaucoma, ICE syndrome

Treatment: penetrating keratoplasty for endothelial decompensation, can recur in graft

Congenital Hereditary Endothelial (CHED)

(see Chapter 5, Pediatrics/Strabismus)

Miscellaneous

Delle(n)

Focal thinning(s) from dehydration due to adjacent area of elevation (i.e., pingueculum, pterygium, filtering bleb)

Treatment: lubrication; may require removal of inciting lesion

Descemetocele

Extreme focal thinning of cornea in which only Descemet's membrane remains

Due to corneal melt (see Corneal melt section)

High risk of perforation

Bullous Keratopathy

Corneal edema with epithelial bullae, thickened stroma, but no guttata

Due to loss or dysfunction of endothelial cells

May develop fibrovascular pannus

Etiology: aphakia, pseudophakia (rigid AC IOL), vitreocorneal touch, iridocorneal touch, sequela of severe or chronic keratitis

Pathology: blister-like elevations of corneal epithelium, damaged hemidesmosomes

DDx of corneal edema: ABK, PBK, inflammation, infection, Fuchs' dystrophy, PPMD, CHED, hydrops, acute angle-closure glaucoma, congenital glaucoma, graft failure, contact lens overwear, hypotony, birth trauma, ICE syndrome, Brown-McLean syndrome, anterior segment ischemia

> ***Brown-McLean Syndrome***: peripheral corneal decompensation in aphakic patients, central cornea clear
>> ETIOLOGY: uncertain, possibly mechanical irritation from floppy peripheral iris

Neurotrophic Keratitis

Corneal anesthesia due to CN 5 lesion

Disruption of reflex arc between CN V_1 and lacrimal gland in anesthetic eye causes epithelial abnormalities

Findings: conjunctival injection, corneal edema, nonhealing epithelial defects, risk of infection and perforation; may have AC reaction

DDx: familial dysautonomia, topical anesthetic abuse, "crack" cornea (anesthesia from smoking crack cocaine)

Diagnosis: decreased corneal sensation (test with cotton-tipped applicator or anesthesiometer)

Treatment: lubrication; consider prophylactic antibiotic, bandage CL, punctal plugs, tarsorrhaphy

Familial Dysautonomia (Riley-Day Syndrome)

(see Chapter 5, Pediatrics/Strabismus)

Exposure Keratopathy

Desiccation of corneal epithelium due to CN 7 lesion (failure to close eyelids)

Findings: epithelial defects; may develop infection, melt, perforation

Treatment: lubrication, moisture chamber goggles, lid taping at bedtime; consider tarsorrhaphy, lid weights

Contact Lens-related Problems

SPK: mechanical or chemical (solutions)

3 and 9 o'clock staining: due to poor wetting of peripheral cornea; refit lens

Abrasion: increased risk of infection in CL wearers
> ***Treatment***: antibiotics, never patch

Infiltrates: hypoxia, antigenic reaction to preservatives in CL solutions, infection
> ***Treatment***: stop CL wear, antibiotics

Edema: epithelial microcystic edema due to altered metabolism; associated with extended wear CL

Treatment: decrease wear time; switch to daily wear lenses

Giant papillary conjunctivitis (GPC): sensitivity to CL material, deposits on CL, or mechanical irritation
Treatment: stop CL wear, topical allergy medication

Superior limbic keratoconjunctivitis (SLK): may be due to hypersensitivity or toxic reaction to thimerosal
Treatment: resolves with discontinuation of lens wear

Neovascularization: superficial, deep, sectoral, or 360°; due to chronic hypoxia
Treatment: refit lens with increased oxygen transmission; stop lens wear if significant vascularization

Corneal warpage: irregular astigmatism related to lens material (hard > rigid gas-permeable [RGP] > soft), fit, and length of time of wear; not associated with corneal edema. Usually asymptomatic; may have contact lens intolerance, blurred vision with glasses, loss of best spectacle-corrected visual acuity, or change in refraction (especially axis of astigmatism); corneal topography is abnormal
Treatment: discontinue lens wear; repeat refraction and corneal topography until stable

Graft Failure

Early (primary): poor tissue or surgery

Late: allograft rejection (delayed onset [at least 2 weeks]); homograft reaction

Risk factors: young age, stromal vascularization, previous graft failure, post chemical burns, inflammatory disease

Symptoms: decreased vision, redness, pain, irritation

Findings:
Epithelial rejection line ("battle" line of host-versus-donor epithelium): occurs in 10%, often precedes more destructive rejection events
Endothelial rejection: anterior chamber reaction, keratitic precipitates, graft edema, Khodadoust rejection line (moves across cornea destroying endothelium, resulting in stromal edema)
Other findings: subepithelial infiltrates, new KP, increased IOP (trabeculitis from AC reaction)

Treatment:
Endothelial rejection: IV steroids (methylprednisone 500 mg; reduces risk of subsequent rejection episodes [33% vs 67% for oral steroids]), topical steroids (40% reversal rate alone), oral steroids
Epithelial rejection or stromal infiltrates with no graft swelling: treat with topical therapy alone

Prognosis: graft survival rate for treating endothelial rejections with a single pulse of IV steroids is 90% when presents within 1 week and 67% when presents later than 1 week (probably due to irreversible damage to endothelial cells despite reversal of rejection)

Epithelial Downgrowth

Can occur following almost any intraocular surgery; increased risk with complicated surgery associated with hemorrhage, inflammation, vitreous loss, or incarcerated tissue

Surface epithelium grows through wound into eye, covering anterior segment structures

Appears as advancing line on corneal endothelium

Epithelium can cover the endothelium (leading to edema) and the angle (resulting in glaucoma); contact inhibition by healthy endothelium may inhibit this

Pathology: multilayered nonkeratinized squamous epithelium; PAS stains conjunctival goblet cells (differentiates between corneal and conjunctival epithelium)

Figure 7-16. Epithelial downgrowth with epithelium present on corneal endothelium, angle, and iris, and into vitreous. (From Yanoff M, Fine BS: *Ocular Pathology*, 5th ed, St. Louis, Mosby, 2002.)

DDx of retrocorneal membrane: mesodermal dysgenesis, ICE syndrome, trauma, posterior polymorphous dystrophy, disciform keratitis (HSV or HZV), alkali burn

Diagnosis: argon laser application to surface of iris produces white burn if iris involved; helps delineate extent of epithelial membrane

Treatment: excision of epithelial membrane and involved tissue with cryotherapy to remaining corneal membrane; high-power laser ablation of entire membrane may occasionally work; complete excision is difficult

Prognosis: poor, often develop secondary glaucoma

Fibrous Ingrowth

Fibrous proliferation through wound into AC

Less progressive and destructive than epithelial downgrowth

Fibroblasts originate from episclera or corneal stroma

Limbal Stem Cell Deficiency

Etiology:
Destruction of stem cells (chemical burn, Stevens-Johnson syndrome, corneal infections)
Dysfunction of stem cells (aniridia, multiple endocrine deficiency, neurotrophic)

Symptoms: decreased vision, photophobia, pain, tearing, blepharospasm

Findings: conjunctivilization, corneal vascularization, poor epithelial integrity, chronic inflammation

Pathology: Bowman's membrane destruction, fibrous tissue ingrowth

Diagnosis: impression cytology (presence of goblet cells on cornea); corneal epithelium takes up fluorescein

Treatment: limbal stem cell transplant (autograft [from other eye if unilateral], allograft [amniotic membrane]); poor candidate for penetrating keratoplasty; risk of recurrent conjunctivilization

Graft-Versus-Host Disease (GVHD)

Ominous complication of bone marrow transplant (BMT)

3 requirements:
Graft must contain immunologically competent cells
Host must possess important transplantation isoantigens lacking in graft (so host appears foreign)
Host must not be able to mount immunologic reaction against graft

3 types of bone marrow transplants:
Autologous: patient's own stored marrow
Syngeneic: marrow from identical twin
Allogeneic: marrow from HLA-matched donor

Complications:
Acute: hemorrhage and infection (first 100 days following BMT [period of aplasia])
Late: GVHD (T-lymphocytes in transplanted marrow recognize antigens of host as foreign, become sensitized, and attack host's organs; minor histocompatability antigens are the inciting antigens, cytotoxic T cells are the effectors)

Occurs primarily in allogeneic grafts: 50% develop acute GVHD (50% mortality); 20% to 40% develop chronic GVHD

Acute GVHD is biggest risk factor for chronic GVHD

Findings:
Conjunctivitis
STAGE 1: hyperemia
STAGE 2: hyperemia and chemosis
STAGE 3: pseudomembranous conjunctivitis
STAGE 4: stage 3 + corneal epithelial slough
Keratoconjunctivitis sicca, cicatricial conjunctivitis (OCP-like appearance with symblepharon), lagophthalmos, entropion, microvascular retinopathy (4%–10%), optic neuropathy (2%; thought to be due to cyclosporine, resolves with discontinuation)

Other findings:
Acute GVHD: maculopapular rash on palms and soles, pruritus, GI involvement (diarrhea), elevated liver enzymes
Chronic GVHD: sclerodermatoid or lichenoid skin changes, Sjögren's-like syndrome

Diagnosis: skin, liver, intestinal biopsy

Treatment: cyclosporine, high-dose systemic steroids; treat ocular complications

Prognosis: Stage 2 or higher occurs in 12% with acute GVHD and has a 90% mortality; chronic GVHD 10-year survival = 40%

Iridocorneal Endothelial Syndrome (ICE)

(see Chapter 10, Anterior Segment)

Multiple Endocrine Neoplasia (MEN)

MEN 1 (Werner's syndrome): Mapped to chromosome 11
Neoplasias of pituitary, parathyroid, and islet cells of pancreas
Findings: visual field defects from pituitary tumors

MEN 2a (Sipple's syndrome) (AD): Mapped to chromosome 10
Medullary thyroid carcinoma, pheochromocytoma, parathyroid adenomas
Findings: prominent corneal nerves
Pathology: thickened conjunctival nerves contain numerous Schwann cells and partially myelinated axons; thickened corneal nerves are due to an increased number of axons per nerve fiber bundle
Diagnosis: elevated calcitonin and vanillylmandelic acid

MEN 2b (Sipple-Gorlin syndrome) (AD): Mapped to chromosome 10
Medullary thyroid carcinoma, pheochromocytoma, mucosal and GI neuromas, marfanoid habitus
Eye findings: prominent corneal nerves, conjunctival neuroma (87%), eyelid neuroma (80%), dry

eye (67%), prominent perilimbal blood vessels (40%)

DDx of prominent corneal nerves: leprosy, *Acanthamoeba*, Down's syndrome, neurofibromatosis, keratoconus, congenital glaucoma, Refsum's disease, Fuchs' endothelial dystrophy, failed corneal graft, keratoconjunctivitis sicca, trauma, advanced age, ichthyosis, posterior polymorphous dystrophy

Tumors

Corneal Intraepithelial Neoplasia (CIN)

(see Conjunctiva section)

Squamous Cell Carcinoma (SCC)

(see Conjunctiva section)

SCLERAL DISORDERS

Episcleritis

Inflammation of episclera

Self-limited, usually young adults

33% bilateral; 67% recurrent

Associated with HZV, RA, gout

Signs: sectoral (70%) or diffuse (30%) injection with mild or no discomfort; may have nodule (20%), chemosis, AC reaction

Pathology: nongranulomatous vascular dilatation, perivascular lymphocytic infiltration; diffuse or nodular (similar to rheumatoid scleritis but limited to episclera); palisade of epithelioid cells bordering central fibrinoid necrosis

Diagnosis: blanches with topical 2.5% phenylephrine

Treatment: topical vasoconstrictor (Naphcon A) or mild topical steroid (FML)

If lasts for >3 weeks, perform systemic workup

Scleritis

Inflammation of sclera

More common in females; onset age 30 to 60 years

>50% bilateral

Etiology: 50% associated with systemic disease
Collagen vascular diseases (RA [20% of all cases of scleritis; only 3% of patients with RA develop scleritis; 75% of RA-related scleritis is bilateral], SLE, polyarteritis nodosa), vascular disease (Wegener's granulomatosis, giant cell arteritis, Takayasu's disease), relapsing polychondritis, sarcoidosis, ankylosing spondylitis, Reiter's syndrome, Crohn's disease, ulcerative colitis, infections (syphilis, TB, leprosy, HSV, HZV), gout, rosacea

Classification:
Anterior: 98%
DIFFUSE (40%): most benign; widespread involvement
PATHOLOGY: sclera thickened, diffuse granulomatous inflammation of scleral collagen
NODULAR (44%): focal involvement; nodule is immobile
PATHOLOGY: zonal necrotizing granuloma, fibrinoid necrosis, chronic inflammation, fusiform thickening, immune complex deposition with complement activation; once collagen has been destroyed, inflammation recedes, uvea herniates into defect
NECROTIZING (14%): associated with life-threatening autoimmune disease (5-year mortality rate = 25%)
WITH INFLAMMATION: focal or diffuse, progressive, pain and redness; vascular sludging and occlusion; underlying blue uveal tissue may be visible giving redness a "violaceous" hue; 40% lose vision; 60% have ocular complications—anterior uveitis, sclerosing keratitis, cataract, glaucoma, peripheral corneal melt, scleral thinning
WITHOUT INFLAMMATION (scleromalacia perforans): minimal symptoms, minimal injection; scleral thinning, marked ischemia; seldom perforate; females with severe rheumatoid arthritis; 8-year mortality rate = 21%
Posterior: 2%; usually unilateral; very painful
Usually no associated systemic disorder
80% have anterior scleritis
FINDINGS: thickened and inflamed posterior sclera, chorioretinal folds, amelanotic fundus mass, ON edema; may have vitritis, macular edema, limitation of motility, ptosis, proptosis, exudative RD, elevated IOP (forward shift of lens-iris diaphragm due to ciliochoroidal detachment)
B-SCAN ULTRASOUND: pocket of fluid in Tenon's space (sclerotenonitis), T sign, thickened sclera
FA: early patchy hypofluorescence, late staining, disc leakage
CT SCAN: thickening of posterior sclera with contiguous involvement of orbital fat (T sign)
DDx: choroidal tumor, orbital pseudotumor (IOI), uveal effusion syndrome, VKH, thyroid-related ophthalmopathy, orbital tumors

Symptoms: pain, redness, photophobia

Findings: diffuse or sectoral area of deep injection (violaceous hue), tender to touch, chemosis, scleral edema; may have scleral nodule, scleral thinning, AC reaction (33%), keratitis (acute stromal keratitis, sclerosing keratitis, marginal keratolysis); chorioretinal folds and serous RD in posterior scleritis

Diagnosis: does not blanch with topical phenyle-phrine

    Lab tests: CBC, ESR, RF, ANA, ANCA, VDRL, FTA-ABS, uric acid, BUN, PPD, CXR

      ANCA (antineutrophil cytoplasmic antibodies): positive in Wegener's; also polyarteritis nodosa, Churg-Strauss, and crescentic glomerulonephritis

      2 TYPES:

        C-ANCA (cytoplasmic; positive in Wegener's)

        P-ANCA (perinuclear; positive in polyarteritis nodosa [PAN])

    Anterior segment fluorescein angiogram: may detect nonperfusion and vaso-obliteration

Treatment: oral NSAID, consider oral steroids or immunosuppressive agents; treat underlying disorder; topical steroids are not effective; sub-Tenon's steroid injection is contraindicated; may require patch graft for perforation

Complications: keratitis, cataract, uveitis, glaucoma

Wegener's Granulomatosis

Necrotizing vasculitis; males > females

Findings (60%): nasolacrimal duct obstruction, proptosis, painful ophthalmoplegia, conjunctivitis, chemosis, KCS, episcleritis, necrotizing scleritis (most common type of ocular involvement), keratitis, cotton-wool spots, arterial narrowing, venous tortuosity, choroidal thickening, CME, CRAO, optic nerve involvement

Other findings: upper respiratory tract (hemoptysis), renal failure (major cause of death), hemorrhagic dermatitis, cerebral vasculitis, weight loss, peripheral neuropathy, fever, arthralgia, saddle nose (destruction of nasal bones)

Diagnosis: ANCA (circulating antineutrophil cytoplasmic antibody)

Treatment: high-dose prednisone and cyclophosphamide

Takayasu's Disease

Narrowing of large branches of aorta

Diminished pulsations in upper extremities

Decreased blood pressure in upper extremities, increased BP in lower extremities

Findings: scleritis, amaurosis fugax, ocular ischemia, AION

Polyarteritis Nodosa

Systemic vasculitis affecting medium-sized and small arteries

Males > females

Findings: necrotizing sclerokeratitis, vascular occlusions, ischemic optic neuropathy, rarely aneurysms of retinal vessels

Other findings: kidneys (nephritic or nephrotic syndrome, hypertension, renal failure), heart (MI, angina, pericarditis), intestines (pain, infarction), arthritis, peripheral neuropathy

Relapsing Polychondritis

Multisystem disorder characterized by recurrent episodes of inflammation in cartilaginous tissues throughout body

Findings (60%): episcleritis, scleritis, iritis, conjunctivitis, KCS, exudative RD, optic neuritis, proptosis, CN 6 palsies

Other findings: migratory polyarthritis, fever, diffuse inflammation of cartilage (nose, ear, trachea, larynx)

Treatment: topical or systemic steroids; dapsone

Discoloration

Blue sclera: sclera appears blue owing to thinning and visualization of underlying uvea

    DDx: Ehlers-Danlos, Hurler's, Turner's, and Marfan's syndromes; osteogenesis imperfecta, scleromalacia perforans, congenital staphyloma

Scleral icterus: yellow sclera caused by hyperbilirubinemia

Ochronosis (alkaptonuria) (AR): homogentisic acid oxidase deficiency

    Homogentisic acid accumulates, metabolized into melanin-like compound with brown pigmentation of cartilage (ear, nose, heart valves) and sclera; excreted in urine (dark)

    Findings: triangular pigment deposits anterior to rectus muscle insertions, pinhead-sized peripheral corneal stromal deposits, pigmentation of tarsus and lids

Cogan's senile scleral plaque: blue-gray hyalinization of sclera anterior to horizontal rectus muscle insertions

SURGERY

Penetrating Keratoplasty (PK; PKP)

Most common indications: bullous keratopathy (pseudophakic, aphakic), Fuchs' dystrophy, keratoconus, graft failure, corneal scar; Peter's anomaly (children)

Success rate: 90% of grafts are clear at 1 year (>90% for keratoconus; 65% for HSV)

Complications: rejection (20%), failure, glaucoma, recurrent pathology, suprachoroidal or expulsive hemorrhage, endophthalmitis, recurrence of pathology

Collaborative Corneal Transplant Treatment Study (CCTS):

ABO blood type incompatability is possible risk factor for rejection

HLA matching is not cost-effective or advantageous

High-risk status: vascularization of cornea in 2 quadrants, history of previous graft rejection, glaucoma, extensive PAS, traumatic or hereditary ocular surface disorders

Donor screening:

Contraindications for donor corneas: septicemia, lymphoma or leukemia, systemic malignancy with ocular metastasis, anterior segment tumors (choroidal melanoma is not a contraindication), Creutzfeldt-Jakob disease, rabies, subacute sclerosing panencephalitis, PML, HIV, hepatitis B and C (neither HIV nor hepatitis C has ever been transmitted)

Tissue preservation:

4°C moist chamber: use within 48 hours

M-K medium (McCarey-Kaufman): TC-199 medium with dextran (5% concentration) and gentamicin stored at 4°C; use within 48 hours

Chondroitin sulfate: acts as antioxidant and membrane growth factor

K-sol (Kaufman): chondroitin sulfate in TC-199 at 4°C; discontinued

Corneal storage media (CSM): from Minnesota Lions Eye Bank researchers plus mercaptoethanol (antioxidant) and chondroitin sulfate; discontinued with introduction of dexsol and optisol

Dexsol: minimal essential medium with chondroitin sulfate and dextran 1% (osmotic agent to keep cornea thin)

Optisol: hybrid of K-sol, dexsol, and CSM, plus vitamins, amino acids, and antioxidants; as effective as dexsol but keeps cornea thinner

Many media contain pH indicators that change color with a change in pH (i.e., microbial contamination)

Keratophakia

Donor lenticule is placed between the cornea and a microkeratome created lamellar section to correct aphakia

Contraindications: thinned corneas, infants, glaucoma

Keratomileusis

Lamellar section is removed, frozen, shaped on a cryolathe, then replaced in stromal bed to correct myopia or hyperopia. Donor lenticule can be used instead

Contraindications: glaucoma

Figure 7-17. Keratomileusis. In a myopic keratomileusis, a corneal button is raised using a microkeratome, and it is reshaped using a cryolathe (*upper part*). When the button is replaced, the central cornea is flattened (*lower part*). (From Chang SW, Azar DT: Automated and manual lamellar surgical procedures and epikeratoplasty. In Yanoff M, Duker JS [eds]: *Ophthalmology*, London, Mosby, 1999.)

| Myopic correction | Donor | Hyperopic correction |

Figure 7-18. Epikeratoplasty. A preshaped donor lenticule is sutured to the recipient stromal bed to correct myopia and hyperopia. (From Chang SW, Azar DT: Automated and manual lamellar surgical procedures and epikeratoplasty. In Yanoff M, Duker JS [eds]: *Ophthalmology*, London, Mosby, 1999.)

Epikeratophakia (Epikeratoplasty)

Figure 7-18

Epithelium is removed and a lathed donor lenticule is placed to correct myopia or hyperopia

Can be performed in children; reversible

Contraindications: blepharitis, dry eye, lagophthalmos

Pathology: 2 Bowman's membranes (donor lenticule and patient)

Astigmatic Keratotomy (AK)

99% depth arcuate or straight incisions typically placed at the 7-mm optical zone (OZ) to correct astigmatism

Various nomograms exist (i.e., Lindstrom ARC-T)

Do not make arcuate incisions >90° (decreased efficacy, increased instability)

When combined with RK, do not cross incisions (creates wound gape and instability)

Radial Keratotomy (RK)

Deep radial corneal incisions to correct low to moderate myopia

Effect dependent on number of incisions, depth of incisions, size of optical zone, patient age
  Number of incisions: the greater the number of incisions, the greater the effect; never use more than 8 incisions (additional incisions have limited effect and cause greater destabilization of the cornea)
  Incision depth: the deeper the incision, the greater the effect; diamond knife is set at 100% of thinnest pachymetry measurement (usually paracentral inferotemporal region; temporal < inferior < nasal < superior)

Optical zone: the smaller the diameter of the OZ (the longer the incision), the greater the effect; do not make OZ <3 mm (visual aberrations [starburst])
Patient age: the older the patient, the greater the effect
Patient sex: greater effect in males than in females

Technique: American (downhill cut [toward limbus], safer but shallower) vs Russian (uphill cut [toward central cornea], deeper but risk of invading OZ); combined technique with special knife gives deep cut with safety

Complications: undercorrection or overcorrection, perforation, infection, scarring, irregular astigmatism, progressive hyperopia (in PERK study, 43% had ≥1.00 D of hyperopia after 10 years), glare/starburst, fluctuating vision

Results: 85% achieved 20/40 or better vision after initial procedure; 96% achieved 20/40 or better after enhancement, 85% achieved 20/25 or better after enhancement

Photorefractive Keratectomy (PRK)

Laser ablation of corneal surface to correct myopia, hyperopia, and astigmatism

Excimer (excited dimer) laser: argon-fluoride (wavelength = 193 nm; far ultraviolet), energy = 64 eV

Functions as a "cold" laser (breaks molecular bonds to ablate tissue; no thermal damage)

Each pulse removes approximately 0.25 μm of corneal tissue

Depth of ablation is related to diameter of optical zone and amount of intended correction

Munnerlyn equation: depth = (refractive error/3) × OZ^2

EXAMPLE: 12 μm for 6 mm OZ and 1 D of myopia

Advantages of PRK: precise removal of tissue, minimal adjacent tissue damage

Disadvantages of PRK: involves visual axis, risk of haze/scarring, regression, requires removal of epithelium

Contraindications: collagen vascular, autoimmune, or immunodeficiency disorders; pregnancy; corneal ectasia; keloid formation; isotretinoin (Accutane), amiodarone, sumatriptan (Imitrex)

Cautions: unstable refraction (change of >0.5 D/year), systemic diseases that affect wound healing (diabetes, atopy, connective tissue diseases, immunocompromised status), herpes keratitis (HSV or HZV), ocular inflammation (keratitis, acne rosacea, pannus that extends into visual axis)

Complications: undercorrection or overcorrection, haze/scarring, delayed reepithelialization, sterile infiltrates, infection, decentered ablation, central island, irregular astigmatism, regression, glare, halos, dry eye, glaucoma or cataract (from steroids)

Corneal haze: risk and severity increases with deeper ablations and ultraviolet (UV) radiation exposure; results in decreased vision with regression of effect. Prevent haze with oral vitamin C 1000 mg/day for 1 week before surgery and 2 weeks postoperatively, and avoidance of UV exposure

Treatment of complications:
Enhancements: it is recommended to wait at least 3 months or until the refraction and corneal topography are stable before performing an enhancement for overcorrection or undercorrection
Haze: treat with topical steroids; consider application of mitomycin C 0.02% for 2 minutes along with scar débridement with either a diamond burr or a superficial excimer laser treatment (PTK). Once the haze is reduced, the refraction can change dramatically, so do not treat residual refractive error at time of haze removal
Irregular astigmatism: rigid gas-permeable contact lens, wavefront-guided retreatment

Laser in Situ Keratomileusis (LASIK)

Combination of keratomileusis and PRK to correct myopia, hyperopia, and astigmatism

Corneal flap created with microkeratome and laser ablation performed on underlying stromal bed

Advantages of LASIK: more rapid healing, less discomfort, less risk of haze, less postoperative medication

Disadvantages of LASIK: microkeratome complications

Complications:
Intraoperative: flap complication (buttonhole, incomplete, or irregular flap, free cap) epithelial abrasion or sloughing, programming error, decentered ablation.
Immediate postoperative: diffuse lamellar keratitis (DLK, sands of Sahara), flap dislocation, flap striae, epithelial ingrowth, central island, irregular astigmatism, dry eye, undercorrection or overcorrection, night vision problems (glare, halos)
Delayed postoperative: dry eye, late DLK, late flap slip, undercorrection or overcorrection, keratectasia

Treatment of complications:
Buttonhole (increased risk with steep corneas), *incomplete or irregular flap*: replace flap, do not perform ablation; when cornea stabilizes, either cut a new flap or perform surface ablation (PRK/PTK)
Free cap (increased risk in cases of flat corneas): place free cap in moisture chamber epithelial side down, perform ablation, then replace cap and let dry
Epithelial slough or corneal abrasion: increased risk with certain microkeratomes and in eyes with epithelial basement membrane dystrophy; increases risk of developing DLK and epithelial ingrowth
Treat with bandage contact lens and close follow-up. If large defect occurs in first eye, consider postponing treatment of second eye
Flap striae or flap dislocation: replace flap and stretch; consider use of epithelial débridement, hypotonic saline or sterile water, ironing with a warm spatula, or suturing (interrupted radials or antitorque)
DLK: inflammation within flap interface; etiology often unknown; increased risk with epithelial defect
Late DLK may result from increased intraocular pressure, epithelial defect, and cornea ulcer. Treat with frequent topical steroids for grades I and II, and flap lifting and interface irrigation for grades III and IV
A short pulse of oral steroids may be considered
Epithelial ingrowth: nests of epithelium growing under the flap; more common in eyes with epithelial basement membrane dystrophy and after enhancements. Ingrowth that is progressive or affects the vision is treated with flap lifting and débridement of the stromal bed and flap undersurface. Consider radial sutures if ingrowth recurs
Irregular ablation (decentered, irregular astigmatism): requires custom or wavefront-guided retreatment
Corneal ectasia (keratectasia): treatment of eyes with a preexisting ectasia (keratoconus, forme fruste keratoconus, pellucid marginal degeneration) or excessive depth of ablation in normal corneas (residual stromal depth <250 μm) can result in progressive myopic astigmatism and corneal ectasia. Treat with a rigid gas-permeable

contact lens. Consider Intacs or corneal transplantation

Dry eye: common problem due to severing of corneal nerves; increased risk with preexisting dry eye condition; superior hinged flap may cause greater dryness than is caused by nasal hinged flap. Treat with frequent lubrication; consider punctal occlusion and topical cyclosporine

Glare/halos: contributing factors include scotopic pupil size larger than treatment optical zone, high corrections, and residual refractive error. Treatment options include pharmacologic miosis (Alphagan-P or Pilocarpine), or retreatment with larger optical zone or blend zone

Infectious keratitis: uncommon but serious complication; most common organisms are Gram-positive cocci and atypical *Mycobacteria*. Suspected infection requires lifting flap and culturing; treat with fortified topical antibiotics (vancomycin and amikacin); may require flap amputation

Laser Assisted Epithelial Keratomileusis (LASEK)

Combination of LASIK and PRK to correct myopia, hyperopia, and astigmatism

Epithelial flap is created with alcohol, excimer laser is applied, and epithelial flap is replaced

Advantages of LASEK: does not require microkeratome, may have less risk of haze than PRK

Disadvantages of LASEK: greater discomfort and longer visual recovery than LASIK

Complications: undercorrection or overcorrection, haze/scarring, delayed reepithelialization, infection, decentered ablation, central island, irregular astigmatism, regression, glare/halos, dry eye

Risk of haze can be reduced with oral vitamin C and avoidance of UV exposure

Phototherapeutic Keratectomy (PTK)

Use of excimer laser to ablate pathology limited to anterior 1/3 of cornea

Indications: superficial scars, dystrophies, irregularities, residual band keratopathy, recurrent erosions

Can use confocal microscopy to determine depth of pathology

Complications: recurrence of pathology, reactivation of HSV, induced hyperopia or irregular astigmatism

Intracorneal Inlays

A thin, contact lens–like, implant placed in the central optical zone beneath a corneal flap to correct myopia, hyperopia, and astigmatism. The thickness and shape of the implant alter the corneal curvature to correct refractive errors without removing corneal tissue

Advantages: reversible, adjustable, no removal of tissue

Complications: undercorrection or overcorrection, irregular astigmatism, glare, halos, flap striae, epithelial ingrowth, DLK, infection, implant decentration or extrusion

Intrastromal Corneal Ring Segments (Intacs)

Ring segment implants placed into peripheral corneal channels outside the visual axis to correct low to moderate myopia. Implants flatten the cornea without cutting or removing tissue from the central optical zone

Advantages: reversible, adjustable, spares visual axis, no removal of tissue; shows potential for treatment of keratoconus

Complications: undercorrection or overcorrection, irregular astigmatism, glare, halos, infection, implant decentration or extrusion, stromal deposits

Figure 7-19. Slit-lamp photograph of the intrastromal corneal ring segments in position in patient's cornea. (Courtesy of Mr. Thomas Loarie. From Friedman NJ, Husain SE, Kohnen T, Koch DD: Investigational refractive procedures. In Yanoff M, Duker JS [eds]: *Ophthalmology*, London, Mosby, 1999.)

Thermokeratoplasty

Thermal energy is applied to the peripheral cornea in a ring pattern to steepen the central corneal and correct low to moderate hyperopia

2 types:

Conductive keratoplasty (CK): a contact probe directly delivers radiofrequency energy

Laser thermokeratoplasty (LTK): a noncontact, holmium:yttrium-aluminum-garnet (Ho:YAG) laser applies thermal burns

Advantages: spares visual axis, no removal of tissue

Complications: undercorrection or overcorrection, irregular astigmatism, regression (LTK > CK)

Figure 7-20. Laser thermal keratoplasty treatment patterns used in some of the Sunrise Clinical Trials. (From Friedman NJ, Husain SE, Kohnen T, Koch DD: Investigational refractive procedures. In Yanoff M, Duker JS [eds]: *Ophthalmology*, London, Mosby, 1999.)

Review Questions *(Answers start on page 363)*

1. Which is the least desirable method for corneal graft storage?
   a. moist chamber at 4°C
   b. glycerin
   c. Optisol
   d. cryopreservation

2. Presently in the United States, phlyctenule is most commonly associated with
   a. HSV
   b. tuberculosis
   c. *Staphylococcus*
   d. fungus

3. Which blood test is most helpful in the evaluation of a patient with Schnyder's crystalline corneal dystrophy?
   a. calcium
   b. uric acid
   c. immunoglobulins
   d. cholesterol

4. Which disease has never been transmitted by a corneal graft?
   a. CMV
   b. Creutzfeldt-Jakob
   c. rabies
   d. *Cryptococcus*

5. Which corneal dystrophy does not recur in a corneal graft?
   a. granular
   b. macular
   c. lattice
   d. PPMD

6. A conjunctival map biopsy is typically used for which malignancy?
   a. squamous cell carcinoma
   b. basal cell carcinoma
   c. sebaceous cell carcinoma
   d. malignant melanoma

7. Corneal clouding does not occur in which mucopolysaccharidosis?
   a. Hunter's
   b. Hurler's
   c. Scheie's
   d. Sly's

8. All of the following may cause follicular conjunctivitis except
   a. *Chlamydia*
   b. *Neisseria*
   c. Iopidine
   d. EKC

9. Which of the following tests is least helpful in determining the etiology of enlarged corneal nerves?
   a. EKG
   b. calcitonin
   c. urinary VMA
   d. acid-fast stain

10. Corneal filaments are least likely to be present in which condition?
    a. Keratoconjunctivitis sicca
    b. Thygeson's SPK
    c. SLK
    d. medicamentosa

11. Which of the following is not an appropriate treatment for SLK?
    a. bandage contact lens
    b. conjunctival resection
    c. silver nitrate stick
    d. conjunctival cautery

12. In what level of the cornea does a Kayser-Fleischer ring occur?
    a. epithelium
    b. Bowman's membrane
    c. stroma
    d. Descemet's membrane

13. Cornea verticillata–like changes are associated with all of the following except
    a. indomethacin
    b. thorazine
    c. chloroquine
    d. amiodarone

14. The least common location for a nevus is
    a. bulbar conjunctiva
    b palpebral conjunctiva
    c. caruncle
    d. lid skin

15. All of the following ions move across the corneal endothelium by both active transport and passive diffusion except
    a. Cl^-
    b. K^+
    c. Na^+
    d. H^+

16. Which organism is associated with crystalline keratopathy?
    a. *S. aureus*
    b. *H. influenzae*
    c. *Enterococcus*
    d. *S. viridans*

17. Which of the following conditions is associated with the best 5-year prognosis for a corneal graft?
    a. PBK
    b. Fuchs' dystrophy
    c. ABK
    d. HSV

18. The best strategy for loosening a tight contact lens is to
    a. increase the diameter
    b. increase the curvature
    c. decrease the diameter
    d. decrease the curvature

19. The type of contact lens that causes the least endothelial pleomorphism is
    a. soft daily wear
    b. soft extended wear
    c. rigid gas permeable
    d. hard/PMMA

20. Which of the following conditions is associated with the worst prognosis for a corneal graft?
    a. PBK
    b. Fuchs' dystrophy
    c. Reis-Bucklers' dystrophy
    d. keratoglobus

21. Which is not a treatment of acute hydrops?
    a. steroid
    b. homatropine
    c. bandage contact lens
    d. corneal transplant

22. Which organism cannot penetrate intact corneal epithelium?
    a. *C. diphtheriae*
    b. *N. gonorrhoeae*
    c. *P. aeruginosa*
    d. *H. aegyptius*

23. Which organism is most commonly associated with angular blepharitis?
    a. *S. epidermidis*
    b. *Moraxella*
    c. *S. aureus*
    d. *Demodex folliculorum*

24. Which of the following medications would be the best choice in the treatment of microsporidial keratoconjunctivitis?
    a. fumagillin
    b. chloramphenicol
    c. galardin
    d. paromomycin

25. All of the following agents are used in the treatment of *Acanthamoeba* keratitis except
    a. paromomycin
    b. natamycin
    c. chlorhexidine
    d. miconazole

26. Goblet cells are most abundant in which location?
    a. fornix
    b. plica
    c. bulbar conjunctiva
    d. limbus

SUGGESTED READINGS

American Academy of Ophthalmology: External Disease and Cornea, vol 8. San Francisco, AAO, 2004.

Arffa RC: Grayson's Diseases of the Cornea, 4th edition. St. Louis, Mosby, 1998.

Brightbill FS: Corneal Surgery Theory, Technique and Tissue, 3rd edition. St. Louis, Mosby, 1999.

Kaufman HE, Barron BA, McDonald MB: The Cornea, 2nd edition. Philadelphia, Butterworth-Heinemann, 1997.

Krachmer JH, Mannis MJ, Holland EJ: Cornea. St. Louis, Mosby, 1995.

Krachmer JH, Palay DA: Cornea Color Atlas. St. Louis, Mosby, 1995.

Leibowitz HM, Waring GO: Corneal Disorders: Clinical Diagnosis and Management, 2nd edition. Philadelphia, WB Saunders, 1998.

Smolin G, Thoft RA: The Cornea: Scientific Foundations and Clinical Practice, 3rd edition. Boston, Little Brown, 1994.

CHAPTER 8

Uveitis

PATHOPHYSIOLOGY

Inflammatory reaction:
  Acute: chemical mediators (histamine, serotonin, kinins, plasmin, complement, leukotrienes, prostaglandins)
  Chronic: cellular infiltrates
    NONGRANULOMATOUS: lymphocytes, plasma cells
    GRANULOMATOUS: epithelioid and giant cells (Langhans', foreign body, Touton)
      3 PATTERNS: diffuse (e.g., VKH syndrome), discrete (e.g., sarcoidosis), zonal (e.g., lens-induced)

Retinal S-antigen:
  Protein found in human retinal photoreceptors and pineal gland
  Most potent uveitic antigen; thought to be an enzyme located in rod outer segments
  In animal model: produces uveitis when injected into nonocular sites (experimental autoimmune uveitis [EAU]; type 4 hypersensitivity); removal of thymus prevents EAU (supports T cell–mediated basis of inflammatory response)

Human diseases that resemble EAU: VKH, sympathetic ophthalmia, birdshot retinochoroidopathy; lymphocytes from these patients develop an in vitro proliferative response to retinal S-antigen, suggesting an autoimmune basis for these diseases

CLASSIFICATION

Pathology: nongranulomatous, granulomatous

Etiology: infection, immune response, malignancy, trauma, chemical, idiopathic

Location: sclerouveitis, keratouveitis, anterior uveitis (iritis), iridocyclitis, lens-induced uveitis, intermediate uveitis, endophthalmitis (infection or inflammation of the vitreous, anterior chamber, ciliary body, and choroid), posterior uveitis (retinitis, choroiditis, vasculitis), panuveitis (endophthalmitis and involvement of the sclera)

ANTERIOR UVEITIS

Inflammation of iris (iritis) and ciliary body (cyclitis)

Most common cause in adults: idiopathic (followed by HLA-B27)

Most common cause of acute, noninfectious, hypopyon iritis: HLA-B27–associated iritis

Etiology:
  Children: JRA, ankylosing spondylitis, psoriatic arthritis, acute interstitial nephritis, Fuchs' heterochromic iridocyclitis, sarcoidosis, postviral, HSV, Lyme disease, trauma, Kawasaki's disease
  50% have posterior component (toxoplasmosis in 50% with posterior component)
  Young adults: HLA-B27 associated, sarcoidosis, syphilis, Fuchs', Behçet's disease, spillover from intermediate or posterior uveitis
  Older adults: idiopathic, sarcoidosis, HZO, masquerade syndromes (peripheral RD, intraocular foreign body, JXG, multiple sclerosis, malignan-

cies [retinoblastoma, leukemia, large cell lymphoma, malignant melanoma])

Classification:

Nongranulomatous:

ACUTE: idiopathic, HLA-B27 associated (5% of general population; associated with acute, recurrent uveitis; usually starts unilaterally; associated with the following 4 disorders: ankylosing spondylitis, Reiter's syndrome, psoriatic arthritis, inflammatory bowel disease), Behçet's disease, glaucomatocyclitic crisis (Posner-Schlossman syndrome), HSV, Kawasaki's disease, Lyme disease, traumatic, postoperative, other autoimmune diseases (lupus, relapsing polychondritis, Wegener's granulomatosis, interstitial nephritis)

CHRONIC (duration >6 weeks): JRA, Fuchs' heterochromic iridocyclitis

Granulomatous:

INFECTIOUS: syphilis, TB, leprosy, brucellosis, toxoplasmosis, *P. acnes*, fungal (*Cryptococcus*, *Aspergillus*), HIV

IMMUNE-MEDIATED: sarcoidosis, VKH syndrome, sympathetic ophthalmia, phacoanaphylactic

Symptoms: pain, photophobia, decreased vision, redness

Findings: conjunctival and episcleral injection, ciliary injection (circumcorneal flush from branches of anterior ciliary arteries), miosis (iris sphincter spasm), AC reaction; may have hypopyon, keratic precipitates, iris nodules, dilated iris vessels (occasionally, rubeosis), synechiae (posterior [iris adhesions to lens; seclusio pupillae is a complete adhesion that can result in iris bombe] or anterior [iris adhesions to cornea and angle])

Keratitic precipitates (KP): aggregates of white blood cells on corneal endothelium; typically located inferiorly and centrally (Figure 8-1)

May occur with any intraocular inflammation, most commonly with uveitis

May be white or pigmented, small or large, nongranulomatous (fine) or granulomatous (mutton fat), diffuse or focal

NONGRANULOMATOUS: composed of lymphocytes and PMNs

GRANULOMATOUS: composed of macrophages, lymphocytes, epithelioid cells, and multinucleated giant cells

DDX OF DIFFUSE KP: Fuchs' heterochromic iridocyclitis, sarcoidosis, syphilis, keratouveitis, toxoplasmosis (rarely)

Iris nodules:

KOEPPE: located at pupil margin; occur in granulomatous and nongranulomatous uveitis

BUSACCA: located on anterior iris surface; occur only in granulomatous uveitis (Figure 8-2)

DDx of hypopyon: HLA-B27 associated, infection (keratitis, endophthalmitis), foreign body, Behçet's

Figure 8-1. Keratic precipitates in anterior uveitis. (From Forster DJ: General approach to the uveitis patient and treatment strategies. In Yanoff M, Duker JS [eds]: *Ophthalmology*, London, Mosby, 1999.)

Figure 8-2. Chronic granulomatous uveitis demonstrating Busacca nodules. (From Forster DJ: General approach to the uveitis patient and treatment strategies. In Yanoff M, Duker JS [eds]: *Ophthalmology*, London, Mosby, 1999.)

disease, VKH syndrome, malignancy (leukemia, retinoblastoma), toxic (rifabutin)

DDx of uveitic glaucoma: HSV, HZV, Posner-Schlossman syndrome, Fuchs' heterochromic iridocyclitis, sarcoidosis; rarely toxoplasmosis, syphilis, sympathetic ophthalmia

Diagnosis:

Minimum: CBC with differential, urinalysis, VDRL and FTA-ABS

Expanded (for recurrent anterior [3 or more attacks], granulomatous, positive review of systems, or posterior involvement): ESR, ACE, ANA, ANCA, IL-10, PPD plus anergy panel, CXR or chest CT; consider Lyme test in endemic areas, HLA typing (25% with HLA-B27 develop sacroiliac disease, so obtain sacroiliac x-ray), HIV Ab test

Targeted approach:

RECURRENT UVEITIS, WITH BACK STIFFNESS UPON AWAKENING: rule out ankylosing spondylitis HLA-B27

Lumbosacral spine imaging (CT)
GRANULOMATOUS UVEITIS: rule out TB and sarcoidosis
CXR
Upper body gallium scan
Angiotensin-converting enzyme ([ACE]; elevated in 60% with sarcoidosis; also in Gaucher's disease, miliary tuberculosis, silicosis)
Lysozyme
Serum calcium
Liver function tests and bilirubin
PPD
CHILD WITH RECURRENT OR CHRONIC IRIDOCYCLITIS: rule out JRA (usually ANA-positive, RF-negative)
ANA
RF
HLA-B8
RETINAL VASCULITIS, RECURRENT APHTHOUS ULCERS, PRETIBIAL SKIN LESIONS: rule out Behçet's disease
Skin lesion biopsy
HLA-B51 and -B27
PARS PLANITIS AND EPISODIC PARESTHESIAS: rule out multiple sclerosis (MS)
Brain MRI
Lumbar puncture
RETINOCHOROIDITIS ADJACENT TO PIGMENTED CR SCAR: rule out toxoplasmosis
Toxoplasma IgM and IgG titers
RETINAL VASCULITIS AND SINUSITIS: rule out Wegener's granulomatosis
ANCA
CXR
Sinus films
Urinalysis
RECURRENT UVEITIS AND DIARRHEA: rule out inflammatory bowel disease (IBD)
GI consult
Endoscopy with biopsy
CHOROIDITIS, EXUDATIVE RD, EPISODIC TINNITUS: rule out Harada's disease/VKH syndrome
FA
Lumbar puncture
Brain MRI
Audiometry
ELDERLY FEMALE WITH VITRITIS: rule out intraocular lymphoma or infection
Vitreal biopsy for culture or cytology
UNILATERAL IRIDOCYCLITIS, FINE WHITE KP, LIGHTER IRIS IN AFFECTED EYE: rule out Fuchs' heterochromic iridocyclitis
IOP
Gonioscopy (fine-angle vessels)

Treatment: topical steroids, cycloplegic; may require systemic steroids, immunosuppressive agents, antibiotics
  Poor response to steroids: Fuchs', syphilis, toxoplasmosis, keratouveitis, Lyme disease, chronic postoperative endophthalmitis, ARN, CMV

Complications: iris atrophy, band keratopathy, cataract, glaucoma, cystoid macular edema

Ankylosing Spondylitis

90% HLA-B27-positive; typically young men

Lower back pain and stiffness with inactivity (upon awakening in morning)

Findings: anterior uveitis (30%; recurrent in 40%), episcleritis, scleritis

Other findings: arthritis (sacroiliac and peripheral joints), heart (aortic insufficiency, heart block), colitis (10%), lungs (restricted chest expansion, apical fibrosis)

Sacroiliac X-ray: sclerosis and narrowing of joint space; ligamentous ossification can occur

Reiter's Syndrome

Triad of conjunctivitis, urethritis, and arthritis

75% HLA-B27; males > females

Associated with infections: *Chlamydia, Ureaplasma urealyticum, Yersinia, Shigella, Salmonella*

Findings: mucopurulent conjunctivitis, keratitis, acute anterior uveitis

Diagnosis: 3 major criteria, or 2 major and 2 minor criteria
  Major:
    Urethritis
    Polyarthritis (knees, sacroiliac joints)
    Conjunctivitis
    Keratoderma blenorrhagicum (scaling skin lesion, often on feet and hands [20%]; similar to pustular psoriasis)
  Minor:
    Plantar fasciitis and Achilles tendinitis
    Circinate balanitis
    Painless mouth ulcers
    Prostatitis
    Cystitis
    Spondylitis/sacroiliitis
    Tendinitis
    Recent history of diarrhea
    Iritis/keratitis

Psoriatic Arthritis

Associated with HLA-B17 and HLA-B27

Uveitis does not occur in psoriasis without arthritis

Findings: conjunctivitis, dry eyes, anterior uveitis

Other findings: arthritis (hands, feet, sacroiliac joints), psoriatic skin and nail changes

Inflammatory Bowel Disease (IBD)

Uveitis occurs in ulcerative colitis (10%) and Crohn's disease (3%)

Findings: conjunctivitis, keratoconjunctivitis sicca, episcleritis, scleritis, anterior uveitis, orbital cellulitis, optic neuritis

Other findings: arthritis, erythema nodosum, pyoderma gangrenosum, hepatitis, sclerosing cholangitis

Fuchs' Heterochromic Iridocyclitis

Occurs in young adults; unilateral

Associated with chorioretinal scars (toxo)

Symptoms: blurred vision

Findings: diffuse small white stellate KP, minimal AC reaction, no posterior synechiae, iris heterochromia (diffuse atrophy of stroma, loss of iris crypts; involved iris is paler; 15% bilateral), fine-angle vessels (may bleed during gonioscopy, cataract surgery, or paracentesis)

Pathology: plasma cells in ciliary body

DDx of iris heterochromia: trauma (intraocular metallic foreign body), inflammation, congenital Horner's syndrome, iris melanoma, Waardenburg's syndrome (iris heterochromia, telecanthus, white forelock, congenital deafness), Parry-Romberg syndrome (iris heterochromia, Horner's syndrome, ocular motor palsies, nystagmus, facial hemiatrophy), glaucomatocyclitic crisis, medication (topical prostaglandin analogues [Xalatan, Lumigan, Travatan]), nevus of Ota

Treatment: poor response to steroids

Complications: glaucoma (60%), cataract (PSC; 50%)

Figure 8-3. Fuchs' uveitis (From Hooper PL: Idiopathic and other anterior uveitis. In Yanoff M, Duker JS [eds]: *Ophthalmology*, London, Mosby, 1999.)

Juvenile Rheumatoid Arthritis (JRA)

(see Chapter 5, Pediatrics/Strabismus)

Kawasaki's Disease

(see Chapter 5, Pediatrics/Strabismus)

Lyme Disease

Borrelia burgdorferi (spirochete)

Ocular involvement is usually bilateral

Affected organ systems: skin, CNS, cardiovascular, musculoskeletal

Findings: follicular conjunctivitis, chronic granulomatous iridocyclitis with posterior synechiae and vitreous cells (can be pars planitis–like), keratitis (multiple stromal infiltrates)

Posner-Schlossman Syndrome (Glaucomatocyclitic Crisis)

Recurrent anterior uveitis and increased IOP; episodes are typically self-limited

Symptoms: unilateral pain

Findings: mild AC reaction, few or no KPs, elevated IOP

Treatment: may require topical glaucoma medications to control IOP, steroids to control inflammation

Phacoanaphylactic Endophthalmitis

Immune complex disease (type 3 hypersensitivity reaction) when normal tolerance to lens protein is lost

Previous rupture of lens capsule in same or fellow eye, followed by latent period; with reexposure to lens protein during surgery, zonal granulomatous uveitis occurs

Associated with trauma (80%)

May develop severe uveitis with hypotony, secondary open-angle glaucoma

Pathology: zonal pattern (PMNs infiltrate central lens material; epithelioid histiocytes and mononuclear cells around nidus)

Treatment: remove lens

Interstitial Nephritis

Rare; can be idiopathic or triggered by allergic reaction to medicines (antibiotics, NSAIDs)

Associated with acute anterior uveitis

Pathology: interstitial edema with mononuclear inflammatory cells; eosinophils can be present

Figure 8-4. Severe idiopathic anterior uveitis with fibrinoid reaction. (From Hooper PL: Idiopathic and other anterior uveitis. In Yanoff M, Duker JS [eds]: *Ophthalmology*, London, Mosby, 1999.)

Figure 8-5. Inferior pars plana snowbank with attached snowballs. (From Zimmerman PL: Pars planitis and other intermediate uveitis. In Yanoff M, Duker JS [eds]: *Ophthalmology*, London, Mosby, 1999.)

INTERMEDIATE UVEITIS

Etiology: pars planitis, multiple sclerosis (5% to 25% have periphlebitis and intermediate uveitis), Lyme disease, sarcoidosis, Fuchs' heterochromic iridocyclitis

Pars Planitis (Figure 8-5)

Most common cause of intermediate uveitis (85% to 90%)

Usually young adults; females > males; 75% bilateral

Accounts for 25% of uveitis in children

Associated with HLA-DR15; MS (5%)

Etiology: unknown; diagnosis of exclusion

Symptoms: floaters, decreased vision

Findings: light flare with a few KPs, anterior vitritis, snowballs (white vitreous cellular aggregates near ora serrata; may coalesce to form peripheral fibrovascular accumulation [snowbank] over inferior pars plana and vitreous base), peripheral retinal periphlebitis, hyperemic disc, no chorioretinitis, no synechiae

Pathology:
  Snowballs: epithelioid cells and multinucleated giant cells
  Snowbank: preretinal membrane of fibroglial and vascular elements
  Peripheral retinal veins: often have perivascular cuff of lymphocytes

DDx: sarcoidosis, toxoplasmosis, toxocariasis, syphilis, Lyme disease, MS
  Multiple sclerosis: bilateral pars planitis can occur (80% bilateral, 20% unilateral); may present with band keratopathy, mild AC reaction, vitreous cells in a young patient; can also have PSC, epiretinal membrane, CME, retinal phlebitis

Treatment (main indication is CME with reduced vision): periocular and oral steroids; consider immunosuppressive agents, vitrectomy, cryotherapy to areas of peripheral NV (controversial; can decrease leakage and macular edema, but can lead to retinal tears)

Prognosis: 10% self-limited, 90% chronic (1/3 with exacerbations)

Complications: cataract, retrolenticular cyclitic membrane, VH (from peripheral retinal neovascularization), tractional RD, CME (primary cause of vision loss, followed by cataract), band keratopathy

POSTERIOR UVEITIS

Most common cause of posterior uveitis in adults is toxoplasmosis (followed by retinal vasculitis)

Signs: vitreous cells, membranes, opacities, inflammatory exudates ("snowballs"), vasculitis (opacification around vessels [sheathing {whole vessel}, cuffing {segment of vessel}]), exudates (candlewax drippings), retinitis, pigmentary changes (due to RPE inflammation), choroiditis (focal, multifocal, or diffuse), choroidal detachment

DDx of vitritis:
  Panuveitis: sarcoidosis, TB, syphilis, VKH, sympathetic ophthalmia, Behçet's disease
  Postsurgical/trauma: Irvine-Gass syndrome
  Endophthalmitis
  Choroiditis: APMPPE, serpiginous, birdshot, multifocal choroiditis, *Toxocara*, POHS
  Retinitis: ARN, CMV, toxoplasmosis, candidiasis, cysticercosis, onchocerciasis
  Vasculitis: Eales disease
  Other infections: nematodes, Whipple's disease, EBV, Lyme disease

Other: amyloidosis, ocular ischemia, masquerade syndromes, spillover from anterior uveitis
Intermediate uveitis: pars planitis, MS

Complications: NV, CME, ON swelling and atrophy
CME: common cause of vision loss in pars planitis, birdshot retinochoroidopathy, retinal vasculitis, and any iridocyclitis (especially chronic, recurrent cases); CME does not occur in VKH

Indications for cytotoxic therapy: Behçet's disease, sympathetic ophthalmia, VKH, pars planitis, Eales disease, retinal vasculitis, serpiginous choroidopathy, OCP, necrotizing scleritis, inflammations unresponsive to maximum steroid therapy

Infections

Toxoplasmosis

(see Chapter 5, Pediatrics/Strabismus)

Toxocariasis

(see Chapter 5, Pediatrics/Strabismus)

Presumed Ocular Histoplasmosis Syndrome (POHS)

(see Chapter 11, Posterior Segment)

Cytomegalovirus (CMV)

Progressive hemorrhagic necrotizing retinitis involving all retinal layers

Occurs in 15% to 40% of all patients who develop AIDS; usually when CD4 count <50 cells/mm³

40% bilateral at presentation

Rare syndrome of neonatal cytomegalic inclusion disease

Symptoms: often asymptomatic; may have floaters, scotoma

Findings: well-circumscribed necrotizing retinitis (2 appearances), mild AC and vitreous reaction
Brushfire: indolent, granular, yellow-white advancing edge with peripheral atrophic "burned out" region
Pizza-pie fundus: thick, yellow-white necrosis; hemorrhage, vascular sheathing

Pathology: infected retinal cells are markedly enlarged, then necrotic, finally atrophic; large owl's eye intranuclear inclusions

Treatment: antiviral therapy (induction during first 2 weeks)
Ganciclovir (Cytovene): virostatic
TOXICITY: neutropenia and thrombocytopenia
INDUCTION: 5–7.5 mg/kg IV bid × 2–4 weeks
MAINTENANCE: 5–10 mg/kg IV qd

INTRAVITREAL INJECTION: 200–2000 µg/0.1 mL 2–3 times a week × 2–3 weeks
Foscarnet: virostatic
TOXICITY: renal
INDUCTION: 90 mg/kg IV bid or 60 mg/kg IV tid × 2 weeks
MAINTENANCE: 90–120 mg/kg IV qd
INTRAVITREAL INJECTION: 2.4 mg/0.1 mL 2–3 times a week × 2–3 weeks, then 1–2 times a week
Cidofovir (Vistide): longer half-life
TOXICITY: renal, uveitis (50%), hypotony
INDUCTION: 3–5 mg/kg IV once a week × 2 weeks
MAINTENANCE: 3–5 mg/kg IV once every 2 weeks
Administered through peripheral line (central line required for ganciclovir and foscarnet)
INTRAVITREAL INJECTION: 165–330 µg once a week × 3 weeks, then every 2 weeks
Associated with lowering of IOP (about 2 mmHg), 20% to 50% develop iritis (about 5 days after last infusion)
Probenecid and hydration with each dose to reduce renal toxicity and decrease iritis
Median time to progression = 120 days
B-scan ultrasound in patients with severe hypotony revealed CB atrophy
Ganciclovir (Vitrasert):
Median time to progression = 194 days (vs 72 days with IV ganciclovir and 15 days with no treatment)
May be increased risk of RD with implantation
Oral ganciclovir: poor bioavailability; only 6% absorbed with food, 9% absorption without food
Surgery: vitrectomy with long-acting tamponade for RD repair

Complications: rhegmatogenous RD

Figure 8-6. Cytomegalovirus retinitis. (From Hudson HL, Boyer DS, Martin DF, Kuppermann BD: Viral posterior uveitis. In Yanoff M, Duker JS [eds]: *Ophthalmology*, London, Mosby, 1999.)

Acute Retinal Necrosis (ARN) (Figure 8-7)

Acute self-limited confluent peripheral necrotizing retinitis due to infection with VZV, HSV, or rarely CMV

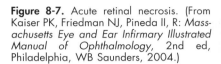

intraretinal hemorrhages   retinal necrosis

Figure 8-7. Acute retinal necrosis. (From Kaiser PK, Friedman NJ, Pineda II, R: *Massachusetts Eye and Ear Infirmary Illustrated Manual of Ophthalmology*, 2nd ed, Philadelphia, WB Saunders, 2004.)

Usually occurs in immunocompetent individuals; 33% bilateral (BARN), commonly in immunosuppressed

Association with HLA-DQw7 (50%)

Symptoms: rapid onset of ocular/periocular pain, pain on eye movement, redness, photophobia, floaters, decreased vision, constriction of visual field

Findings: diffuse episcleral injection, mild iritis with granulomatous KP, vitritis; "thumbprint" nummular infiltrates posterior to equator with isolated peripheral patches of necrotizing retinitis that becomes confluent; sawtooth demarcation line between necrotic and healthy retina, generalized obliterative retinal arteritis (with peripheral vaso-occlusion), pale disc edema; within 2 months, retinitis gradually resolves and necrotic retina sloughs; coarse salt and pepper pigmentation

Pathology: necrosis occurs from virally induced cytolysis, arteriolar and choriocapillaris occlusion; necrotic cells slough into vitreous, leaving large areas devoid of retina

FA: focal areas of choroidal hypoperfusion early; late staining

Treatment: acyclovir (IV × 5–10 days, then oral × 6 weeks; decreases risk of development of ARN in fellow eye by approximately 50%; ganciclovir is an alternative); oral steroids; aspirin to inhibit vascular thrombosis

Prognosis: watch fellow eye closely (usually develops ARN within 4 weeks)

65% to 90% develop rhegmatogenous RD (usually within 3 months)

Progressive Outer Retinal Necrosis (PORN)

Variant of ARN in AIDS but painless with minimal intraocular inflammation

Often have history of cutaneous zoster

74% unilateral at presentation, 70% become bilateral

Findings: multiple discrete peripheral or central areas of retinal opacification/infiltrates (deep with very rapid progression), "cracked mud" appearance after resolution; vasculitis is not prominent

Treatment: combination of foscarnet and ganciclovir; poor response to antivirals

Prognosis: 67% become NLP within 4 weeks; RD in 90%

Figure 8-8. Progressive outer retinal necrosis, early stage. (From Hudson HL, Boyer DS, Martin DF, Kuppermann BD: Viral posterior uveitis. In Yanoff M, Duker JS [eds]: *Ophthalmology*, London, Mosby, 1999.)

Herpes Zoster

Uveitis typically develops during convalescence from acute *Varicella* infection

Reactivated uveitis (anterior and/or posterior), may have keratitis (epithelial or stromal)

Rubella

Sensorineural hearing loss, salt and pepper retinopathy; may develop cataract or glaucoma (rare to have both)

Vision and electrophysiologic testing are usually normal

Live virus in an infant is found in the lens, as well as conjunctival swab, pharyngeal swab, and urine cultures

Figure 8-9. Rubella retinopathy. (Courtesy of George S. Novalis, MD. From Hudson HL, Boyer DS, Martin DF, Kuppermann BD: Viral posterior uveitis. In Yanoff M, Duker JS [eds]: *Ophthalmology*, London, Mosby, 1999.)

Measles

Pigmentary retinopathy due to infection acquired in utero

Acute blindness 6–12 days after measles rash appears

Findings: keratoconjunctivitis, retinal edema, vascular attenuation, macular star, no hemorrhages; Koplik's spots in mouth

Treatment: none; most infants recover, some develop pigmentary degeneration

Subacute sclerosing panencephalitis (SSPE): fatal measles slow virus infection of CNS
   Findings: macular or perimacular chorioretinitis, pigmentary changes with bone spicules, papilledema, optic atrophy, nystagmus, cortical blindness
   Other findings: personality or behavioral changes, dementia, seizures, myoclonus
   Pathology: eosinophilic nuclear inclusions in neuronal and glial cells

Candidiasis

Yeast-like form (blastoconidia), or pseudohyphae or elongated branching structures (pseudomycelia)

Occurs in debilitated patients on hyperalimentation and in IV drug abusers

Most cases occur without positive blood cultures or ongoing fungemia

Approximately 10% with candidemia develop endophthalmitis

Findings: anterior uveitis, retinal hemorrhages, perivascular sheathing, chorioretinitis with fluffy white lesions (puff balls; may be joined by opaque vitreous stands ["string of pearls"]), vitreous abscess; may have subretinal abscess

Culture: blood agar or Sabaraud's glucose (large, creamy white colonies)

DDx of pale subretinal mass: metastasis, amelanotic melanoma, choroidal osteoma, old subretinal hemorrhage, granuloma

Treatment: IV amphotericin B

Prognosis: 70% mortality within 1 year

Pneumocystis Choroiditis

Due to *Pneumocystis carinii*

Choroiditis with multifocal orange nummular lesions; lesions contain cysts of *Pneumocystis carinii*

Associated with use of inhaled pentamidine (which is prophylaxis for pulmonary *Pneumocystis* only)

Figure 8-10. Multiple choroidal lesions in *Pneumocystis* choroiditis. (From Cowan CL: Sarcoidosis. In Yanoff M, Duker JS [eds]: *Ophthalmology*, London, Mosby, 1999.)

Cysticercosis

Due to infection with pork tapeworm *Taenia solium* or *T. saginata*; humans are definitive host, pigs are intermediate host

Adult worm lives in small intestine; larvae travel to eye, producing cystic subretinal or intravitreal lesion (cysticercus)

Findings: mass lesion or exudative RD

Treatment: vitrectomy required for posterior segment disease (Figure 8-11)

Leprosy

Due to *Mycobacterium leprae*

5–15 million infected; 250,000 blind

Findings:
   Lids: lagophthalmos, madarosis, blepharochalasis, nodules, trichiasis, entropion, ectropion, reduced blinking

Figure 8-11. Cysticercus in the eye. (From Cowan CL: Sarcoidosis. In Yanoff M, Duker JS [eds]: *Ophthalmology*, London, Mosby, 1999.)

Lacrimal: acute and chronic dacryocystitis

Cornea: anesthesia, exposure keratopathy, band keratopathy, corneal leproma, interstitial keratitis, thickened nerves, superficial stromal keratitis

Sclera: episcleritis, scleritis, staphyloma, nodules

Iris: miosis, iritis, synechiae, seclusio pupillae, atrophy, iris pearls, leproma

Ciliary body: loss of accommodation, hypotony, phthisis

Fundus: peripheral choroidal lesions, retinal vasculitis

Complications: cataract, glaucoma

Diffuse Unilateral Subacute Neuroretinitis (DUSN)

Due to infection with small roundworm in subretinal space: dog hookworm (*Ancylostoma caninum*) or racoon nematode (*Baylisascaris procyonis*)

Findings: deep, gray-white retinal lesions; optic nerve swelling; vitreous cells; late findings include retinal vascular narrowing, diffuse RPE pigmentary changes, optic atrophy; results in unilateral "wipe-out" syndrome

ERG: decreased

Treatment: laser nematode

Cat-Scratch Disease

Due to *Bartonella henselae* (also causes oculoglandular syndrome)

Findings: retinal granuloma or neuroretinitis

Treatment: oral antibiotics (doxycycline 100 mg bid, and rifampin 300 mg bid × 4–6 weeks)

Onchocerciasis (River Blindness)

Due to Onchocerca volvulus: larvae mature in humans, forming adult worms that live in fibrous, subcutaneous nodules (usually in joints); female worms (100 cm long, live for up to 20 years) and male worms (5 cm long, live for much shorter time) reproduce sexually, females give birth to ~2000 microfilariae/day; microfilariae (300 microns long, live for 1–2 years) migrate all over body by direct invasion and hematogenous spread, prefer skin and eyes; live microfilariae induce little or no inflammation; death of organism causes severe granulomatous inflammation and scarring

Transmitted by black fly: breeds along fast-moving streams; bites infected host and acquires microfilariae, which mature into infectious larvae; transmits larvae to humans with bite; 17 million infected; 1–2 million blind (Africa and Latin America)

Second leading cause of corneal blindness in world (trachoma is first)

Findings: intraocular microfilariae (in AC), anterior uveitis, SPK, sclerosing keratitis, scleritis, chorioretinitis, optic neuritis and atrophy; may develop cataract, PAS, and glaucoma

Other findings: pruritus, pigmentary changes (leopard-skin appearance), chronic inflammation, scarring, maculopapular rash, subcutaneous nodules

Diagnosis: skin snip (place piece of skin in tissue media, 20–100 microfilariae emerge)

Treatment: ivermectin, suramin, DEC

Figure 8-12. Sclerosing keratitis as a result of onchocerciasis. (Courtesy of Professor HR Taylor. From Cowan CL: Sarcoidosis. In Yanoff M, Duker JS [eds]: *Ophthalmology*, London, Mosby, 1999.)

Whipple's Disease

Due to *Tropheryma whipplei*; Gram-positive bacillus, Actinomycetes family; found intracellularly and extracellularly

Findings: uveitis, retinal vasculitis

Other findings: malabsorption (diarrhea, steatorrhea), migratory arthralgias

Pathology: PAS-positive macrophages within lamina propria of "clubbed" (abnormal) microvilli of intestinal wall, or vitreous biopsy

Treatment: Bactrim may be helpful; may require a year of therapy as shorter courses lead to relapses

Propionibacterium Acnes

Gram-positive rod; anaerobic

May become sequestered in capsular bag following cataract surgery

Findings: delayed onset, chronic granulomatous uveitis, often with fibrin or hypopyon; white plaque on posterior capsule is characteristic

Treatment: intravitreal antibiotics (vancomycin, cephalosporins; resistant to aminoglycosides); alone rarely works; usually requires partial or total removal of capsular bag with/without IOL removal/exchange

Ophthalmomyiasis

Due to direct ocular invasion by fly larvae (maggots) that can invade AC, posterior segment, or subretinal space

Subretinal invasion: larvae travel through fundus, leaving criss-crossing tracks of atrophied RPE; death of organism causes ocular inflammation

Inflammations (Table 8-1)

Acute Posterior Multifocal Placoid Pigment Epitheliopathy (APMPPE)

Occurs in young, healthy adults; female = male; usually bilateral

Acute, self-limited; may be nonspecific choroidal hypersensitivity reaction

Possible HLA-B7 association

Associated with cerebral vasculitis

Flu-like prodrome (33%) followed by decreased vision

Findings: multiple creamy yellow-white plaque-like lesions (usually <1 DD) at level of RPE or choriocapillaris (possibly due to choroidal hypoperfusion); lesions fade over 2–6 weeks, leaving geographically shaped RPE changes (hypopigmentation and hyperpigmentation); may have vitreous cells, mild AC reaction; rarely vascular sheathing, disc edema, CNV

Other findings: thyroiditis, erythema nodosum, cerebral vasculitis, regional enteritis

FA: initial blockage with late hyperfluorescence; window defects in old cases

Figure 8-13. Acute posterior multifocal placoid pigment epitheliopathy demonstrating multiple posterior pole lesions. (From Kaiser PK, Friedman NJ, Pineda II, R: *Massachusetts Eye and Ear Infirmary Illustrated Manual of Ophthalmology*, 2nd ed, Philadelphia, WB Saunders, 2004.)

Figure 8-14. Fluorescein angiogram of same patient as shown in Figure 8-13 demonstrating early hypofluorescence of the lesions. (From Kaiser PK, Friedman NJ, Pineda II, R: *Massachusetts Eye and Ear Infirmary Illustrated Manual of Ophthalmology*, 2nd ed, Philadelphia, WB Saunders, 2004.)

Figure 8-15. Fluorescein angiogram of same patient as shown in Figure 8-14 demonstrating late staining of the lesions. (From Kaiser PK, Friedman NJ, Pineda II, R: *Massachusetts Eye and Ear Infirmary Illustrated Manual of Ophthalmology*, 2nd ed, Philadelphia, WB Saunders, 2004.)

Table 8-1. **White Dot Syndromes**

	APMPPE	MEWDS	Serpiginous	Birdshot	Multifocal Choroiditis with Panuveitis	PIC
Age	20–40	20–50	30–50	40–60	20–50	20–40
Sex	F = M	F > M	F = M	F > M	F > M	Female
Laterality	Bilateral	Unilateral	Bilateral	Bilateral		
HLA	B7, DR2	None	B7	A29	None	None
Vitritis	Mild	Mild	Mild	Chronic, moderate	Chronic, moderate	None
Lesions	Large, geographic, gray-white; shallow pigmented scars within 1–2 weeks	Small, soft, gray-white dots; no scarring	Active, geographic, gray-white patches; deep scars with fibrosis	Deep, creamy spots; indistinct margins; yellow scars without pigmentation	50–350 µm gray-white yellow spots; mixture of old scars and new spots	100–300 µm yellow or gray spots; punched-out scars
Macula	Rare CNV	Granularity Rare CNV	Subretinal scars 25% CNV	CME Rare CNV	CME 35% CNV	Atrophic scars 40% CNV
Prognosis	Good	Good	Poor	Fair	Fair	Good
Treatment	None	None	Steroids Laser CNV	Steroids Cyclosporine	Steroids Laser CNV	None Laser CNV

Treatment: none

Prognosis: vision recovers in most patients to >20/40; rarely recurs

Multiple Evanescent White Dot Syndrome (MEWDS)

Onset ages 14–50 years old; female > male; unilateral > bilateral

Symptoms: decreased vision, dark spots in the periphery (peripheral scotomas), shimmering photopsias

Findings: granular retinal appearance with small (100–200 µm) white spots in posterior pole at level of RPE; may have vitreous cells, RAPD, mild optic disc swelling

VF: enlarged blind spot

FA: early hyperfluorescence in wreathlike configuration; late staining of lesions and optic nerve

ERG: reduced a-wave (involvement of RPE and outer retina)

multiple evanescent white dot syndrome

Figure 8-16. Multiple evanescent white dot syndrome demonstrating faint white spots. (From Kaiser PK, Friedman NJ, Pineda II, R: *Massachusetts Eye and Ear Infirmary Illustrated Manual of Ophthalmology*, 2nd ed, Philadelphia, WB Saunders, 2004.)

dot syndrome   early hyperfluorescence

Figure 8-17. Same patient as shown in Figure 8–16 demonstrating early fluorescein angiogram appearance. (From Kaiser PK, Friedman NJ, Pineda II, R: *Massachusetts Eye and Ear Infirmary Illustrated Manual of Ophthalmology*, 2nd ed, Philadelphia, WB Saunders, 2004.)

Prognosis: vision recovers over weeks but may be permanently decreased due to pigmentary changes in fovea; 10% have recurrent episodes in same or fellow eye

Serpiginous Choroidopathy

Chronic, recurrent, indolent disease of unknown etiology

Onset ages 40–60 years; female = male; usually bilateral

Affects inner chorioretinal pigment epithelium

Symptoms: painless loss of vision

Findings: geographic (map-like) pattern of scars with active edges (yellow-gray, edematous), usually beginning in posterior pole (often extending from disc); active areas become atrophic over weeks to months; new lesions occur contiguously or elsewhere (often in snakelike pattern); may have mild AC reaction, vitritis, vascular sheathing, RPE detachment, NVD, CNV (rare)

VF: absolute scotomas corresponding to atrophic scars

FA: acute lesions stain

Treatment: may respond to oral steroids, immunosuppressive drugs

Prognosis: fair to poor; commonly recurs months to years later

Figure 8-18. Fundus view of the right eye of a 57-year-old woman has early serpiginous choroiditis. (From Moorthy RS, Jampol LM: Posterior uveitis of unknown cause. In Yanoff M, Duker JS [eds]: *Ophthalmology*, London, Mosby, 1999.)

Birdshot Choroidopathy (Vitiliginous Chorioretinitis)

Occurs after 4th decade of life; female > male; usually bilateral

Associated with HLA-A29 (90%)

Symptoms: decreased vision, nyctalopia, decreased color vision, peripheral visual field loss

Findings: cream-colored depigmented spots scattered throughout fundus; may have mild AC reaction, vitritis, retinal vasculitis, disc edema, optic atrophy, CME, epiretinal membrane, CNV

FA: pronounced perifoveal capillary leakage with CME

ERG: diminished scotopic response (rod dysfunction)

Figure 8-19. Birdshot retinochoroidopathy. (From Moorthy RS, Jampol LM: Posterior uveitis of unknown cause. In Yanoff M, Duker JS [eds]: *Ophthalmology*, London, Mosby, 1999.)

Multifocal Choroiditis with Panuveitis

Onset ages 20–50 years, female > male

Findings: multiple gray-white to yellow lesions (50–350 μm) at level of choroid or RPE; vitreous and AC cells; chronic lesions become atrophic with punched-out margins, variable amounts of pigmentation, and occasionally fibrosis (Figure 8-20)

FA: acute lesions block or fill early and stain late; older lesions behave like window defects with early hyperfluorescence and late fading

Treatment: steroids

Complications: CNV (most common cause of vision loss), CME

Punctate Inner Choroidopathy (PIC)
(Figure 8-21)

Healthy, moderately myopic women, ages 20–40 years

Symptoms: acute scotomas and photopsias

Findings: small (100–300 μm) yellow or gray inner choroidal lesions; resolve over weeks to form atrophic scars that may enlarge and become pigmented; new lesions do not appear; may have

Figure 8-20. Fundus view of the left eye of a 50-year-old woman who has progressive subretinal fibrosis and uveitis syndrome. (From Moorthy RS, Jampol LM: Posterior uveitis of unknown cause. In Yanoff M, Duker JS [eds]: *Ophthalmology*, London, Mosby, 1999.)

Figure 8-21. Punctate inner choroidopathy. (From Moorthy RS, Jampol LM: Posterior uveitis of unknown cause. In Yanoff M, Duker JS [eds]: *Ophthalmology*, London, Mosby, 1999.)

Figure 8-22. Retinal pigment epitheliitis. (From Moorthy RS, Jampol LM: Posterior uveitis of unknown cause. In Yanoff M, Duker JS [eds]: *Ophthalmology*, London, Mosby, 1999.)

Figure 8-23. "Frosted branch angiitis" secondary to cytomegalovirus retinitis. (From Hudson HL, Boyer DS, Martin DF, Kuppermann BD: Viral posterior uveitis. In Yanoff M, Duker JS [eds]: *Ophthalmology*, London, Mosby, 1999.)

serous RDs; 40% risk of CNV; no AC or vitreous cells

Treatment: none

Acute Retinal Pigment Epitheliitis (Krill's Disease) (Figure 8-22)

Rare, occurs in young adults; usually unilateral

Symptoms: sudden decrease in vision

Findings: clusters of hyperpigmented spots (300–400 μm) in macula surrounded by yellow-white halos; with resolution, the spots lighten or darken, but halos remain; no vitritis

DDx: central serous retinopathy, acute macular neuroretinopathy (wedge-shaped or cloverleaf dark red perifoveal dots; paracentral scotoma; normal ERG)

FA: blockage of spots with halos of hyperfluorescence

Treatment: none

Prognosis: resolves completely in 6–12 weeks

Frosted Branch Angiitis (Figure 8-23)

White spots along retinal arterioles

DDx: CMV retinitis, toxoplasmosis (Kyrieleis' plaques)

Acute Zonal Occult Outer Retinopathy (AZOOR)

Usually bilateral; females > males

Symptoms: rapid loss of function in 1 or more regions of visual field, photopsias

Findings: minimal changes initially; retinal degeneration/pigmentary changes late

DDx: MEWDS, acute macular neuroretinopathy, multifocal choroiditis

VF: scotomas (may enlarge)

ERG: decrease rod and cone

Idiopathic Uveal Effusion Syndrome

Occurs in healthy, middle-aged males

Chronic, recurrent disorder

Symptoms: decreased vision, metamorphopsia, scotomas

Findings: serous retinal, choroidal, and ciliary body detachments; mild vitritis, RPE changes (leopard spots), conjunctival injection; key finding of shifting subretinal fluid

B-scan ultrasound: thickened sclera, serous RD, choroidal detachments

FA: no discrete leakage

Treatment: steroids and immunosuppressive agents are not effective; consider scleral resection in nanophthalmic eyes, or quadrantic partial-thickness scleral windows

ENDOPHTHALMITIS

Inflammation involving 1 or more coats of the eye and adjacent ocular cavities

Etiology: infectious or sterile; must rule out infection

Symptoms: pain, decreased vision

Findings: lid edema, chemosis, AC reaction, hypopyon (pink hypopyon = *Serratia*), vitritis

Classification:
Acute postoperative (<6 weeks after surgery; 90% in 1st week):
RISK FACTORS: blepharitis, wound leak, iris prolapse, vitreous loss, contaminated IOL, diabetes, chronic alcoholism
ORGANISMS: *S. epidermidis*, *S. aureus*, *Streptococci*, *Pseudomonas*
INCIDENCE:
ECCE or ICCE (with or without IOL): 0.072%
Secondary IOL: 0.3%
PPV: 0.51%
PK: 0.11%
Glaucoma filter: 0.061% (*S. faecalis*, *Streptococci* [57%], *H. influenzae* [23%])
PREVENTION:
TREAT BLEPHARITIS: 85% of responsible organisms (*S. epidermidis* and *S. aureus*) are found on lids; hot compresses, lid hygiene, Polysporin ointment × 1 week preop; add

doxycycline 100 mg bid × 1 week for acne rosacea or seborrheic dermatitis
STERILIZE OPERATIVE FIELD: 5% povidine iodine (Betadine); preoperative topical antibiotics (fluoroquinolone)
AVOID INOCULATION: drape eyelashes
ANTIBIOTICS: intracameral (injection or in irrigating solution) controversial; topically postop for 4–7 days; consider oral fluoroquinolone with broken posterior capsule or vitreous loss
Delayed postoperative:
Propionibacterium acnes (anaerobic gram + rod) or fungal
Trauma:
RISK FACTORS: penetrating trauma (2%–7%), retained intraocular FB (7%)
25% CULTURE POSITIVE: *Bacillus* (30%), *S. epidermidis* (25%), *Streptococci* (13%), *S. aureus* (8%), Gram-negative and mixed flora
Poor visual outcome
Endogenous:
RISK FACTORS: immunosuppression, indwelling venous catheters, IVDA, following intra-abdominal surgery
30% of patients with *Candida* septicemia develop endophthalmitis
Sterile: culture negative

Treatment: rule out infection (AC and vitreous taps)
Intravitreal antibiotics: vancomycin 1 mg/0.1 mL, ceftazidime 2.25 mg/0.1 mL (consider intravitreal dexamethasone 400 μg/0.1 mL)
Systemic antibiotics: in severe cases, most traumatic cases, and endogenous bacterial cases; vancomycin 1 g IV q12 hours or cefazolin 1 g IV q8 hours; ceftazidime 1 g IV q12 hours
Topical fortified antibiotics: vancomycin 25–50 mg/mL, ceftazidime 50 mg/mL q1 hour
Topical steroids and cycloplegics

MAJOR CLINICAL STUDY

Endophthalmitis Vitrectomy Study (EVS)

Objective: to evaluate the treatment of acute postoperative (<6 weeks) endophthalmitis (cataract or secondary IOL surgery) with immediate vitrectomy vs "tap and inject," and whether intravenous antibiotics (ceftazidime and amikacin) are necessary

Methods: Patients with clinical evidence of acute postoperative (<6 weeks) endophthalmitis (cataract or secondary IOL surgery) and visual acuity of LP or better, and sufficient clarity to see at least some part of the iris were randomly assigned to emergent AC and vitreous taps alone or with vitrectomy and with injection of intravitreal antibiotics (0.4 mg amikacin and 1.0 mg vancomycin). Patients were also given subconjunctival injections of antibiotics (25 mg vancomycin,

100 mg ceftazidime, and steroid [6 mg dexamethasone phosphate]), topical fortified antibiotics (50 mg/mL vancomycin and 20 mg/mL amikacin) and steroid (prednisolone acetate), and oral steroid (prednisone 30 mg bid × 5–10 days). Patients were also randomly assigned to receive systemic IV antibiotics (2 g ceftazidime IV q8 hours and 7.5 mg/kg amikacin IV followed by 6 mg/kg q12 hours) or no systemic antibiotics. Intravitreal steroids were not used

Results: 420 patients enrolled

On average, signs and symptoms occurred 6 days after surgery (75% presented within 2 weeks of surgery)

69% had positive cultures; 94% were Gram-positive bacteria (70% coagulase-negative *Staphylococcus*, 10% *S. aureus*, 9% *Streptococci* species)

IV antibiotics were of no benefit

Immediate vitrectomy had significant benefits only when patients presented with light perception vision or worse

Conclusions:

For endopthalmitis after cataract or secondary IOL surgery, perform emergent treatment with AC tap and injection of intravitreal antibiotics when vision is better than LP

Vitrectomy should be reserved for patients presenting with light perception vision or worse

IV antibiotics do not improve the outcome

PANUVEITIS

Sarcoidosis

Multisystem granulomatous disease characterized by noncaseating granulomas; unknown etiology

Females > males; more common among African Americans (10 : 1)

25% to 50% have systemic sarcoidosis

Ocular disease: 30% unilateral, 70% bilateral; 40% acute, 60% chronic

Findings (25%–30%): uveitis in 60% of patients with ocular involvement; 66% of uveitis is anterior (2 forms: acute granulomatous [responds well to corticosteroids] and chronic recurrent [difficult to control with corticosteroids]), KP, iris nodules, lacrimal gland infiltration (25%; painless bilateral enlargement), conjunctival follicles, keratoconjunctivitis sicca, episcleritis and scleritis with nodules, choroiditis with yellow or white nodules, retinal periphlebitis with candlewax drippings (granulomas along retinal venules), pars planitis, vitritis, retinal neovascularization, optic nerve granuloma; secondary cataracts, glaucoma, and band keratopathy

Other findings: pulmonary (50%), constitutional (40%; malaise, fever, weight loss), skin (15%), lymphadenopathy (20%) (see Box 8-1)

Figure 8-24. Sarcoidosis demonstrating conjunctival granuloma with giant cells surrounded by lymphocytes and plasma cells. (From Yanoff M, Fine BS: *Ocular Pathology*, 5th ed, St, Louis, Mosby, 2002.)

Pathology: noncaseating granulomas (caseating granulomas occur in TB) with Langhans' multinucleated giant cells

Diagnosis:

Lab tests: angiotensin-converting enzyme (ACE; elevated in any diffuse granulomatous disease affecting the lung), serum lysozyme (more sensitive than ACE, but less specific)

Chest X-ray or chest CT: hilar adenopathy (Figure 8-25)

Gallium scan: look for parotid, lacrimal, or pulmonary involvement

Biopsy: skin lesion, conjunctival nodule, lymph node, salivary or lacrimal gland, lung; if elevated ACE and positive CXR, 60% to 70% of blind conjunctival biopsies will be positive

Treatment: topical, periocular, and systemic steroids, immunosuppressive therapy

Lofgren's Syndrome

Hilar lymphadenopathy, erythema nodosum, anterior uveitis, arthralgia

Figure 8-25. Bilateral hilar adenopathy in a patient without pulmonary symptoms. (From Cowan CL: Sarcoidosis. In Yanoff M, Duker JS [eds]: *Ophthalmology*, London, Mosby, 1999.)

Mikulicz's Syndrome

Lacrimal & parotid gland swelling, sicca syndrome
   Etiology: sarcoidosis, TB, lymphoma/leukemia

Heerfordt's Syndrome

Fever, parotid gland enlargement, anterior uveitis, facial nerve palsy

Behçet's Disease (Figure 8-26)

Chronic recurrent multisystem condition characterized by relapsing inflammation and occlusive vasculitis

Figure 8-26. Fundus view of a patient who has Behçet's disease. (From Yanoff M, Fine BS: *Ocular Pathology*, 5th ed, St, Louis, Mosby, 2002.)

Triad of oral ulcers, genital ulcers, and inflammatory eye disease

Associated with HLA-B51; males > females, usually young adults; more common in Japan and Mediterranean countries

Findings (75%): recurrent, explosive inflammatory episodes with active episodes lasting 2–4 weeks

Uveitis (posterior more common than anterior); can present with nongranulomatous anterior uveitis (usually bilateral; may have transient hypopyon); occasionally, conjunctivitis, episcleritis, or keratitis can occur; posterior involvement with recurrent vascular occlusions, retinal hemorrhages, exudates, CME, vitritis, traction RD, ischemic optic neuropathy; may develop glaucoma and cataract

Other findings: oral (aphthous) ulcers, genital ulcers, skin lesions (erythema nodosum, acne-like lesions, folliculitis), arthritis (50%; especially wrists and ankles), thrombophlebitis, large vessel occlusion; GI pain, diarrhea, constipation; CNS involvement (25%; meningoencephalitis, strokes, palsies, confusional states)

Pathology: obliterative vasculitis with activation of both cellular and humoral limbs of immune system; circulating immune complexes in >50%

Diagnosis:
   Clinical: (see Box 8-2)
   Behcetine skin test (cutaneous hypersensitivity): intradermal puncture; positive test = pustule formation within minutes
   HLA-B51

BOX 8-2. Criteria for Behçet's Disease

Major criteria
1. Oral aphthous ulcers (round, discrete borders; heal without scarring)
2. Genital ulcers
3. Skin lesions (erythema nodosum)
4. Ocular disease (75%): nongranulomatous iridocyclitis with sterile hypopyon, necrotizing retinal vasculitis (may cause vascular occlusion), posterior synechiae, glaucoma (pupillary block, uveitic), cataract, TRD

Minor criteria
1. Arthritis (50%)
2. GI lesions
3. Occlusive vascular lesions of major vessels (vena cava)
4. Migratory thrombophlebitis (33%)
5. CNS involvement (25%; neuro-Behçet's; meningoencephalitis, involvement of brain stem, spinal cord, peripheral nerves)
6. Pulmonary artery aneurysm (pathognomonic CXR finding)
7. Interstitial lung changes

Treatment: systemic steroids, cytotoxic agents (chlorambucil most effective for retinal vasculitis, meningoencephalitis), colchicine (prevents recurrences), cyclosporine; plasmapheresis

Vogt-Koyanagi-Harada Syndrome (VKH)

Uveoencephalitis: bilateral diffuse granulomatous panuveitis, serous RDs, disc edema, meningeal irritation, skin pigmentary changes, and auditory disturbance

Harada's disease if only eye findings

Presumed autoimmune process against melanocytes

Typically occurs in Asians, American Indians, and Hispanics between ages 30 and 50 years; female > male

Associated with HLA-DR4

Symptoms: decreased vision, pain, redness, photophobia, stiff neck, headache, deafness, tinnitus, vertigo

Findings: bilateral diffuse granulomatous panuveitis, exudative RDs, vitritis, exudative choroiditis, CB detachment, CME, ON hyperemia and edema, poliosis; later develop perilimbal vitiligo (Sugiura's sign), Dalen-Fuchs nodules (yellow-white retinal spots), sunset fundus (RPE disturbance with focal areas of atrophy and hyperpigmentation [healing phase])

Other findings: temporary deafness, tinnitis, vertigo, meningeal irritation, skin changes (30%; alopecia, vitiligo, poliosis)

Clinical course:
  Prodrome: headache, meningismus, seizures, bilateral decreased vision with pain, redness, photophobia
  Syndrome: uveitis with serous RDs
  Chronic stage: sunset fundus, Dalen-Fuchs nodules, perilimbal vitiligo
  Recurrent stage: AC reaction, pigment changes; 60% retain vision >20/30

Pathology: inflammation of choriocapillaris and retina; Dalen-Fuchs nodules (epithelioid cells between Bruch's membrane and RPE) (Figure 8-27)

DDx: sympathetic ophthalmia, posterior scleritis, syphilis, lupus choroiditis, hypotony, uveal effusion syndrome

Diagnosis:
  LP: CSF pleocytosis
  FA: multiple focal areas of subretinal leakage ("1000 points of light")

Treatment: steroids (6 months), cycloplegic, immunosuppressive agents

Prognosis: 60% retain vision >20/30

Complications: cataracts (25%), glaucoma (33%), CNV (10%)

Figure 8-27. VKH demonstrating granulomatous inflammation in choroid extending into choriocapillaris and through RPE. (From Yanoff M, Fine BS: *Ocular Pathology*, 5th ed, St, Louis, Mosby, 2002.)

Sympathetic Ophthalmia

Bilateral granulomatous panuveitis following penetrating eye trauma

Due to immune sensitization to melanin or melanin-associated proteins in uveal tissues; 10 days to 50 years after injury

T cell mediated (delayed hypersensitivity reaction); latency of 2 weeks to 46 years

Incidence: 0.1% to 0.3% of penetrating injuries; 0.015% of intraocular surgery

Findings: Koeppe nodules, mutton fat KP, retinal edema, Dalen-Fuchs nodules; may have disc edema

Dalen-Fuchs nodules

Figure 8-28. Dalen-Fuchs nodules in a patient with sympathetic ophthalmia. (From Kaiser PK, Friedman NJ, Pineda II, R: *Massachusetts Eye and Ear Infirmary Illustrated Manual of Ophthalmology*, 2nd ed, Philadelphia, WB Saunders, 2004.)

Pathology: diffuse lymphocytic infiltration of choroid with ill-defined patchy accumulations of epithelioid (giant) cells that contain phagocytosed uveal pigment; inflammation can extend into optic nerve, causing granulomatous optic neuritis; Dalen-Fuchs nodules (epithelioid giant cells between Bruch's membrane and RPE that appear as small, round, yellow depigmented spots in peripheral retina [also seen in VKH, sarcoidosis, TB]); no involvement of choriocapillaris

Figure 8-29. SO demonstrating thickened choroid with epithelioid cells and lymphocytes; the choriocapillaris is spared. (From Yanoff M, Fine BS: *Ocular Pathology*, 5th ed, Philadelphia, Mosby, 2002.)

FA: multiple hyperfluorescent sites of leakage

Treatment: steroids, immunosuppressive agents; consider enucleation of injured eye within 10–14 days if NLP vision, but once inflammation has started in fellow eye, removal of inciting eye is controversial

Prognosis: Many patients retain very good vision

Syphilis (Figure 8-31)

Panuveitis ("great mimic") due to infection with spirochete *Treponema pallidum*

Acquired:
  Findings (secondary and tertiary): panuveitis, iris papules and gummata (yellow-red nodules), chorioretinitis (salt and pepper changes), optic neuritis, optic atrophy, Argyll-Robertson pupil, ectopia lentis, interstitial keratitis
  Other findings:
    SECONDARY: chancre, rash, lymphadenopathy, condyloma lata
    TERTIARY: CNS, aortic aneurysm, gummas
  Diagnosis: serology (VDRL or RPR, and FTA-ABS); must rule out neurosyphilis with LP
    FALSE-POSITIVE VDRL: rheumatoid arthritis, anti-cardiolipin antibody, SLE
  Treatment: as for neurosyphilis
    Penicillin G 12–24 million units/day IV × 2 weeks, followed by penicillin G 2.4 million units/week IM × 3 weeks
    In penicillin-allergic patients: doxycycline, erythromycin

Congenital:
  Findings: interstitial keratitis (new vessels meet in center of cornea [salmon patch]); then atrophy (ghost vessels), anterior uveitis, ectopia lentis, Argyll-Robertson pupil, optic atrophy, chorioretinitis (salt and pepper fundus)

Figure 8-30. Higher magnification of Figure 8-29 shows a Dalen-Fuchs nodule between RPE and Bruch's membrane. (From Yanoff M, Fine BS: *Ocular Pathology*, 5th ed, Philadelphia, Mosby, 2002.)

Figure 8-31. Extensive chorioretinal damage with hyperplasia of retinal pigment epithelium due to syphilis. (From Dugel PU: Syphilitic uveitis. In Yanoff M, Duker JS [eds]: *Ophthalmology*, London, Mosby, 1999.)

Other findings: death (in utero or perinatal), inflammation of internal organs, dental abnormalities (Hutchinson's teeth), facial deformities (saddle nose), saber shins

Tuberculosis

Due to infection with *Mycobacterium tuberculosis*

Findings: lupus vulgaris on eyelids, phlyctenule, primary conjunctival TB, interstitial keratitis, scleritis, lacrimal gland involvement, orbital periostitis, granulomatous panuveitis, secondary glaucoma and cataract, chorioretinal plaque or nodule (tuberculoma), exudative RD, cranial nerve palsies (often due to basal meningitis)

Treatment: isoniazid, rifampin, ethambutol, pyrazinamide; systemic steroids may cause a flare-up; ethambutol and isoniazid can cause a toxic optic neuropathy

MASQUERADE SYNDROMES

Conditions that present as uveitis: peripheral RD, intraocular foreign body, JXG, multiple sclerosis, malignancies (retinoblastoma, leukemia [ALL], large cell lymphoma, malignant melanoma), RP

Retinoblastoma

Findings: pseudohypopyon, vitreous cells

Diagnosis:
AC tap: LDH levels, cytology
B-scan ultrasound: calcifications

Malignant Melanoma

Necrotic tumor may seed tumor cells into the vitreous and anterior segment, causing an inflammatory response

Findings: AC reaction, iris heterochromia, vitreous hemorrhage; may have brown pseudohypopyon (melanin-laden macrophages) and melanomalytic glaucoma

Diagnosis: FA, B-scan ultrasound

Primary Intraocular Lymphoma (Reticulum Cell Sarcoma)

Findings: bilateral vitreous cells, retinal hemorrhage and exudates, retinal and choroidal infiltrates

Diagnosis: cytology (aqueous and vitreous)

Treatment: radiation therapy (ocular and CNS), intrathecal chemotherapy

Leukemia

Retina is most common ocular tissue affected clinically

Choroid is most common ocular tissue affected histopathologically

Findings: AC reaction, iris heterochromia, Roth spots, retinal hemorrhages, cotton wool spots, peripheral NV, serous RDs, vascular dilation and tortuosity, optic nerve infiltration

Diagnosis: bone marrow, peripheral blood smear, aqueous cytology
FA with serous retinal detachment: multiple areas of hyperfluorescence (similar to VKH)

Multiple Sclerosis

Findings: periphlebitis, pars planitis, optic neuritis

Diagnosis: neurologic examination, head MRI

Juvenile Xanthogranuloma

Findings: small fleshy iris tumors, AC reaction, spontaneous hyphema

Diagnosis: skin lesions, iris biopsy

Intraocular Foreign Body

Findings: AC reaction; may have signs of ocular trauma, visible FB, iris heterochromia

Diagnois: X-ray, B-scan ultrasound

Retinitis Pigmentosa

Findings: vitreous cells

Diagnosis: ERG, EOG, visual fields

DIFFERENTIAL DIAGNOSIS OF UVEITIS AND ASSOCIATED SIGNS

Band keratopathy: JRA, sarcoidosis, multiple myeloma

Hyphema: Fuchs' heterochromic iridocyclitis, trauma, JXG, HZV

Vitreous hemorrhage: VKH, POHS

Iris nodules: TB, syphilis, sarcoidosis, leprosy

Bell's palsy (bilateral): Lyme disease, sarcoidosis

Urinary disorder: Reiter's syndrome, gonococcal disease, Behçet's disease

Jaundice: leptospirosis, inflammatory bowel disease (IBD), CMV, schistosomiasis

Liver enlargement: toxocariasis, toxoplasmosis, CMV

CNS involvement: TB meningitis, VKH, congenital toxoplasmosis, congenital CMV, Behçet's disease, large cell lymphoma

Skin rash: secondary syphilis, sarcoidosis, Behçet's disease, psoriasis, Reiter's syndrome, VKH, POHS

Erythema nodosum: sarcoidosis, TB, IBD, POHS, Behçet's disease, AMPPE

Oral ulcers: Behçet's disease, Reiter's syndrome, HSV, IBD, OCP, SJS, SLE

Genital ulcers: syphilis, Reiter's syndrome, Behçet's disease, OCP

Pulmonary involvement: TB, sarcoidosis, Churg-Strauss, *Toxocara*, aspergillosis, coccidioidomycosis, POHS, Wegener's granulomatosis

SURGERY AND UVEITIS

Usually wait at least 3 months for cataract surgery, 6 months for corneal transplant

JRA: no IOL
Can develop cyclitic membranes and CB detachments
Consider lensectomy with partial vitrectomy

Pars planitis: increased risk of complications
Vitreous opacities may limit vision; therefore, consider lensectomy with pars plana vitrectomy
Higher risk for CME

Fuchs' heterochromic iridocyclitis: cataract surgery is safe; increased risk of transient postoperative hyphema

Review Questions (Answers start on page 364)

1. The most effective antibiotic for the treatment of *P. acnes* endophthalmitis is
   a. amikacin
   b. gentamicin
   c. vancomycin
   d. ceftazidime

2. For the diagnosis of granulomatous inflammation, which cell type must be present?
   a. Langhans' cell
   b. lymphocyte
   c. Touton giant cell
   d. epithelioid histiocyte

3. All of the following are true concerning sarcoidosis except
   a. Touton giant cells are common
   b. lymphocytes surround the granuloma
   c. histiocytes are abundant
   d. necrosis is rare

4. Which of the following is not characteristic of Fuchs' heterochromic iridocyclitis?
   a. iris neovascularization
   b. cataract
   c. posterior synechiae
   d. vitreous opacities

5. The most common organism causing endopthalmitis following cataract surgery is
   a. *S. pneumoniae*
   b. *H. influenzae*
   c. *S. aureus*
   d. *S. epidermidis*

6. MEWDS can be differentiated from APMPPE by
   a. age of onset
   b. female predilection
   c. paracentral scotomas
   d. viral prodrome

7. All of the following disorders are correctly paired with their HLA associations except
   a. POHS, B9
   b. Behçet's disease, B51
   c. Birdshot retinochoroidopathy, A29
   d. Reiter's syndrome, B27

8. Decreased vision in a patient with intermediate uveitis is most likely due to
   a. cataract
   b. macular edema
   c. papillitis
   d. glaucoma

9. A 71-year-old woman with a 6-month history of fatigue, anorexia, and 10-pound weight loss is found to have left-sided weakness, visual acuity of 20/80 OD and 20/60 OS, and vitreous cells. The most helpful workup is
   a. LP and vitrectomy
   b. ESR and temporal artery biopsy
   c. CBC and lymph node biopsy
   d. PPD and chest x-ray

10. The most common organisms causing endophthalmitis following trauma are
    a. *Enterococcus* species and *S. aureus*
    b. *Bacillus* species and *S. epidermidis*
    c. *Pseudomonas* species and *S. aureus*
    d. *S. aureus* and *S. epidermidis*

11. All of the following are features common to both sympathetic ophthalmia and Vogt-Koyanagi-Harada syndrome except
    a. serous retinal detachments
    b. Dalen-Fuchs nodules
    c. pathology localized to choroid
    d. vitritis

12. Which disorder is more common in males?
    a. MEWDS
    b. uveal effusion syndrome
    c. APMPPE
    d. Birdshot choroidopathy

13. EVS findings include all of the following except
    a. vitrectomy was beneficial only in patients with LP vision
    b. intravitreal corticosteroids were helpful
    c. IV antibiotics were not helpful
    d. the most common organism was *S. epidermidis*

14. Which of the following is not characteristic of MEWDS?
    a. enlargement of the blind spot
    b. bilaterality
    c. flulike illness
    d. female preponderance

15. The most common cause of posterior uveitis is
    a. sarcoidosis
    b. syphilis
    c. CMV
    d. toxoplasmosis

16. All of the following are causes of HLA-B27–associated uveitis except
    a. ankylosing spondylitis
    b. ulcerative colitis
    c. Crohn's disease
    d. psoriasis

17. Which of the following is not part of the classic triad of findings in Reiter's syndrome?
    a. iritis
    b. arthritis
    c. keratitis
    d. urethritis

18. Which of the following laboratory tests is most commonly found in JRA-related iritis?
    a. RF–, ANA–
    b. RF+, ANA–
    c. RF–, ANA+
    d. RF+, ANA+

19. Phacoantigenic endophthalmitis is characterized by which pattern of granulomatous inflammation?
    a. zonal
    b. diffuse
    c. discrete
    d. necrotizing

20. Which combination of findings is least likely to occur in rubella?
    a. retinopathy and cataract
    b. glaucoma and cataract
    c. glaucoma and retinopathy
    d. cataract and deafness

21. A 35-year-old man with decreased vision OD is found to have optic nerve edema and a macular star. The causative organism is most likely
    a. *Onchocerca volvulus*
    b. *Bartonella henselae*
    c. *Treponema pallidum*
    d. *Borrelia burgdorferi*

22. Which is least helpful for the diagnosis of toxocariasis?
    a. ELISA test
    b. AC tap
    c. vitrectomy
    d. stool examination

23. A person living in which area of the US would be most likely to develop POHS?
    a. southwest
    b. northwest
    c. midwest
    d. southeast

24. All of the following are true of birdshot choroidopathy except
    a. more common in males
    b. usually bilateral
    c. CME is common
    d. associated with HLA-A29

25. Which of the following is least commonly associated with *Treponema pallidum* infection?
    a. interstitial keratitis
    b. chorioretinitis
    c. ectopia lentis
    d. glaucoma

SUGGESTED READINGS

American Academy of Ophthalmology: Intraocular Inflammation and Uveitis, vol 9. San Francisco, AAO, 2004.

Foster CS, Vitale AT: Diagnosis and Treatment of Uveitis. Philadelphia, WB Saunders, 2002.

Jones NP: Uveitis: An Illustrated Manual. Philadelphia, Butterworth-Heinemann, 1998.

Michelson JB: Color Atlas of Uveitis, 2nd edition. St. Louis, Mosby, 1992.

Nussenblatt RB, Whitcup SM, Palestine AG: Uveitis: Fundamentals and Clinical Practice, 2nd edition. Philadelphia, Mosby, 2003.

Tabbara KF, Nussenblatt RB: Posterior Uveitis Diagnosis and Management. Philadelphia, Butterworth-Heinemann, 1994.

CHAPTER 9

Glaucoma

ANATOMY/PHYSIOLOGY

Ciliary Body (CB)

6-mm-wide structure located between the scleral spur anteriorly and the ora serrata posteriorly; composed of the pars plicata (anterior 2 mm with ciliary processes) and the pars plana (posterior 4 mm, flat)

Pars plicata consists of
Ciliary muscle: longitudinal fibers (insert into scleral spur and affect outflow facility), circular fibers (anterior inner fibers oriented parallel to limbus and affect accommodation), and radial fibers (connect longitudinal and circular fibers)
Ciliary vessels: major arterial circle of the iris (in CB near iris root) formed by anastomosis of branches of anterior and long posterior ciliary arteries
Ciliary processes: 70 finger-like projections composed of pigmented and nonpigmented epithelial cell bilayer, capillaries, and stroma

Functions:
Suspends and alters shape of lens: zonular fibers that originate between the ciliary processes of the pars plicata, attach to the crystalline lens, and suspend it. Helmholtz's theory of accommodation explains the changes in lens shape and thus refractive power with contraction and relaxation of the ciliary muscle. Contraction of the longitudinal fibers pulls the lens forward, shallowing the anterior chamber. Contraction of the circular fibers relaxes the zonules making the lens more spherical with greater focusing power. Relaxation of circular fibers (or cycloplegia) tightens the zonules, stretching the lens and making it thinner with less focusing power.
Produces aqueous humor: production of aqueous is primarily by active secretion (also diffusion and ultrafiltration); both an Na^+/K^+ pump and carbonic anhydrase are involved. β-blockers act through adenylcyclase to inhibit the NA^+/K^+ pump; glucose enters by passive diffusion.
Rate = 2–3 µL/min, AC volume = 250 µL, posterior chamber volume = 60 µL (AC volume turnover is approximately 1%/min). Rate measured by fluorophotometry (direct optical measurement of decreasing fluorescein concentration) or tonography (indirect calculation from outflow measurement). Diurnal production of aqueous (may be related to cortisol levels) decreases with sleep (45%), age (2%/decade; counterbalanced by the decreased outflow with age), inflammation, surgery, trauma, and drugs
AQUEOUS COMPOSITION: slightly hypertonic and acidic (pH 7.2) compared with plasma; 15× more ascorbate than plasma; low protein (0.02% vs 7% in plasma); lower calcium and phosphorus (50% of the level in plasma); chloride and bicarbonate vary (from 25% above or below plasma levels); sodium, potassium, magnesium, iron, zinc, and copper levels similar to those in plasma
FUNCTIONS OF AQUEOUS: maintains intraocular pressure, provides metabolic substrates (glucose, oxygen, electrolytes) to the cornea and lens, and removes metabolic waste (lactate, pyruvate, carbon dioxide)
Affects aqueous outflow: contraction of ciliary muscle causes traction on the trabecular meshwork, increasing outflow

Synthesizes acid mucopolysaccharide component of vitreous: occurs in nonpigmented epithelial cells of pars plana and enters vitreous body at its base

Maintains blood-aqueous barrier: within the ciliary processes, plasma enters from thin fenestrated endothelium of capillary core → passes through stroma → 2 layers of epithelium with apposing apical surfaces (which forms the ciliary epithelial bilayer):

OUTER PIGMENTED LAYER: continuous with the RPE (basal lamina continuous with Bruch's membrane) contains zonula occludens

INNER NONPIGMENTED LAYER: equivalent to the sensory retina (basal lamina continuous with ILM), site of active secretion.

Both layers have basal basement membranes with their apices facing each other. During passage from the bloodstream to the posterior chamber, a molecule must pass through capillary basement membrane, pigmented epithelium basement membrane, pigmented epithelium, nonpigmented epithelium, nonpigmented epithelium basement membrane

Cryodestruction and inflammation cause loss of barrier function (tight junctions open), resulting in flare (proteins in aqueous); atropine reduces flare by closing tight junctions

Outflow Pathways

Trabecular meshwork (traditional pathway): represents major aqueous drainage system; uveoscleral meshwork → corneoscleral meshwork → juxtacanalicular connective tissue → Schlemm's canal → collector channels → aqueous veins → episcleral and conjunctival veins → anterior ciliary and superior ophthalmic veins → cavernous sinus

The pore size of the meshwork decreases towards Schlemm's canal:

Uveal meshwork: collagenous core surrounded by endothelial cells; pore size up to 70 μm; linked to ciliary muscle

Corneoscleral meshwork: sheet-like beams insert into scleral spur; pore size up to 30 μm.

Juxtacanalicular tissue: links corneoscleral trabeculae with Schlemm's endothelium; pore size = 4–7 μm; site of greatest aqueous outflow resistance

Canal of Schlemm is lined by a single layer of endothelial cells (mesothelial cells) and connects to the venous system by 30 collector channels

Uveoscleral outflow (15%–20% of total outflow): aqueous passes through face of ciliary body in the angle, enters the ciliary muscle and suprachoroidal space, and is drained by veins in the ciliary body, choroid, and sclera

Cyclodialysis cleft increases aqueous outflow through the uveoscleral pathway (without reducing aqueous production); cycloplegics and prostaglandin analogues increase uveoscleral outflow; miotics decrease uveoscleral outflow and increase trabecular meshwork outflow

Angle Structures

Visible only by gonioscopy because of total internal reflection at the air/cornea interface (Figure 9-1)

Schwalbe's line: peripheral/posterior termination of Descemet's membrane, which corresponds to apex of corneal light wedge (optical cross section of the cornea with narrow slit beam reveals 2 linear reflections, 1 from external and 1 from internal corneal surfaces, which meet at Schwalbe's line)

Trabecular meshwork (TM): anterior nonpigmented portion appears as a clear white band; posterior pigmented portion has variable pigmentation (usually darkest inferiorly). Increased pigmentation of trabecular meshwork occurs with pseudoexfoliation syndrome (Sampaolesi's line), pigment dispersion syndrome, uveitis, melanoma, trauma, surgery, hyphema, darkly pigmented individuals, and increasing age

Schlemm's canal: usually not visible or only faintly visible as a light gray band at the level of posterior TM; elevated venous pressure or pressure from the edge of the gonioscopy lens may cause blood to reflux, making Schlemm's canal visible as a faint red band

DDx of blood in Schlemm's canal: elevated episcleral venous pressure, oculodermal melanocytosis (nevus of Ota), neurofibromatosis, congenital ectropion uveae, hypotony, secondary to gonioscopy

Scleral spur (SS): narrow white band that corresponds to the site of insertion of longitudinal fibers of ciliary muscle to sclera

Ciliary body (CB): pigmented band that represents the anterior face of the ciliary body; iris processes may be seen as lacy projections crossing this band but not the scleral spur (occur in 33% of population)

Angle Abnormalities

Peripheral anterior synechia (PAS): any pigmented structure that crosses scleral spur

Etiology: angle-closure, uveitis, neovascularization, flat anterior chamber, ICE syndrome, ciliary body tumors, mesodermal dysgenesis

Normal vessels: radial iris vessels, portions of arterial circle of CB, and rarely, vertical vessels deep in CB; do not branch or cross the scleral spur; present in 7% of patients with blue irides and 10% with brown

Abnormal vessels: fine, often branch, no orientation, cross-scleral spur

Schwalbe's line
Trabecular meshwork
Schlemm's canal
Scleral spur
Ciliary body

Grade 4 pigment   Grade 2 pigment   No pigment

Schwalbe's line
Trabecular meshwork (anterior nonpigmented and posterior pigmented)
Scleral spur
Ciliary body

Longitudinal muscle   Circular muscle   Ciliary processes

Figure 9-1. Composite drawing of the microscopic and gonioscopic anatomy. (From Becker B, Shaffer RN: Diagnosis and Therapy of the Glaucomas. St. Louis, CV Mosby Co, 1965.)

DDx: neovascularization (rubeosis iridis), iris neoplasm, Fuchs' heterochromic iridocyclitis (sparse, faint, and delicate; bleed easily on decompression of AC)

Angle recession: tear between longitudinal and circular fibers of the ciliary muscle. Because longitudinal fibers are still attached to the scleral spur, miotics still work, but because they decrease uveoscleral outflow, IOP may actually increase. Breaks in posterior TM result in scarring and a nonfunctional TM; aqueous drains primarily through uveoscleral outflow; 60% to 90% of patients with traumatic hyphemas have angle recession; 5% of eyes with angle recession will develop glaucoma

> ***Gonioscopic findings***: widened ciliary body band, increased visibility of scleral spur, torn iris processes, sclera visible through disrupted ciliary body tissue, marked variation in CB width in different quadrants of same eye

Cyclodialysis cleft: separation of ciliary body from scleral spur; often from trauma. Results in direct communication between AC and suprachoroidal space causing hypotony; spontaneous closure may occur (unlikely after 6 weeks) with marked IOP rise; shortly thereafter, the TM should begin to function normally again

> ***Gonioscopic findings***: cleft at junction of scleral spur and CB band
> ***Treatment***: cycloplegic to relax ciliary body in an attempt to close cleft (avoid pilocarpine, which

may open the cleft through ciliary muscle traction); laser (argon induces inflammation to close the cleft; spot size = 50–100 μm, duration = 0.1–0.2 second; power = 0.5–1.0 watts to uvea and 1–3 watts to sclera); cryotherapy; suture CB to sclera (direct cyclopexy); intravitreal air bubble for a superior cleft; YAG laser can be used to open a closed cleft

Iridodialysis: tear/disinsertion of iris root. If large or symptomatic, consider surgical repair with mattress sutures.

Optic Nerve (Figure 9-2)

Approximately 1.2 million axons; cell bodies of ganglion cells are located in the ganglion cell layer

4 layers of optic nerve head based on blood supply:
> ***Nerve fiber***: supplied by branches of central retinal artery
> ***Prelaminar***: supplied by capillaries of the short posterior ciliary arteries
> ***Laminar*** (lamina cribrosa): supplied by dense plexus from short posterior ciliary arteries
> ***Retrolaminar***: supplied by both ciliary (via recurrent pial vessels) and retinal (via centripetal branches from pial region) circulations

Optic nerve blood flow is influenced by mean blood pressure, IOP, blood viscosity, blood vessel caliber, and blood vessel length

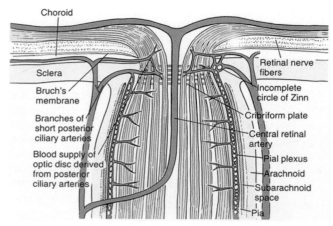

Figure 9-2. Vascular supply and anatomy of the anterior optic nerve. (From Hart WM Jr: In Podos SM, Yanoff M [eds]: *Textbook of Ophthalmology*, vol 6, London, Mosby, 1994.)

TESTING

Intraocular Pressure

Goldmann equation: IOP = F/C + EVP relates 3 factors important in determination of IOP

  F = rate of aqueous formation = 2–3 µL/min

  C = facility of outflow = 0.28 µL/min/mm Hg; <0.20 is abnormal; decreases with age, increases with medication; measured by tonography

  EVP = episcleral venous pressure = 8–12 mm Hg; increases with venous obstruction or A-V shunt; measured by manometry

IOP = 8–21 mm Hg is considered normal; average = 16 +/–2.5 mm Hg; distribution is not Gaussian and is skewed to higher IOPs

IOP is influenced by age (may increase with age), genetics, race (higher in African Americans), season (higher in winter, lower in summer), blood pressure, obesity, exercise (lower after exercise), Valsalva, time of day (diurnal variation [2–6 mm/day]; peak in morning), posture (higher when lying down vs sitting), various hormones, and drugs. Also ocular factors: refractive error (higher in myopes) and eyelid closure

Tonometry

IOP measurement can be performed with a variety of devices (tonometers)

Indentation:

  Schiøtz tonometer: known weight indents cornea and displaces a volume of fluid within the eye; amount of indentation estimates pressure; falsely low readings occur with a very elastic eye (low scleral rigidity as with high myopia, buphthalmos, retinal detachment, treatment with cholinesterase inhibitors, thyroid disease, and previous ocular surgery) or a compressible

intraocular gas (e.g., SF_6 and C_3F_8); falsely high readings occur with scleral rigidity and hyperopia

Applanation: based on the Imbert-Fick principle: P = F/A (for an ideal thin-walled sphere, pressure inside sphere equals force necessary to flatten its surface divided by the area of flattening). The eye is not an ideal sphere: the cornea resists flattening, and capillary action of the tear meniscus pulls the tonometer to the eye. However, these 2 forces cancel each other when the applanated diameter is 3.06 mm

  Goldmann tonometer: biprism attached to a spring; fluorescein semicircles align when area applanated has a diameter = 3.06 mm; unaffected by ocular rigidity; error can occur with squeezing, Valsalva, irregular or edematous cornea, corneal thickness (thick corneas overestimate IOP [~5 mm Hg per 70 µm], and thin corneas underestimate IOP [~5 mm Hg per 70 µm]), amount of fluorescein, external pressure on or restriction of globe, and astigmatism >1.5 D (must align red mark on tip with axis of MINUS cylinder)

  Perkins tonometer: portable form of Goldmann device

  Mackay-Marg tonometer: applanates small area; good for corneal scars and edema. Examples of this style tonometer include the tonopen and the pneumotonometer

    TONOPEN: probe indents cornea, and microprocessor calculates IOP and reliability

    PNEUMOTONOMETER: central sensing device is controlled by air pressure

Noncontact:

  Air puff tonometer: noncontact device; time required for air jet to flatten cornea is proportional to IOP; varies with cardiac cycle

Gonioscopy

Classification systems:

  Scheie:

    Grade I = wide open (CB visible)

    Grade II = SS visible; CB not visible

    Grade III = only anterior TM visible

    Grade IV = closed angle (TM not visible)

  Schaffer: opposite of Scheie (Grade 0 is closed; Grade IV is wide open) (Figure 9-3)

    Grade I = 10% open

    Grade II = 20% open

    Grade III = 30% open

    Grade IV = 40% open

  Spaeth: most descriptive; 4 elements

    FIRST ELEMENT: level of iris insertion (capital letter A–E)

    A = Anterior to TM

    B = Behind Schwalbe's line or at TM

    C = At scleral spur

    D = Deep angle, CB visible

    E = Extremely deep, large CB band

  Perform indention gonioscopy: if true insertion is more posterior, place original impression

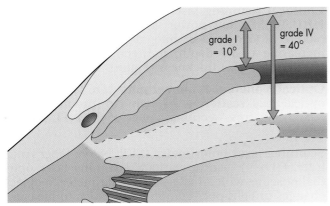

Figure 9-3. Shaffer's angle-grading system. (From Fran M, Smith J, Doyle W: Clinical examination of glaucoma. In Yanoff M, Duker JS [eds]: *Ophthalmology*, 2nd ed, St. Louis, Mosby, 2004.)

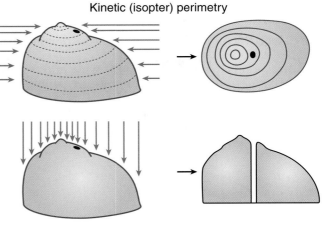

Figure 9-4. Kinetic and static perimetry. (From Bajandas FJ, Kline LB: *Neuro-Ophthalmology Review Manual*, 3rd ed, Thorofare, NJ, Slack, 2004.)

in parentheses followed by true insertion location

SECOND ELEMENT: number that denotes the iridocorneal angle width in degrees from 5–45

THIRD ELEMENT: peripheral iris configuration (lower case letter r, s, or q)

r = regular (flat)

s = steep (convex)

q = queer (concave)

FOURTH ELEMENT: pigmentation of posterior TM (graded from 0 [none] to 4 [maximal])

EXAMPLE: (A)B15 r, 1+ (appositionally closed 15° angle that opens to TM with indentation, regular iris configuration, and mildly pigmented posterior TM)

Types of lenses:

Koeppe lens: direct view

Goldmann 3-mirror lens: requires coupling solution (Goniosol)

Zeiss, Posner, and Sussman 4-mirror lenses: can perform indentation gonioscopy to determine whether angle closure is appositional or synechial

Visual Fields

Perimetry measures the "island of vision" or topographic representation of differential light sensitivity. Peak = fovea; depression = blind spot; extent = 60° nasally, 60° superiorly, 70–75° inferiorly, and 100–110° temporally

Central field tests points only within a 30° radius of fixation

2 types: (Figure 9-4)

Kinetic: uses a moving stimulus of constant intensity to produce an isopter or points of equal sensitivity (horizontal cross section of the hill of vision)

Static: uses a fixed stimulus with constant or variable intensity to produce a profile (vertical cross section of the hill of vision)

Goldmann (kinetic and static):

Test distance: 0.33 m

Test object size: I–V (each increment doubles the diameter [quadruples the area] of test object; III4e test object will have 2× the diameter and 4× the area of II4e)

Light filters: 1–4 (increments of 5 db), a–e (increments of 1 db)

Humphrey (static):

Test distance = 0.33 m; background illumination = 31.5 apostilbs (asb); stimulus size = III; stimulus duration = 0.2 s; various programs (i.e., central 30°, 24°, 10°, neuro fields, ptosis fields, etc.)

Reliability indices:

FIXATION LOSS: patient responds when a target is displayed in blind spot

FALSE-POSITIVE: patient responds when there is no stimulus (nervous or trigger-happy; causes white areas)

FALSE-NEGATIVE: patient fails to respond to a superthreshold stimulus at a location that would be expected to be seen (indicates loss of attention or fatigue; causes cloverleaf pattern)

Global indices:

MEAN DEVIATION (MD): average departure of each test point from the age-adjusted normal value

PATTERN STANDARD DEVIATION (PSD): standard deviation of the differences between the threshold and expected values for each test point

SHORT-TERM FLUCTUATION (SF): variability in responses when the same point is retested; measure of consistency

CORRECTED PATTERN STANDARD DEVIATION (CPSD): adjustment of the PSD by subtracting out the component due to the SF

Tangent screen (usually kinetic): test distance is 1 m, test object may vary in size and color; tests only central field. Magnifies scotoma and is of low cost; however, poor reproducibility and lack of standardization

VF defect: a scotoma is an area of partial or complete blindness

Corresponds to a defect that is 3° wide and 6 decibels (dB) deep; also 1 point on Humphrey testing that is depressed >10 dB or at least 2 points that are depressed at least 5 dB

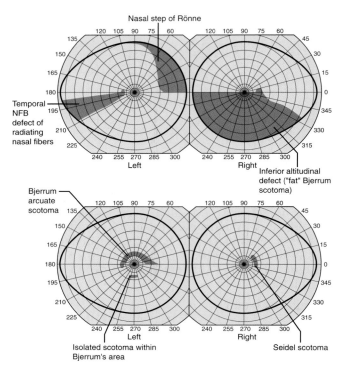

Figure 9-5. Composite diagram depicting different types of field defects. (From Bajandas FJ, Kline LB: *Neuro-Ophthalmology Review Manual*, 3rd ed, Thorofare, NJ, Slack, 2004.)

Typical localized glaucomatous scotomas:
PARACENTRAL: within central 10°
ARCUATE (Bjerrum): isolated, nasal step of Rönne and Seidel (connected to blind spot)
TEMPORAL WEDGE
Glaucomatous scotomas do not respect the vertical meridian (vs neurologic VF defects, which do)
VF should correlate with optic nerve appearance; otherwise, consider refractive error, level of vision, media opacities, pupil size, and other causes of VF defects (tilted ON head, ON head drusen, retinal lesions, etc.)

Optic Nerve Head (ONH) Analyzers
(Figure 9-6)

Various digital and video cameras that capture ONH image; computer then calculates cup area in an attempt to objectively quantify ONH appearance

Confocal scanning laser ophthalmoscopy (CSLO; HRT; TopSS): low-power laser produces digital 3D picture of ON head by integrating coronal scans of increasing tissue depth; indirectly measures nerve fiber layer (NFL) thickness (Figures 9-7 and 9-8)

Optical coherence tomography (OCT): measures optical backscattering of light to produce high-resolution, cross-sectional image of the NFL (Figure 9-9)

Scanning laser polarimetry (SLP; Nerve Fiber Analyzer, GDx™): uses a confocal scanning laser ophthalmoscope with an integrated polarimeter to detect changes in light polarization from axons to measure the NFL thickness; quantitative analysis of NFL thickness to detect early glaucomatous damage (Figure 9-10)

Optic nerve blood flow measurement: color Doppler imaging and laser Doppler flowmetry (Figure 9-11)

PATHOLOGY

Glaucoma

Dropout of ganglion cells, replacement of NFL with dense gliotic tissue and some glial cell nuclei; partial preservation of inner nuclear layer with loss of Müller's and amacrine cells (normal 8–9 cells high; in glaucoma, 4–5 cells high); earliest histologic changes occur at level of lamina cribrosa; advanced cases may show backward bowing of lamina or "beanpot" appearance (Figures 9-12 and 9-13)

Schnabel's Cavernous Optic Atrophy

Histologic finding in eyes with increased IOP or atherosclerosis and normal IOP; hyaluronic acid infiltration of nerve from vitreous due to imbalance between perfusion pressure in the posterior ciliary arteries and IOP; also occurs in eyes with ischemic optic neuropathy

Pathology: atrophy of neural elements with cystic spaces containing hyaluronic acid (mucopolysaccharides derived from vitreous), which stains with colloidal iron (Figure 9-14)

Gliosis of the Optic Nerve

With optic atrophy, glial cells replace nerve cells and assume a random distribution throughout the optic nerve

DISORDERS

Childhood Glaucoma

(see Chapter 5, Pediatrics/Strabismus)

Technique	Equipment needed	Governing principles	Advantages	Disadvantages
Ophthalmoscopy	Direct ophthalmoscope or slit lamp and 78D or 90D lens Red-free light	Nerve fiber layer visibility is enhanced with short-wavelength light	Easy to perform using readily available equipment	May be difficult without clear media Nerve fiber layer not easily seen in lightly pigmented fundi
Red-free, high-contrast fundus photography	Fundus camera with red-free filter High contrast black-and-white film and paper	Nerve fiber layer visibility is enhanced with short-wavelength light	Nerve fiber layer defects may be easy to detect	Requires skilled photographer and dilated pupil Requires dilated pupil Limitations of ophthalmoscopy apply
Retinal contour analysis	Scanning laser ophthalmoscope that can perform tomographic topography	Three-dimensional construction of retinal surface can measure retinal height above a reference plane – height is related to nerve fiber layer thickness	Easy to perform through undilated pupil No discomfort to patient Can image through most media opacities unless very dense	Equipment is expensive Height measurements depend upon location of reference plane Retinal thickness may not be true indirect measure of nerve fiber layer thickness
Optical coherence tomography	Optical coherence tomography unit	Uses reflected and backscattered light to create images of various retinal layers (analogous to the use of sound waves in ultrasonography)	Can differentiate layers within the retina, including the nerve fiber layer, with a $10\mu m$ resolution Correlates with known histology	Equipment is expensive Requires dilated pupil Resolution may not be high enough to detect small changes
Scanning laser polarimetry	Scanning laser polarimeter	Birefringent properties of the nerve fiber layer cause a measurable phase shift of an incident polarized light proportional to the tissue thickness	Easy to perform through undilated pupil No discomfort to patient Can image through most media opacities, unless very dense Resolution limited to size of a pixel (possibly as small as $1\mu m$) Reproducibility $5–8\mu m$	Equipment is expensive Measurements not correlated histologically in humans Requires compensation for other polarizing media, e.g. cornea

Figure 9-6. Summary of techniques for retinal nerve fiber layer analysis. (From Chopin NT: Retinal nerve fiber layer analysis. In Yanoff M, Duker JS [eds]: *Ophthalmology*, London, Mosby, 1999.)

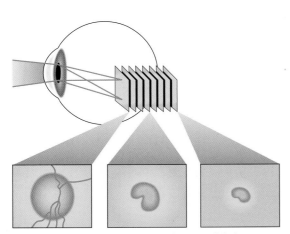

Figure 9-7. Confocal scanning laser ophthalmoscopy. (Adapted from Schuman JS, Noeker RJ: Imaging of the optic nerve head and nerve fiber layer in glaucoma. *Ophthalmol Clin North Am* 8:259–279, 1995.)

Figure 9-8. Confocal scanning laser ophthalmoscopy printed report. (From Zangwill L, de Souza K, Weinrob RN: Confocal scanning laser ophthalmoscopy to detect glaucomatous optic neuropathy. In Shuman JS [ed]: *Imaging in Glaucoma*, Thorofare, NJ, Slack, 1997.)

A

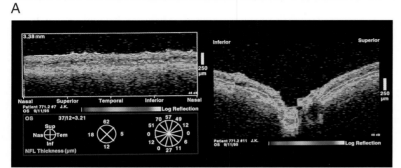

B

Figure 9-9. Optical coherence tomography. (From Pedut-Kloizman TP, Schuman JS: Disc analysis. In Yanoff M, Duker JS [eds]: *Ophthalmology*, London, Mosby, 1999.)

Figure 9-10. Printout from the GDx software of the Nerve Fiber Analyzer; normal eye. (From Chopin NT: Retinal nerve fiber layer analysis. In Yanoff M, Duker JS [eds]: *Ophthalmology*, London, Mosby, 1999.)

NERVE FIBER ANALYSIS

	Actual value	Status	Probability
Symmetry	0.97	Within normal	
Superior ratio	2.30	Within normal	
Inferior ratio	2.36	Within normal	
Superior/nasal	2.12	Within normal	
Maximum modulation	1.36	Within normal	
Ellipse modulation	2.13	Within normal	
The number	10		
Average thickness	64	Within normal	
Ellipse average	69	Within normal	
Superior average	78	Within normal	
Inferior average	80	Within normal	
Superior integral	0.227	Within normal	

Figure 9-11. Color Doppler imaging of the ophthalmic artery. (From O'Brien C, Harris A: Optic nerve blood flow measurement. In Yanoff M, Duker JS [eds]: *Ophthalmology*, London, Mosby, 1999.)

Figure 9-12. POAG demonstrating cupping of the optic nerve head. (From Yanoff M, Fine BS: *Ocular Pathology*, 5th ed, St. Louis, Mosby, 2002.)

A   **B**

Figure 9-13. POAG demonstrating atrophy of the inner retinal layers. **A**, low power, **B**, higher magnification. (From Yanoff M, Fine BS: *Ocular Pathology*, 5th ed, St. Louis, Mosby, 2002.)

Figure 9-14. Schnabel's cavernous optic atrophy demonstrating cystic spaces in optic nerve parenchyma. **A**, H&E stain, **B**, colloidal iron stain. (From Yanoff M, Fine BS: *Ocular Pathology*, 5th ed, St. Louis, Mosby, 2002.)

Primary Open-Angle Glaucoma (POAG)

Progressive, bilateral, optic neuropathy with open angles, typical pattern of nerve fiber bundle visual field loss, and increased intraocular pressure (IOP >21 mm Hg) not caused by another systemic or local disease

Epidemiology: second leading cause of blindness in US; most common form of glaucoma (60%–70%); 7% of population has ocular hypertension; 3% of population in Baltimore Eye Study had glaucomatous VF defects. If damage in one eye, untreated fellow eye has 29% risk over 5 years. Steroid responders have 31% risk of developing glaucoma within 5 years

Genetics: juvenile-onset POAG has been mapped to chromosome 1q21-q31 (GLC1A, MYOC/TIGR). Adult POAG has been mapped to chromosomes 2qcen-q13 (GLC1B), 3q21-q24 (GLC1C), 8q23 (GLC1D), 10p14 (GLC1E, OPTN [optineurin]). A mutation in the OPTN gene accounts for ~17% of POAG

Risk factors: increased IOP, increased cup-to-disc ratio, thinner central corneal thickness (less than ~550 μm), positive family history (6× increase in first-degree relatives), age (increased in patients >60 years old; 15% of those >80 years old have glaucoma), race (6× increase in African Americans vs Caucasians); other possible risk factors include DM, myopia, hypertension, migraines

Pathogenesis: unknown
Theories of optic nerve damage:
  Mechanical: resistance to outflow, trabecular meshwork dysfunction
  Vascular: poor optic nerve perfusion; ischemia occurs with systemic hypotension; also, increased IOP reduces blood flow to optic nerve. Possible contribution of vasospasm
  Ganglion cell necrosis or apoptosis: excitotoxicity (glutamate), neurotrophin starvation, autoimmunity, abnormal glial-neuronal interactions (TNF), defects in endogenous protective mechanisms (heat shock proteins)

Findings: increased IOP, large cup-to-disc ratio (especially vertical elongation of optic cup; notching of rim; asymmetry of C/D ratio), nerve fiber layer loss (evaluate with red-free light), disc splinter hemorrhage (often followed by notching in region of hemorrhage), characteristic visual field defects. Peripapillary atrophy is not a sign of glaucoma damage.
  With optic nerve damage, loss of yellow-blue color axis occurs first
  Combined sensitivity of tonometry and disc exam = 67%

Visual fields: sensitivity (% of diseased properly identified) = 85%; specificity (% of normals properly identified) = 85%. Risk of initial field loss is 1% to 2%/year for ocular hypertensive patients, risk of field loss increases with increasing IOP

Secondary Open-Angle Glaucoma

Mechanism/Etiology
  Clogging of TM: RBCs (hyphema, sickle cell, ghost cells), macrophages (hemolytic, phacolytic, melanocytic, melanomalytic), neoplastic cells (malignant tumors, neurofibromatosis, juvenile xanthogranuloma), pigment (pigmentary glaucoma, pseudoexfoliation, chronic uveitis, malignant melanoma), lens protein (lens-particle glaucoma), photoreceptor segments (Schwartz's syndrome), zonular fragments (alpha-chymotrypsin induced), viscoelastic
  Toxic/medication: steroid-induced, siderosis, chalcosis
  Inflammation: Posner-Schlossman syndrome, Fuchs' heterochromic iridocyclitis, uveitis, IK, UGH syndrome
  Increased episcleral venous pressure
  Trauma: angle recession, chemical injury, hemorrhage, postoperative

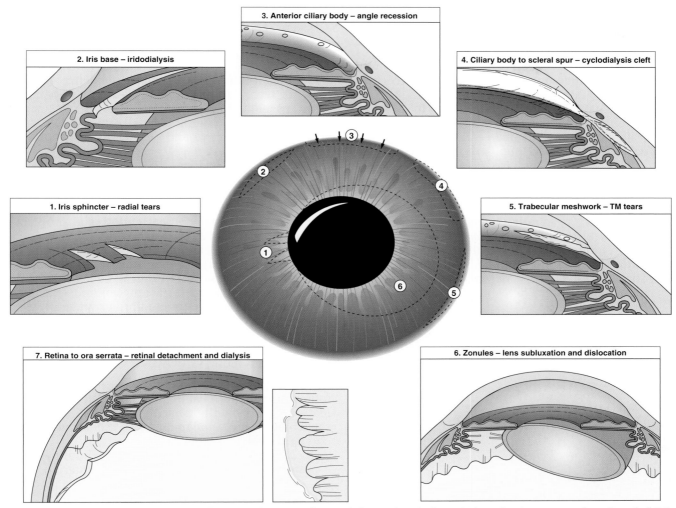

Figure 9-15. Seven areas of traumatic ocular tears (shown in yellow) with the resultant findings. (Adapted with permission from Campbell DG: Traumatic glaucoma. In Shingleton BJ, Hersh PS, Kenyon KR [eds]: *Eye Trauma*, St. Louis, Mosby, 1991.)

Hyphema: 27% risk of glaucoma if hyphema >50% of AC volume; 52% risk with total hyphema

Surgical intervention for uncontrolled IOP, corneal blood staining, prolonged presence of clot (>15 days), rebleed, 8-ball hyphema (see Chapter 10, Anterior Segment)

Sickle cell: sickled cells are rigid; therefore, even small hyphemas can obstruct TM and raise IOP; acetazolamide (Diamox) contraindicated (increases ascorbic acid in AC causing greater sickling, also causes hemoconcentration and systemic acidosis, both of which favor sickling)

Ghost cells: weeks to months after vitreous hemorrhage, degenerated RBCs pass through hyaloid face. These khaki-colored, spherical cells are less pliable than RBCs and do not pass through trabecular meshwork; layer of cells forms a pseudohypopyon

Lytic glaucomas: macrophages laden with various material

Hemolytic: hemosiderin-laden macrophages deposit in TM

Phacolytic: denatured lens proteins escape from hypermature or morgagnian cataract; proteins and macrophages that have ingested lens material clog the outflow tract; appears as milky substance in AC; requires surgical removal of lens. Reduce the inflammation preoperatively with topical steroid, cycloplegic, and ocular hypotensive medications

Melanomalytic: melanin from malignant melanoma is engulfed by macrophages, which clog TM

Melanocytomalytic: melanin from necrotic melanocytoma

Tumor cells: deposition of tumor cells, inflammatory cells, and cellular debris; also macrophages laden with melanin from melanomas, direct infiltration of trabecular meshwork, or neovascularization with subsequent intraocular hemorrhage or NVG. 45% of anterior uveal melanomas and 15% of choroidal melanomas are associated with glaucoma. Retinoblastoma causes glaucoma in 25% to 50% from NVG, pupillary block, or tumor material. Also lymphoma

Pigmentary glaucoma (PG) (AD): Mapped to chromosome 7q35-q36 (GLC1F) (Figure 9-16)

Typically young myopic males; up to 50% of patients with pigment dispersion syndrome (PDS) develop glaucoma

Mechanism: reverse pupillary block bows iris against zonules, and iris movement results in pigment liberation. Pigment obstructs TM

Findings: halos and blurry vision with IOP spikes (pigment may be released with exercise); Krukenberg's spindle (melanin phagocytized by corneal endothelium); heavy TM pigmentation; iridodonesis; iris transillumination defects (radial midperipheral spoke-like appearance)

Associated with lattice degeneration (20%) and retinal detachment (5%)

Figure 9-16. Gonioscopic view of pigmentary glaucoma. (From Ball SF: Pigmentary glaucoma. In Yanoff M, Duker JS: *Ophthalmology*, London, Mosby, 1999.)

Treatment: miotics minimize iris-zonule touch; very good response to laser trabeculoplasty Laser peripheral iridotomy helps reduce posterior bowing of iris

Pseudoexfoliation (PXG): high incidence (up to 50%) of secondary open-angle glaucoma in patients with pseudoexfoliation syndrome (PXS); more common among Scandinavians. Amyloid-like substance deposits in eye and clogs TM, also found in other organs (Figure 9-17)

Findings: iridopathy (blood-aqueous barrier defect, pseudouveitis, iris rigidity, posterior synechiae, poor pupillary dilation), keratopathy (reduced endothelial cell count, endothelial decompensation, corneal endothelial proliferation over trabecular meshwork), Sampaolesi's line (scalloped band of pigmentation anterior to Schwalbe's line), weak zonules (phacodonesis, risk of lens dislocation during cataract surgery, and angle closure from anterior movement of lens), lens capsule (white fibrillar material)

Treatment: very good response to laser trabeculoplasty. PXS usually presents with higher initial IOP and is more difficult to control with medical treatment alone vs POAG

Lens-particle glaucoma: lens material blocks TM following trauma or cataract surgery. Greater inflammation than with phacolytic; PAS, posterior synechiae, and inflammatory membranes are common. IOP can be very high

Treatment: cycloplegics, steroids (careful because steroids slow absorption of lens material), and ocular hypotensive medications

Schwartz's syndrome: high IOP associated with rhegmatogenous RD. Photoreceptor outer segments migrate transvitreally into aqueous and block trabecular meshwork. Outflow obstruction is also due to pigment released from RPE and glycosaminogly-

A

B

Figure 9-17. Pseudoexfoliative syndrome demonstrating exfoliative material on lens capsule. (From Samuelson TW, Shah G: Pseudoexfoliative glaucoma. In Yanoff M, Duker JS: *Ophthalmology*, London, Mosby, 1999.)

cans released from photoreceptors. Usually resolves after repair of RD

Alpha-chymotrypsin induced: zonular fragments accumulate in trabecular meshwork after intracapsular cataract extraction (ICCE) with enzymatic zonulysis. Alpha-chymotrypsin itself does not cause damage

Corticosteroid-induced: risk factors include open-angle glaucoma, family history of glaucoma, diabetes, and high myopia. Topical steroids have greater pressure-raising effects than do systemic steroids:
   In response to topical dexamethasone 0.1% qid for 6 weeks, 65% had IOP rise of <5 mm Hg, 30% had a rise of 5–14 mm Hg, and 5% had a rise of at least 15 mm Hg
   Fluorometholone, rimexolone (Vexol), and loteprednol etabonate (Lotemax) are less likely to increase IOP

Siderosis (iron) or chalcosis (copper): TM toxicity and scarring from intraocular foreign body

Glaucomatocyclitic crisis (Posner-Schlossman syndrome): episodic trabeculitis (mononuclear cells in TM) with high IOP for hours to weeks; minimal inflammatory signs

Fuchs' heterochromic iridocyclitis: 15% to 60% develop high IOP (glaucoma occurs more commonly in patients with bilateral disease and spontaneous hyphema); may persist after resolution of uveitis

Uveitic glaucoma: normally, a decrease in aqueous production by the ciliary body occurs due to inflammation (trabeculitis); however, aqueous outflow is acutely impaired by the disruption of the blood-aqueous barrier and inflammatory cells. Chronic inflammation may cause TM scarring. Glaucoma occurs in about 20% of JRA-associated uveitis cases

Uveitis-glaucoma-hyphema syndrome: nongranulomatous inflammation. IOL physically irritates iris and ciliary body

Chemical burn: can damage trabecular meshwork or uveal circulation, or cause shrinkage of scleral collagen

After vitrectomy: most common complication is glaucoma; caused by intraocular gas, hyphema, ghost cells, uveitis, silicone oil

Elevated episcleral venous pressure: causes resistance to aqueous outflow
   Etiology: carotid-cavernous sinus fistula, cavernous sinus thrombosis, Sturge-Weber syndrome, neurofibromatosis, orbital mass (tumor, varices), thyroid-related ophthalmopathy (false elevation of IOP can be caused by IR fibrosis with increased resistance in upgaze), superior vena cava obstruction, mediastinal tumors and syndromes, idiopathic. May see blood in Schlemm's canal

Primary Angle-Closure Glaucoma

Glaucoma caused by peripheral iris obstructing the trabecular meshwork, most commonly due to pupillary block; classified as acute, intermittent, or chronic. Plateau iris syndrome is a form of primary angle-closure without pupillary block

Mechanism of pupillary block: in susceptible patients, iridolenticular touch causes resistance of aqueous flow from posterior to anterior chamber, causing increased posterior pressure. When the pupil is mid-dilated (i.e., stress, low ambient light levels, sympathomimetic or anticholinergic medications), the elevated posterior chamber pressure causes peripheral iris tissue to bow forward and occlude the TM

Epidemiology: acute form is most common in Eskimos and Asians, followed by Caucasians, then African Americans; highest risk is between age 55 and 65 years old; more common in women only among Caucasians. Chronic form is more common in African Americans than Asians, who have a higher risk than Caucasians. 5% of population older than 60 years of age have angles that can be occluded; 0.5% of these individuals develop angle closure. Usually bilateral (75% risk in untreated fellow eye within 5 years)

Anatomic features predisposing to angle closure: small anterior segment (hyperopia, nanophthalmos, microcornea, microphthalmos); hereditary narrow angle; anterior iris insertion (Eskimos, Asians, and African Americans); shallow AC (large lens, plateau iris configuration, loose or dislocated lens)

Acute angle closure:
   Symptoms: blurred vision, colored halos around lights, pain, redness, nausea and vomiting, headache
   Findings: high IOP, corneal epithelial edema, conjunctival injection, mid-dilated pupil, shallow anterior chamber, mild AC cell and flare, closed angle (perform indentation gonioscopy to differentiate between appositional and synechial angle closure; glycerin can be used to clear corneal edema; evaluate angle in other eye), ON swelling and hyperemia; with rapid rise in IOP, may see arterial pulsations (retinal ischemia can occur)
   Sequelae of ischemia: segmental iris atrophy (focal iris stroma necrosis), dilated irregular pupil (sphincter and dilator necrosis), glaukomflecken (focal anterior lens epithelial necrosis)
   Late findings: decreased vision, PAS, chronic corneal edema
   Provocative tests: prone test, dark-room test, prone dark-room test, pharmacologic pupillary dilation; positive if IOP rises >8 mm Hg

Thymoxamine test: α-adrenergic antagonist used to distinguish angle closure from glaucoma with narrow angles; thymoxamine blocks iris dilator muscle producing miosis; however, it does not affect trabecular meshwork and normally does not decrease IOP; therefore, decrease in IOP suggests miosis has removed iris from the outflow channel reversing angle closure

Treatment of acute angle-closure glaucoma: peripheral iridotomy or iridectomy (PI, definitive treatment); compression gonioscopy (may force aqueous through block and open angle); pilocarpine (may not be effective at IOP >40 mm Hg due to sphincter ischemia; may also cause lens-iris diaphragm to move forward, worsening pupillary block); reduce IOP with β-blocker, α$_2$-agonist, topical or oral CAI, or hyperosmotic agent (isosorbide, glycerin [contraindicated in diabetics], or IV mannitol [risk of cardiovascular adverse effects]); topical steroids for inflammation; laser PI in fellow eye (75% chance of attack in untreated fellow eye; pilocarpine lowers risk to 40% but may lead to chronic angle closure)

If attack of angle closure is broken medically, consider waiting a few days before performing laser PI because corneal edema, iridocorneal touch, and iris congestion make the procedure more difficult

Persistently increased IOP following laser PI may be due to PAS, incomplete iridotomy, underlying open-angle glaucoma, or secondary angle closure

Intermittent angle closure: 2 : 1 ratio of nonacute-to-acute presentations; may be asymptomatic or have similar presentation as acute angle closure but less severe, and occurs over days to weeks; often complain of headaches, episodes resolve spontaneously, especially by entering a well-lit area (induces miosis); IOP may be normal, glaukomflecken and PAS are evidence of previous attack. Treat with laser PI

Chronic angle closure: gradual closure of angle by apposition or development of PAS leads to slow rise in IOP; variable IOP, but less than with acute angle closure. Often asymptomatic; cornea usually clear due to gradual rise in IOP, but can have large visual field loss

Plateau iris:
  Configuration: angle anatomy resulting in deep central AC and shallow peripheral AC
  Syndrome: angle closure in an eye with plateau iris configuration; usually occurs in 4th to 5th decade of life, and in individuals with less hyperopia than typical angle-closure patient
  Findings: may present with acute or chronic angle closure; anteriorly positioned ciliary processes force the peripheral iris more anteriorly than normal; deep chamber centrally; flat iris contour

with sharp dropoff peripherally; with dilation, peripheral iris folds into the angle and occludes TM; with compression gonioscopy, angle is more difficult to open and does not open as widely as in primary angle closure
  Treatment: laser peripheral iridotomy, laser iridoplasty, and miotics; plateau iris appearance remains

Grading system of flat anterior chamber:
  Grade I: Contact between cornea and peripheral iris
  Grade II: Contact between cornea and iris up to pupil (consider reforming AC with BSS or viscoelastic)
  Grade III: Contact between cornea and crystalline lens (surgical emergency)

Secondary Angle-Closure Glaucoma

Mechanism/Etiology
  With pupillary block:
    Phacomorphic (lens enlargement in elderly; urgent surgery needed to remove lens); dislocated lens; seclusio pupillae; nanophthalmos; aphakic and pseudophakic pupillary block; silicone oil (prevent by performing an inferior PI because oil is lighter than water)
  Without pupillary block:
    POSTERIOR "PUSHING" MECHANISM (mechanical/anterior displacement of lens-iris diaphragm)
      Anterior rotation of ciliary body: inflammation (scleritis, uveitis, after scleral buckle or panretinal photocoagulation [PRP]), congestion (postscleral buckling, nanophthalmos), choroidal effusion (hypotony; uveal effusion), suprachoroidal hemorrhage
      Aqueous misdirection (malignant glaucoma)
      Pressure from posterior segment: tumor, expanding gas, exudative retinal detachment (RD)
      Persistent hyperplastic primary vitreous (PHPV)
      Retinopathy of prematurity (ROP)
    ANTERIOR "PULLING" MECHANISM (adherence of iris to trabecular meshwork/membranes over TM)
      Epithelial: epithelial downgrowth, fibrous ingrowth
      Endothelial: iridocorneal endothelial (ICE) syndrome, posterior polymorphous dystrophy (PPMD)
      Neovascular: neovascular glaucoma (NVG)
      Peripheral anterior synechiae (PAS)
      Adhesion from trauma

Angle closure associated with RD surgery: anterior rotation of CB around the scleral spur secondary to swelling from excessive PRP or tight scleral buckle

Treatment: cycloplegics, PI, consider cutting encircling band

Nanophthalmos: >10 D hyperopia; small eye (<20 mm) with small cornea (mean diameter = 10.5 mm), shallow AC, narrow angle, and high lens/eye volume. Pupillary block or uveal effusion produces angle-closure glaucoma. Thick sclera (about 2× thicker than normal) may impede vortex venous drainage, as well as decrease uveoscleral outflow, and can also result in spontaneous uveal effusion with anterior rotation of CB leading to angle closure

> ***Treatment***: weak miotics, cycloplegics (if no angle crowding), laser PI, laser iridoplasty, trabeculectomy after prophylactic sclerotomy. Because there is a high complication rate with surgery (uveal effusion), first use medical therapy, then laser

> Increased risk of complications with cataract surgery (RD, choroidal effusion, angle-closure glaucoma, flat AC, CME, corneal decompensation, malignant glaucoma, IOL miscalculations). If shallow AC and thickened choroid preoperatively, perform prophylactic anterior sclerotomies with surgery

Malignant glaucoma (aqueous misdirection syndrome, ciliolenticular or ciliovitreal block):

> ***Mechanism***: tips of ciliary processes rotate forward against lens (ciliolenticular block); can also have a trapdoor tear in the anterior hyaloid; causes anterior displacement of lens-iris diaphragm

> ***Risk factors***: uveitis, angle closure, nanophthalmos, hyperopia; occurs postoperatively (usually 5 days) following a variety of laser or incisional surgeries; usually in patients with PAS or chronic angle closure following intraocular surgery if the hyaloid face has not been broken (follows 2% of surgical cases for angle closure); can also occur in unoperated eye when mydriatics are stopped or miotics are added

> ***Findings***: entire AC shallow (versus angle closure in which the AC is deeper centrally than peripherally), IOP higher than expected, presence of patent iridectomy, absence of suprachoroidal fluid or blood

> ***DDx***: pupillary block (no patent iridectomy; moderate depth of central AC), suprachoroidal hemorrhage (acute severe pain and choroidal elevation), choroidal effusion (usually low IOP and choroidal elevation), annular peripheral choroidal detachment

> ***Treatment***:

>> MEDICAL: cycloplegic (relaxes ciliary muscle and pulls lens-iris diaphragm posteriorly; continued indefinitely to prevent recurrence), aqueous suppressants, peripheral iridotomy in both eyes (eliminate any component of pupillary block); miotics are contraindicated

>> 50% resolve within 5 days with medical therapy alone

>> SURGICAL: argon laser photocoagulation of ciliary processes (requires shrinkage of at least 2–4 ciliary processes), Nd:YAG laser rupture of hyaloid face (for pseudophakic and aphakic patients; 4–6 mJ; best to perform peripherally [through PI]), vitrectomy (for phakic patients; debulk vitreous and overdeepen AC with air)

Intraocular tumors: can push angle closed from posteriorly

> Malignant melanoma of the anterior uveal tract can cause glaucoma by direct extension of tumor into trabecular meshwork, inducing neovascularization of the angle, obstructing TM with melanin-laden macrophages (melanomalytic), or seeding of tumor cells in outflow channels

> Other mechanisms include pigment dispersion, inflammation, and hemorrhage

PHPV: contraction of retrolenticular membrane and swelling of cataract can cause angle closure

> ***Treatment***: remove lens and membrane via limbal approach (pars plana approach may be dangerous in that retina can extend up to the pars plicata)

ROP: due to contraction of retrolental tissue

Epithelial downgrowth: due to epithelium growing over angle

Fibrous ingrowth: due to fibrous proliferation through wound into AC

ICE syndrome: due to descemetization of TM and angle closure from contraction of endothelial membrane; PAS are prominent but less responsible for glaucoma

PPMD: due to abnormal corneal endothelial cells that migrate into angle causing glaucoma (15%)

NVG: due to widespread retinal or ocular ischemia; clinically transparent fibrovascular membrane flattens anterior iris surface; myofibroblasts provide motive force for angle closure and ectropion uveae

> ***Etiology***: proliferative retinopathy (diabetes [33% of all forms of NVG], ischemic CRVO [33%], carotid occlusive disease [13%], ciliary artery occlusion, sickle cell, Norrie's disease, ROP); intraocular inflammation (uveitis, postoperative); neoplasms (retinoblastoma [50% develop NVG], malignant melanoma, large cell lymphoma [reticulum cell sarcoma], metastatic); chronic retinal detachment

> ***Treatment***: aqueous suppressants and hyperosmotics; increase uveoscleral outflow (atropine; avoid miotics); panretinal photocoagulation; peripheral retinal cryotherapy (if poor visualization of retina; 50% develop phthisis with cyclocryotherapy); glaucoma drainage implant (70% success rate)

Normal Tension Glaucoma (NTG)

Glaucoma with open angles and IOP <22 mm Hg

Proposed mechanisms:

Nocturnal systemic hypotension: diurnal curve of BP similar to IOP. 66% of patients will have a BP drop of greater than 10% during early morning hours ("dippers"); patients with HTN have an even greater swing in BP (26% average drop); patients with HTN treated with β-blockers can have diastolic BP <50 mm Hg, which may compromise blood supply to optic nerve

Autoimmune: increased incidence of proteinemia and autoantibodies in patients with NTG

Vasospasm

Previous hemodynamic crisis: excessive blood loss or shock

DDx: POAG with large diurnal variation, "burned-out" secondary open-angle glaucoma, chronic angle closure. Must rule out intracranial processes and other causes of optic neuropathy

Cupping can occur with neurologic disease: AION (arteritic 50%; nonarteritic 10%), chiasmal compressive lesions (5%), optic neuritis (<5%), methanol toxicity. These entities are more likely to have early loss of central vision and color vision; pallor may be worse than cupping

Diagnosis: diurnal curve, neurologic workup (CBC, ESR, ANA, VDRL and FTA-ABS, carotid evaluation, brain neuroimaging)

VF: defects in NTG have steeper slopes, greater depths, and closer proximity to fixation than in POAG; splinter hemorrhages are more common; more difficult to treat

TREATMENT

Generally, medications are tried first, followed by laser treatment, and then surgery; however, the choice and timing of various treatment modalities are dependent on the type of glaucoma, severity of optic nerve damage, level of control, and many other factors. Therapy must also be directed to any pre-existing or underlying process

Medication

Ocular hypotensive agents (see Chapter 2, Pharmacology)

Laser

Argon laser trabeculoplasty (ALT): power 400–1200 mW; spot size 50 μm; duration 0.1 second; titrate power to generate small bubble at junction of non-pigmented and pigmented TM; 50 applications/180°; average of 30% reduction in IOP; can be repeated

Iopidine immediately postoperatively to avoid pressure spike, and treat with steroids for 1 week. Assess efficacy of treatment at 6 weeks postoperatively

Anterior burns have poor effect; posterior burns more likely to develop PAS

Results: 25% fail to control IOP at 1 year; 10% per year failure rate thereafter. Repeating ALT may provide IOP control in 33% to 50%, but sustained elevation in 10%

Best predictor of success is type of glaucoma: PXG (best) > PG > POAG > NTG > aphakic (worst)

The greater the amount of pigment in the angle, the better the result; poorer response in patients <50 years of age. ALT is ineffective (and may worsen IOP) in inflammatory glaucoma, angle recession, angle-closure glaucoma (membranes in angles), congenital glaucoma, and steroid-induced glaucoma. Contraindicated in patients with large amounts of PAS

Complications: IOP spike (increases with energy and number of laser burns), iritis, PAS (Figure 9-18)

Selective laser trabeculoplasty (SLT): time and spot size (400 μm) are fixed, power 0.7–0.9 mJ; 50 confluent applications/180°, straddling TM

Produces less tissue destruction than ALT, and is repeatable

Laser iridotomy: perform prophylactically in eyes with narrow angles, iris bombe, synechial angle closure, pigmentary glaucoma (due to configuration of iris), plateau iris, and malignant glaucoma

YAG: power 1–12 mJ; bleed more, but close less than with argon

Argon: reaction is pigment-related and requires more energy and total applications than with YAG; less bleeding because of thermal effect; extensive tissue destruction at margins of treatment; iritis more pronounced

Iridoplasty: for narrow angles; aim at peripheral iris; stretch iris away from angle; power 200–400 mW; spot size 500 μm; duration 0.5–1.0 second

Surgery

Trabeculectomy:

Consider use of antimetabolite in patients at risk for bleb failure

Risk factors for bleb failure: previous surgical failure, darker skin pigmentation, history of keloid formation, neovascular changes, younger age, intraocular inflammation, scarred conjunctiva, high hyperopia, inability to use corticosteroids, shallow AC

Antimetabolites:

MITOMYCIN-C (MMC): antineoplastic antibiotic (isolated from *Streptomyces caespitosus*)

MECHANISM: intercalates with DNA and prevents replication; suppresses fibrosis and

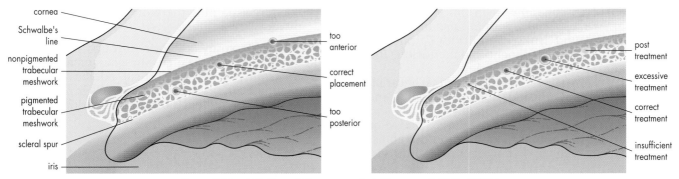

Figure 9-18. ALT. (From Schwartz et al: *J Glaucoma* 2:329, 1993.)

Table 9-1. Treatment of shallow or flat anterior chamber following trabeculectomy

Bleb Height	IOP	DDx	Treatment
Elevated	Low	Excessive filtration	Bleb revision
Flat	Low	Choroidal detachment	Cycloplegic, steroid, drainage
		Bleb leak	Antibiotic, aqueous suppressants, stop steroid, AC reformation, pressure patch, Simmons' scleral compression shell, large diameter soft contact lens, trichloroacetic acid, glue, laser, or autologous blood injection. Consider surgical intervention (drainage of choroidals and repair of wound) for impending failure of bleb, flat anterior chamber with corneal decompensation, kissing choroidals, progressive cataract
Flat	Elevated	Suprachoroidal hemorrhage	Drainage
		Pupillary block	Cycloplegic, steriod, PI
		Malignant glaucoma	Cycloplegic, aqueous suppressants, PI, YAG anterior vitreolysis or vitrectomy
Elevated	Elevated	Encapsulated bleb	Needling, aqueous suppressants, bleb revision

vascular ingrowth after exposure to the filtration site. Toxic to fibroblasts in all stages of cell cycle; 100× more potent than 5-FU

TOXICITY: intraocular causes corneal decompensation (damages endothelium), AC inflammation, and necrosis of ciliary body and iris; can develop scleral necrosis; retinal toxicity with intravitreal injection

5-FU: specifically affects the S-phase of the cell cycle; requires postoperative injections (30–35 mg in 5-mg doses over 1–3 weeks); corneal epithelial toxicity may occur

Complications:

In hyperopia, nanophthalmos, or chronic angle closure, the ciliary processes can roll anteriorly and block ostium during surgery

TREATMENT: suture wound and reinflate eye allowing ciliary processes to revert to normal position

If still present, use cautery to remove the processes

HIGH IOP IMMEDIATELY POSTOPERATIVELY: attempt digital massage or laser suture lysis

SHALLOW OR FLAT AC: (Table 9-1)

BLEBITIS: red eye, photophobia, discharge, marked conjunctival injection around an opalescent filtering bleb; often Seidel-positive, moderate AC cells and flare, but no involvement of the vitreous. Organism usually *Staphylococcus*

TREATMENT: intensive topical antibiotics, repair wound leak, observe daily for endophthalmitis

BLEB-ASSOCIATED ENDOPHTHALMITIS: pain, decreased vision, AC cells and flare, hypopyon, and vitreous cells; often Seidel-positive. Organism usually *Streptococcus* species or *H. flu*

TREATMENT: emergent, as for endophthalmitis

SUPRACHOROIDAL HEMORRHAGE: usually occurs several days after trabeculectomy surgery with acute pain, often while straining; also, nausea, vomiting, and decreased vision

MECHANISM: progressive serous choroidal detachment, stretching the long posterior ciliary artery until it ruptures

RISK FACTORS: aphakia, hypertension, cardiovascular disease, and increased age

HYPOTONY: generally seen in young myopic patients, especially with antimetabolites

DDx: wound leak, overfiltration, iridocylitis, cyclodialysis, ciliochoroidal effusion, RD

TREATMENT: wound revision

COMPLICATIONS: corneal edema, cataract, choroidal effusion, optic disc edema, chorioretinal folds, maculopathy

EXUBERANT BLEB: bleb can enlarge, spread onto cornea, and interfere with vision due to astigmatism, dellen, or encroachment into visual axis

TREATMENT: recess or amputate bleb; usually a cleavage plane is present

Drainage implants (setons/tubes):

Seton is from Latin "seta" or bristle (original surgery used horse hair)

Types:

NONVALVE: Molteno (single- or double-plate), Schocket, Baerveldt; must temporarily occlude tube lumen with suture or biodegradable collagen plug

VALVE: Ahmed (1-way valve maintains IOP at 8 mm Hg or higher), Krupin, and Baerveldt (pressure-sensitive valve)

Anterior chamber glaucoma drainage implant: for patients with scleral buckles who do not have adequate scleral surface for placement of a seton; a silicone implant shunts fluid from AC or PC to the fibrous capsule surrounding the episcleral encircling element

Goniosynechialysis: Direct lysis of PAS with cyclodialysis spatula or other microinstrument; consider for angle-closure glaucoma of less than 12 months duration

Cyclophotocoagulation: Laser treatment of ciliary body with argon (transpupillary or endoprobe), Nd:YAG (contact or noncontact), or diode (contact); useful in many types of refractory glaucomas, including aphakic, neovascular, and inflammatory, and in eyes with failed filtering blebs

Mechanism: reduced aqueous production by destruction of ciliary epithelium

Procedure is painful; therefore, requires peribulbar or retrobulbar block

Cyclocryotherapy:

First treatment: 2.5 mm cryo tip, with anterior edge 1 mm from inferior limbus and 1.5 mm from superior limbus. Provide 6 freezes on the clock hours of the inferior 180°. Maintain each freeze for 60 seconds at –80°C. The iceball will encroach upon cornea for about 0.5 mm. Wait 1 month for the IOP to reach new baseline

Second treatment: if first treatment does not lower IOP sufficiently, treat superior temporal quadrant with 2–4 freezes. Always leave at least 1 quadrant (usually superonasal) free to prevent hypotony. Give subconjunctival steroid postoperatively

Procedure is painful; therefore, requires peribulbar or retrobulbar block

Surgical iridectomy: perform through 3 mm clear corneal wound for angle-closure glaucoma

Indications: if severe corneal edema precludes adequate iris visualization, AC is extremely shallow, or patient is unable to cooperate for laser iridotomy

MAJOR GLAUCOMA CLINICAL STUDIES

Advanced Glaucoma Intervention Study (AGIS)

Objective: to evaluate argon laser trabeculoplasty (ALT) vs trabeculectomy as the initial surgery in patients with advanced open-angle glaucoma not controlled by medical treatment

Main outcome variable was visual function (field and acuity)

Results:

After 7 years:

In African Americans, the best results were obtained when ALT was performed 1st, followed by trabeculectomy (ATT sequence)

In Caucasians, the best results occurred when trabeculectomy was performed 1st, followed by ALT, and finally by a 2nd trabeculectomy (TAT sequence)

Visual field defects were more severe in African American patients

Eyes with IOP <18 mm Hg at all visits had almost no progression of VF loss

Trabeculectomy increased the risk of cataract by 78% (47% if no complications occurred vs 104% if complications occurred, especially severe inflammation and flat anterior chamber)

Conclusions:

In patients with advanced POAG, ALT should be considered as the first surgical treatment in African American patients; trabeculectomy should be considered first in Caucasians

Risk factors for ALT failure are younger age and higher IOP

Risk factors for trabeculectomy failure are younger age, higher IOP, diabetes, and postoperative complications (particularly elevated IOP and marked inflammation)

Risk factors for bleb encapsulation include male sex and previous ALT (but this was not statistically significant)

Low IOP reduces VF deterioration

Trabeculectomy is associated with an increased risk of cataract formation

Ocular Hypertension Treatment Study (OHTS)

Objective: to evaluate the effect of topical medication in delaying or preventing POAG in patients with ocular hypertension (IOP between 24 and 32 mm Hg in one eye and between 21 and 32 mm Hg in the fellow eye; normal visual fields and optic nerves)

The goal in the treatment group was to reduce the IOP by at least 20% from baseline and obtain a target pressure of ≤24 mm Hg

The primary outcome variable was visual field loss or optic nerve damage

Results:

Mean IOP reduction in the medicine group was 22.5% vs 4.0% in the observation group

At 5 years, the cumulative risk of developing POAG was 4.4% in the medicine group vs 9.5% in the observation group

Conclusions:

Topical ocular hypotensive medication is effective in delaying or preventing POAG in eyes with ocular hypertension

Predictive factors for developing POAG include baseline IOP, age, cup-to-disc ratio, and central corneal thickness (CCT ≤555 µm)

Collaborative Initial Glaucoma Treatment Study (CIGTS)

Objective: to evaluate medicine (stepped regimen) vs trabeculectomy (with or without 5-fluorouracil) for the treatment of newly diagnosed open-angle glaucoma (primary, pigmentary, or pseudoexfoliative)

The primary outcome variable was progression of visual field loss

Secondary outcomes were quality of life, visual acuity, and intraocular pressure

Results:

5-year data:

VF loss was not significantly different with either treatment

Surgery had an initially increased risk of significant visual loss, but by 4 years, the average VA was equal in the 2 groups

IOP averaged 17–18 mm Hg in the medicine group vs 14–15 mm Hg in the surgery group

The rate of visually significant cataract was greater in the surgery group

Conclusions:

Initial treatment of open-angle glaucoma with medicine or surgery results in similar VF outcome

Although VA loss was initially greater in the surgery group, the differences converged with time

Early Manifest Glaucoma Trial (EMGT)

Objective: to evaluate the effectiveness of reducing IOP (vs no treatment) on the progression of newly diagnosed open-angle glaucoma

The treatment group received argon laser trabeculoplasty plus topical betaxolol

The primary outcome measures were progression of visual field loss and optic disc changes

A secondary aim was to assess risk factors for progression

Results:

6-year data:

53% of patients progressed

Treatment reduced the IOP on average 5.1 mm Hg (25%)

Progression was less common in the treatment group (45% vs 62%) and occurred later

Each 1 mm Hg of IOP lowering from baseline to the first follow-up visit (3 months) reduced the risk of progression by approximately 10%

Increased nuclear lens opacity occurred with treatment

Conclusions:

Treatment of early glaucoma halves the risk of progression

Risk factors for progression included higher baseline IOP, exfoliation, bilateral disease, older age, and frequent disc hemorrhages

Glaucoma Laser Trial (GLT)

Objective: to evaluate the efficacy and safety of starting treatment for POAG with ALT vs topical medication (timoptic 0.5% bid)

Results:

Eyes treated initially with ALT had lower IOP and better VF and optic nerve status than fellow eyes treated initially with topical medication

Conclusions:

Initial treatment of POAG with ALT is at least as efficacious as initial treatment with Timoptic

Review Questions *(Answers start on page 365)*

1. Which form of glaucoma is associated with Down's syndrome?
   a. congenital
   b. pigmentary
   c. Axenfeld-Rieger
   d. POAG

2. What is the most appropriate initial treatment of pupillary block in a patient with microspherophakia?
   a. Diamox
   b. laser iridotomy
   c. pilocarpine
   d. cyclopentolate

3. Which of the following statements is true? Uveoscleral outflow is
   a. inversely proportional to intraocular pressure
   b. measured clinically by fluorophotometry
   c. increased by atropine
   d. responsible for about 10% of total outflow

4. Risk factors for angle-closure glaucoma include all of the following except
   a. pseudoexfoliation
   b. myopia
   c. Eskimo ancestry
   d. nanophthalmos

5. Which of the following would cause the greatest elevation in IOP?
   a. blinking
   b. decreased blood cortisol levels
   c. change from supine to sitting position
   d. darkening the room

6. The most likely cause of a large filtering bleb and a shallow chamber is
   a. aqueous misdirection
   b. bleb leak
   c. pupillary block
   d. overfiltration

7. A change in Goldmann visual field stimulus from I4E to II4E is equivalent to
   a. 1 log
   b. 2 log
   c. 3 log
   d. 4 log

8. An Amsler grid held at 33 cm measures approximately how many degrees of central vision?
   a. 5
   b. 10
   c. 20
   d. 30

9. The most decreased sensitivity in an arcuate scotoma occurs in which quadrant?
   a. inferotemporal
   b. superonasal
   c. superotemporal
   d. inferonasal

10. The best gonioscopy lens for distinguishing appositional from synechial angle closure is
    a. Goldmann 3-mirror
    b. Zeiss
    c. Koeppe
    d. Goldmann 1-mirror

11. Which is not a risk factor for POAG?
    a. myopia
    b. CVO
    c. diabetes
    d. CRAO

12. ALT would be most effective in a patient with which type of glaucoma?
    a. congenital
    b. inflammatory
    c. pigmentary
    d. aphakic

13. In which direction should a patient look to aid the examiner's view of the angle during Zeiss gonioscopy?
    a. up
    b. toward the mirror
    c. away from the mirror
    d. down

14. The best parameter for determining the unreliability of a Humphrey visual field is
    a. fixation losses
    b. false-positives
    c. false-negatives
    d. fluctuation

15. Which of the following does not cause angle-closure glaucoma?
    a. ICE syndrome
    b. PHPV
    c. RD
    d. choroidal effusion

16. Factors producing increased IOP 2 days postoperatively include all of the following except
    a. retained viscoelastic
    b. red blood cells
    c. macrophages
    d. steroid drops

17. Treatment of malignant glaucoma may include all of the following except
    a. laser iridotomy
    b. pilocarpine
    c. atropine
    d. vitrectomy

18. The most common organism associated with bleb-related endophthalmitis is
    a. *Streptococcus* species
    b. *S. epidermidis*
    c. *H. influenzae*
    d. Gram-negative organisms

19. Which visual field defect is least characteristic of glaucoma?
    a. paracentral scotoma
    b. nasal defect
    c. central scotoma
    d. enlarged blind spot

20. The type of tonometer most greatly affected by scleral rigidity is
    a. Goldmann
    b. tonopen
    c. Schiøtz
    d. pneumotonometer

21. Which of the following conditions is not associated with an increased incidence of glaucoma?
    a. aniridia
    b. nanophthalmos
    c. Axenfeld-Rieger syndrome
    d. cornea plana

22. As compared with plasma, aqueous has a higher concentration of

a. calcium
b. protein
c. ascorbate
d. sodium

23. The rate of aqueous production per minute is approximately
    a. 0.2 μL
    b. 2 μL
    c. 20 μL
    d. 200 μL

24. The location of the greatest resistance to aqueous outflow is
    a. corneoscleral meshwork
    b. uveal meshwork
    c. juxtacanalicular connective tissue
    d. Schlemm's canal

25. Facility of aqueous outflow is best measured by
    a. tonography
    b. manometry
    c. tonometry
    d. fluorophotometry

SUGGESTED READINGS

American Academy of Ophthalmology: Glaucoma, vol 10. San Francisco, AAO, 2004.

Anderson DR, Patella VM: Automated Static Perimetry, 2nd edition. St. Louis, Mosby, 1999.

Campbell DG, Netland PA: Stereo Atlas of Glaucoma. St. Louis, Mosby, 1998.

Higginbotham EJ, Lee DA: Clinical Guide to Glaucoma Management. Amsterdam, Butterworth-Heinemann, 2003.

Netland PA, Mandal AK: Pediatric Glaucoma. Philadelphia, Butterworth-Heinemann, 2003.

Ritch R, Shields MB, Krupin T: The Glaucomas, 2nd edition. St. Louis, Mosby, 1996.

Shields MB: Textbook of Glaucoma, 4th edition. Philadelphia, Lippincott Williams and Wilkins, 1998.

Weber J, Caprioli J: Atlas of Computerized Perimetry. Philadelphia, WB Saunders, 2000.

Zimmerman TJ, Kooner KS: Clinical Pathways in Glaucoma. New York, Thieme Medical Publishers, 2001.

CHAPTER 10

Anterior Segment

IRIS, CILIARY BODY, AND ANTERIOR CHAMBER ANGLE

Anatomy

Limbus

Transition zone between cornea and sclera; 1 to 2 mm wide

Conjunctiva and Tenon's capsule are fused over this area; contains corneal epithelial stem cells, goblet cells, lymphoid cells, Langerhans' cells, mast cells

Definitions:
  Anatomist's: termination of Descemet's and Bowman's membranes

  Pathologist's: anterior limbus corresponds to termination of Bowman's and Descemet's membranes, and posterior limbus corresponds to line between iris root and Schlemm's canal

  Surgeon's: anterior blue zone (1 mm) and posterior white zone (1 mm); a perpendicular incision through the conjunctival insertion enters the AC through Descemet's membrane; a perpendicular incision through the posterior aspect of the limbus will enter the AC through the trabecular meshwork (Figure 10-1)

Ciliary Body and Angle Structures

(see Chapter 9, Glaucoma)

Disorders

Trauma

Hyphema

Blood in anterior chamber

Etiology: trauma, surgery (incisional or laser), spontaneous (neovascularization, Fuchs' heterochromic iridocyclitis, intraocular tumors, juvenile xanthogranuloma), clotting abnormalities (leukemia, hemophilia, anemia, coumadin, aspirin, ethanol)

Findings: layer of blood and/or clot with suspended RBCs in AC; called microhyphema if only suspended cells; damage to other structures may be seen

Diagnosis: sickle prep, consider hemoglobin electrophoresis, rule out ruptured globe, gonioscopy (wait 4–6 weeks in traumatic cases)

Treatment: cycloplegic, topical steroid, control IOP (avoid miotics); consider amicar, protective shield; elevate head, bed rest, no aspirin-containing products, control systemic BP, antiemetics (if needed); may require surgery (AC washout)
  Indications for surgical intervention: large hyphema that persists for longer than 10 days, total hyphema that persists for longer than 5 days, corneal blood staining, uncontrolled IOP,

Anterior limbal border
Blue zone
White zone
Posterior limbal border
Scleral spur

Termination of Bowman's membrane

Termination of Descemet's membrane (Schwalbe's line)

Trabecular meshwork

Schlemm's canal

Iris root

Figure 10-1. Anatomy of the surgical limbus.

8-ball hyphema; best to perform washout 4 to 7 days after injury (clot has time to solidify, reducing rate of rebleed)

Complications:
8-Ball hyphema: hyphema that has clotted and taken on a black or purple color because of impaired aqueous circulation and deoxygenated blood, which prevents resorption; total hyphema is differentiated from 8-ball hyphema by retention of bright red color, which indicates aqueous circulation
Corneal blood staining: passage of erythrocyte breakdown products into stroma, creates yellow-brown discoloration; occurs in about 5%, especially with recurrent hemorrhage, compromised endothelial cell function, large hyphemas that remain for extended periods, elevated IOP
Recurrent hemorrhage: usually larger than initial hyphema; incidence 5% to 35% with greatest risk at 2 to 5 days
Secondary glaucoma:
EARLY: due to TM obstruction, pupillary block by clot, hemolytic, steroid-induced
LATE: due to angle recession, ghost cell, PAS formation, posterior synechiae with iris bombe
Central retinal artery occlusion

Sickle cell and hyphema: higher elevation in IOP (sickled RBCs cannot pass through TM), and higher risk of central retinal artery occlusion and optic nerve infarction due to vascular sludging

Factors that increase sickling: acidosis, hypoxia, hemoconcentration
Ocular hypotensive medications in sickle cell: β-blockers are safe; avoid CAIs (increases concentration of ascorbic acid in aqueous, decreasing pH and leading to sickling), epinephrine and α-agonists (cause vasoconstriction with subsequent deoxygenation and sickling); hyperosmotics (lead to hemoconcentration with vascular sludging and sickling)

Angle Trauma (see Figure 9-15)

Iris sphincter tear: small tear at pupillary margin; asymptomatic

Traumatic mydriasis: dilated, poorly reactive pupil; may cause glare or photophobia; consider cosmetic contact lens or surgical repair

Iridodialysis: tear in iris root; consider cosmetic contact lens or surgical repair if large or symptomatic

Angle recession: tear in anterior face of ciliary body between the longitudinal and circular ciliary muscles; most common source of hemorrhage in blunt trauma, occurs in more than 60% of hyphemas; 10% of patients with greater than 180° of angle recession will develop chronic glaucoma

Cyclodialysis: separation of ciliary body from scleral spur; allows free passage of aqueous into suprachoroidal space; can result in hypotony; treat with atropine, laser, and/or surgical repair

Open Globe/Intraocular Foreign Body

Full-thickness defect in cornea or sclera

Usually due to trauma (penetrating or blunt), may also occur from melt (chemical injury, autoimmune disorder, infection)

Penetration: entrance wound only

Perforation: entrance and exit wounds (double penetrating injury)

Risk of infectious endophthalmitis (3%–7%) increases if retained foreign body, delayed surgery (>24 hours), rural setting (soil contamination), and lens disruption

S. aureus is most common organism to cause post-traumatic endophthalmitis; *Bacillus cereus* is also common and causes severe damage

Findings: wound with positive Seidel test, hemorrhage (conjunctiva, hyphema, vitreous, retina), decreased IOP, shallow or flat AC, peaked pupil (toward wound), cataract, retinal tear/detachment, prolapsed intraocular contents (uvea, vitreous), foreign body (small high-velocity FB may cause self-sealing wound or intermittently positive Seidel; iris transillumination defect, capsule/lens disruption)

Types of foreign bodies:
　Inert: glass, plastic, sand, stone, ceramic, gold, platinum, silver, aluminum
　Reactive:
　　COPPER: severity of inflammation is directly proportionate to amount of copper in foreign body (≥85% copper causes severe endophthalmitis; <85% causes chalcosis; <70% is relatively inert)
　　　CHALCOSIS: mild intraocular inflammation, deposition of copper in anterior lens capsule (sunflower cataract) and Descemet's membrane (Kayser-Fleisher ring), retinal degeneration, iris may become green and sluggishly reactive to light
　　　ERG: decreased amplitude (suppressed by copper ions)
　　IRON (siderosis): iris heterochromia (hyperchromatic on involved side), mid-dilated minimally reactive pupil, lens discoloration (brown-orange dots from iron deposition in lens epithelium, generalized yellowing from involvement of cortex), vitritis, pigmentary RPE degeneration with sclerosis of vessels, retinal thinning, and atrophy
　　　ERG: initial a-wave increased, may eventually become flat
　　WOOD: significant inflammation; plant matter has higher risk of endophthalmitis

Treatment: rule out FB with CT or MRI (contraindicated for metallic FB); surgical exploration and repair, remove reactive material as soon as possible
　Prophylactic antibiotics: IV (aminoglycoside plus cephalosporin or vancomycin; consider clindamycin) and intravitreal (vancomycin [1 mg/0.1 mL], amikacin [0.4 mg/0.1 mL], or ceftazidime [2.25 mg/0.1 mL]) reduces risk of endophthalmitis; consider intravitreal dexamethasone 0.4 mg/0.1 mL

Prognosis: variable; poor if endophthalmitis or PVR develops (7–21 days later)

Congenital Abnormalities

(see Chapter 5, Pediatrics/Strabismus)

Mesodermal Dysgenesis Syndromes

(see Chapter 5, Pediatrics/Strabismus)

Other Disorders

Corectopia

Displacement of pupil

Isolated or associated with Axenfeld-Rieger syndrome, ICE syndrome, uveitis, trauma, or ectopia lentis et pupillae

Iris Heterochromia

Iris of different colors

May be congenital or acquired, unilateral (heterochromia iridis) or bilateral (heterochromia iridum)

DDx:
　Congenital:
　　INVOLVED IRIS HYPOCHROMIC: Horner's syndrome, Waardenburg's syndrome, Hirschsprung's disease, Parry-Romberg hemifacial atrophy
　　INVOLVED IRIS HYPERCHROMIC: ocular or oculodermal melanocytosis, iris pigment epithelium hamartoma
　Acquired:
　　INVOLVED IRIS HYPOCHROMIC: Horner's syndrome, Fuchs' heterochromic iridocyclitis, iris atrophy, metastatic carcinoma, juvenile xanthogranuloma
　　INVOLVED IRIS HYPERCHROMIC: iris nevus or melanoma, ICE syndrome, rubeosis, siderosis, hemosiderosis, medication (prostaglandin analogues)

Treatment: rule out tumor or intraocular foreign body

Rubeosis Iridis

Neovascularization of the iris

Etiology: ischemia (usually PDR, CRVO, carotid occlusive disease; also CRAO, sickle cell retinopathy, anterior segment ischemia), tumor, uveitis, chronic RD.

Findings: abnormal iris vessels; perform gonioscopy to assess presence of angle neovascularization; may have elevated IOP (neovascular glaucoma [NVG])

Treatment: often requires panretinal photocoagulation (PRP) for ischemia; NVG often needs glaucoma drainage implant for IOP control

Pigment Dispersion Syndrome

Pigment liberation from posterior iris surface (due to contact with zonules)

More common in young Caucasian males

Associated with myopia and lattice degeneration (20%)

Findings: pigment deposits on lens capsule, anterior iris, angle structures, and corneal endothelium (Krukenberg's spindle); midperipheral, radial, iris transillumination defects; pigmentary glaucoma may develop

Iridocorneal Endothelial (ICE) Syndrome

Nonhereditary, progressive abnormality of corneal endothelium

Abnormal corneal endothelium grows across angle and iris, producing membrane that obstructs trabecular meshwork, distorts iris, and may contract around iris stroma to form nodules

Unilateral, mostly women, occurs during middle age

Findings: fine, beaten metal appearance of endothelium; secondary angle-closure glaucoma may develop due to angle endothelialization and PAS

3 syndromes: common features of iris distortion, corneal edema, secondary angle-closure glaucoma
  Iris nevus (Cogan-Reese) syndrome: flattening and effacement of iris stroma, pigmented iris nodules (pseudonevi) composed of normal iris cells that are bunched up from the overlying membrane, corectopia, ectropion uveae
  Chandler's syndrome: corneal edema often with normal IOP, mild or no iris changes (minimal corectopia, iris atrophy, peripheral anterior synechiae)
  Essential iris atrophy: proliferating endothelium produces broad PAS, corectopia, ectropion uveae, and iris holes (stretch holes [area away from maximal pull of endothelial membrane is stretched so thin that holes develop] and melting

holes [holes in areas without iris thinning due to iris ischemia])

Pathology: growth of endothelium and Descemet's membrane over trabecular meshwork and onto iris

DDx: posterior polymorphous dystrophy, mesodermal dysgenesis syndromes

Iridoschisis

Separation of iris stroma due to senile changes

Bilateral; onset in 6th to 7th decade of life

Glaucoma in 50%

Iris Nodules

Brushfield's Spots

(see Chapter 5, Pediatrics/Strabismus)

Juvenile Xanthogranuloma (JXG)

(see Chapter 5, Pediatrics/Strabismus)

Epithelial Invasion, Serous Cyst, Implantation Membrane, Solid or Pearl Cyst

Serous or solid cysts after surgery or injury

Koeppe Nodules

Along pupillary border in granulomatous uveitis

Pathology: inflammatory cells and debris

Busacca Nodules

On anterior surface of the iris in granulomatous uveitis

Pathology: inflammatory cells and debris

Iris Nevus Syndrome (Cogan-Reese)

(see above)

Iris Tumors

Perform transillumination to differentiate cyst from solid tumor

Freckle

No distortion of iris architecture

Nevus

Localized or diffuse variably pigmented lesion of stroma; obscures crypts

Pathology: usually low-grade spindle cells

Small risk of transformation into melanoma (~5% of suspicious iris lesions grow during first 5 years after detection)

Melanocytosis

Congenital ocular: usually unilateral with diffuse iris nevus causing iris heterochromia

Oculodermal (nevus of Ota): ocular plus periorbital skin involvement

Melanocytoma

Form of nevus; darkly pigmented, very discohesive (like black, wet sand)

May have necrotic center

5% risk of melanoma

Malignant Melanoma

Elevated, vascular, darkly pigmented or amelanotic lesion; usually located inferiorly

Can be diffuse (appearing as iris heterochromia) and associated with glaucoma, localized, annular, or tapioca (dark tapioca appearance)

Common in Caucasians with light irides

Findings suggestive of melanoma: growth (only 6.5% of iris melanomas enlarge over 5-year period), spontaneous hyphema, large size, vascularity, ectropion uveae, iris heterochromia, elevated IOP, angle involvement, glaucoma, sector cataract

Pathology: low-grade spindle B cells; epithelioid cells are rare

Treatment: resection (sector iridectomy), may require enucleation if extensive

Prognosis: 4% to 10% mortality; 14% overall risk of metastasis (associated with tumor extension into TM, glaucoma, older age, poorly defined margins)

Tumors of Iris Pigment Epithelium

Adenoma (benign) or adenocarcinoma (malignant)

Rare compared with melanomas

Deeply pigmented, circumscribed or multinodular mass; can cause secondary glaucoma by involvement of angle

Treatment: chemotherapy, radiation, or excision

Lisch Nodules

Benign, tan, iris hamartomas; associated with neurofibromatosis type 1

Metastasis

Most commonly, breast, lung, lymphoma

Findings: fluffy, friable iris mass; may have pseudo-hypoyon, anterior uveitis, hyphema, rubeosis, and glaucoma

Leiomyoma

Well localized or pedunculated, often diffuse and flat

Pathology: very similar to amelonotic spindle cell melanoma

Leukemia

Rare nodular or diffuse milky lesions with intense hyperemia

Findings: iris thickening with loss of normal architecture; iris heterochromia and pseudohypopyon

Cystic Lesions

IPE: can be AD; flocculi around pupillary margin; associated in certain families with aortic dissection; midperipheral cysts, peripheral cysts (usually clear; can push iris forward)

Stroma: congenital or acquired (after trauma or surgery)

Ciliary Body Tumors

Melanoma

Pigmented mass

May be very large before detection, producing lenticular astigmatism, cataract, or shallow AC; may have classic sentinel vessel or nodule of extrascleral extension

Pathology: spindle, epithelioid, or mixed cells

Treatment: local resection, XRT, enucleation

Ciliary Body Leiomyoma

Similar to fibroid; myogenic origin

Schwannoma

Looks like amelanotic melanoma

Ciliary Body Adenoma or Adenocarcinoma

Arises from neuroepithelial cells

Occurs during adulthood

May metastasize

Fuchs' Adenoma (Fuchs' Reactive Hyperplasia, Benign Ciliary Epithelioma)

Proliferation of basement membrane material (type IV collagen and laminin) and nonpigmented ciliary body epithelial cells located at ciliary crest

Occurs in 25% of older patients

Rarely causes localized occlusion of anterior chamber angle

Medulloepithelioma

(see Chapter 5, Pediatrics/Strabismus)

LENS

Anatomy/Physiology

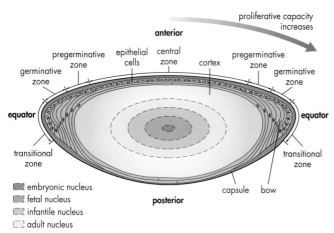

Figure 10-2. Gross anatomy of the adult human lens. (From Saxby LA: Anatomy. In Yanoff M, Duker JS [eds]: *Ophthalmology*, London, Mosby, 1999.)

Lens capsule: basement membrane secreted by epithelium; thickest peripherally near the equator, thinnest posteriorly. Thickening of lens capsule can occur with anterior chamber inflammation or pathologic proliferation of lens epithelium

Figure 10-3. Thickness of the lens capsule. (From Saxby LA: Anatomy. In Yanoff M, Duker JS [eds]: *Ophthalmology*, London, Mosby, 1999.)

Epithelium: present anteriorly, ending just posterior to the lens equator. Derived from cells of original lens vesicle. In the germinative zone, just anterior to equator, lens epithelial cells divide, elongate, and differentiate into lens fibers. During this transformation, epithelial cells lose their nuclei and most organelles. Lens fibers do not contain nuclei except in rubella, Lowe's syndrome, and trisomy 13. The embryonal nucleus develops by proliferation and migration of epithelial cells from the equator. Acute IOP elevation may cause patches of epithelium degeneration and necrosis beneath the capsule, which appear as white flecks (glaukomflecken). Chronic iritis may cause liquefaction of the nucleus, peripheral cortical changes, and degeneration and necrosis, as well as proliferation of anterior lens epithelium

Sutures: upright Y-suture anteriorly and inverted Y-suture posteriorly represent the ends of lens fibers; sutures appear during the 2nd month of gestation because of unequal growth of new lens fibers

Zonules: attach from pars plicata to anterior and posterior lens capsule in midperiphery (inserting more centrally on anterior capsule). During the 5th month of gestation, nonpigmented ciliary epithelium of ciliary body secretes collagen fibers that become zonules. Equatorial zonules are lost with aging

Tunica vasculosa lentis: vascular network that surrounds lens during embryogenesis; derived from hyaloid and long ciliary arteries. Remnants of tunica vasculosa lentis include Mittendorf's dot, epicapsular star, persistent pupillary membrane, and capsular whorls

Properties of the crystalline lens:
Composed of proteins: highest protein content in body (up to 60% wet weight and most of dry weight)
WATER SOLUBLE:
ALPHA CRYSTALLINS: largest of all water-soluble proteins, composed of 4 subunits; approximately 35% of lens protein by weight; involved in transforming epithelial cells into lens fibers
BETA CRYSTALLINS: most abundant lens protein by weight; composed of 3 subunits; approximately 55% of lens protein by weight; first appears in cortex
GAMMA CRYSTALLINS: smallest lens protein
WATER INSOLUBLE:
MAIN INTRINSIC POLYPEPTIDE: correlates with nuclear brunescence
Potassium-rich tissue: due to Na^+/K^+ pumps found on lens epithelial cells, which pump Na^+ out and K^+ in; concentrations of Na^+ and K^+ in aqueous are inverse to those in lens (10× as much Na^+ in aqueous as in lens)
Grows throughout life: weight at maturity is 3 × that at birth, anterior-posterior diameter increases from 3.5 mm at birth to 5 mm at matu-

rity, equatorial length increases from 6.4 mm at birth to 9.0 mm at maturity; also increase in curvature with greater refractive power

Refractive index: increase in lens curvature and thickness with age is offset by change in gradient of refractive index due to increased concentration of main intrinsic polypeptide; associated with increased brunescence, resulting in greater absorption of blue and violet wavelengths, as well as UV light (aiding in retinal protection)

Metabolism: anaerobic; 80% of glucose metabolized by glycolysis, 10% metabolized by pentose phosphate pathway, 5% reduced to sorbitol, and 5% converted to glucuronic acid; highest metabolic rate is in cortex; energy is required for ion transport and glutathione production

Lens fiber structure: fibers contain few intracellular organelles and no nuclei; appear hexagonal in cross section

Average lens power: at birth = 37 diopters (D), at age 2 years = 23 D, at adulthood = 20 D

Protective mechanisms against free radical damage and oxidation: glutathione peroxidase, superoxide dismutase, catalase, and vitamins C and E

Accommodation: parasympathetic fibers of CN 3

Generally accepted theory is that of von Helmholtz: ciliary muscle contraction causes zonules to relax, allowing the lens to become more spherical and increasing its focusing power; presbyopia is therefore due to loss of lens elasticity with age

Disorders

Congenital Anomalies

(see Chapter 5, Pediatrics/Strabismus)

Cataracts

Congenital Cataracts

(see Chapter 5, Pediatrics/Strabismus)

Acquired Cataracts

Classified by location or etiology

Cortical: lens fiber fragments, degenerated protein, liquefaction

Spokes and vacuoles: radial lines and dots

Mature: completely white

Hypermature: leakage of degenerated cortical material, wrinkled capsule; may have calcium deposits

Morgagnian: total liquefaction of lens cortex; nucleus floats freely within capsule; lens material can leak through intact capsule

Pathology: hydropic swelling of lens fibers; morgagnian globules (eosinophilic, globular material between lens fibers)

Figure 10-4. Cortical cataract. (From Collin J: The morphology and visual effects of lens opacities. In Yanoff M, Duker JS [eds]: *Ophthalmology*, London, Mosby, 1999.)

Figure 10-5. Morgagnian cataract. (From Collin J: The morphology and visual effects of lens opacities. In Yanoff M, Duker JS [eds]: *Ophthalmology*, London, Mosby, 1999.)

Nuclear sclerosis: increased nuclear density, then opacification occurs with aging; lenticular myopia results from increased index of refraction; "second sight" (presbyopes can often read again without spectacles)

Cataract brunescens (poor blue discrimination), cataract nigrans, calcium oxalate crystals in nucleus

Pathology: inwardly sequestered lens fibers degenerate (analogous to desquamating skin); homogenous loss of cellular laminations

Posterior subcapsular (PSC): posterior migration of lens epithelium, and bladder (Wedl) cell formation (eosinophilic globular cells with nuclei; swell to 5–6 × normal size)

Etiology: age, trauma, steroids, inflammation, ionizing radiation, retinitis pigmentosa, atopic dermatitis, Werner's syndrome, Rothmund's syndrome, diabetes

Symptoms: glare and poor vision from bright lights; affects near vision more than distance vision

Pathology: posterior migration of lens epithelial cells, which swell along posterior capsule (swollen cells are called Wedl cells)

Anterior subcapsular (ASC): fibrous plaque beneath folded anterior capsule, secreted by irritated metaplastic anterior epithelial cells (due to trauma or uveitis)

Pathology: cells surrounded by basement membrane

Glaukomflecken: necrosis of lens epithelial cells due to ischemia from elevated IOP (angle closure); appears as central subcapsular small white dots and flecks

Traumatic and toxic cataracts:

Contusion: petalliform or rosette pattern due to separation of lens fibers around lens sutures

Vossius' ring: with blunt injury, pigment from pupillary ruff is imprinted onto anterior lens capsule

Soemmering's ring: doughnut of residual equatorial cortex; after cataract surgery or trauma; can be associated with an adherent leukoma

Siderosis lentis: iron deposits in lens epithelium; anterior subcapsular orange deposits; photoreceptor and RPE degeneration resulting in pigmentary retinopathy with peripheral visual field loss; iris heterochromia (involved iris darker)

Chalcosis lentis: copper deposits in lens capsule; green discoloration of anterior lens capsule and cortex in petaloid configuration occurs in Wilson's disease, forming a sunflower cataract; also Kayser-Fleischer ring (copper deposition in peripheral Descemet's membrane); can also occur in multiple myeloma and lung carcinoma

Other intraocular foreign bodies: gold, silver, platinum, aluminum are inert; lead and zinc may cause mild nongranulomatous reaction

COPPER: if concentration ≥85%, an acute inflammatory reaction occurs; if concentration between 70% and 85%, chalcosis develops; lesser concentrations are relatively inert

Mercurial lentis: mercury deposits in lens capsule (occupational)

Electrical: lens vacuoles in anterior midperiphery; linear opacities (stellate pattern) in anterior subcapsular cortex; burns >200 volts cause conjunctival hyperemia, iritis, hyphema, iris atrophy, sphincter changes

Argon laser: blue light absorbed by yellow sclerotic nucleus

Nonionizing radiation: infrared causes true exfoliation (glassblower's cataract) with splitting and scrolling of anterior lens capsule; ultraviolet produces nuclear sclerosis

Ionizing radiation: a threshold level of radiation is required to induce cataract development (PSC)

Medications:

CORTICOSTEROIDS: PSC from long-term use of any form of steroids, most commonly topical; develop in 33% of patients on long-term daily dose of 10 mg; also associated with inhaled steroids

MIOTICS: echothiophate iodide and demecarium bromide cause anterior subcapsular vacuoles in adults (not children)

PHENOTHIAZINES AND AMIODARONE: pigmented deposits in anterior lens capsule; axial, spoke-like configuration; dose and duration dependent

BUSULFAN: PSC

Cataracts associated with systemic disease:

Atopic dermititis: ASC shield–like plaque

Also associated with chronic keratoconjunctivitis, keratoconus, vernal keratoconjunctivitis

Diabetes: osmotic cataract due to high glucose levels and aldose reductase, which results in high sorbitol levels

Snowflake cataract (punctate white subcapsular opacities) can occur rapidly with high blood sugar

Myotonic dystrophy (AD): Mapped to chromosome 19

FINDINGS: characteristic presenile "Christmas tree" cataract consisting of polychromatic cortical crystals; ptosis, lid lag, light-near dissociation, mild pigmentary retinopathy; ERG—low voltage

OTHER FINDINGS: myotonia (bilateral facial weakness, difficulty relaxing grip, muscle wasting), testicular atrophy, frontal baldness, cardiac abnormalities, mental retardation; excessive contractility of muscles

Neurofibromatosis type 2: presenile PSC opacities

Werner's syndrome: syndrome of premature aging, scleroderma-like matting of skin, and bilateral cataracts in 3rd to 4th decade of life

Wilson's disease (hepatolenticular degeneration): deficiency of ceruloplasmin (alpha-2 globulin)

FINDINGS: green sunflower cataract due to deposition of copper in anterior lens capsule and cortex in petaloid configuration; Kayser-Fleischer ring (copper in peripheral Descemet's membrane)

OTHER FINDINGS: cirrhosis, renal impairment, degeneration of basal ganglia

TREATMENT: penicillamine to lower serum copper

Lens Capsule Abnormalities

True Exfoliation

Delamination/schisis of anterior lens capsule, forming scrolls; often due to infrared radiation (glassblowers), can be an aging change; not associated with glaucoma

Pseudoexfoliation Syndrome (PXS)

Material produced by lens epithelial cells and extruded through lens capsule

Appears to be an ocular sign of systemic elastosis; also found in conjunctiva, skin, lung, and liver

Usually elderly, Caucasian females; increased incidence in Scandinavians and with increasing age

Findings: white fibrillar material on anterior lens capsule, iris, ciliary body, zonules, anterior vitreous with characteristic pattern of deposition on lens surface (central disc, clear zone, then peripheral annulus, often with bridging strands to central disc); may see flakes on pupillary margin; Sampaolesi's line (pigment band anterior to Schwalbe's line) on gonioscopy; 10% develop glaucoma (PXG); poor dilation due to iris muscle degeneration or lack of iris stromal elasticity; peripupillary trans-illumination defects; weak zonules (increased incidence of complications during and after cataract surgery [vitreous loss, IOL and capsular dislocation])

Posterior Capsular Opacification (PCO; Secondary Cataract)

Proliferation of residual lens epithelial cells (Elschnig's pearls) and fibrosis

Incidence: up to 50% of patients within 2 years of extracapsular cataract surgery; influenced by optic material (acrylic < silicone < PMMA) and edge design (square edge < round edge); with newer IOLs, the incidence has decreased to <10%. Incidence approaches 100% in children and patients with uveitis

Treatment: Nd:YAG laser posterior capsulotomy when visually significant

  In young children, primary posterior capsulotomy and anterior vitrectomy are performed at the time of cataract surgery

Ectopia Lentis

Displacement of lens

Subluxation: partial displacement, remains in pupillary axis

Dislocation (luxation): complete displacement from pupil

Findings: decreased vision, astigmatism, monocular diplopia, iridodonesis, phacodenesis, malpositioned lens

DDx: trauma (most common acquired cause), Marfan's syndrome, homocystinuria, aniridia, congenital glaucoma, megalocornea, Ehlers-Danlos syndrome, hyperlysinemia, sulfite oxidase deficiency, hereditary ectopia lentis (AD ≫ AR; bilateral; may not present until 3rd to 5th decade), ectopia lentis et pupillae (AR; lens and pupil are displaced in opposite directions; bilateral, asymmetric), tertiary syphilis, Weill-Marchesani syndrome, medulloepithelioma, Stickler's syndrome, pseudoexfoliation (rare)

Marfan's Syndrome (AD)

Mapped to chromosome 15q; defect in fibrillin (elastic microfibrillar glycoprotein, major constituent of zonules); 15% have no family history

Findings: ectopia lentis (65%; usually superotemporal); glaucoma, keratoconus, cornea plana, axial myopia, retinal degeneration (salt and pepper fundus), high risk of retinal detachment

Other findings: tall stature, spidery digits, arm span is larger than height, cardiac disease, dissecting aneurysm of the aorta

Homocystinuria (AR)

Deficiency of cystathionine β-synthase, which converts homocysteine to cystathionine; methionine and homocysteine accumulate; zonules are deficient in cysteine and weakened because of reduced sulfhydryl cross-linkage; degeneration of entire zonule occurs

Findings: bilateral ectopia lentis (90%; usually inferonasal; 30% in infancy, 80% by age 15), enlarged globe, myopia, peripheral RPE degeneration, increased risk of retinal detachment after cataract surgery, early loss of accommodation due to disintegration of zonules

Other findings: blonde, tall (marfinoid habitus with arachnodactyly), osteoporosis, fractures, seizures, mental retardation (50%), cardiomegaly, platelet abnormality with hypercoagulability (risk of thromboembolic problems, especially with general anesthesia); infants appear normal at birth; 75% mortality by age 30 years

Hyperhomocystinemia occurs in patients heterozygous for homocystinemia: high serum homocysteine increases risk of arterial and venous thrombosis (CRAO and CVO) and cardiovascular disease, especially in type 2 diabetic patients. In nondiabetic patients younger than 55 years of age who have had a stroke or MI, 25% have elevated homocysteine levels (5% in normal population)

Diagnosis: increased urinary excretion of homocysteine (nitroprusside urine test), amino acid assays; check renal function (homocysteine levels rise with elevated creatinine levels); subnormal or low levels of folate are associated with elevated levels of homocysteine

Treatment: vitamin B_6 (folate), methionine-restricted diet, supplementary cysteine (this diet can reduce lens dislocation); certain medications (methotrexate, phenytoin, carbamazepine) can elevate homocysteine levels by interfering with folate metabolism

Weill-Marchesani Syndrome (AR)

Findings: ectopia lentis (usually inferiorly or anteriorly), microspherophakia, high lenticular myopia, cataract, microcornea, glaucoma (pupillary block)

Other findings: short stature; short, stubby fingers with broad hands; hearing defects; inflexible joints; mental retardation

Ehlers-Danlos Syndrome
(AD, AR, or X-Linked)

Defect in type III collagen; at least 9 types

Findings: ectopia lentis, easy lid eversion (Metenier's sign), epicanthal folds, myopia, microcornea, blue sclera, keratoconus, angioid streaks, retinal detachment

Other findings: hyperextensible joints and skin, poor wound healing, easy bruising

Sulfite Oxidase Deficiency (AR)

Enzymatic defect causing molybdenum deficiency and increased urinary sulfite

Findings: ectopia lentis (50%), enophthalmos, Brushfield's spots

Other findings: seizures, mental retardation, frontal bossing

Hyperlysinemia (AR)

Deficiency of lysine dehydrogenase

Findings: ectopia lentis, microspherophakia

Other findings: growth, motor and mental retardation

Surgery

Nd : YAG Laser

Posterior Capsulotomy

Open visually significant posterior capsule opacity

Power: 1.0 to 2.0 mJ; make an opening equal to the size of the pupil in ambient light

Treatment: pretreat with iopidine, then topical steroid qid × 1 week

Complications: increased IOP (glaucoma patients–17% have rise after 2 hours; 14% with high IOP at 1 week; nonglaucoma patients—6% have rise after 2 hours, 3% with high IOP at 1 week), retinal detachment (RD), cystoid macular edema (CME), rupture of the anterior hyaloid face, IOL dislocation, iritis, pitting of IOL, corneal or retinal burn

Vitreolysis

Disrupt anterior vitreous face in aphakic and pseudophakic eyes with malignant glaucoma
  Power: 3 to 11 mJ, focused on anterior hyaloid; deepening of anterior chamber signifies success
  Treatment: topical steroid qid × 1 week and cycloplegic; vitrectomy if regimen described here fails and in phakic eyes

Relieve CME due to vitreous wick
  Power: 5- to 10-mJ bursts, often best to aim near wound or pigmented area of incarcerated vitreous; success occurs with a change in the pupil shape back to round
  Treatment: pretreat with pilocarpine to induce miosis and stretch the strand, then topical steroid × 1 week

Cataract Surgery

Indications: altered vision (based on patient's functional impairment; when patient is having visual difficulty performing tasks and does not achieve adequate improvement from corrective lenses), also medical indications (phacolytic glaucoma, phacomorphic glaucoma, phacoantigenic uveitis, dense cataract that obscures view of fundus in patients who require regular retinal evaluation [ie, diabetes, glaucoma])

IOL Calculations (see Chapter 1, Optics)

Formulas: rough estimation, use IOL power (D) = A constant of IOL – 2.5 (axial length) – 0.9 (average keratometry)
  ACD (anterior chamber depth) approximately 3.5 mm
  First generation: ACD is constant
  Second generation: ACD is based on axial length (AL)
  Third generation (Holladay 1, Hoffer Q, SRK/T): ACD is based on AL and keratometry (K)
  Fourth generation (Holladay 2): variables include AL, K, corneal diameter, ACD, lens thickness, refraction, and patient age

Most accurate formulas according to axial length
  Long eyes (AL > 26.5 mm): SRK/T
  Medium-long eyes (AL 24.5–26.5 mm): Holladay 1
  Normal eyes (AL 22.0–24.5 mm): Hoffer Q, Holladay 1, SRK/T
  Short eyes (AL < 22.0 mm): Hoffer Q

A-scan: error of 0.1 mm = 0.3 D error in lens power; however, the shorter the axial length, the greater the effect of a measurement error

Myopia: 1.75 D error per mm of AL error

Emmetropia: 2.35 D error per mm of AL error

Hyperopia: 3.75 D error per mm of AL error

Ultrasound waves travel faster through lens (1640 m/sec) than either aqueous or vitreous (1532 m/sec)

To correct any AL, use the formula: $AL_{corrected} = AL_{measured} \times (V_{correct}/V_{measured})$

Average measurements:

Axial length: 23.5 mm (22.0–24.5 mm)

Keratometry: 43.0 to 44.0 D

Anterior chamber depth (ACD): 3.25 mm

Lens thickness: 4.6 mm

Ultrasound speeds:

PHAKIC EYE = 1550 m/sec

APHAKIC EYE = 1534 m/sec

PSEUDOPHAKIC EYE (depends on IOL material and thickness) = 1556 m/sec for PMMA lens, 1487 m/sec for silicone lens, and 1549 m/sec for acrylic lens

More accurate method for calculating pseudophakic AL is to measure at 1532 m/sec and to use correction factors:

PMMA: $AL_{corrected} = AL_{1532} + 44\%$ IOL thickness + 0.04

SILICONE: $AL_{corrected} = AL_{1532} - 56\%$ IOL thickness + 0.04

ACRYLIC: $AL_{corrected} = AL_{1532} + 75\%$ IOL thickness + 0.04

SILICONE OIL = 980 to 1040 m/sec (this is only for the portion of the eye containing silicone); thus to find the correct AL, the previous formula can be used, or the eye can be measured using an average velocity: phakic eye with silicone oil = 1140 m/sec

If silicone oil is to be left in the eye, the index of refraction of the oil will cause a hyperopic refraction; therefore, adjust the IOL power by adding 3.0 to 3.5 D

Immersion technique is more accurate than contact because of corneal compression (0.1–0.2 mm) for the later method

Contact A-scan: 5 spikes corresponding to beam reflection from interfaces: cornea, anterior lens surface, posterior lens surface, retina, sclera (Figure 10-6)

Causes of falsely long axial length:

Posterior staphyloma in high myopia; fovea may be located more anteriorly than the staphyloma

Measurement of the sclera rather than the retina

Wrong ultrasonic velocity (too fast)

Causes of falsely short axial length:

Excessive indentation of cornea with contact probe

Nonperpendicular measurement

Figure 10-6. A-scan pattern of a phakic eye with the initial spike removed from the screen display. Identified are the 2 corneal peaks (C1 and C2), the anterior lens spike (L1), the posterior lens spike (L2), and the retinal spike (R). (From Shammas HJ: Intraocular lens power calculations. In Azar DT [ed]: *Intraocular Lenses in Cataract and Refractive Surgery*, Philadelphia, WB Saunders, 2001.)

Choroidal thickening or effusion

Vitreous opacity

Keratometry in patient following refractive surgery: need to determine accurate central corneal curvature; keratometer measures at 3 mm from center of cornea

Methods:

CLINICAL HISTORY: K = preopK + (refraction preop – refraction postop)

Convert for vertex distance: refraction (corneal surface) = refraction (spectacle plane)/ (1–0.012 refraction [spectacle plane])

CONTACT LENS: use plano rigid gas-permeable contact lens with known base curve

K = base curve of CL + power + refraction (with CL) – refraction (without CL)

Convert for vertex distance

CORNEAL TOPOGRAPHY: use central 1 mm effective power reading from the Holladay diagnostic summary map (not sim K readings)

Presence of cataract may induce myopia, causing error in first method, and may cause poor vision with inability to perform adequate CL overrefraction; therefore, a variety of methods should be used, then take flattest K to use in IOL calculation and consider using a final IOL 1 to 2 D stronger to avoid a hyperopic result

Piggyback IOL

Hyperopia (1.5 D per 1.0 D of hyperopia): if patient is +6.00, place a +9.00 D piggyback IOL.

Myopia (1.0 D per 1.0 D of myopia): if patient is –6.00, place a –6.00 D piggyback IOL

Interface membranes have been reported between piggyback lenses

Viscoelastic Device (Ophthalmic Viscosurgical Device [OVD])

Variety of clear gel–like materials composed of sodium hyaluronate and chondroitin sulfate

Used intraocularly to maintain and preserve space, displace and stabilize tissue, and coat and protect corneal endothelium

Vary in molecular weight, viscosity, clarity, ease of removal, and potential for IOP spike if retained in eye (peak usually 4–6 hours postoperatively)

Classification:
  Cohesive agent (ability to adhere to itself): long-chain, high-molecular-weight, high surface tension (low coating capability), high degree of pseudoplasticity (ability to transform from high viscosity at rest [zero shear rate] to lower viscosity at high shear rate)
    ADVANTAGES: capsulorrhexis, insert IOL, ease of viscoelastic removal

  EXAMPLES: Healon™, Healon GV™, Amvisc™, Amvisc Plus™, Provisc™

  Dispersive agent: short-chain, low-molecular-weight, low surface tension (high coating ability), low to moderate pseudoplasticity
    ADVANTAGES: corneal coating, less IOP rise if retained, maintain space, move tissue

  EXAMPLES: Viscoat™, Vitrax™, Ocucoat™

  Viscoadaptive agent: ultrahigh-molecular-weight, superviscous and cohesive at low shear rates, more dispersive at increasing shear rates; thus combines the advantages of cohesive and dispersive agents

  EXAMPLE: Healon 5™

Phacodynamics

Irrigation: rate of fluid delivery; determined by bottle height above eye (34–110 cm); not adjusted by machine; depends on aspiration rate and wound leakage; maintains anterior chamber depth

Flow (aspiration rate [AFR]): rate of fluid removal (0–60 mL/min); determines how quickly vacuum is created; attracts material to tip

Vacuum (aspiration level): negative pressure created at tip by pump (0–500 mm Hg); holds material onto occluded tip

Pump systems:
  Flow-based: independent, direct control of AFR and vacuum; vacuum rise requires tip occlusion; physically contacts and regulates aspiration line fluid
    PERISTALTIC: rollers compress tubing; AFR not smooth because of peristaltic wave; less accurate, especially at higher vacuum levels
    SCROLL: scroll element orbits against housing; more accurate; can act clinically like Venturi pump
  Vacuum-based: direct control of vacuum only; AFR indirectly controlled by vacuum level; vacuum not affected by changes in tip occlusion; indirectly contacts aspiration line fluid by the induced vacuum in rigid drainage cassette between line and pump
    VENTURI: compressed air flows through tube; rapid, precise aspiration and vacuum response; requires external air supply
    DIAPHRAGM: flexible membrane moves like a piston; outmoded, large noisy system
    ROTARY VANE: wheel with vanes rotates; does not require external air supply
  Hybrid: programmable like peristaltic or Venturi

Vacuum rise time: time for vacuum to reach preset limit; affected by aspiration rate; requires tip occlusion with peristaltic pump

Postocclusion surge (vacuum rush): collapse of AC due to increase in aspiration rate to level of pump speed; during occlusion, vacuum builds to preset level, no flow occurs, and tubing collapses; when occlusion breaks, pump pulls fluid at preset rate and rebound of tubing pulls additional fluid through tip. Prevented by venting, rigid tubing, microprocessor in pump

Followability: ability to bring material to tip; function of flow and vacuum

Holdability: ability to keep material at tip; function of vacuum and power

Phaco power (0%–100%): depends on frequency and stroke length; surgeon (linear) or panel control; pushes material away from tip; generates heat.
  Power factors: amplitude (fixed vs linear) and duration (continuous vs intermittent)
  Power modulation: pulse, burst, bimodal, dual linear

Ultrasound effect:
  Fragmentation: mechanical (jackhammer effect)
  Cavitation: sound waves expand and compress liquid, creating shock wave and microbubbles, which implode, forming cavity and dissolving nucleus in front of needle tip

Ultrasound instrument:
  Handpiece: produces vibration of needle
    MAGNETORESTRICTIVE: converts magnetic energy into motion
    PIEZOELECTRIC CRYSTAL: converts electricity into motion
  Needle: oscillation produces phaco power

FREQUENCY: rate of oscillation (25–62 kHz)

STROKE LENGTH: distance of travel (0.002–0.004 inch)

BEVEL: occlusion vs cutting (0°–45°)

SHAPE: straight, angled

INNOVATIONS: microflow, microseal, aspiration bypass (ABS), flared

Footpedal: usual settings; can be programmed differently

KICK LEFT: reflux

POSITION 0: resting

POSITION 1: irrigation

POSITION 2: aspiration

POSITION 3: ultrasound

Audible clues:

METALLIC CLICK: irrigation (plunger opens)

HUMMING: aspiration

BUZZING: ultrasound (harmonic overtones)

BELLS: occlusion (no flow)

Customized tones

Alternative systems: Sonic, Fluid, Laser, Catarex, PhacoTmesis

Complications of Cataract Surgery

Preoperative (retrobulbar/peribulbar injection):
Globe perforation
Retrobulbar hemorrhage
Strabismus (inferior rectus fibrosis or myotoxicity)
Central anesthesia

Intraoperative:
Wound burn
Iris prolapse
Iris damage
Descemet's membrane detachment
Posterior capsular rupture
Retained material (nucleus, cortex)
Vitreous loss
Choroidal effusion
Suprachoroidal hemorrhage
Phototoxicity

Postoperative:
Wound leak
Inadvertent filtering bleb
Epithelial downgrowth
Corneal edema
Corneal melt
Secondary glaucoma
UGH syndrome
Sputtering hyphema (vascularization of posterior wound lip; malpositioned IOL)
Pupillary capture of IOL
IOL decentration
Capsular block syndrome
Anterior capsular contraction syndrome
Posterior capsular opacification (PCO)
Cystoid macular edema (CME)
Retinal detachment (RD)
Endophthalmitis
Mydriasis
Ptosis

Retrobulbar Hemorrhage

May occur following retrobulbar injection or trauma; risk of CRAO as orbital pressure rises

Findings: marked proptosis, rapid orbital swelling and congestion, limited extraocular motility, hemorrhagic chemosis, lid ecchymosis and edema

Treatment: consider emergent surgical decompression with lateral canthotomy and cantholysis, hyperosmotic agents to lower IOP

Strabismus

Due to inferior rectus damage

Paralysis or fibrosis result from anesthetic injection

Central Anesthesia Following Retrobulbar Block

Agent spreads along meningeal cuff of optic nerve to enter CSF

Increased risk with 4% lidocaine

Findings: mental confusion, dysphagia, dyspnea, apnea, amaurosis of fellow eye

Wound Burn

Thermal injury from phaco needle due to lack of irrigation

Etiology: excessively tight incision, low or empty infusion bottle, low-flow settings, occluded phaco tip (with dispersive viscoelastic agent or impaled nucleus), phaco needle without thermal protective design

Findings: wound whitening, distortion, and astigmatism

Treatment: scleral relaxing incision, horizontal suture, bandage contact lens; if severe, may require astigmatic surgery after stabilization or patch graft

Iris Prolapse During Phaco

Wound too large or too posterior, bottle too high, posterior pressure, suprachoroidal hemorrhage

Descemet's Membrane Detachment

Due to inadvertent stripping of Descemet's from instrument insertion during surgery or viscoelastic injection; causes corneal edema or decompensation

Treatment: air or gas bubble, may require suture repair

Expulsive Suprachoroidal Hemorrhage

May occur during intraocular surgery or days later; incidence of 0.5%

Risk factors: elderly patient, hypertension, atherosclerosis, diabetes, sudden drop in IOP during surgery, high myopia, vitreous loss or previous vitrectomy, previous expulsive hemorrhage in fellow eye, glaucoma, aphakia, postoperative Valsalva maneuver

Findings: forward movement of intraocular contents during surgery and loss of red reflex (ominous sign), subretinal hemorrhage, choroidal detachment, and extrusion of intraocular contents; delayed hemorrhage presents with severe eye pain, nausea, vomiting, and rapid loss of vision

Treatment: close wound rapidly; may require surgical drainage

Prevention: decompress eye preoperatively, small wound, control BP during surgery, prevent bucking in patients under general anesthesia

Phototoxicity

Occurs in up to 39% for surgical time >100 minutes

Prevention: dim light, oblique light, pupil shield

Corneal Edema

Etiology: trauma to endothelium, elevated IOP, endothelial chemical toxicity, Descemet's detachment, decompensation in patient with Fuchs' corneal endothelial dystrophy

Corneal Ulceration and Melting

Occurs most commonly after cataract surgery in patients with keratoconjunctivitis sicca and rheumatoid arthritis; melting several weeks after uncomplicated cataract surgery due to collagenase release from surrounding inflammatory cells

Uveitis-Glaucoma-Hyphema (UGH) Syndrome

Due to repeated trauma to angle structures and iris by IOL; scarring and degeneration occur

Treatment: atropine, topical steroids, ocular hypotensive medications; consider argon laser of bleeding site; usually requires IOL explantation

Hyphema

Result of fine neovascularization of incision (Swan syndrome) or mechanical trauma from IOL haptics

Occurs with more posteriorly located incisions

IOP can become dangerously elevated

Pupillary Capture

Portion of IOL optic anterior to iris

Risk factors: large or incomplete capsulorrhexis, sulcus haptic placement, nonangulated IOL, upside-down IOL placement, vitreous pressure

Treatment: observe if long-standing and stable without symptoms; dilate and place patient supine if occurs early postoperatively; may require lens repositioning with microhook

IOL Decentration

Causes diplopia or polyopia because of prismatic effect

Sunset syndrome: inferior displacement of IOL within capsular bag; occurs with unrecognized zonular dialysis, capsular tears, or asymmetric IOL haptic implantation (1 in bag and other in sulcus)

Sunrise syndrome: asymmetric IOL haptic placement

Treatment: consider pilocarpine; IOL repositioning or exchange may be required

Capsular Block Syndrome

Due to retained viscoelastic behind IOL

Causes myopic shift

Treatment: Nd:YAG laser anterior capsulotomy

Anterior Capsular Contraction Syndrome (Capsular Phimosis)

Due to small capsulorrhexis with retention of lens epithelial cells

Treatment: Nd:YAG laser radial anterior capsulotomies

CME (Irvine-Gass Syndrome)

More common with intracapsular (ICCE) than extracapsular cataract extraction (ECCE)

50% angiographically for ICCE vs 15% for ECCE

Clinically significant (visual loss) in <1% of patients with ECCE

Risk factors: capsular rupture, dislocated IOL, iris-supported IOL, iris tuck, vitreous adhesion to pupil or wound

FA: petalloid hyperfluorescence, late leakage; late staining of optic nerve helps to differentiate postoperative CME from other forms of CME

Treatment: topical steroid and NSAID, consider posterior sub-Tenon's steroid injection with kenalog

Endophthalmitis

(see Chapter 8, Uveitis)

Rhegmatogenous Retinal Detachment

Incidence: 1% to 2%

Risk factors: high myopia, lattice degeneration, history of RD in fellow eye, vitreous loss

Mydriasis

Due to sphincter damage (mechanical from iris stretching or ischemic from elevated IOP)

Ptosis

Due to trauma from lid speculum

Review Questions *(Answers start on page 366)*

1. The most helpful test for evaluating macular function in a patient with advanced cataract is
   a. blue field entoptic phenomenon
   b. 2-light separation
   c. red-light discrimination
   d. directional light projection

2. Ectopia lentis is least likely to be associated with
   a. cleft palate
   b. pectus excavatum
   c. short stature
   d. mental retardation

3. Anterior segment signs of ciliary body melanoma include all of the following except
   a. corneal edema
   b. increased IOP
   c. astigmatism
   d. cataract

4. Which of the following is least characteristic of ICE syndrome?
   a. corneal edema
   b. increased IOP
   c. ectropion uveae
   d. PAS

5. The crystalline lens is formed from which embryologic tissue?
   a. neural crest
   b. ectoderm
   c. mesoderm
   d. endoderm

6. A stellate anterior subcapsular cataract is most likely to be found in a patient with
   a. Fabry's disease
   b. atopic dermatitis
   c. myotonic dystrophy
   d. electrical injury

7. The most useful diagnostic test in an infant with an oil-droplet cataract is
   a. urine amino acids
   b. calcium
   c. TORCH titers
   d. urine reducing substances

8. Which of the following does not occur in siderosis bulbi?
   a. glaucoma
   b. retinal atrophy
   c. sunflower cataract
   d. fixed pupil

9. A patient has a history of increased IOP with exercise; which finding is associated with this condition?
   a. Krukenberg's spindle
   b. PAS
   c. phacodenesis
   d. pars plana snowbank

10. Separation between the longitudinal and circumferential fibers of the ciliary muscle is called
    a. iridoschisis
    b. angle recession
    c. iridodialysis
    d. cyclodialysis

11. Characteristics of pigment dispersion syndrome include all of the following except
    a. increased IOP with exercise
    b. Krukenberg's spindle
    c. phacodenesis
    d. radial iris transillumination defects

12. Genetics of aniridia are best summarized as
    a. 1/3 AR, 2/3 AD
    b. 1/3 sporadic, 2/3 AR
    c. 1/3 AD, 2/3 sporadic
    d. 1/3 sporadic, 2/3 AD

13. Blood in Schlemm's canal is not associated with
    a. Fuchs' heterochromic iridocyclitis
    b. thyroid-related ophthalmopathy
    c. hypotony
    d. Sturge-Weber syndrome

14. A sickle cell patient with a hyphema develops increased IOP; which of the following treatment choices is best?
    a. pilocarpine
    b. Diamox
    c. hyperosmotic
    d. timoptic

15. A pigmentary retinopathy occurs in which mesodermal dysgenesis syndrome?
    a. Axenfeld's anomaly
    b. Alagille's syndrome
    c. Rieger's syndrome
    d. Peter's anomaly

16. Of the following causes of iris heterochromia, the involved iris is hyperchromic in

a. ICE syndrome
b. Horner's syndrome
c. Waardenburg's syndrome
d. Fuchs' heterochromic iridocyclitis

17. Which of the following iris lesions is a true tumor?
    a. Kunkmann-Wolffian body
    b. Koeppe nodule
    c. Lisch nodule
    d. juvenile xanthogranuloma

18. At which location is the lens capsule thinnest?
    a. anterior capsule
    b. posterior capsule
    c. equatorial capsule
    d. anterior paracentral capsule

19. The iris sphincter is derived from what embryologic tissue?
    a. neural crest cells
    b. surface ectoderm
    c. neural ectoderm
    d. mesoderm

20. Which of the following is not associated with sunset syndrome?
    a. asymmetric IOL haptic placement
    b. polyopia
    c. pseudoexfoliation
    d. hyphema

SUGGESTED READINGS

Abelson MB: Allergic Diseases of the Eye. Philadelphia, WB Saunders, 2001.

American Academy of Ophthalmology: Lens and Cataract, vol 11. San Francisco, AAO, 2004.

Boruchoff SA: Anterior Segment Disorder: A Diagnostic Color Atlas. Boston, Butterworth-Heinemann, 2001.

Elander RE, Rich LF, Robin JB: Principles and Practice of Refractive Surgery. Philadelphia, WB Saunders, 1997.

Jaffe NS, Jaffe MS, Jaffe GF: Cataract Surgery and Its Complications, 6th edition. St. Louis, Mosby, 1997.

Mackie IA: External Eye Disease. Boston, Butterworth-Heinemann, 2003.

Watson P, Hazleman B, Pavesio C: Sclera and Systemic Disorders. Philadelphia, Butterworth-Heinemann, 2003.

CHAPTER 11

Posterior Segment

ANATOMY

Vitreous

Figures 11-1 and 11-2

Composed of 99% water and a few collagen fibers; viscous, gel-like quality from mucopolysaccharide and hyaluronic acid that is folded into coiled chains and holds water like a sponge; volume ~4 cm³; syneresis (liquefaction) occurs with aging

Vitreous base: portion of vitreous that attaches to peripheral retina and pars plana; width of 6 mm; straddles ora serrata; avulsion is pathognomonic for trauma

Vitreoretinal junctions: arise from footplates of Müller's cells at internal limiting membrane; provide firm vitreoretinal attachment, especially at vitreous base, macula, optic nerve, and retinal vessels; also at edge of lattice degeneration, chorioretinal scars, degenerative remodeling, enclosed oral bays; weak attachments at fovea and disc, and over areas of lattice

Retina (Figure 11-3)

Neurosensory Retina (9 Layers)

1. **Internal limiting membrane** (ILM): foot processes of Müller's cells (PAS-positive basement membrane); true basement membrane; clinically visible as small yellow-white spots (Gunn's dots) at ora serrata; continuous with inner bordering membrane of ciliary body

2. **Nerve fiber layer** (NFL): unmyelinated ganglion cell axons; also contains glial cells (astrocytes); myelination by oligodendrites occurs at lamina cribrosa; axons synapse with nuclei of cells in LGB

3. **Ganglion cell layer**: usually a single cell layer with cells packed tightly near the optic disc and more scattered in the periphery; nuclei are multilayered in macula

4. **Inner plexiform layer**: synaptic processes between bipolar and ganglion cells, as well as amacrine with bipolar cells; outermost layer completely nourished by retinal arteries

5. **Inner nuclear layer**: outermost retinal layer nourished by retinal vasculature, receives 33% of its nourishment from retinal arteries; contains cell bodies of bipolar, amacrine (confined to inner surface), horizontal (confined to outer surface), and Müller's (span from ILM [foot processes] to ELM [microvilli, which point toward RPE]) cells

6. **Outer plexiform layer**: synaptic processes between photoreceptors and dendritic processes of bipolar cells
   Middle limiting membrane: synapses; forms approximate border of vascular inner portion and avascular outer portion of the retina
   Central retinal artery supplies retina internally (MLM to ILM)
   Choriocapillaris supplies retina externally (MLM to RPE)

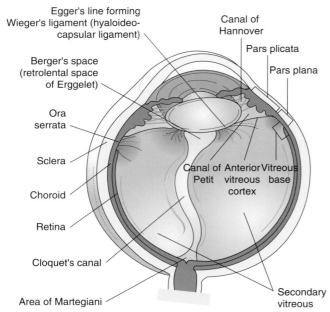

Figure 11-1. Vitreous anatomy according to classic anatomic and histologic studies. (From Schepens CL, Neetens A: *The Vitreous and Vitreoretinal Interface,* New York, Springer-Verlag, 1987.)

Figure 11-2. Ultrastructure of hyaluronan-collagen interaction in the vitreous. (Courtsey of Dr. Akiko Asakura. From Askura A: Histochemistry of hyaluronic acid of the bovine vitreous body as studied by electron micoscopy. *Acta Soc Ophthalmol Jpn* 89:179–191, 1985.)

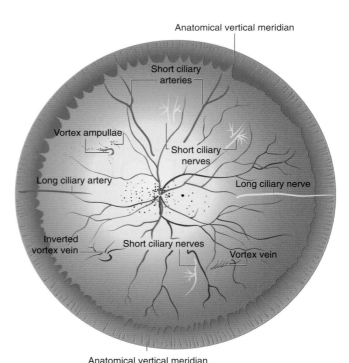

Figure 11-3. Normal fundus as seen through indirect ophthalmoscope. (A Manual for the Beginning Ophthalmology Resident. 3e, edited by James M. Richard. 1980, p. 122 Figure 60.)

Interior to MLM: dendrites of bipolar cells along with horizontally coursing processes of horizontal cells

External to MLM: basal aspect of photoreceptors
In macula, outer plexiform layer is called Henle's fiber layer; radial orientation of fibers (responsible for macular star configuration and cystic spaces in cystoid maular edema)

7. Outer nuclear layer: photoreceptor nuclei; most cone nuclei lie in single layer immediately internal to ELM

8. External limiting membrane (ELM): fenestrated intercellular bridges, situated external to photoreceptor nuclei; interconnects photoreceptor cells to Müller's cells; not a true basement membrane but an illusion caused by tight junctions between Müller's cells and photoreceptors

9. Photoreceptor layer: rods and cones; number equal in macula
　　120 million rods: rhodopsin; density maximal in a ring 20° to 40° around fovea; when dark adapted, rods are 1000 times more sensitive than cones
　　6 million cones (50% in macula): 3 types of visual pigment; density maximal in fovea (Figure 11-4)

Peripheral Retina

Extends from macula to ora serrata, nonpigmented epithelium is contiguous with pars plana; defined as any area of the retina with a single layer of ganglion cells (Figure 11-5)

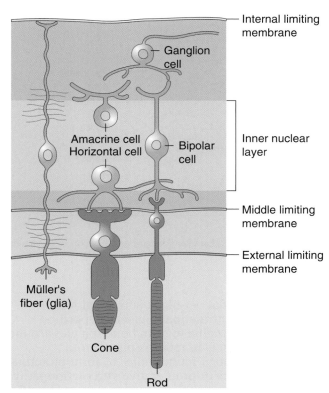

Figure 11-4. Neuronal connections in the retina and participating cells. (From Schubert HD: Structure and function of the neural retina. In Yanoff M, Duker JS [eds]: *Ophthalmology*, London, Mosby, 1999.)

Figure 11-5. Transition of neural retina to nonpigmented epithelium at the ora serrata. (From Schubert HD: Structure and function of the neural retina. In Yanoff M, Duker JS [eds]: *Ophthalmology*, London, Mosby, 1999.)

Macula

(Figures 11-6 and 11-7)

Area of retina in which ganglion cell layer is more than 1 cell thick (5–6 mm in diameter)

Centered 4 mm temporal and 0.8 mm inferior to optic nerve

Differentiation of the macula does not occur until age 4 to 6 months old

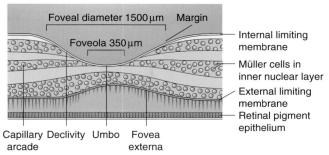

Figure 11-6. Foveal margin, foveal declivity, foveola, and umbo. (From Schubert HD: Structure and function of the neural retina. In Yanoff M, Duker JS [ed]: *Ophthalmology*, London, Mosby, 1999.)

Fovea

Central depression of inner retinal surface (1.5 mm in diameter) within macula

Corresponds to the macular avascular zone

Contains taller RPE cells and xanthophyll pigment

Initially, ganglion cell nuclei are present in fovea but are gradually displaced peripherally, leaving fovea devoid of accessory neural elements

Foveola

Central area of fovea (350 μm in diameter)

Absence of ganglion cells and other nucleated cells; avascular

Mechanisms to prevent foveal detachment:
  Microvilli of RPE, which surround tips of photoreceptors
  Viscous mucopolysaccharides, which bathe photoreceptors and RPE
  Intraocular pressure

Intercellular Junctions

Blood-retinal barrier:
  Inner barrier: tight junctions (zonula occludens) between retinal vascular endothelial cells
  Outer barrier: tight junctions between RPE cells

Other intercellular junctions:
  Zonula adherens (external limiting membrane): no barrier to passage of fluids
  Macula adherens (desmosomes): no barrier to passage of fluids

Clinical Correlation

Collateral vessels: occur at site of obstruction, across horizontal raphe, and at disc

Hemorrhages:
  Flame or splinter: superficial; blood tracks along NFL
  Blot or dot: deep; blood confined by axons oriented perpendicular to Bruch's membrane

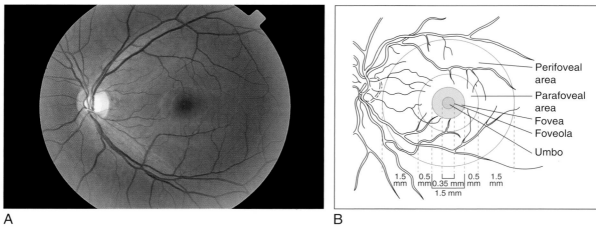

Figure 11-7. Normal fundus with macula encompassed by major vascular arcades. (From Schubert HD: Structure and function of the neural retina. In Yanoff M, Duker JS [eds]: *Ophthalmology*, London, Mosby, 1999.)

Boat-shaped (scaphoid):
  SUB-ILM: hemorrhagic detachment of ILM
  SUB-HYALOID: blood between ILM and posterior hyaloid
Dark hemorrhage: sub-RPE; can be confused with choroidal melanoma

RPE

Monolayer of hexagonal cells with apical microvilli and basement membrane at base

RPE and outer segments of photoreceptors have apex-to-apex arrangement, resulting in a potential subretinal space

Functions:
  Helps with development of photoreceptors during embryogenesis
  Involved in vitamin A cycle (uptake, transport, storage, metabolism, and isomerization)
  Provides nourishment for outer half of retinal cells
  Receives waste products: phagocytoses photoreceptor outer segments; photoreceptors renew outer segments every 10 days
  Forms outer blood-retinal barrier (tight junctions between RPE cells)
  Secretes basement membrane material (deposits on inner basal lamina of Bruch's membrane)
  Produces melanin granules in 6th week of gestation (first cells of body to melanize); melanization may induce further differentiation of retinal layers (may explain why macula fails to develop properly in albinism); melanin helps absorb excess light; macular RPE cells contain larger and a greater number of melanosomes than those in periphery
  Contributes to adhesion of sensory retina
  ATP-dependent Na^+/K^+ pump on apical surface maintains environment of subretinal space

RPE cells may undergo hypertrophy, hyperplasia, migration, and metaplasia

Hypertrophy: flat, jet-black subretinal lesion
Hyperplasia: intraretinal pigment deposition
  Migrate into retina to form bone spicules around blood vessels in retinitis pigmentosa
  Migrate through retinal holes to form preretinal membranes in proliferative vitreoretinopathy
Metaplasia: nonspecific reaction, observed most often in phthisis; fibrous (component of disciform scars in ARMD) or osseous (intraocular ossification)

Bruch's Membrane

Permeable to small molecules

5 layers:
  1. Basement membrane (inner basal lamina of RPE)
  2. Collagen
  3. Elastic tissue
  4. Collagen
  5. Basement membrane (outer basal lamina of choriocapillaris)

RPE and Bruch's membrane are continuous with the pigmented ciliary epithelium

Neuroglial Cells

Astrocytes: branching neural cells in retina and CNS; proliferation leads to gliosis; cell of origin for optic nerve glioma; provide structural support to optic nerve and retina; contribute to nourishment of neuronal elements; foot processes ensheath blood vessels within nerve, contributing to blood-brain barrier

Müller's cells: modified astrocytes; footplates form ILM, nuclei in inner nuclear layer; provide skeletal support; contribute to gliosis; extend from ILM to ELM

Microglia: phagocytic cells of the CNS

Figure 11-8. Human choriocapillaris, retinal view. (From Fryczkowski AW: Anatomical and functional choroidal lobuli. *Int Ophthalmol* 18:131–141, 1994.)

Arachnoidal cells: cell of origin for meningioma

Oligodendrocytes: produce myelin in the CNS; cell of origin for oligodendroglioma

Schwann cells: produce myelin in peripheral nervous system

Choroid

Attached to sclera at optic nerve, scleral spur, vortex veins, and long and short posterior ciliary vessels

4 layers:
1. Bruch's membrane
2. Choriocapillaris
3. Stroma
4. Suprachoroidal space

Blood supply from posterior ciliary arteries

Endothelium is permeable to large molecules

Choriocapillaris arranged in segmental pattern; major source of nutrition for RPE and outer retinal layers (Figure 11-8)

PHYSIOLOGY

Visual pigments: 4 types, each composed of 11-cis-retinal (vitamin A aldehyde) + a protein (opsin)
3 cone pigments and 1 rod pigment (Table 11-1)

Rod photoreceptor membranes: lipid bilayer in which rhodopsin is an integral component

Chromophore 11-cis-retinaldehyde is oriented parallel to the lipid bilayer (perpendicular to the path of photons)

Bleaching releases all-*trans*-retinaldehyde from the visual pigment (opsin) with conversion to all-*trans*-retinol; this initiates an electrical impulse that travels to visual cortex; rhodopsin is then resynthesized, and vitamin A is stored in liver and transported to RPE by serum retinol–binding protein and prealbumin

Rods shed outer segments during the day

Cones shed outer segments during the night

Luminosity curves:
  Light-adapted: cone peak sensitivity is to light of 555 nm; yellow, yellow-green, and orange appear brighter than blue, green, and red
  Dark-adapted: rod peak sensitivity is to light of 505 nm (blue)
  Purkinje shift: shift in peak sensitivity that occurs from light- to dark-adapted states

Table 11-1. **Visual Pigments**

Photoreceptor	Pigment	Peak Sensitivity
Rod	Rhodopsin	505 nm
Red cones	Erythrolabe	575 nm
Green cones	Chlorolabe	545 nm
Blue cones	Cyanolabe	445 nm

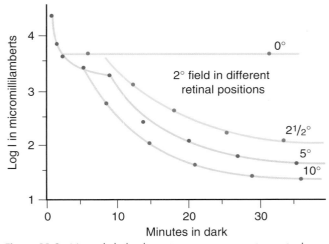

Figure 11-9. Normal dark-adaptation curves measuring retinal sensitivity to a small spot of light whose intensity is varied until the threshold value is found; a 2° test spot was placed at different distances from the foveal center. Note the cone-rod break at 9 minutes, middle graph. (From Hecht S, Haig C, Wald G: The dark adaptation of retinal fields of different size and location. *J Gen Physiol* 19:321–337, 1935.)

ELECTROPHYSIOLOGY

Electroretinogram (ERG)

Measures mass retinal response; useful for processes affecting large areas of retina

Photoreceptors, bipolar and Müller's cells contribute to flash ERG; ganglion cells do not

Light is delivered uniformly to entire retina, and electrical discharges are measured with a corneal contact lens electrode

Components: (Figure 11-10)

a-wave: photoreceptor cell bodies (negative waveform)

b-wave: Müller's and bipolar cells (positive waveform)

Amplitude: bottom of a-wave to top of b-wave; measured in microvolts

Measures response of entire retina; proportionate to area of functioning retina

Decreased in anoxic conditions (diabetes, CRAO, ischemic CVO)

Implicit time: time from light flash to peak of b-wave; measured in milliseconds

Increased in various hereditary conditions

Oscillatory potential: wavelets on ascending b-wave of scotopic and photopic bright flash ERG

Generated in middle retinal layers (inner plexiform layer): may be inhibitory potentials from amacrine cells

Reduced in conditions of retinal hypoxia or microvascular disease

c-wave: RPE; late (2–4 seconds) positive deflection; occurs in dark-adapted state

Early receptor potential (ERP): outer segments of photoreceptors; completed within 1.5 msec

Represents bleaching of visual pigment; requires intense stimulus in dark-adapted state (Figure 11-11)

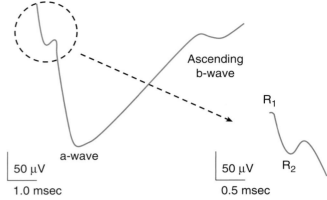

Figure 11-11. Normal human early receptor potential (ERP). This rapid response is complete within 1.5 msec and is believed to be generated by the outer segments. An intense, bright stimulus in the dark-adapted state is needed for an ERP to be obtained. (Redrawn from Berson EL, Goldstein EG: Early receptor potential in dominantly inherited retinitis pigmentosa. *Arch Ophthalmol* 83:412–420, 1970. From Samovits TL: *Basic and Clinical Science Course: Section 12: Orbit, Eyelids, and Lacrimal System.* San Francisco, American Academy of Ophthalmology, 1993.)

Ganglion cells are not measured; therefore, flash ERG is not useful in glaucoma

Photopic (light adapted): measures cone funtion; light adapted to bleach out rods

Flicker ERG: flashing light at 30 flashes/sec isolates cone response

Small wave follows each flash

Cone response because rods cannot recycle rhodopsin this quickly

Poor response at 30 cycles/sec indicates abnormal cone function; rods can respond up to 20 Hz

Cones also respond to repetitive light

Scotopic (dark adapted): measures rod function; dark adapted for 30 min

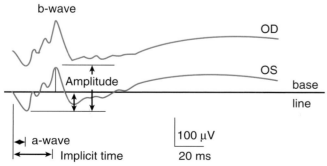

Figure 11-10. The photopic (cone-mediated) ERG is a light-adapted, bright flash–evoked response from the cones of the retina; the rods do not respond in the light-adapted state. (From Slamovits TL: *Basic and Clinical Science Course: Section 12: Orbit, Eyelids, and Lacrimal System.* San Francisco, American Academy of Ophthalmology, 1993.)

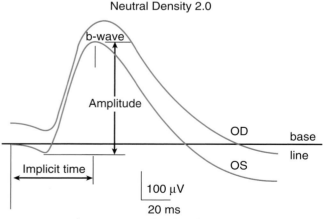

Figure 11-12. The scotopic (rod-mediated) ERG is a dark-adapted, dim flash (below cone threshold)–evoked response that records the signal from the rods. The test should be performed after at least 30 minutes of dark adaptation. (From Slamovits TL: *Basic and Clinical Science Course: Section 12: Orbit, Eyelids, and Lacrimal System.* San Francisco, American Academy of Ophthalmology, 1993. In Yanoff M, Duker JS [eds]: *Ophthalmology.* London, Mosby, 1999.)

Dim white or blue flash below cone threshold

At low intensity: small a- and b-waves

At increasing intensity: implicit time shortens, b-wave amplitude increases

Bright-flash ERG (in scotopic state; measures combined maximal rod and cone response): deep a-wave and large b-wave; oscillatory potentials are present (Figure 11-13)

Indications:

Diagnose generalized retinal degeneration

Assess family members for heritable retinal degeneration

Assess decreased vision and nystagmus present at birth

Assess retinal function in presence of opaque ocular media or vascular occlusion

Evaluate functional visual loss

Disease states: (Figure 11-14 and Table 11-2)

CRAO: normal a-wave (perfused by choroid), absent b-wave

Ischemic CVO: reduced b-wave amplitude, reduced b : a-wave ratio, prolonged b-wave implicit time

Retinitis pigmentosa: early, reduced amplitude (usually b-wave) and prolonged implicit time; later, extinguished with no rod or cone response to bright flash

Female carriers of X-linked RP: prolonged photopic b-wave implicit time, reduced scotopic b-wave amplitude

Sector RP: normal b-wave implicit time

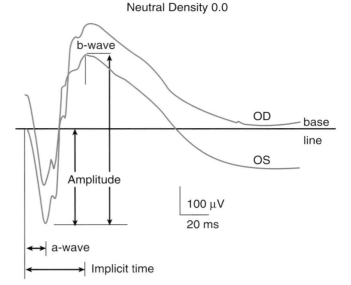

Figure 11-13. The bright flash, dark-adapted ERG stimulates both the cone and rod systems and gives large A and B waves, with oscillatory potentials in the ascending B wave. Some testing centers call this a "scotopic ERG," but the rods are not isolated by this method. (From Slamovits TL: *Basic and Clinical Science Course; Section 12: Orbit, Eyelids, and Lacrimal System.* San Francisco, American Academy of Ophthalmology, 1993. In Yanoff M, Duker JS [eds]: *Ophthalmology.* London, Mosby, 1999.)

Figure 11-14. Electroretinogram patterns. (From Samovits TL: *Basic and Clinical Science Course: Section 12: Orbit, Eyelids, and Lacrimal System.* San Francisco, American Academy of Ophthalmology, 1993.)

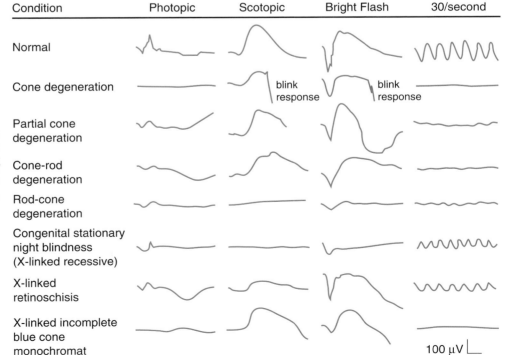

Table 11-2. **ERG Patterns for Various Ocular Diseases**

Extinguished ERG	Normal a-wave, Reduced b-wave	Abnormal Photopic, Normal Scotopic ERG
RP	CSNB; Oguchi's disease	Achromotopsia
Ophthalmic artery occlusion	X-linked juvenile retinoschisis	Cone dystrophy
DUSN	CVO	
Metallosis	CRAO	
RD	Myotonic dystrophy	
Drug toxicity (phenothiazine; chloroquine)	Quinine toxicity	
Cancer-associated retinopathy		

Cone dystrophy: abnormal photopic and flicker, normal scotopic

X-linked foveal retinoschisis: normal a-wave until late, reduced b-wave (especially scotopic)

Retinal detachment: reduction in amplitude corresponds to extent of neurosensory loss
50% decrease in amplitude = 50% of neurosensory retina is functionally detached

Diffuse progressive retinal disease: increased b-wave implicit time

Nonprogressive retinal disease: decreased b-wave amplitude

MEWDS: reduced a-wave

Chalcosis: reduced amplitude (suppressed by intraocular copper ions)

Retinal microvascular disease (diabetes, hypertension, CVO): loss of oscillatory potentials

Achromotopsia: absent cone function; normal rod function

Leber's congenital amaurosis: flat ERG

CSNB: normal a-wave, poor b-wave

Congenital rubella: normal ERG

Glaucoma: normal ERG

Optic neuropathy/atrophy: normal ERG

Pattern ERG (PERG): waveform similar to flash ERG, but different test to measure ganglion cell activity; stimulus is an alternating checkerboard pattern that gives a constant illumination to the retina (Figure 11-15)
Normal response is composed of 3 waves:
N_{35}: cornea-negative wave at 35 msec
P_{50}: cornea-positive wave peak at 50 msec
N_{95}: negative trough at 95 msec

Electro-oculogram (EOG) (Figure 11-16)

Indirect measure of standing potential of eye (voltage difference between inner and outer retina)

Depolarization of basal portion of RPE produces light peak; normal result requires that both RPE and sensory retina be normal

Figure 11-15. Pattern ERG with components labeled. This waveform measures retinal ganglion cell function and is not related to the flash ERG test. (After Treat GL: The pattern electroretinogram in glaucoma and ocular hypertension. In Heckenlively JR, Arden GB [eds]: *Principles and Practice of Clinical Electrophysiology of Vision*. St. Louis, Mosby-Yearbook, 1991.)

Arden ratio: ratio of light-to-dark peak (2 : 1 is normal; <1.65 is abnormal); decreased ratio is due to photoreceptor or RPE disorder

Procedure: light adapt, dark adapt × 20 min, light adapt × 10 min
Dark adaptation causes progressive decrease in response reaching a trough at 8 to 12 minutes
Light adaptation causes progressive rise in amplitude over 6 to 9 minutes
Measure lowest voltage with dark adaptation and highest voltage with light adaptation
Amplitude is higher with light adaptation than dark adaptation

ERG is abnormal in all cases in which EOG is abnormal except:
Best's disease and carriers: normal ERG but abnormal EOG

Figure 11-16. Diagram illustrating technique used in recording the electro-oculogram test; the patient is positioned so that the eyes will traverse a 30° arc between 2 blinking red lights. The skin electrodes are positioned at the lateral and inner canthi. The standing potential is measured as the patient moves his eyes between the lights, first in the dark and then in the light. The maximum amplitude from the light condition is compared with minimum value from the dark to give a light peak-to-dark trough ratio. (From Heckenlively JR: *Retinitis Pigmentosa.* Philadelphia, JB Lippincott, 1988.)

Viewing screen

(Background is lighted second half of test)

← 30° arc →

$$\text{Arden ratio} = \frac{\text{Largest potential in light}}{\text{Lowest potential in dark}} \times 100$$

Tracing of standing potential in dark

Tracing of standing potential light-adapted

Recorder

OD

OS

←12 min→   ←12 min→

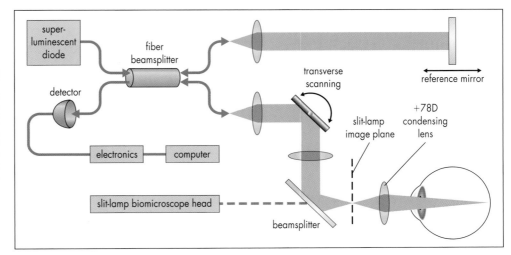

Figure 11-17. Optical coherence tomography principle. (Adapted from Shuman JS, Hee MR, Puliafito CA et al: Quantification of nerve fiber layer thickness in normal and glaucomatous eyes using optical coherence tomography. *Arch Ophthalmol* 113:586–596, 1995; from Yanoff M, Duker JS [eds]: *Ophthalmology.* London, Mosby, 1999.)

super-luminescent diode

fiber beamsplitter

detector

transverse scanning

reference mirror

slit-lamp image plane

+78D condensing lens

electronics   computer

slit-lamp biomicroscope head

beamsplitter

Pattern dystrophies
Chloroquine toxicity

Abnormal ERG, normal EOG: conditions with abnormal bipolar region but normal rods

 CSNB
 X-linked retinoschisis

RETINAL IMAGING

Optical Coherence Tomography (OCT)

Creates cross-sectional image of retina

Provides retinal thickness measurements and cross-sectional retinal imaging to ~10 µm

Diode mounted on slit lamp fires beam of infrared light through fiberoptic Michelson interferometer at both the eye and a reference mirror; the reflected light from the retina is compared with the light from the reference mirror and analyzed so that the tissue reflectivity (similar to ultrasound) and density can be determined

Useful for macular pathology (edema, hole, pucker); can compare thickness in cases of macular edema from one visit to next; can diagnose stage 1 macular hole vs full-thickness hole (≥stage 2) vs pseudohole, or lamellar holes (Figures 11-17 and 11-18)

Heidelberg Retinal Tomograph (HRT)

Laser tomography

Confocal scanning laser produces 3-dimensional sections of optic nerve and retina through undilated pupil

670-nm diode laser that is periodically deflected by oscillating mirrors; laser scans retina, and instrument measures reflectance and constructs series of 2-dimensional images at different depths, which are combined to create a multilayer 3D topographic image

Measures surface height to within 20 µm

A

B

Figure 11-18. Stage 2 macular hole. **A**, fundus photograph, **B**, OCT. (From Yanoff M, Duker JS [eds]: *Ophthalmology*. London, Mosby, 1999.)

Retinal Thickness Analyzer (RTA)

Creates thickness contour map

HeNe laser scans central 2 × 2 mm area; receives 2 reflections, 1 from ILM and 1 from RPE, then maps distance between these layers

Scanning Laser Ophthalmoscope (SLO)

Modulated red light laser (633 nm)

Performs funduscopy and automated perimetry simultaneously

Ultrasound

Acoustic imaging of globe and orbit

A-scan: 1-dimensional display (time/amplitude)

B-scan: 2-dimensional display

Reflectivity: height of spike on A-scan and signal brightness on B-scan
   Internal reflectivity refers to amplitude of echoes within a lesion or tissue

medium internal reflectivity

Figure 11-20. A-scan ultrasound demonstrating medium internal reflectivity. (From Kaiser PK, Friedman NJ, Pineda R II: *Massachusetts Eye and Ear Infirmary Illustrated Manual of Ophthalmology*, 2nd ed, Philadelphia, Saunders, 2004.)

low internal reflectivity

Figure 11-21. A-scan ultrasound demonstrating low internal reflectivity. (From Kaiser PK, Friedman NJ, Pineda R II: *Massachusetts Eye and Ear Infirmary Illustrated Manual of Ophthalmology*, 2nd ed, Philadelphia, Saunders, 2004.)

Internal structure: degree of variation in histologic architecture within a mass lesion
   Regular internal structure indicates homogenous architecture (minimal or no variation in the heights of spikes in A-scan and uniform appearance of echoes on B-scan)

high internal reflectivity

Figure 11-19. A-scan ultrasound demonstrating high internal reflectivity. (From Kaiser PK, Friedman NJ, Pineda R II: *Massachusetts Eye and Ear Infirmary Illustrated Manual of Ophthalmology*, 2nd ed, Philadelphia, Saunders, 2004.)

Table 11-3. **Ultrasound Characteristics of Various Lesions**

Pathology	Location	Shape	Internal Reflectivity	Internal Structure	Vascularity
Melanoma	Choroid and/or CB	Dome or collar button	Low to medium	Regular	Yes
Choroidal hemangioma	Choroid; posterior pole	Dome	High	Regular	Yes
Metastasis	Choroid; posterior pole	Diffuse, irregular	Medium to high	Irregular	No
Choroidal nevus	Choroid	Dome or flat	High	Regular	No
Choroidal hemorrhage	Choroid	Dome	Variable	Variable	No
Disciform lesion	Macula	Dome, irregular	High	Variable	No

Table 11-4. **Ultrasound Characteristics of Different Types of Detachments**

Pathology	Topographic (B-scan)	Quantitative (A-scan)	After Movement
Retinal detachment	Smooth or folded surface Open or closed funnel Inserts at ON and ora serrata May see intraretinal cysts	Steep spike (100% high)	Moderate to none
Posterior vitreous detachment	Smooth surface Open funnel With or without ON or fundus insertion Inserts at ora serrata or ciliary body	Variable spike height (<100%)	Marked to moderate
Choroidal detachment	Smooth, dome, or flat surface No ON insertion Inserts at ciliary body and vortex veins	Steeply rising, thick, double-peaked spike (100% high)	Mild to none

Sound attenuation: occurs when acoustic wave is scattered, reflected, or absorbed by tissue

Decrease in strength of echoes within or posterior to lesion; may produce a void posterior to lesion called "shadowing" (caused by dense substances [bone, calcium, foreign body])

After movement: dynamic features of lesionechoes

Observe B-scan echoes for motion after cessation of eye movements (i.e., rapid movement of vitreous hemorrhage distinguished from slower, undulating movement of rhegmatogenous retinal detachment)

Vascularity: spontaneous motion of echoes within lesion corresponds to blood flow; may be visualized with Color doppler

Specific lesions: (Tables 11-3 and 11-4) (Figures 11-22 to 11-27)

Asteroid hyalosis:

A-SCAN: medium to high internal reflectivity

B-SCAN: bright echoes in vitreous due to calcium soaps; area of clear vitreous usually present between opacities and posterior hyaloid face

Intraocular foreign body:

B-SCAN: high reflectivity when ultrasound probe is perpendicular to reflective surface of foreign

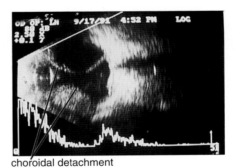

choroidal detachment

Figure 11-22. B-scan ultrasound demonstrating choroidal detachment. (From Kaiser PK, Friedman NJ, Pineda R II: *Massachusetts Eye and Ear Infirmary Illustrated Manual of Ophthalmology*, 2nd ed, Philadelphia, Saunders, 2004.)

body; bright echo persists when gain turned down; shadowing often present

Intraocular calcification:

A-SCAN: high amplitude peak due to strong acoustic interface

B-SCAN: white echoes; partial or complete shadowing

DDx: tumors (retinoblastoma, choroidal osteoma, optic nerve meningioma, choroidal hemangioma, choroidal melanoma), *Toxocara* granuloma, chronic retinal detachment, optic

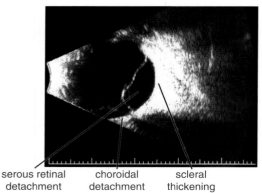

serous retinal   choroidal   scleral
detachment   detachment   thickening

Figure 11-23. B-scan ultrasound demonstrating serous retinal detachment with shifting fluid, shallow peripheral choroidal detachment, and diffuse scleral thickening. (From Kaiser PK, Friedman NJ, Pineda R II: *Massachusetts Eye and Ear Infirmary Illustrated Manual of Ophthalmology*, 2nd ed, Philadelphia, Saunders, 2004.)

scleral thickening   T-sign

Figure 11-24. B-scan ultrasound demonstrating scleral thickening and the characteristic peripapillary T sign. (From Kaiser PK, Friedman NJ, Pineda R II: *Massachusetts Eye and Ear Infirmary Illustrated Manual of Ophthalmology*, 2nd ed, Philadelphia, Saunders, 2004.)

choroidal hemangioma

Figure 11-25. B-scan ultrasound demonstrating elevated mass with underlying thickened choroid. (From Kaiser PK, Friedman NJ, Pineda R II:: *Massachusetts Eye and Ear Infirmary Illustrated Manual of Ophthalmology*, 2nd ed, Philadelphia, Saunders, 2004.)

choroidal malignant melanoma

Figure 11-26. B-scan ultrasound demonstrating dome-shaped choroidal mass. (From Kaiser PK, Friedman NJ, Pineda R II: *Massachusetts Eye and Ear Infirmary Illustrated Manual of Ophthalmology*, 2nd ed, Philadelphia, Saunders, 2004.)

serous retinal detachment   choroidal metastasis

Figure 11-27. B-scan ultrasound of a patient with choroidal metastasis demonstrating elevated choroidal mass with irregular surface and overlying serous retinal detachment. (From Kaiser PK, Friedman NJ, Pineda R II: *Massachusetts Eye and Ear Infirmary Illustrated Manual of Ophthalmology*, 2nd ed, Philadelphia, Saunders, 2004.)

nerve head drusen, vascular occlusive disease of optic nerve, phthisis bulbi, intumescent cataractous lens

Fluorescein Angiogram (FA)

Phases: choroidal filling, arterial, venous, recirculation

Dye enters choroidal circulation via short posterior ciliary arteries 10 to 15 seconds after injection; choroidal flow is very rapid; choriocapillaris filling is usually completed in the AV or early venous phase; cilioretinal artery is filled at time of choroidal filling; central retinal artery takes more circuitous route, resulting in dye arriving 1 to 2 seconds after choroidal filling; AV phase occurs 1 to 2 seconds after arterial phase; veins fill in 10 to 12 seconds (Figures 11-28 to 11-32)

Blue light stimulates fluorescein to emit yellow-green light: fluorescein absorbs light at 490 nm, emits at 530 nm

80% bound to albumin and other serum proteins

90% excreted from kidney

Death occurs in 1 per 220,000

Figure 11-28. FA demonstrating choroidal and early arterial filling.

Figure 11-31. FA demonstrating peak AV transit.

Figure 11-29. FA demonstrating arterial phase.

Figure 11-32. FA demonstrating late phase.

Figure 11-30. FA demonstrating early venous phase with laminar filling.

Characteristics:

Hyperfluorescence: leakage (fenestrated choriocapillaris, iris vessels), staining (structures such as collagen), pooling (pockets of fluid), window defects (RPE defects)

Hypofluorescence: blockage (by RPE, blood, xanthophyll), ischemia

Macular dark spot is due to blockage by xanthophyll in outer plexiform layer and tall RPE cells with increased melanin and lipofuscin

Fluorescein passes through Bruch's membrane, cannot pass through RPE or retinal capillaries

Choroidal filling: choroidal lesions (malignant melanoma, cavernous hemangioma) and cilioretinal artery

Arterial phase filling: retinal lesions (capillary hemangioma, NVD)

A   B

Figure 11-33. Serous retinal pigment epithelial detachment seen on FA (A) with associated hot spot seen on ICG (B). (From Reichel E: Indocyanine green angiography. In Yanoff M, Duker JS [eds]: *Ophthalmology*, London, Mosby, 1999.)

Indocyanine Green (ICG)

Absorbs light at 805 nm, emits at 835 nm (near infrared), which penetrates RPE to greater extent than visible light

98% bound to serum proteins; therefore, leaks very slowly from choroidal circulation CNV and appears as hot spot (bright area; occurs within 3–5 min, lasts 20 min) (Figure 11-33)

DISORDERS

Vitreous Abnormalities

Asteroid Hyalosis

Refractile particles (calcium soaps) suspended in vitreous

More common in older patients and those with diabetes; 25% bilateral

Rarely affects vision

Pathology: gray spheres with "Maltese cross" birefringence on polarization

Synchisis Scintillans (Cholesterol Bulbi)

Cholesterol crystals derived from old vitreous hemorrhage

Rare, unilateral

Occurs after blunt or penetrating trauma in blind eyes

Crystals sink to bottom of globe because no fixed vitreous framework

Primary Amyloidosis

Vitreous involvement in familial amyloidotic polyneuropathies

Amyloid enters via retinal vessels

Patients have cardiac disease and amyloid neuropathy

Posterior Vitreous Detachment (PVD)

Separation of posterior hyaloid face from retina

Mechanism: vitreous syneresis (liquefaction) and contraction with age

Symptoms: floaters; may see flashes (due to traction on retina)

Findings: PVD; may have retinal tear (10%–15% of acute symptomatic PVDs), vitreous hemorrhage (hemorrhagic PVD; 7.5% of PVDs) if vessel is torn during vitreous separation (70% risk of retinal tear), retinal detachment (RD)

Vitreous Hemorrhage (VH)

Etiology: diabetes (most common), other proliferative retinopathies, trauma, PVD, Terson's syndrome (blood from subarachnoid hemorrhage travels along optic nerve and into eye), ruptured retinal arterial macroaneurysm, retinal angioma; in children, consider child abuse, pars planitis, X-linked retinoschisis

Ochre membrane: results from chronic hemorrhage accumulating on posterior surface of detached vitreous

Persistent Hyperplastic Primary Vitreous (PHPV)

(see Chapter 5, Pediatrics/Strabismus)

Congenital Abnormalities of the Retina

(see Chapter 5, Pediatrics/Strabismus)

Trauma

Commotio Retinae (Berlin's Edema)

Figure 11-34. Berlin's edema (commotio retinae) in a patient after blunt ocular trauma. (From Rubsamen PE: Posterior segment ocular trauma. In Yanoff M, Duker JS [eds]: *Ophthalmology*. London, Mosby, 1999.)

Transient retinal whitening at level of deep sensory retina due to disruption (probably photoreceptor outer segments) with photoreceptor loss and thinning of outer nuclear and plexiform layers

Pigmentary changes can occur (RPE hyperplasia); traumatic macular hole may develop; usually resolves without sequelae

Contusion of RPE

Blunt trauma can cause RPE edema with overlying serous RD

Choroidal Rupture

Tear in choroid, Bruch's membrane, and RPE due to blunt or penetrating trauma

Mechanism: mechanical deformation results in rupture of choroid; sclera is resistant due to high tensile strength, retina is resistant due to elasticity; Bruch's membrane is less elastic and breaks with choroid and RPE

Direct: occurs anteriorly at site of impact; oriented parallel to ora serrata

Indirect: occurs posteriorly away from site of impact; usually crescent-shaped, concentric with and temporal to optic disc; often associated with VH

Findings: choroidal neovascular membrane (CNV) can develop during healing process (months to years after trauma; can regress spontaneously), scar forms

by 3 to 4 weeks, hyperplasia of RPE at margin of lesion

Figure 11-35. Choroidal rupture after blunt trauma. (From Rubsamen PE: Posterior segment ocular trauma. In Yanoff M, Duker JS [eds]: *Ophthalmology*. London, Mosby, 1999.)

Retina Sclopetaria (Figure 11-36)

Trauma to retina and choroid caused by transmitted shock waves from high-velocity projectile

Findings: rupture of choroid and retina with hemorrhage and commotio; vitreous hemorrhage can occur; lesion heals with white fibrous scar and RPE changes

Low risk of RD in young patients with formed vitreous; posterior vitreous face usually intact; choroid and retina tightly adherent

Traumatic Retinal Tear

Most patients are young with formed vitreous that tamponades the tear

As vitreous liquefies over time, fluid passes through breaks, causing retina to detach

Trauma is associated with 10% to 20% of all phakic RDs

4 types of traumatic retinal breaks: horseshoe tear, operculated tear, retinal dialysis, macular hole (rare)

Dialysis: most common type of retinal tear associated with traumatic RD; usually inferotemporal (31%) or superotemporal (22%); 50% have demarcation line; 10% of dialysis-related RDs are present on initial examination, 30% occur within 1 month, 50% within 8 months, 80% within 2 years

Avulsion of vitreous base: separation of vitreous base from ora serrata; pathognomonic for trauma

Oral tear: at ora serrata; due to split of vitreous; fish-mouth appearance

Preoral tear: anterior border of vitreous base; most often superotemporal

Figure 11-36. Gunshot wound to the periocular region demonstrating appearance of retina sclopetaria A) acute, B) chronic. (From Rubsamen PE: Posterior segment ocular trauma. In Yanoff M, Duker JS [eds]: *Ophthalmology*. London, Mosby, 1999.)

Treatment: laser therapy or cryotherapy for horseshoe tear, operculated tear, and retinal dialysis without RD; vitrectomy with gas for macular hole; scleral buckle for RD due to retinal tear; PVR is uncommon

Purtscher's Retinopathy (Figure 11-37)

Due to head trauma or compressive injury to trunk

Unilateral or bilateral

Findings: retinal whitening, hemorrhages, cotton wool spots, papillitis; may have positive RAPD

DDx: pancreatitis, fat emboli, lupus, leukemia, amniotic fluid emboli, dermatomyositis

FA: leakage from retinal vasculature, late venous staining

May take up to 3 months to resolve

Terson's Syndrome

Vitreous hemorrhage following subarachnoid or subdural hemorrhage due to intracranial hypertension blocking venous return from eye

Figure 11-37. Purscher's retinopathy. (From Regillo CD: Distant trauma with posterior segment effects. In Yanoff M, Duker JS [eds]: *Ophthalmology*. London, Mosby, 1999.)

20% of patients with spontaneous or traumatic subarachnoid hemorrhage will present with vitreous hemorrhage; bleeding can also occur between ILM and retina

Figure 11-38. Terson's syndrome. (From Regillo CD: Distant trauma with posterior segment effects. In Yanoff M, Duker JS: *Ophthalmology*. London, Mosby, 1999.)

Valsalva Retinopathy

Rise in intrathoracic or intra-abdominal pressure against a closed glottis (Valsalva maneuver) causes superficial veins to rupture with hemorrhage under ILM

Preretinal hemorrhage in macula causes sudden decreased vision

Fat Emboli Syndrome

Follows fracture of medullated bones; occurs in 5% of patients with long bone fractures

Affects multiple organ systems

Findings (in 50%): cotton wool spots, small blot hemorrhages; rarely intravenous fat or CRAO

20% mortality

Whiplash Retinopathy

Associated with severe flexion/extension of head and neck without direct eye injury

Findings: mild reduction in vision (to 20/30); gray swelling of fovea, foveal pit (50–100 μm)

FA: may have tiny focal area of early hyperfluorescence

Macular Diseases

Epiretinal Membrane (Cellophane Maculopathy, Macular Pucker)

Proliferations at vitreoretinal junction, may contract and cause retinal folds

12% prevalence in individuals 43 to 86 years old; 20% bilateral; 2% associated with retinal folds (decreased vision)

Associated with diabetes, retinal vascular occlusions, PVD, high myopia, retinal hole/tear, previous ocular or laser surgery, and increasing age

OCT: epiretinal membrane visible on surface of retina, distortion of retinal surface may be evident

Treatment: consider surgery for decreased vision (<20/50), marked retinal distortion, or metamorphopsia

Macular Hole

Due to tangential traction on foveal region by posterior cortical vitreous

Most commonly idiopathic (senile); may develop after trauma, surgery, CME, or inflammation

Female > male; bilateral in 25% to 30%; prevalence = 0.33%; average age of onset is 67 years; risk of developing in fellow eye <1% (no risk if PVD present)

Macular cyst may be precursor

Gass classification:
1. Premacular or impending hole with foveal detachment and macular cyst (yellow spot [1a] or ring [1b])
2. Full-thickness eccentric hole
3. Full-thickness hole with operculum, cuff of subretinal fluid, yellow deposits at base, positive Watzke-Allen sign
4. Full-thickness hole with PVD

Figure 11-39. Optical coherence tomography scans demonstrating cross-sectional image of all stages of macular hole formation and the full-thickness retinal defect characteristic of stage 3 and 4 holes. (From Kaiser PK, Friedman NJ, Pineda R II: *Massachusetts Eye and Ear Infirmary Illustrated Manual of Ophthalmology*, 2nd ed, Philadelphia, Saunders, 2004.)

Often have rim of SRF

Watzke-Allen sign: shine narrow-slit beam over macular hole, positive if patient perceives "break" in slit beam

DDx: epiretinal membrane with pseudohole, lamellar hole, vitreomacular traction/detachment; for stage 1: drusen, CME, CSR

FA: window defect (hyperfluorescence during choroidal filling)

OCT: differentiates between various stages and other disease, hole evident on scan (Figure 11-39)

Treatment: stage 1 may close spontaneously; consider vitrectomy with peeling of posterior hyaloid and gas tamponade for stage 2 through stage 4
  Complications of surgery: increased size of hole, RPE mottling, light toxicity, cataract, retinal tear, retinal detachment

Prognosis: good if recent onset, poor if >1 year duration

Traumatic macular hole: rare (5%); due to disruption and necrosis of retinal photoreceptors with subsequent loss of retinal tissue; results from preexisting commotio retinae in macula

Solar Retinopathy

Photochemical retinal damage can occur after ~90 seconds or longer of sungazing, thought to be caused by blue (441 nm) and near UV light (325–250 nm)

With foveal fixation, retinal image of sun is 160 μm and is usually within the foveola and FAZ

Associated with solar eclipse, psychiatric disorders, religious rituals, or ingestion of hallucinogens

Symptoms: vision can range from normal to 20/100; usually returns to 20/20 to 20/40 within 6 months

Findings: yellow-white spot in fovea; later, red foveolar depression or lamellar hole

FA: intense staining of damaged RPE, particularly in acute phase of injury, but no leakage; as RPE heals, window defects develop (Figure 11-41)

Figure 11-41. Fluorescein angiography of solar retinopathy in the left eye. (Courtesy of William E.Benson. From Baumal CR: Light toxicity and laser burns. In Yanoff M, Duker JS [eds]: *Ophthalmology*. London, Mosby, 1999.)

A

B

Figure 11-40. Solar retinopathy of both eyes. (Courtesy of William E. Benson. From Baumal CR: Light toxicity and laser burns. In Yanoff M, Duker JS [eds]: *Ophthalmology*. London, Mosby, 1999.)

Findings: blurred vision, micropsia, paracentral scotoma; poor color vision; induced hyperopia, absent foveal reflex; after resolution, may have yellow subretinal deposits, RPE changes

DDx: AMD, VKH syndrome, uveal effusion syndrome, toxemia of pregnancy, optic nerve pit, pigment epithelial detachment from other causes (CNV)

FA: small focal hyperfluorescent dot (leakage of dye from choroid through RPE); later, dye accumulates beneath neurosensory detachment; "smokestack" appearance in 10%; expanding dot of hyperfluorescence in 80%, diffuse leakage in the rest

OCT: sensory retinal elevation, may have PED

ICG: can be useful in helping to distinguish atypical diffuse CSR in older patients from occult CNV in exudative AMD and idiopathic polypoidal choroidal vasculopathy

Central Serous Retinopathy/ Chorioretinopathy (CSR)/Idiopathic Central Serous Choroidopathy (ICSC)

Serous detachment of macula ± retinal pigment epithelium

Males (80%), typically in 4th to 5th decade

Associated with hypertension and type A personality

pigment epithelial detachment

Figure 11-42. Idiopathic central serous retinopathy with large serous retinal detachment. (From Kaiser PK, Friedman NJ, Pineda R II: *Massachusetts Eye and Ear Infirmary Illustrated Manual of Ophthalmology*, 2nd ed, Philadelphia, Saunders, 2004.)

pigment epithelial
detachment

"smokestack"
leakage

Figure 11-43. Fluorescein angiogram demonstrating classic smoke-stack appearance. (From Kaiser PK, Friedman NJ, Pineda R II: *Massachusetts Eye and Ear Infirmary Illustrated Manual of Ophthalmology*, 2nd ed, Philadelphia, Saunders, 2004.)

Treatment: observation, consider laser
Laser indications:
1. Persistent serous detachment (>4 months)
2. Previous episode of CSR, with permanent vision reduction
3. Episode in fellow eye with vision loss
4. Demand for rapid recovery of binocular function for occupational reasons
Laser accelerates resolution of fluid but does not result in better final vision or reduce rate of recurrence; may rarely cause CNV

Prognosis: 90% spontaneous resorption in 1 to 6 months; 50% recur; 66% achieve 20/20; 14% with bilateral vision loss over 10 years

Retinal Pigment Epithelial Detachment (PED)

Appears as discrete, blister-like elevation; sometimes outlined by orange-pink rim of subretinal fluid

DDx:
In patient <50 years old: probably due to central serous retinopathy

In patient >50 years old: PED associated with drusen may indicate occult CNV, especially if PED has a notch

FA: discrete early hyperfluorescence of entire serous PED with late pooling into PED

Complications: 33% develop CNV (FA shows slower, more homogenous filling with sharp border)

Age-Related Macular Degeneration (ARMD, AMD)

Leading cause of central visual loss in patients >60 years old in the United States

Risk factors: age, heredity, sex (female), race (white), smoking, nutrition, photic exposure, hypertension, light iris color, hyperopia

Symptoms: decreased vision, central scotoma, metamorphopsia

2 forms:
1. *Nonexudative or dry* (80–90%): drusen, pigment changes, RPE atrophy (Figures 11-44 to 11-47)
2. *Exudative, neovascular, or wet* (10–20%): CNV (vision <20/200 in 90%) (Figures 11-48 to 11-50)

Drusen: clinical marker for sick RPE; PAS-positive, mildly eosinophilic hyaline excrescences of abnormal basement membrane material between RPE basement membrane and inner Bruch's membrane

Types of drusen:
Hard (nodular/cuticular/hyaline): small yellow-white spots 50 μm in diameter
Soft: larger, less dense, more fluffy, with tapered edges; may resemble PED; associated with thickened inner Bruch's membrane and wet AMD
Basal laminar: diffuse, confluent
Calcific: sharply demarcated, glistening; associated with RPE atrophy

A   B   C

Figure 11-44. Nodular "hard" drusen. (From Edwards MG, Bressler NM, Raja SC: Age-related macular degeneration. In Yanoff M, Duker JS [eds]: *Ophthalmology*. London, Mosby, 1999.)

Figure 11-45. Dry, age-related macular degeneration demonstrating drusen and pigmentary changes (category 3). (From Kaiser PK, Friedman NJ, Pineda R II: *Massachusetts Eye and Ear Infirmary Illustrated Manual of Ophthalmology*, 2nd ed, Philadelphia, Saunders, 2004.)

Figure 11-46. Advanced, atrophic, nonexudative, age-related macular degeneration demonstrating subfoveal geographic atrophy (category 4). (From Kaiser PK, Friedman NJ, Pineda R II: *Massachusetts Eye and Ear Infirmary Illustrated Manual of Ophthalmology*, 2nd ed, Philadelphia, Saunders, 2004.)

Figure 11-47. Fluorescein angiogram of same patient as in Figure 11-46, demonstrating well-defined window defect corresponding to the area of geographic atrophy. (From Kaiser PK, Friedman NJ, Pineda R II: *Massachusetts Eye and Ear Infirmary Illustrated Manual of Ophthalmology*, 2nd ed, Philadelphia, Saunders, 2004.)

Figure 11-48. Exudative age-related macular degeneration, demonstrating subretinal hemorrhage from classic choroidal neovascular membrane. (From Kaiser PK, Friedman NJ, Pineda R II: *Massachusetts Eye and Ear Infirmary Illustrated Manual of Ophthalmology*, 2nd ed, Philadelphia, Saunders, 2004.)

Figure 11-49. Fluorescein angiogram of same patient as in Figure 11-48, demonstrating leakage from the CNV and blockage from the surrounding subretinal blood. (From Kaiser PK, Friedman NJ, Pineda R II: *Massachusetts Eye and Ear Infirmary Illustrated Manual of Ophthalmology*, 2nd ed, Philadelphia, WB Saunders, 2004.)

Drusen size classification:
Small: <64 μm in diameter
Intermediate: 64–124 μm in diameter
Large: ≥125 μm in diameter

DDx of yellow foveal spot: solar maculopathy, adult vitelliform dystrophy, Best's disease, stage 1a macular hole, CSR, old subfoveal hemorrhage, CME, pattern dystrophy

FA: hyperfluorescence of drusen due to window defects (from degeneration of overlying RPE) and uptake of dye within drusen (staining)

Signs of CNV: subretinal blood, fluid, and/or lipid; RPE detachment (PED); gray-green subretinal discoloration

Types of CNV: defined by appearance of leakage on FA

A   **B**   **C**

Figure 11-50. Neovascular, age-related macular degeneration. (From Edwards MG, Bressler NM, Raja SC: Age-related macular degeneration. In Yanoff M, Duker JS [eds]: *Ophthalmology*. London, Mosby, 1999.)

Classic:
> EARLY PHASE: bright, fairly uniform hyperfluorescence that progressively intensifies throughout the transit phase
> LATE PHASE: progressive leakage of dye that extends beyond the margins of the CNV seen in early stages

Occult (2 types):
> FIBROVASCULAR PED:
>> EARLY PHASE: irregular mottled hyperfluorescence at level of RPE
>> LATE PHASE: stippled hyperfluorescent leakage that is not as bright or extensive as classic lesions
> LATE LEAKAGE OF UNDETERMINED ORIGIN:
>> EARLY PHASE: no apparent leakage
>> LATE PHASE: stippled hyperfluorescence at level of RPE

Location of CNV:
> *Extrafoveal*: posterior border of CNV is 200 to 2500 μm from center of foveal avascular zone (FAZ)
> *Juxtafoveal*: 1 to 199 μm from center of FAZ, or CNV 200 to 2500 μm from center of FAZ with blood or blocked fluorescence within 200 μm of FAZ center
> *Subfoveal*: under center of FAZ

ICG: helpful for visualizing CNV that is not well seen on FA; CNV appears as focal hot spots or plaque of late hyperfluorescence; can demonstrate CNV under thin hemorrhage that would be blocked on FA; high-speed ICG useful to delineate feeder vessels of CNV

Treatment: follow Amsler grid, low-vision aids, vitamin supplements, consider laser or PDT for CNV
> *Age-related Eye Disease Study* (AREDS):
>> Supplements with high-dose antioxidants and zinc are helpful in reducing vision loss and the progression of disease in patients with category 3 and 4 AMD

Macular Photocoagulation Study (MPS):
> Treatment of well-demarcated extrafoveal or juxtafoveal CNV with uniform laser. After 5 years, 64% of untreated eyes had >6 lines of vision loss; 46% of treated eyes had >6 lines of vision loss; >50% recurrence rate. However, many patients do not qualify owing to subfoveal CNV and occult lesions

Treatment of Age-Related Macular degeneration with Photodynamic Therapy (TAP) Trial:
> Photodynamic therapy with verteporfin (Visudyne) can prevent vision loss in eyes with subfoveal, predominantly classic and occult, with no classic CNV

Verteporfin in Photodynamic Therapy (VIP) Trial:
> Photodynamic therapy with verteporfin (Visudyne) can prevent vision loss in eyes with occult and no classic CNV, especially if less than 4 MPS DA in size or baseline vision worse than 20/50

Macugen: anti-vascular endothelial growth factor (VEGF) aptamer, that blocks $VEGF_{165}$, has been shown to decrease visual loss in all CNV subtypes

Combination treatment: adjunctive antiangiogenic or angiostatic agents may be effective

Surgery: in certain cases, consider submacular surgery (being evaluated in the Submacular Surgery Trials) to remove CNV or macular translocation (experimental)

Prognosis:
> *Risk of CNV in fellow eye at 5 years*: if drusen is present
> Hard (nodular) = 10%
> Soft = 30%
> Pigmented = 30%
> Soft and pigmented = 60%
> *Risk of fellow eye developing CNV*: 4% to 12% per year; increased risk with multiple soft drusen, RPE clumping, densely packed drusen, PED

MAJOR AGE-RELATED MACULAR DEGENERATION CLINICAL STUDIES

Macular Photocoagulation Study (MPS)

Objective: to evaluate efficacy of laser photocoagulation in preventing visual loss from CNV

Methods: Patients were randomly assigned to laser photocoagulation vs observation in the following groups:

Extrafoveal Study: well-demarcated CNV due to AMD or OHS, or idiopathic, that was 200 to 2500 μm from center of foveal avascular zone (FAZ) with vision better than 20/100. Patients who received previous photocoagulation were excluded. Patients randomly assigned to argon blue-green treatment to the entire CNV and 100 to 125 μm beyond the borders of the lesion vs observation

Juxtafoveal (Krypton) Study: well-demarcated CNV due to AMD or OHS, or idiopathic, that was 1 to 199 μm from center of foveal avascular zone (FAZ), or with a CNV more than 200 μm with blood or pigment extending within 200 μm and with vision better than 20/400. Patients randomly assigned to Krypton red treatment of entire CNV and 100 μm beyond the borders of the lesion except on the foveal side of the lesion vs observation

Subfoveal, New CNV AMD Study: well-demarcated CNV due to AMD under the center of foveal avascular zone (FAZ) with vision between 20/40 and 20/320. The entire lesion had to measure less than 3.5 MPS disc areas in size and could be classic or occult CNV. Patients randomly assigned to argon green or krypton red treatment of entire CNV and 100 μm beyond the borders of the lesion vs observation

Subfoveal Recurrent CNV Study: well-demarcated CNV due to AMD under the center of foveal avascular zone (FAZ) contiguous with previous laser treatment scar and with vision between 20/40 and 20/320. The entire lesion had to measure less than 6 MPS disc areas in size and could be classic or occult CNV. Patients randomly assigned to argon green or krypton red treatment of entire CNV and 100 μm beyond the borders of the lesion vs observation

DEFINITIONS:
  EXTRAFOVEAL: 200 to 2500 μm from center of foveal avascular zone (FAZ)
  JUXTAFOVEAL: 1 to 199 μm from center of FAZ
  SUBFOVEAL: extends beneath center of fovea
MAIN OUTCOME MEASURES: visual acuity, contrast sensitivity, reading speed, persistent and/or recurrent CNV, treatment complications

Results:
Extrafoveal Study:
  AFTER 18 MONTHS:
    AMD: 25% of treated vs 60% of untreated eyes had lost ≥6 lines of vision (a quadrupling of the visual angle [i.e., 20/50 to 20/200])

    POHS: 9.4% of treated vs 34.2% of untreated eyes had lost ≥6 lines of vision
    IDIOPATHIC: sample size (67) was too small to reach clinical significance, but trend was similar to results for AMD and POHS
    Recurrence of CNV after argon laser was 52% with AMD, 28% with POHS, 28% with idiopathic CNV
  AFTER 3 YEARS:
    Relative risk of severe vision loss (≥6 lines) for no treatment vs treatment was 1.4 for AMD, 5.5 for POHS, and 2.3 for idiopathic CNV
  AFTER 5 YEARS:
    AMD: treated eyes lost 5.2 lines of vision vs 7.1 lines in untreated eyes; recurrence in 54% of treated eyes; 26% developed CNV in fellow eye
    POHS: treated eyes lost 0.9 line of vision vs 4.4 lines in untreated eyes; recurrence in 26% of treated eyes
    IDIOPATHIC: treated eyes lost 2.7 lines of vision vs 4.4 lines in untreated eyes; recurrence in 34% of treated eyes
Juxtafoveal Study:
  AFTER 3 YEARS:
    POHS: 4.6% of treated vs 24.6% of untreated eyes had lost ≥6 lines of vision
    IDIOPATHIC: 10% of treated vs 37% of untreated eyes had lost ≥6 lines of vision
  AFTER 5 YEARS:
    Relative risk of severe vision loss (≥6 lines) for no treatment vs treatment was 1.2 for AMD (hypertensive patients had little or no benefit), 4.26 for POHS, and intermediate between AMD and POHS for idiopathic CNV
Subfoveal New AMD Study:
  AFTER 3 MONTHS:
    AMD: 20% of treated vs 11% of untreated eyes had lost ≥6 lines of vision
  AFTER 2 YEARS:
    AMD: 20% of treated vs 37% of untreated eyes had lost ≥6 lines of vision; recurrence in 51% of treated eyes
  AFTER 4 YEARS:
    AMD: 22% of treated vs 47% of untreated eyes had lost ≥6 lines of vision
Subfoveal Recurrent AMD Study:
  AFTER 3 YEARS: 12% of treated vs 36% of untreated eyes had lost ≥6 lines of vision

Conclusions:
Treat extrafoveal CNV in patients with AMD, POHS, and idiopathic lesions
Patients with juxtafoveal CNV (AMD, POHS, and idiopathic) benefit from krypton laser photocoagulation, except for hypertensive AMD patients
AMD patients with subfoveal CNV (new or recurrent) benefit equally from argon green or krypton red laser treatment
For unilateral CNV, large drusen and focal hyperpigmentation are risk factors for development of CN in fellow eye

Treatment of AMD patients with juxtafoveal CNV is beneficial when the lesion is classic, even though CNV recurs; treatment of classic CNV alone in lesions with both classic and occult CNV was not beneficial

Treatment of Age-Related Macular Degeneration with Photodynamic Therapy Trial (TAP)

Objective: to evaluate verteporfin (Visudyne) ocular photodynamic therapy (OPT) in the management of subfoveal CNV with some classic characteristics

Methods: Patients with evidence of AMD, age >50 years, evidence of new or recurrent subfoveal "classic" (can have occult features) CNV by fluorescein angiography with greatest linear dimension of CNV <5400 μm (9 MPS disc areas), ETDRS visual acuity of 20/40 to 20/200, and the ability to return every 3 months for 2 years. Patients were excluded who had other ocular diseases that could compromise visual acuity, history of previous experimental treatment for CNV, porphyrin allergy, liver problems, or intraocular surgery within the previous 2 months. Two thirds of patients in both studies were randomly assigned (2 : 1 randomization scheme) to receive verteporfin (Visudyne 6 mg/m^2) and one third to control vehicle (D$_5$W IV infusion) infused over a 10-minute period. All patients were then irradiated with the use of a 689-nm diode laser (light dose: 50 J/cm^2; power density: 600 mW/cm^2; duration: 83 seconds) 15 minutes after the start of the infusion

Results: Enrollment included 609 patients (311 in Study A and 298 in Study B). Vision was stabilized or improved in 61.4% of patients treated with Visudyne™ OPT compared with 45.9% treated with placebo at 12 months. The difference was sustained at 24 and 60 (TAP Extension Study) months. In subgroup analysis, the visual acuity benefit was most pronounced for lesions in which the area of classic CNV occupied more than 50% of the entire area of the lesion (predominantly classic). Specifically, 33% of the Visudyne™-treated eyes compared with 61% of the placebo-treated eyes sustained moderate visual loss. No difference in visual acuity was noted when the area of classic CNV was greater than 0% but less than 50% of the entire lesion (minimally classic). Sixteen percent of patients experienced an improvement in vision (1 or more lines) in the Visudyne™-treated group compared with 7.2% in the control group. Overall, the Visudyne™ group was 34% more likely to retain vision. Most patients required periodic retreatments with an average of 3.4 (of a possible 4) being required in the first year, 2.1 in the second year (5.5 total over 24 months), and 1.5 in the third year (7 total over 36 months)

Conclusions: Visudyne™ ocular photodynamic therapy is recommended for subfoveal, predominantly classic, CNV

Verteporfin in Photodynamic Therapy (VIP) Trial Verteporfin in Photodynamic Therapy–Pathologic Myopia (VIP-PM) Trial

Objective: To evaluate Visudyne™ ocular photodynamic therapy (OPT) in the management of subfoveal CNV not included in the original TAP investigation

Methods: Patients with evidence of AMD, age >50 years, evidence of subfoveal "occult" only CNV by FA with recent disease progression defined as evidence of hemorrhage, loss of ≥1 line of vision, or increased size of the lesion by 10% during the preceding 3 months, and ETDRS visual acuity ≥20/100; or subfoveal "classic" CNV with ETDRS visual acuity of ≥20/40, greatest linear dimension of CNV <5400 μm (9 MPS disc areas), and the ability to return every 3 months for 2 years. Patients were excluded who had other ocular diseases that could compromise visual acuity, history of previous experimental treatment for CNV, porphyrin allergy, liver problems, or intraocular surgery within the previous 2 months. Two thirds of the patients in both studies were randomly assigned (2 : 1 randomization scheme) to receive verteporfin (Visudyne™ 6 mg/m^2) and one third to control vehicle (D$_5$W IV infusion) infused over a 10-minute period. All patients were then irradiated with the use of a 689-nm diode laser (light dose: 50 J/cm^2; power density: 600 mW/cm^2; duration: 83 seconds) 15 minutes after the start of the infusion

Results: 459 patients enrolled. The 1-year results showed no statistically significant difference between the Visudyne™-treated patients and placebo (difference 4.2%). However, by 24 months, a statistically significant difference was seen that was due to a decline in vision in the control group (difference 13.7%). Moreover, this difference was most pronounced in patients with "occult" only CNV lesions measuring <4 MPS disk areas in size at baseline, or who had a baseline visual acuity of 20/50 or worse

Few ocular or other systemic adverse events were seen with Visudyne™ therapy. In 4.4% of patients, an immediate severe visual decrease within 7 days of treatment was observed

Conclusions: Visudyne™ ocular photodynamic therapy (OPT) is recommended in the management of subfoveal occult but not classic CNV when there is evidence of recent disease progression, especially if the baseline lesion size is smaller than 4 MPS DA, or the baseline vision is worse than 20/50

Age-Related Eye Disease Study (AREDS)

Objective: to evaluate the effect of high-dose supplements on the progression of AMD, and on the development and progression of cataracts

Methods: patients received antioxidants (vitamin C [500 mg], vitamin E [400 IU], beta-carotene [vitamin A, 15 mg]), zinc (80 mg plus 2 mg copper), both, or placebo

Categorized into 4 groups:

Category 1: fewer than 5 small (<63 μm) drusen

Category 2 (mild AMD): multiple small drusen or single or nonextensive intermediate (63–124 μm) drusen, or pigment abnormalities

Category 3 (intermediate AMD): extensive intermediate-sized drusen, or 1 or more large (>125 μm) drusen, or noncentral geographic atrophy

Category 4 (advanced AMD): vision loss (<20/32) due to AMD in 1 eye (due to either central/subfoveal geographic atrophy or exudative macular degeneration)

Primary outcomes:

Progression to advanced AMD: treatment for CNV or photographic evidence (geographic atrophy of center of macula, non-drusenoid RPE detachment, serous or hemorrhagic RD, subretinal hemorrhage or fibrosis)

Moderate vision loss: ≥15-letter loss (doubling of visual angle)

Development and progression of lens opacities

Results: 4753 patients enrolled

Antioxidants plus zinc: reduced the risk of progression to advanced AMD and vision loss over 6 years in 25% of high-risk patients

HIGH-RISK PATIENTS: intermediate AMD (many intermediate drusen [63–124 μm] or 1 large drusen [≥125 μm] in 1 or both eyes) or advanced AMD (in 1 eye only)

Zinc alone: reduced risk of vision loss by 21%

Antioxidants alone: reduced risk of vision loss by 17%

Conclusions:

High-dose supplements are beneficial in reducing the risk of vision loss in patients with high-risk AMD (categories 3 and 4). Caution should be exercised in smokers or recent smokers in the use of high-dose beta-carotene because of the possible increased risk of lung cancer

Treatment is of no benefit in patients with no AMD or early AMD (several small or intermediate drusen)

Treatment does not affect development or progression of cataract

Other Disorders Associated with Choroidal Neovascular Membrane (CNV)

Presumed Ocular Histoplasmosis Syndrome (POHS)

Age of onset commonly 20 to 45 years; no sex predilection; mostly in eastern and midwestern United States; rare in Europe; rare among African Americans

Associated with HLA-B7, DRw2

Primary target tissue is choroid

Findings: triad of peripapillary atrophy, multiple punched-out chorioretinal scars ("histo spots," may enlarge, 5% to 10% develop new spots), CNV (different from that in AMD in that vessels penetrate Bruch's membrane and extend over RPE; a second layer of RPE forms [basal side up] and attempts to encircle the CNV; the surrounded CNV is more easily removed with surgery); no vitritis

Risk of CNV: 1% with normal disc and macula; 25% risk over 4 years if not normal

CXR: calcifications

Treatment: consider laser or submacular surgery for extrafoveal and juxtafoveal lesions (MPS showed that laser treatment for juxtafoveal and extrafoveal CNV was beneficial); subfoveal lesions treated with verteporfin ocular photodynamic therapy

Figure 11-51. POHS demonstrating peripapillary scarring and macular, juxtafoveal choroidal neovascular membrane with surrounding subretinal hemorrhage. (From Noorthy RS, Fountain JS: Fungal uveitis. In Yanoff M, Duker JS [eds]: *Ophthalmology*. London, Mosby, 1999.)

Angioid Streaks

Peripapillary linear cracks in thickened, degenerated, and calcified Bruch's membrane

Subretinal hemorrhage can occur with minor trauma

Etiology: 50% associated with systemic condition, 50% idiopathic

Mnemonic **PEPSI**:

Pseudoxanthoma elasticum (PXE) (AR ≫ AD): female > male; peau d'orange appearance to retina; redundant skin with waxy, yellow, papule-like lesions ("plucked chicken" skin); increased elastic tissue; vascular malformations; abnormal mucosal vasculature may cause GI bleeds; may have optic nerve head drusen; angioid streaks present in 85%

Ehlers-Danlos syndrome (fibrodysplasia hyperelastica) (AD): hyperextensible skin due to deficient collagen matrix; other eye findings include subluxed lens, high myopia, keratoconus, blue sclera, retinal detachment

Paget's disease: increased bone production and destruction; increased serum alkaline phosphatase; prone to basal skull and long bone fractures; other bone disorders (acromegaly, calcinosis)

Sickle cell: risk for autoinfarction of spleen and thrombotic episodes; other hematologic diseases (thalassemia, hereditary spherocytosis, acanthocytosis [Bassen-Kornzweig syndrome]); angioid streaks present in 1%

Idiopathic: 50%

DDx: lacquer cracks in myopia

Figure 11-52. Peripapillary angioid streaks. (From Vander JF: Angioid streaks. In Yanoff M, Duker JS [eds]: *Ophthalmology*. London, Mosby, 1999.)

Pathologic Myopia

Axial length >26 mm; >6 D of myopia; approximately 2% of US population; female > male

Findings: long, oval disc, may be tilted, cup usually shallow; temporal crescent; posterior staphyloma; tigroid fundus with visible choroidal vessels; lacquer cracks (breaks in Bruch's membrane); Fuchs' spot (macular hemorrhage); cataract; retinal holes and rhegmatogenous RD

Lacquer crack: sudden decrease in vision, metamorphopsia, often in teenagers; focal subretinal hemorrhage, dense, round, deep, and often centered on fovea; blood may obscure crack

Complications: CNV often near fovea (65%); worse prognosis; 60% with vision <20/200 at 2 years

Other Causes of Macular CNV

Idiopathic, optic nerve head drusen, choroidal rupture, choroidal nevus, sympathetic ophthalmia, Vogt-Kayanagi-Harada disease, serpiginous choroiditis, other posterior uveitides (choroidal inflammation may enhance production of angiogenic factors; when coupled with RPE–Bruch's membrane disruption, CNV can develop)

Retinal Vascular Diseases

Damage to vessel walls causes leakage of serum and blood into plexiform layers, causing edema, exudates, and hemorrhages

Edema: histologically appears as clear cystoid spaces

Lipid: appears as yellow lesion; histologically, hard exudates are eosinophilic and PAS-positive

DDx: diabetes, hypertensive retinopathy CNV, vein occlusion, parafoveal telangiectasia, Coats' disease, radiation retinopathy, CSR, trauma, macroaneurysm, papilledema, angiomatosis retinae

Microaneurysm: fusiform outpouching of capillary wall

Cotton wool spot: microinfarction of NFL (usually secondary to occlusion of retinal arteriole) with cessation of axoplasmic flow, mitochondria accumulate (resemble a nucleus, so lesion appears like a cell ["cytoid body"])

Hemorrhage: shape of intraretinal blood depends on layer in which it occurs (dot/blot in plexiform layer where cells are oriented vertically; flame-shaped/feathery border in NFL where cells are oriented horizontally)

Roth spot: white-centered hemorrhage

DDx: ischemia (anemia, anoxia, carbon monoxide poisoning), elevated venous pressure (birth trauma, shaken baby syndrome, intracranial hemorrhage), capillary fragility (hypertension, diabetes), infection (bacterial endocarditis, HIV), leukemia, collagen vascular disease

Neovascularization: growth of new vessels on vitreous side of ILM; new vessels grow along posterior hyaloid

Vascular tortuosity: may be congenital (arterial and venous) or acquired (venous)

DDx: hypertension, high venous pressure (occlusion), papilledema, high viscosity, AV fistula; associated with fetal alcohol syndrome, Peter's anomaly, optic nerve hypoplasia

Retinal Vasculitis

Involvement of retinal arterioles (arteritis), veins (phlebitis), or both (periphlebitis)

Findings: sheathing of vessels, hemorrhage

DDx: temporal arteritis, polyarteritis nodosa, lupus, Behçet's disease, inflammatory bowel syndrome, multiple sclerosis, pars planitis, Wegener's granulomatosis, Eales disease, sarcoidosis, syphilis, toxoplasmosis, viral retinitis (HSV, HZV), IV drug abuse, Lyme disease, tuberculosis

Cystoid Macular Edema (CME)

Intraretinal edema in honeycomb-like spaces; flower-petal pattern due to Henle's layer

Etiology: mnemonic **DEPRIVEN**
Diabetes
Epinephrine
Pars planitis
RP
Irvine-Gass syndrome
Venous occlusion
E$_2$ prostaglandin
Nicotinic acid maculopathy
  Others: XRT, parafoveal telangiectasia, CNV (rare), juvenile retinoschisis, Goldmann-Favre, Xalatan, vitreous wick

Pathophysiology: abnormal perifoveal retinal capillary permeability; initial fluid accumulation may be within Müller's cells (rather than in spaces of outer plexiform and inner nuclear layers)

Findings: CME, optic nerve swelling, vitreous cells

FA: multiple small focal fluorescein leaks early; late pooling of dye in cystoid spaces; classically, flower-petal ("petalloid") pattern; staining of optic nerve

OCT: cystic intraretinal spaces

intraretinal cysts   disc edema

Figure 11-53. Cystoid macular edema with decreased foveal reflex, cystic changes in fovea, and intraretinal hemorrhages. (From Kaiser PK, Friedman NJ, Pineda R II: *Massachusetts Eye and Ear Infirmary Illustrated Manual of Ophthalmology*, 2nd ed, Philadelphia, Saunders, 2004.)

DDx of cystic macular changes (looks like CME clinically, but no fluorescein filling of cysts):
1. Juvenile retinoschisis
2. Goldmann-Favre
3. Some types of RP
4. Nicotinic acid maculopathy

petalloid leakage   disc leakage

Figure 11-54. Fluorescein angiogram of same patient as in Figure 11-53, demonstrating characteristic petalloid appearance with optic nerve leakage. (From Kaiser PK, Friedman NJ, Pineda R II: *Massachusetts Eye and Ear Infirmary Illustrated Manual of Ophthalmology*, 2nd ed, Philadelphia, Saunders, 2004.)

cystoid macular edema

Log reflection

Figure 11-55. Optical coherence tomography of cystoid macular edema, demonstrating intraretinal cystoid spaces and dome-shaped configuration of fovea. (From Kaiser PK, Friedman NJ, Pineda R II: *Massachusetts Eye and Ear Infirmary Illustrated Manual of Ophthalmology*, 2nd ed, Philadelphia, Saunders, 2004.)

Treatment: depends on etiology; focal laser treatment, topical steroid and NSAID, oral Diamox, sub-Tenon's steroid injection

Retinal Telangiectases Coats' Disease (Leber's Miliary Aneurysms)

(see Chapter 5, Pediatrics/Strabismus)

Parafoveal/Juxtafoveal Telangiectasia (PFT, JXT)

Microaneurysmal and saccular dilation of parafoveal vessels

Classification:
  Type 1: unilateral, male > female (10 : 1); onset during middle age; in spectrum of Coats' disease
    TYPE 1A: congenital; confined to temporal half of fovea; macular edema and exudation (lipid)

TYPE 1B: idiopathic; capillary telangiectasia confined to 1 clock hour at edge of FAZ; minimal leakage on FA; occasional hard exudates; vision usually better than 20/25; can be treated with laser

Type 2 (most common): bilateral, acquired; male = female; 5th to 6th decade of life; symmetric, involving area <1 DD; minimal macular edema; occasionally, superficial glistening white dots (Singerman's spots); right-angle retinal venules dive deep into choroid; eventual develop RPE hyperplasia; occasionally, yellow lesion measuring 1/3 DD centered on FAZ (pseudovitelliform macular degeneration); may develop macular edema that is due to ischemia (not amenable to laser treatment)

FA: parafoveal capillary leakage; risk of CNV

Type 3: bilateral, idiopathic; male = female; capillary occlusion predominates

Structural abnormalities in types 2 and 3 are similar to diabetic microangiopathy (but no risk of NVE)

DDx: diabetes, vein occlusion, radiation retinopathy, Coats' disease, Eales disease, Best's disease, sickle cell, Irvine-Gass syndrome, ocular ischemia

Complications: macular edema, exudates, CNV

A

B

Figure 11-56. Macroaneurysm with surrounding dilated and telangiectatic capillary bed. **A**, fundus photograph, **B**, FA. (Courtesy Susan Fowell, MD. From Mittra RA, Mieler WF, Pollack JS: Retinal arterial macroaneurysms. In Yanoff M, Duker JS [eds]: *Ophthalmology.* London, Mosby, 1999.)

Retinal Arterial Macroaneurysm (RAM)
(Figure 11-56)

May bleed, then autoinfarcts

Usually, elderly females; most common along temporal arcades

Mechanism: arteriosclerosis (fibrosis, thinning, decreased elasticity of vessel wall), hypertension (increased pressure on thin wall)

Findings: blood in every retinal layer, lipid exudate, artery occlusion downstream (especially following laser treatment), CME

DDx of blood in every retinal layer (subretinal, intraretinal, and preretinal): macroaneurysm, trauma, sickle cell retinopathy, choroidal melanoma, vein occlusion (rare), CNV (rare)

Pathology: overall thickening of vessel wall with hypertrophy of muscularis

Treatment: observation; consider focal laser (risk of hemorrhage)

Hypertensive Retinopathy

Focal or generalized vasoconstriction, breakdown of blood-retinal barrier with subsequent hemorrhage and exudate

Associated with microaneurysms or macroaneurysms

Findings:
Retinopathy: AV nicking, "copper or silver wire" arterial changes, hemorrhages, exudates, cotton wool spots

Choroidopathy: fibrinoid necrosis of choroidal arterioles; may have Elschnig's spots (zone of nonperfusion of choriocapillaris; pale white or red patches of RPE) and exudative RD; due to acute hypertensive episode (preeclampsia, eclampsia, or pheochromocytoma); FA shows early hypoperfusion and late staining

Optic neuropathy: florid disc edema with macular exudate

Pathology: thickening of arteriolar walls leads to nicking of venules; endothelial hyperplasia

Complications: retinal vein occlusion, retinal macroaneurysm, nonarteritic AION, ocular motor nerve palsies, worsening of diabetic retinopathy

Diabetic Retinopathy (DR)

Leading cause of new blindness in United States, adults aged 20 to 74 years

Classification:

Background or nonproliferative (BDR, NPDR): hemorrhages, exudates, cotton wool spots, microaneurysms (MA), intraretinal microvascular abnormalities (IRMA), venous beading

Severe NPDR ("4-2-1 rule"):
Defined as any one of the following:
4 quadrants of hemorrhages/MAs
2 quadrants of venous beading
1 quadrant of IRMA

Very severe NPDR:
Defined as 2 or more of the above

Proliferative (PDR): neovascularization (NV) of disc or elsewhere

High risk proliferative (HR-PDR):
Defined as any one of the following:
1. NVD ≥ 1/4 to 1/3 disc area
2. Any NVD with vitreous hemorrhage
3. NVE ≥ 1/2 disc area with vitreous hemorrhage

Epidemiology:

Type 1 DM:
AT DIAGNOSIS: no BDR
AT 5 YEARS: 25% BDR, PDR rare
AT 20 YEARS: 98% BDR, 60% PDR, 30% CSME

Type 2 IDDM:
AT DIAGNOSIS: 30% BDR
AT 5 YEARS: 40% BDR, 2% PDR
AT 20 YEARS: 90% BDR, 25% PDR, 40% CSME

Type 2 NIDDM:
AT DIAGNOSIS: 20% BDR
AT 5 YEARS: 30% BDR, 2% PDR
AT 20 YEARS: 50% BDR, 10% PDR, 20% CSME

Findings: cotton wool spots, lipid exudates (may appear as circinate exudate [ring of hard exudate surrounding leaky focus] or macular star [pattern reflects radial orientation of Henle's fibers]), hemorrhages (blot [outer plexiform layer], flame [tracks along NFL]), microaneurysms, IRMA (intraretinal microvascular abnormalities; shunts [arteriole to venule]), venous beading and loops, neovascularization (disc [NVD], elsewhere in retina [NVE], iris [NVI]) (Figures 11-57 to 11-60)

Clinically significant macular edema (CSME) definition: one of the following
1. Thickening within 500 μm of the foveal avascular zone (FAZ)
2. Hard exudate within 500 μm of the FAZ with associated thickening of adjacent retina
3. Zone of retinal thickening 1 disk *area* in size, any part of which is within 1 disk *diameter* of the foveal center

Asymmetric diabetic retinopathy usually due to carotid disease (on either side)

Figure 11-57. Nonproliferative diabetic retinopathy.

lipid exudate   intraretinal hemorrhages

Figure 11-58. Severe nonproliferative diabetic retinopathy with extensive hemorrhages, microaneurysms, and exudates. (From Kaiser PK, Friedman NJ, Pineda R II: *Massachusetts Eye and Ear Infirmary Illustrated Manual of Ophthalmology*, 2nd ed, Philadelphia, Saunders, 2004.)

neovascularization   neovascularization
of the disc   elsewhere

Figure 11-59. Proliferative diabetic retinopathy demonstrating florid neovascularization of the disc and elsewhere. (From Kaiser PK, Friedman NJ, Pineda R II: *Massachusetts Eye and Ear Infirmary Illustrated Manual of Ophthalmology*, 2nd ed, Philadelphia, Saunders, 2004.)

neovascularization   capillary nonperfusion

Figure 11-60. Fluorescein angiogram of a patient with proliferative diabetic retinopathy, showing extensive capillary nonperfusion, neovascularization elsewhere, and vascular leakage. (From Kaiser PK, Friedman NJ, Pineda R II: *Massachusetts Eye and Ear Infirmary Illustrated Manual of Ophthalmology*, 2nd ed, Philadelphia, Saunders, 2004.)

Main cause of vision loss in NPDR: macular edema or ischemia

Main causes of vision loss in PDR: tractional RD (TRD), neovascular glaucoma (NVG), vitreous hemorrhage (VH)

Other sequelae:

    Diabetic cataract: aldose reductase pathway converts glucose into sorbitol and fructose; causes osmotic effect; aldose reductase also converts galactose into galactitol (which causes cataracts in galactosemia)

    Diabetic iridopathy: iris NV; lacy vacuolization of iris pigment epithelium in 40%; glycogen-filled cysts in iris pigment epithelium (PAS+)

    Papillitis: acute disc swelling; vision usually ≥20/50; 50% bilateral; may have VF defect; most recover to ≥20/30

    Isolated cranial nerve palsies: CN 3, 4, 6 (including pupil-sparing CN 3 palsy)

    Pupillary abnormalities: light-near dissociation

    Fluctuation in refractive error: due to osmotic effect on crystalline lens from unstable blood sugar levels

Pathology: loss of pericytes, no endothelial cells or pericytes in nonperfused areas; thickening of capillary basement membrane; breakdown of blood-retinal barrier; lacy vacuolization of iris pigment epithelium; intraepithelial vacuoles contain glycogen; gitter cells (lipid-laden macrophages) (Figures 11-61 and 11-62)

DDx: ocular ischemic syndrome, radiation retinopathy, hypertensive retinopathy, retinal vein occlusion, proliferative retinopathies (sarcoidosis, sickle cell), juxtaoveal telangiectasia

FA: indications

    Identify macular ischemia

    Localize microaneurysms to guide focal laser treatment

    Identify areas of NVE

    Identify areas of capillary nonperfusion

Figure 11-61. Lacy vacuolization of iris pigment epithelium. (Modified from Yanoff M et al: *Am J Ophthalmol*, 69:201, 1970. (From Yanoff M, Fine BS: *Ocular Pathology*, 5th ed, St. Louis, Mosby, 2004.)

Figure 11-62. Microaneurysms, pericyte dropout, and acellular capillaries are seen. (From Benson WE: Diabetic retinopathy. In Yanoff M, Duker JS [eds]: *Ophthalmology*. London, Mosby, 1999.).

Treatment:

    Based on results of several important studies

    Early Treatment Diabetic Retinopathy Study (ETDRS):

        Focal laser decreases vision loss from macular edema by 50%

        No benefit from aspirin

    Diabetic Retinopathy Study (DRS):

        PRP reduces incidence of severe vision loss in high-risk PDR by 60%

    Diabetic Retinopathy Vitrectomy Study (DRVS):

        Early Vitrectomy for VH in type 1 diabetics only, can defer in type 2

    Diabetes Control and Complications Trial (DCCT):

        Tight control of blood sugar slows progression of retinopathy, diabetic macular edema, and visual loss in type 1 diabetic patients; patients with HbA1c <8% had a significantly reduced risk of retinopathy

        Rapid normalization and tight control of blood sugar after a period of prolonged hyperglycemia can lead to worsening of retinopathy

United Kingdom Prospective Diabetes Study (UKPDS):

Tight control of blood sugar and blood pressure slows progression of retinopathy and development of macular edema in type 2 diabetic patients

Focal laser: for CSME (visual acuity is not part of treatment criteria); argon green preferred; yellow (577 nm) also used because well absorbed by hemoglobin within microaneurysms; reexamine every 3 to 4 months

Panretinal photocoagulation (PRP):

CRITERIA: HR-PDR

1. NVD ≥1/4 to 1/3 disc area
2. Any NVD with vitreous hemorrhage
3. NVE ≥1/2 disc area with vitreous hemorrhage

COMPLICATIONS: decreased night vision (destruction of extramacular rods), angle-closure glaucoma (choroidal effusion), retinal detachment (regression of NV fronds can cause contracture, leading to retinal tear and rhegmatogenous or traction RD), central scotoma (worsening of CSME), progression of cataract

Up to 33% of patients will not respond to PRP

Vitrectomy:

INDICATIONS:

Nonclearing vitreous hemorrhage

Combined tractional-rhegmatogenous RD

Traction retinal detachment of the fovea. If tractional detachment is extramacular, watch closely; if macula is threatened or detaches, perform vitrectomy

Anterior hyaloidal fibrovascular proliferation

Refractory macular edema: patients with taut posterior hyaloid face can have chronic macular edema that does not resolve with laser. Chronic traction of vitreous face on macula appears to produce persistent leakage; can resolve after traction is relieved with vitrectomy

Progressive fibrovascular proliferation despite complete PRP

Ghost cell glaucoma

Prognosis: risk of progression without treatment from preproliferative to proliferative DR over 2 years is 50%

Severe NPDR has 50% risk of progression to proliferative disease in 12 to 18 months

Conditions that exacerbate diabetic retinopathy: hypertension, puberty, pregnancy (at conception, if no BDR, 88% have no retinopathy; if mild BDR, 47% worsen, 5% develop PDR; if PDR, 46% have progression), renal disease, anemia

Follow HbA1c (serum glycosylated hemoglobin [provides 3-month view of blood sugar levels])

MAJOR DIABETIC RETINOPATHY CLINICAL STUDIES

Diabetic Retinopathy Study (DRS)

Objective: to evaluate whether photocoagulation prevents severe visual loss in eyes with diabetic retinopathy

Methods: patients had PDR in at least 1 eye or severe NPDR in both eyes, or 20/100 or better vision in each eye, and were randomly assigned to treatment with scatter laser photocoagulation (randomly assigned to either xenon arc [200–400, 4.5° spots] or argon blue-green laser [800–1600, 500 μm spots]) in 1 eye and no treatment in the fellow eye (protocol later amended to allow deferred laser photocoagulation). Surface neovascularization (NVE) treated directly with confluent burns, and NVD treated directly only in argon laser–treated eyes. Patients were excluded if they had previous panretinal photocoagulation or a traction retinal detachment threatening the macula

Severe NPDR defined as having at least 3 of the following:

Cotton wool spots

Venous beading

Intraretinal microvascular abnormalities (IRMA) in ≥2 of 4 contiguous overlapping photographic fields

Moderate to severe retinal hemorrhages and/or microaneurysms in ≥1 standard photographic field

Results: 1727 patients enrolled

PRP reduced the risk of severe vision loss (VA <5/200 on 2 consecutive visits 4 months apart) by 50% to 60% in patients with high-risk characteristics (see later)

Conclusions: perform PRP for patients with high-risk proliferative retinopathy (HR-PDR) regardless of vision

NVD (new vessels on or within 1 disc diameter of the disc) ≥1/4 to 1/3 of disc area (standard photo 10A)

Any NVD with vitreous or preretinal hemorrhage

NVE (new vessels elsewhere) ≥1/2 of disc area (standard photo 7) with vitreous or preretinal hemorrhage

PRP is also indicated for NVI

DRS did not report a clear benefit for immediate PRP in patients with severe nonproliferative diabetic retinopathy and proliferative diabetic retinopathy without high-risk characteristics. However, older-onset diabetic patients should be considered for earlier PRP

Early Treatment Diabetic Retinopathy Study (ETDRS)

Objective: to evaluate

1. Whether photocoagulation is effective for diabetic macular edema

2. Effect of aspirin on the course of diabetic retinopathy
3. When to initiate PRP treatment for diabetic retinopathy

Methods: patients had mild, moderate, or severe NPDR or early PDR (does not meet high-risk criteria of PDR) in both eyes, and 20/200 or better vision in each eye, and were randomly assigned to receive 650 mg daily aspirin or not AND 1 of the following:

1. Moderate to severe NPDR or early PDR with no macular edema = immediate PRP (further randomly assigned to full [1200–1600, 500 μm spots] scatter or mild [400–650, 500 μm spots] scatter PRP) vs deferred PRP until high-risk characteristics developed
2. Mild or moderate NPDR and macular edema = immediate laser (further randomly assigned to immediate focal laser photocoagulation and deferred full scatter or mild scatter when high-risk characteristics developed; or immediate mild or full scatter PRP and deferred focal laser photocoagulation) vs deferred laser photocoagulation
3. Severe NPDR or early PDR and macular edema = immediate laser (further randomly assigned to immediate mild or full PRP and immediate or deferred focal laser photocoagulation) vs deferred laser photocoagulation

Patients were excluded if they had high-risk proliferative diabetic retinopathy

Mild diabetic retinopathy defined as:
At least 1 microaneurysm, but not enough to qualify as moderate NPDR

Moderate diabetic retinopathy defined as:
Extensive intraretinal hemorrhages and/or microaneurysms, cotton wool spots, IRMA, venous beading, but not enough to qualify as severe NPDR

Severe diabetic retinopathy defined with "4-2-1 rule" as any one of the following:
Intraretinal hemorrhages and/or microaneurysms in all 4 quadrants
Venous beading in at least 2 quadrants
IRMA in at least 1 quadrant

CSME defined as one of the following:
1. Retinal thickening at or within 500 μm of the foveal avascular zone (FAZ)
2. Hard exudates at or within 500 μm of the foveal avascular zone (FAZ) with associated thickening of the adjacent retina
3. Retinal thickening ≥1 disc *area* in size ≤1 disc *diameter* from the center of the fovea

Results: 3711 patients enrolled
Immediate focal laser decreased moderate vision loss in patients with clinically significant macular edema by ~50%
Early PRP reduced the risk of development of high-risk PDR in patients with NPDR and early PDR, but difference in severe visual loss was minimal
Immediate focal laser and deferred scatter PRP reduced moderate visual loss by 50% in patients with mild or moderate NPDR and macular edema
Immediate focal laser and scatter PRP reduced severe visual loss by 50% in patients with severe NPDR or early PDR and macular edema
Aspirin had no effect on progression or complications of diabetic retinopathy

Conclusions: treat all patients with CSME regardless of vision
Immediate PRP should be reserved for patients with high-risk PDR and possibly those with severe NPDR in both eyes
No benefit from aspirin (650 mg/day)

Diabetic Retinopathy Vitrectomy Study (DRVS)

Objective: to observe patients with severe DR in type 1 and type 2 diabetes over 2 years to determine visual outcomes

Methods: patients with severe NPDR or early PDR (do not meet high-risk criteria of PDR) were placed into 1 of 3 groups
Group N: natural history study with 744 eyes of 644 patients enrolled
Group NR: to evaluate early surgical intervention vs delayed surgery (for at least 1 year) in eyes with severe diabetic retinopathy and active neovascularization or fibrovascular proliferation but without severe visual loss (vision better than 10/200). 370 eyes enrolled. Amount of new vessel severity was quantified
NVC-1 (least severe): new vessel severity no worse than moderate in only 1 photographic field
NVC-2 (moderately severe): moderate new vessels in 2 or more fields, but not severe in any field
NVC-3 (severe): severe NVD or NVE in at least 1 field
NVC-4 (very severe): severe NVD and NVE in at least 1 field
Group H: to evaluate early surgical intervention (within days) vs delayed surgery (for at least 1 year, unless TRD of macula detected on ultrasound examination) in eyes with severe diabetic retinopathy and active neovascularization or fibrovascular proliferation, with history of sudden visual loss from severe vitreous hemorrhage within 6 months (vision worse than 5/200, not NLP). 616 eyes enrolled. (Note: endophotocoagulation was not used in the DRVS)
Patients were excluded if they had a previous vitrectomy, photocoagulation within 3 months, IOP >29 mm Hg on medications, severe iris neovasularizataion, or neovascular glaucoma

Results:
Group NR:
4-YEAR RESULTS: patients in the early vitrectomy group had better vision than those in the deferral group

Up to 18 months, the early vitrectomy group had a higher risk of no light perception vision; this was not seen at later time points

Type 1 diabetic patients had an increased chance of obtaining good vision with early vitrectomy

Previous PRP increased chances of good vision

With increasing severity of vessels, early intervention was better than deferred intervention

Group H:

2-YEAR RESULTS: patients in the early vitrectomy group had better vision than those in the deferral group

Patients with type 1 DM had superior outcomes from early vitrectomy, no advantage seen in type 2 DM

Conclusions: early vitrectomy for eyes with severe visual loss due to nonclearing vitreous hemorrhage (at least 1 month) is helpful in type 1 diabetic patients and monocular patients despite the type of diabetes. Early vitrectomy is also recommended for eyes with useful vision and advanced active PDR, especially when extensive neovascularization is present. NLP was seen in 20% of eyes regardless of intervention once a severe vitreous hemorrhage had occurred. Eyes with traction retinal detachment not involving the fovea can be observed until the fovea becomes detached, provided that the fibrovascular proliferation is not severe

Diabetes Control and Complications Trial (DCCT)

Objective: to evaluate effect of tight vs conventional control of blood sugar on diabetic complications in type 1 diabetic patients

Methods: patients with insulin dependence defined by C-peptide secretion were randomly assigned to either

Intensive therapy: 3 or more daily insulin injections or implantation of an insulin pump

Self-monitoring of glucose levels at least 4 times a day

Adjust insulin dose based on glucose level

Preprandial glucose = 70 to 120 mg/dL (3.9 and 6.7 mmol/L)

Postprandial glucose <180 mg/dL (10.0 mmol/L)

Weekly 3 AM glucose >65 mg/dL (3.6 mmol/L)

Monthly HbA1c <6.05% (nondiabetic range)

Conventional therapy: 1 or 2 daily insulin injections

Daily self-monitoring of glucose levels

Did not adjust insulin dose daily

Education about diet and exercise

Followed every 3 months

No glycosuria or ketonuria

Absence of hyperglycemic or hypoglycemic symptoms

Results: 1441 patients included, study stopped after average follow-up of 6.5 years by independent safety and monitoring committee

Average difference in HbA1c was >2% between groups; however, <5% of intensive group kept <6.05%

Incidence of DR was the same up to 36 months

At baseline, 726 patients had no retinopathy, and 715 had mild retinopathy. After 5 years, the incidence of retinopathy was approximately 50% less with intensive therapy

Patients with HbA1c <8% had significantly reduced risk of retinopathy

Intensive control:

Reduced the risk of development of DR by 76%

Slowed the progression of DR by 54% and reduced the development of severe NPDR or PDR by 47%

Reduced the risk of macular edema by 23%

Reduced the risk of laser treatment by 56%

Reduced albuminuria by 54%

Reduced clinical neuropathy by 60%

Adverse effect: 2 to 3× increase in severe hypoglycemia

Conclusions: tight control is beneficial; however, rapid normalization and tight control of blood sugar after a period of prolonged hyperglycemia can lead to an initial worsening of retinopathy

Epidemiology of Diabetes Interventions and Complications (EDIC) Trial

Objective: to gain further follow-up of patients from the DCCT

Methods: 1208 patients from DCCT, all of whom received intensive therapy and were followed for an additional 4 years

Results: intensive therapy reduced the risk of

Progression of retinopathy by 75%

Any macular edema by 58%

Laser treatment by 52%

Conclusions: tight control is still beneficial

United Kingdom Prospective Diabetes Study (UKPDS)

Objective: to compare the effects on the risk of microvascular and macrovascular complications of intensive blood glucose control with oral hypoglycemics and/or insulin and conventional treatment with diet therapy

Methods: 4209 newly diagnosed patients with type 2 diabetes, median age 54 years (range, 25–65 years), were randomly assigned to intensive therapy with a sulfonylurea (chlorpropamide, glibenclamide, or glipizide) or with insulin, or conventional therapy using diet control

Results: after a median duration of therapy of 11 years, intensive treatment with sulfonylurea, insulin, and/or metformin was equally effective in reducing fasting plasma glucose concentrations.

Over 10 years, HbA1c was 7.0% (range, 6.2–8.2) in the intensive group compared with 7.9% (range, 6.9–8.8)

in the conventional group—an 11% reduction. No difference in HbA1c was seen among agents in the intensive group.

Compared with the conventional group, the risk in the intensive group was 12% lower for any diabetes-related end point; 10% lower for any diabetes-related death; and 6% lower for all-cause mortality.

The reduction in HbA1c was associated with a 25% overall reduction in microvascular complications, including retinopathy (21% reduction) and nephropathy (34% reduction). 37% of patients had microaneurysms in 1 eye at diagnosis and random assignment

Conclusions: type 2 diabetic patients benefit from intensive glycemic control, as do type 1 diabetic patients

The United Kingdom Prospective Diabetes Study—Hypertension in Diabetes Study (UKPDS-HDS)

Objective: to compare the effects of intensive blood pressure control on the risk of microvascular and macrovascular complications

Methods: 1148 patients with type 2 diabetes and mild to moderate hypertension to determine if "tight blood pressure control (150/85 mm Hg)" using an angiotensin-converting enzyme (ACE) inhibitor or a β-blocker vs "less tight control (<180/105 mm Hg)" would prevent diabetic complications.

Patients were randomly assigned to captopril (ACE inhibitor) or atenolol (β-blocker) and followed for a median of 8.4 years.

Results: tight control of blood pressure in patients with hypertension and type 2 diabetes reduced the risk of death related to diabetes by 32%.

In addition, there was a 34% reduction in risk of deterioration of retinopathy by 2 or more ETDRS steps from baseline, and a 47% reduction in risk of deterioration of visual acuity by 3 ETDRS lines with tight blood pressure control.

Lowering of blood pressure with captopril or atenolol was similarly effective in reducing the incidence of diabetic complications, suggesting that blood pressure reduction in itself may be more important than the treatment used

Conclusions: tight blood pressure control reduced the risk of complications from diabetic retinopathy

Sickle Cell Retinopathy

Proliferative retinopathy, usually equatorial or pre-equatorial

Most severe in HbSC disease; SC > S Thal > SS > SA

Incidence in African American population: SS = 1%; sickle trait = 8%; SC <0.5%;

20% to 60% autoinfarct

Findings: salmon patch (intraretinal hemorrhage following peripheral retinal arteriolar occlusion), black sunburst (chorioretinal scar with RPE proliferation due to old hemorrhage), sea fan (peripheral NV), refractile spots (old, resorbed hemorrhages), silver wiring of peripheral vessels, angioid streaks, vascular occlusions (macular arteriolar occlusions [wedge sign], CRAO, RVO, choroid; CRAO can develop in patients with hyphema), venous tortuosity, comma-shaped conjunctival vessels, vitreous hemorrhage, rhegmatogenous RD (due to contracture of NV fronds)

Figure 11-63. An equatorial "salmon patch" intraretinal hemorrhage with periarteriolar hemorrhage. (Courtesy of William Tasman, MD. From Ho AC: Hemoglobinopathies. In Yanoff M, Duker JS [eds]: *Ophthalmology*. London, Mosby, 1999.)

Figure 11-64. A black "sunburst" retinal lesion. (From Ho AC: Hemoglobinopathies. In Yanoff M, Duker JS [eds]: *Ophthalmology*. London, Mosby, 1999.)

Figure 11-65. A sea fan in a sickle SC patient. (From Ho AC: Hemoglobinopathies. In Yanoff M, Duker JS [eds]: *Ophthalmology*. London, Mosby, 1999.)

Stage 1: Peripheral arterial occlusions
Stage 2: Peripheral anastomoses
Stage 3: Neovascularization (sea fan)
Stage 4: Vitreous hemorrhage
Stage 5: Vitreous traction with RD

Diagnosis: sickle cell prep, Hgb electrophoresis

FA: capillary nonperfusion, AV anastomoses, neovascularization

Figure 11-66. Fluorescein angiography of sea fans with peripheral nonperfusion. (From Ho AC: Hemoglobinopathies. In Yanoff M, Duker JS: [eds] *Ophthalmology*. London, Mosby, 1999.)

Treatment: laser (PRP) or consider cryotherapy (controversial) for neovascularization; surgery for RD and chronic VH

Eales Disease

Idiopathic retinal perivasculitis and peripheral nonperfusion with NV

Occurs in healthy young men; 90% bilateral

More common in Middle East and India

Increased risk of BVO

Findings: NV (80%, NVD or NVE), recurrent VH, rubeosis, neovascular glaucoma, cataract, vascular sheathing (80%) with leakage on FA, vascular tortuosity, collateral formation around occluded vessels, peripheral nonperfusion; may have AC reaction, KP, vitreous cells, macular edema
    Stage 1: sheathing of retinal venules, retinal edema, hemorrhages
    Stage 2: more severe involvement and vitreous haze
    Stage 3: peripheral NV
    Stage 4: proliferative retinopathy with VH and TRD

Other findings: vestibulocochlear involvement (sensorineural hearing loss and vestibular dysfunction), PPD-positive, cerebral vasculitis (rare)

DDx of peripheral neovascularization: hemoglobinopathies, diabetes, retinal vein occlusions, ROP, FEVR, retinal emboli (talc), hyperviscosity syndromes, carotid-cavernous sinus fistula, ocular ischemia, sarcoidosis, lupus, inflammatory bowel disease, retinal vasculitis, uveitis, VKH syndrome, pars planitis, Norrie's disease, incontinentia pigmenti

Retinopathy of Prematurity (ROP; Retrolental Fibroplasia)

(see Chapter 5, Pediatrics/Strabismus)

Familial Exudative Vitreoretinopathy (FEVR)

(see Chapter 5, Pediatrics/Strabismus)

Branch Retinal Vein Occlusion (BVO)

Site of occlusion is at AV crossing (usually artery compresses vein); generally superotemporal (63%)

Associated with atherosclerosis, hypertension, diabetes, age (>50 years old), glaucoma, papilledema, increased IOP, optic disc drusen

2 types:
    Nonischemic: <5 DD of capillary nonperfusion
    Ischemic: ≥5 DD of capillary nonperfusion

Findings: numerous deep and superficial hemorrhages (in a wedge-shaped distribution with the tip pointing toward the etiologic crossing), cotton wool spots, CME, disc edema (Figures 11-67 and 11-68)

Treatment: sector PRP for NV and VH, grid laser for macular edema when vision <20/40 for at least 3 months and no macular ischemia on FA
    Branch Vein Occlusion Study (BVOS):
    Perform grid argon laser for macular edema and vision <20/40 for >3 months (treated eyes more likely to have improved vision)

Figure 11-67. BVO. Early leakage.

Figure 11-68. BVO. Late leakage.

Perform PRP for ≥5 DD of nonperfusion if neovascularization develops (treated eyes less likely to develop NV and VH)

Prognosis: >50% maintain vision better than 20/40 after 1 year; 10% have episode in fellow eye

Complications:
  Nonischemic BVO: macular edema can develop
  Ischemic BVO: macular edema, ischemic maculopathy, neovascularization, vitreous hemorrhage, tractional or rhegmatogenous RD; 40% risk of developing NV (NVI rare)

Central Retinal Vein Occlusion (CVO)

Occlusion occurs at level of the lamina cribrosa

2 types:
  Perfused/nonischemic (70%): vision >20/200, 16% progress to nonperfused; 50% resolve completely without treatment; defined as <10 DD of capillary nonperfusion

Figure 11-69. Nonischemic central retinal vein occlusion. (From Heier JS, Morley MG: Venous obstructive disease of the retina. In Yanoff M, Duker JS [eds]: *Ophthalmology*. London, Mosby, 1999.)

  Nonperfused/ischemic (30%): ≥10 DD nonperfusion; patients are older and have worse vision; 60% develop iris NV; up to 33% develop neovascular glaucoma (NVG; "90-day" glaucoma)

Figure 11-70. Ischemic central retinal vein occlusion. (From Heier JS, Morley MG: Venous obstructive disease of the retina. In Yanoff M, Duker JS [eds]: *Ophthalmology*. London, Mosby, 1999.)

10% combined with BRAO (usually cilioretinal artery due to low perfusion pressure of choroidal system)

Risk factors: age (>50 years old), hypertension (61%), diabetes, heart disease, glaucoma, syphilis, sarcoidosis, vasculitis, increased intraorbital or intraocular pressure, hyphema, hyperviscosity syndromes (multiple myeloma, Waldenström's macroglobulinemia, leukemia), high homocysteine levels, sickle cell, HIV

Findings: venous dilation and tortuosity, hemorrhages in all 4 quadrants, may have disc edema and macular edema

> **High-risk characteristics**: marked vision loss, numerous cotton wool spots, positive RAPD, dense central scotoma with peripheral field changes on VF, widespread capillary nonperfusion on FA, reduced b-wave–to–a-wave ratio on ERG

Pathology: marked retinal edema, focal retinal necrosis, gliosis; subretinal, intraretinal, and preretinal hemorrhages

Treatment: follow every month for first 6 months, including gonioscopy

> **Central Vein Occlusion Study** (CVOS):
> No benefit from early PRP (to prevent iris NV) in ischemic CVO; therefore, wait until first sign of NV
> No benefit from focal laser for macular edema

Complications: iris NV (more common than NVD or NVE), NVG, TRD, VH, and macular edema

Hemiretinal Vein Occlusion (HRVO)

Risk factors: hypertension, diabetes, glaucoma

Ischemic HRVO: higher risk of NVD (30%) or NVE (40%) than with either an ischemic CVO or a BVO; NVI in 10%

MAJOR RETINAL VEIN OCCLUSION CLINICAL STUDIES

Branch Vein Occlusion Study (BVOS)

Objective: to evaluate photocoagulation in patients with branch vein occlusion (BVO) for
1. Prevention of neovascularization
2. Prevention of vitreous hemorrhage
3. Improvement of vision in eyes with macular edema, reducing vision to 20/40 or worse

Methods:

> **Group I** (at risk for neovascularization): patients with BVO occurring within 3 to 18 months with an area of retinal involvement at least 5 DD in size, with no neovascularization present and vision better than 5/200, were randomly assigned to peripheral scatter laser photocoagulation vs observation
>
> **Group II** (at risk for vitreous hemorrhage): patients with BVO occurring within 3 to 18 months with disc or peripheral neovascularization and vision better than 5/200 were randomly assigned to peripheral scatter laser photocoagulation vs observation
>
> **Group III** (at risk for vision loss due to macular edema): patients with BVO occurring within 3 to 18 months with macular edema involving the fovea and vision worse than 20/40 were randomly assigned to grid pattern laser photocoagulation with argon laser vs observation

> **Group X** (at high risk for neovascularization): patients with BVO occurring within 3 to 18 months with at least 5 DD of capillary nonperfusion were followed. Note: This group was recruited after group I recruitment had ended

Results:

> **Group 1** : 319 patients enrolled. After an average follow-up of 3.7 years, the development of neovascularization was significantly less in laser-treated eyes. Treated eyes were less likely to develop NV (12% vs 24% of untreated)
>
> **Group II**: 82 eyes enrolled. After an average follow-up of 2.8 years, the development of vitreous hemorrhage was significantly less in the laser-treated eyes. Treated eyes were less likely to develop VH (29% vs 61% of untreated)
>
> **Group III**: 139 patients enrolled. After an average follow-up of 3.1 years, treated eyes were more likely to have improved vision (gain of ≥2 lines in 65% vs 37% of untreated), vision >20/40, and final average vision better than untreated eyes
>
> **Group X**: eyes with ≥5 DD of nonperfusion were considered nonperfused and showed a greater risk of developing neovascularization

Conclusions:

> Grid pattern laser photocoagulation recommended for eyes with a BVO of 3 to 18 months duration if visual acuity is 20/40 or worse *and* if fluorescein angiography documents macular edema without foveal hemorrhage as the cause of visual loss
>
> Perform PRP if retinal neovascularization develops, especially if ≥5 DD of nonperfusion exists

Central Vein Occlusion Study (CVOS)

Objective: to evaluate patients with central retinal vein occlusion (CVO) for
1. Natural history of eyes with perfused (<10 disc areas of nonperfusion) CVO
2. Improvement of vision in eyes with perfused macular edema
3. Eyes with nonperfused CVO; does early PRP prevent NVI?
4. Eyes with nonperfused CVO; is early PRP more effective than delayed PRP in preventing NVG?

Methods:

> **Group P** (perfused): patients with CVO occurring for less than 1 year with intraretinal hemorrhages in all 4 quadrants and with capillary nonperfusion less than 10 DD in size and with no iris or angle neovascularization. These patients were observed. 547 patients enrolled
>
> **Group N** (nonperfused): patients with CVO occurring for less than 1 year with intraretinal hemorrhages in all 4 quadrants and with capillary nonperfusion greater than 10 DD in size and with no iris or angle neovascularization were randomly assigned to immediate PRP or observation. 180 patients enrolled

Group I (indeterminate): patients with CVO occurring for less than 1 year with intraretinal hemorrhages in all 4 quadrants and with retinal hemorrhages that prevent measurement of the area of capillary nonperfusion and with no iris or angle neovascularization. These patients were followed. 52 eyes enrolled

Group M (macular edema): patients with CVO occurring for at least 3 months with macular edema that involves the fovea and with visual acuity of 20/50 to 5/200 were randomly assigned to grid pattern laser photocoagulation or observation. 155 eyes enrolled

Results:

Group P: 34% became nonperfused at 3 years

RISK FACTORS FOR PROGRESSION TO NONPERFUSED: CVO of less than 1 month duration, visual acuity less than 20/200, presence of greater than 5 disc areas of nonperfusion

Group N: prophylactic PRP did not prevent iris or angle NV (18 of 90 eyes [20%] with prophylactic PRP developed iris or angle NV, vs 32 of 91 eyes [35%] that did not receive prophylactic PRP), eyes prophylactically treated with PRP did not respond well to supplemental PRP (18 of 32 [56%] observation eyes responded to PRP following development of iris or angle NV, vs 4 of 18 eyes [22%] that received prophylactic PRP responded to supplemental PRP).

RISK FACTORS FOR DEVELOPING NVI: amount of nonperfused retina, extent of retinal hemorrhages, male sex, CVO of less than 1 month duration

Group M: grid pattern photocoagulation did not preserve or improve visual acuity (but reduced angiographic evidence of macular edema)

Conclusions:

No benefit from early PRP in nonperfused CVO; therefore, wait until first sign of NVI before initiating PRP

PRP for nonperfused CVO when 2 clock hours of NVI or any angle NV present

Monthly follow-up with gonioscopy during first 6 months after CVO

No benefit from focal laser for treatment of macular edema after CVO

Branch Retinal Artery Occlusion (BRAO)

90% caused by emboli (cholesterol, calcium, fibrin, platelets)

Most commonly at retinal arterial bifurcations

10% risk of episode in fellow eye

Central Retinal Artery Occlusion (CRAO)

Most common cause of cherry red spot (thin transparent foveal tissue surrounded by opacified ischemic retina)

Etiology:

Atherosclerosis: of CRA at lamina cribrosa

Emboli: cholesterol (73%), platelet fibrin (15%) from carotid plaque, calcific (from heart), tumor (atrial myxoma), lipid emboli (pancreatitis), talc

Vasculitis: GCA in elderly patient (always check ESR)

Trauma: retrobulbar injection, orbital surgery, penetrating injury

Coagulopathy: oral contraceptives, pregnancy, sickle cell (especially after hyphema), platelet or factor abnormalities, homocystinuria, hyperhomocysteinemia, protein S deficiency, antiphospholipid antibody (check anticardiolipid antibody panel; also at risk for DVT, pulmonary embolism, cardiac vessel blockage, and spontaneous abortion; treat with coumadin; steroids do not decrease risk of thromboembolism)

Ocular abnormalities: optic disc drusen, prepapillary loops, elevated IOP

Collagen vascular disease: lupus, polyarteritis nodosa, Wegener's granulomatosis

Migraine: in young patients; 90% present with vision of LP to CF; 10% recover vision (usually from cilioretinal artery [in 25% of population]), 18% have vision ≥20/40, 66% have vision ≤20/400

Orbital mucor

Fibromuscular hyperplasia

Behçet's disease

Leukemia

Findings: retinal whitening in posterior pole with cherry red spot, box-carring (interuption of blood column), emboli, RAPD; whitening resolves after 4 to 6 weeks, and pale disc and attenuated vessels develop

Pathology: atrophy of inner retinal layers (those supplied by retinal circulation)

DDx: ophthalmic artery occlusion, inadvertent intraocular injection of gentamicin, arteritic AION

DDx of cherry red spot: sphingolipidosis (Tay-Sachs, Niemann-Pick, Gaucher's, Farber's disease), quinine toxicity, commotio retinae, macular hole with surrounding RD, macular hemorrhage, subacute sclerosing panencephalitis, ocular ischemia, methanol toxicity

Diagnosis:

Lab tests: CBC, ESR, complete cardiovascular workup; consider workup for clotting disorders: serum protein electrophoresis, protein C, activated protein C resistance (factor 5 Lieden deficiency), protein S, antithrombin III, anticardiolipin antibodies, lupus anticoagulant, plasma homocysteine, C-ANCA

FA: delayed filling, increased AV transit time, focal staining at obstruction, collateral or retrograde flow

Retinal edema   Patent
cilioretinal
artery

Figure 11-71. Cilioretinal artery-sparing central retinal artery occlusion with patent cilioretinal artery, allowing perfusion (thus no edema) in a small section of the macula. (From Kaiser PK, Friedman NJ, Pineda R II: *Massachusetts Eye and Ear Infirmary Illustrated Manual of Ophthalmology*, 2nd ed, Philadelphia, Saunders, 2004.)

Patent   Absent flow
cilioretinal
artery

Figure 11-72. Fluorescein angiogram of the same patient as in Figure 11-71, demonstrating no filling of retinal vessels except in cilioretinal artery and surrounding branches. (From Kaiser PK, Friedman NJ, Pineda R II: *Massachusetts Eye and Ear Infirmary Illustrated Manual of Ophthalmology*, 2nd ed, Philadelphia, Saunders, 2004.)

ERG: depressed b-wave (inner retina), normal/supernormal a-wave, loss of oscillatory potentials

Treatment: irreversible damage occurs after 90 minutes; therefore, emergent lowering of IOP to allow arterial pressure to reestablish blood flow: paracentesis, ocular massage, carbogen (95% O_2, 5% CO_2) or breath into paper bag, oral and topical ocular hypotensive agents may be tried

Prognosis: <5% develop neovascular glaucoma; 1% with bilateral disease; 10% risk of episode in fellow eye

Complications: rubeosis (15%)

Ophthalmic Artery Occlusion

NLP vision and no cherry red spot; RPE pigmentary changes develop

May occur with orbital mucormycosis

FA: absent choroidal and retinal filling

ERG: absent a-wave

Ocular Ischemic Syndrome

Reduced blood flow to globe produces anterior and/or posterior segment ischemia

Etiology: carotid occlusion (most common), carotid dissection, arteritis (rare)

Associated with diabetes (56%), hypertension (50%), coronary artery disease (38%), CVA/TIA (31%)

Symptoms: amaurosis fugax, gradual or sudden visual loss, dull pain; may experience transient visual loss, sometimes precipitated by exposure to bright light (due to impaired photoreceptor regeneration)

Findings:
  Anterior segment: chronic conjunctivitis, rubeosis, PAS, AC cells and flare, corneal edema, cataract, altered IOP, hypopyon (rare)
  Posterior segment: vitreous cells, NV, optic disc pallor (40%), optic nerve swelling (8%), superficial hemorrhages in midperiphery, CME, cherry red spot (18%), altered vessels (attenuated, box-carring, dilated, nontortuous veins)

Figure 11-73. Retinal vascular changes in ocular ischemic syndrome. (From Fox GM, Sivalingham A, Brown CG: Ocular ischemic syndrome. In Yanoff M, Duker JS [eds]: *Ophthalmology*. London, Mosby, 1999.)

DDx: aortic arch disease, Takayasu's disease

Diagnosis: digital pressure on eye causes arterial pulsation
  FA: delayed filling (retina and choroid), diffuse leakage
  Ophthalmodynamometry
  Carotid ultrasound: severe stenosis (>80%)

Treatment: lower IOP to increase perfusion pressure, carotid surgery; PRP (controversial because anterior segment ischemia can possibly be due to uveal ischemia without retinal ischemia)

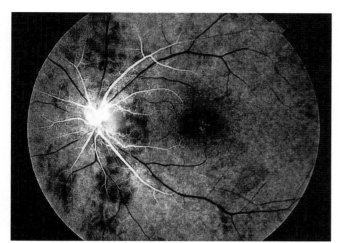

Figure 11-74. Fluorescein angiography, ocular ischemic syndrome. (From Fox GM, Sivalingham A, Brown CG: Ocular ischemic syndrome. In Yanoff M, Duker JS [eds]: *Ophthalmology*. London, Mosby, 1999.)

Radiation Retinopathy

Slowly progressive microangiopathy following exposure to radiation (6 months to 3 years after radiation treatment)

Threshold dose is 300 rads; occurs 4 to 32 months following plaque brachytherapy with mean dose of 15,000 rads; occurs 36 months after external beam radiation with mean dose of 5000 rads

Findings: hemorrhage, exudate, microaneurysms, capillary nonperfusion, cotton wool spots, NV, optic disc swelling, optic neuropathy; gradual occlusion of larger retinal vessels, eventually proliferative retinopathy

Pathology: vascular decompensation with focal loss of capillary endothelial cells and pericytes; radiation-induced optic neuropathy: ischemic demyelination with obliterative endarteritis of nerve sheath vasculature

Treatment: focal laser for macular edema, PRP for NV; hyperbaric O$_2$ (controversial)

Certain types of chemotherapy can worsen radiation retinopathy

Hypercoagulable States

Etiology: antiphospholipid antibodies (lupus anticoagulant) and anticardiolipins, Waldenström's macroglobulinemia, leukemia

Findings: cotton wool spots, blot hemorrhages, boxcarring, capillary nonperfusion, arteriolar attenuation

Disseminated Intravascular Coagulation

May cause fibrinoid necrosis of choriocapillaris, serous retinal detachments, and multiple areas of RPE changes

Phakomatoses

(see Chapter 5, Pediatrics/Strabismus)

Inflammatory/Immune Disease

(see Chapter 8, Uveitis)

Infections

(see Chapter 8, Uveitis)

Neuroretinitis

Usually unilateral

50% have viral prodrome

Symptoms: decreased vision; colors appear washed out; rarely, retrobulbar pain, pain associated with eye movement, or headache

Findings: optic nerve swelling (optic atrophy can develop), peripapillary NFL hemorrhages, serous RD; iritis, vitritis, and/or scleritis (rare); vascular occlusions may develop

Etiology:
  Noninfectious: cerebral AV malformation, elevated ICP, malignant hypertension, ischemic optic neuropathy, polyarteritis nodosa, Leber's idiopathic stellate neuroretinitis
    LEBER'S IDIOPATHIC STELLATE NEURORETINITIS (LISN):
      Affects individuals age 8 to 55 years old (usually in 3rd decade); male = female; >70% unilateral
      Viral prodrome in 5%
      FINDINGS: decreased vision; RAPD (75%); cecocentral or central scotoma; vitreous cells; optic disc edema (resolves over 8–12 weeks); optic atrophy is rare; macular star develops in 2nd week; exudative peripapillary RD can occur; RPE defects late; rarely develop chorioretinitis with elevated yellow-white spots in deep retina
      FA: hot disc; no perifoveal capillary leakage or macular abnormalities
      PROGNOSIS: excellent
  Infectious (suggested by multiple areas of retinitis): syphilis, Lyme disease, viral (influenza A, mumps, coxsackie B, EBV), cat-scratch disease (*Bartonella henselae*), TB, *Salmonella typhi*, parasites (*Toxocara, Toxoplasma*, DUSN)

DIFFUSE UNILATERAL SUBACUTE NEURORETINITIS (DUSN):

Due to subretinal nematode: *Ancylostoma caninum* (dog hookworm), *Baylisascaris procyonis* (raccoon worm)

Chronic course

Does not have characteristic neuroretinitis appearance

FINDINGS: multifocal pigmentary changes due to movement of the worm, minimal intraocular inflammation, decreased vision (typically out of proportion to findings); may have RAPD. Late findings include visual field defects, optic nerve pallor, chorioretinal atrophy, and narrowed retinal vessels

DIAGNOSIS: stool for ova and parasites, CBC with differential (eosinophilia sometimes present); LDH and SGOT sometimes elevated

FA: early hypofluorescence and late staining of lesions, perivascular leakage, and disc staining; multifocal window defects in late disease

ERG: subnormal, loss of b-wave

TREATMENT: laser photocoagulation of the worm; rarely subretinal surgery to remove worm (controversial)

Systemic antihelmintic medications (thiabendazole, diethylcarbamazine, pyrantel pamoate) are controversial and often not effective; steroids usually are added because worm death may increase inflammation

PROGNOSIS: poor without treatment; variable if worm can be killed with treatment

DDx of optic nerve swelling and macular star: Leber's idiopathic stellate neuroretinitis, syphilis, hypertension, trauma, acute febrile illness (measles, influenza), TB, coccidiomycosis, cat-scratch disease, papillitis, papilledema, AION (macular star rare), DUSN (macular star rare)

Diagnosis:

Lab tests: ESR, VDRL, FTA-ABS, Lyme titer, *Bartonella* serology, *Toxoplasma* and *Toxocara* titers, PPD

FA: diffuse leakage from disc, peripapillary capillary staining; 10% have disc leakage in fellow eye; no leakage in macula

Treatment: treat underlying disease, observe idiopathic form; most recover ≥20/50 after 3 months; only 3% to 5% have permanent severe visual loss

HIV Retinopathy

Microangiopathy in up to 50% of HIV-infected individuals

Asymptomatic, nonprogressive

Findings: cotton wool spots, Roth spots, hemorrhages, and microaneurysms in posterior pole; many HIV-positive patients have early presbyopia caused by inflammation of ciliary body with loss of accommodative amplitude

Diagnosis: HIV antibody test, CD4 count, HIV viral load

Treatment: none; spontaneous resolution within 1 to 2 months

Toxic Retinopathies

Chloroquine (Aralen)/ Hydroxychloroquine (Plaquenil)

Binds to melanin in RPE; ganglion cells are also directly affected

Toxic dose: chloroquine >3.5 mg/kg/day or 300 g total; hydroxychloroquine >6.5 mg/kg/day or 700 g total; <400 mg/day appears safe

Findings: early, mild mottling of perifoveal RPE with decreased foveal reflex; progresses to bull's-eye maculopathy; peripheral pigmentary retinopathy and cornea verticillata may develop

DDx of bull's-eye maculopathy: cone dystrophy, ARMD, Stargardt's disease, fundus flavimaculatus, Spielmeyer-Vogt disease, albinism, fenestrated sheen macular dystrophy, central areolar choroidal dystrophy, benign concentric annular macular dystrophy, clofazimine toxicity, fucosidosis

VF: decreased; small scotoma to red test object on tangent screen

ERG: enlarged a-wave, depressed b-wave

EOG: depressed

Progression of retinopathy can occur after cessation of medication

Thioridazine (Mellaril) (Figure 11-75)

RPE damage, decreased vision, nyctalopia, and sometimes altered color vision

Toxic dose: >1200 mg/day

Findings: peripheral pigmentary retinopathy, pigment deposition in eyelids, cornea, and lens

ERG: depressed a- and b-waves

Progression of retinopathy can occur after cessation of medication

Chlorpromazine (Thorazine)

Toxic dose: 1200 to 2400 mg/day for at least 12 months

Findings: pigment deposition in eyelids, cornea, lens, and retina

Figure 11-75. Thioridazine retinopathy associatd with chronic use (nummular retinopathy). (From Weinberg DV, D'Amico DJ: Retinal toxicity of systemic drugs. In Albert DM, Jakobiec FA [eds]: *Principles and Practice of Ophthalmology*, Philadelphia, WB Saunders, 1994.)

Figure 11-76. Severe tamoxifen retinopathy. (From McKeown CA, Swartz M, Blom J et al: Tamoxifen retinopathy, *Br J Ophthalmol*, 65:177–179, 1981.)

Chloramphenicol

Atrophy of maculopapillar bundle

VF: cecocentral scotoma

Quinine

Findings: fine RPE mottling, retinal vascular attenuation, disc pallor

Toxicity causes blurred vision, visual field loss, photophobia, sometimes transient blindness; patient may become comatose

Acute toxicity (single dose of 4 g): blurred vision, nyctalopia, nausea, loss of hearing, drowsiness, dilated pupils, retinal opacification with cherry red spot, dilated retinal vessels; after acute phase resolves, vision can improve

Tamoxifen

Occurs with doses >30 mg/day

Asymptomatic

Findings: fleck-like crystalline retinopathy with refractile retinal deposits, typically in ring around macula; may develop pigmentary retinal changes and mild CME (Figure 11-76)

FA: macular edema

Canthaxanthine

Occurs with cumulative dose >35 g

Asymptomatic, or mild metamorphopsia

Findings: refractile yellow deposits in a ring around the fovea; "gold-dust" retinopathy (Figure 11-77)

Figure 11-77. Canthaxanthine retinopathy. (From Weinberg DV, D'Amico DJ: Retinal toxicity of systemic drugs. In Albert DM, Jakobiec FA [eds]: *Principles and Practice of Ophthalmology*, Philadelphia, WB Saunders, 1994.)

Methoxyflurane

Crystalline retinopathy due to oxalate crystals

Methoxyflurane is metabolized to oxalate, which binds with calcium to form insoluble calcium oxalate salt

Crystals are permanent

Talc

Particles deposit in blood vessels of IV drug users; appear as tiny crystals

Talc deposits in lungs, with prolonged abuse pulmonary AV shunts develop and talc passes into systemic circulation

Talc emboli can cause arteriolar occlusions, resulting in ischemic maculopathy, retinal NV, and VH

Treatment: consider PRP for neovascularization

Nicotinic Acid Maculopathy

Atypical nonleaking CME due to intracellular edema of Müller's cells

Blurred vision with metamorphopsia

FA: CME does not leak

Digoxin

Direct effect on cones; causes visual disturbance with minimal fundus changes

Findings: xanthopsia (yellow vision), blurred vision, poor color vision, paracentral scotomas, and reduced vision with increased background light

Ergotamine

Vasoconstriction of retinal vessels, CME, CVO, papillitis, optic disc pallor; orthostatic hypotension, postpartum hemorrhages

Oral Contraceptives

Associated with thromboembolic disease

May develop CME, retinal hemorrhages, vascular occlusions

Sulfa

Induced myopia ranging from 1 to 5 D, reversible with cessation of medication

Other drugs that induce myopia: tetracyclines, promethazine, corticosteroids, ampicillin, acetaminophen

Gentamicin

Intraocular injection can cause rapid macular ischemia, optic atrophy, RPE changes, neovascular glaucoma

Macular infarction can occur with 400 micrograms

Interferon

Presumed to be due to immune complex deposition in retinal vasculature followed by white blood cell infiltration with eventual vascular closure

Findings: cotton wool spots, hemorrhages, macular edema, capillary nonperfusion, vascular occlusions

May exacerbate autoimmune thyroiditis and poly-arthropathy

Sildenafil (Viagra)

May cause transient blue hue to vision 1 to 2 hours after ingestion, possibly by changing the transduction cascade in photoreceptors

Occurs in 3% of individuals taking a dose of 25 to 50 mg, 11% of patients taking 100 mg dose, and in 50% taking >100 mg

Inherited Retinal Diseases

(see Chapter 5, Pediatrics/Strabismus)

Metabolic Diseases

(see Chapter 5, Pediatrics/Strabismus)

Vitreoretinal Disorders

(see Chapter 5, Pediatrics/Strabismus)

Retinal Degenerations

Table 11-5. **Classification of Retinal Degenerations**

Benign	Predisposing to RD
White without pressure	Lattice degeneration
Pigment clumping	Snail track degeneration
Diffuse chorioretinal atrophy	Zonuloretinal traction tufts
Peripheral microcystoid changes	Snowflake degeneration
Pavingstone degeneration	
Oral pigmentary degeneration	
Degenerative "senile" retinoschisis	

Oral Bay

Oval island of pars plana epithelium immediately posterior to ora serrata (Figure 11-78)

Meridional Fold

Elevated fold of retina in upper nasal quadrant

20% prevalence

Retinal break may occur (Figure 11-79)

Meridional Complex

Meridional fold extending to posterior aspect of a ciliary process

Retinal break may occur

Normal variation of anatomy at ora serrata

Figure 11-78. Enclosed oral bays. (From Tasman WS: Peripheral retinal lesions. In Yanoff M, Duker JS [eds]: *Ophthalmology*. London, Mosby, 1999.)

risk of RD, therefore no prophylactic treatment; associated with 10% of RDs; second to lattice degeneration as visible peripheral retinal lesion associated with RD

Zonular traction tuft: thin strand of fibroglial tissue extending from peripheral retina anteriorly to a zonule; usually nasal; present at birth; break occurs in 2% to 10%

Pars Plana Cyst

Clear cystoid space between pigmented and nonpigmented ciliary epithelium of pars plana; filled with mucopolysaccharides (hyaluronic acid)

Not a true cyst (not lined with epithelium)

Occurs in 17% of autopsied eyes

Analagous to detachment of sensory retina from underlying RPE; caused by traction by vitreous base and zonules; no increased risk of RD

Stains with Alcian blue

Also seen in conditions with formation of abnormal proteins (multiple myeloma)

Figure 11-79. Meridional fold with a small break at the base of the fold. (From Tasman WS: Peripheral retinal lesions. In Yanoff M, Duker JS [eds]: *Ophthalmology*. London, Mosby, 1999.)

Figure 11-80. Pars plana cysts. (Courtesy of Dr. Ralph Eagle. From Tasman WS: Peripheral retinal lesions. In Yanoff M, Duker JS [eds]: *Ophthalmology*. London, Mosby, 1999.)

Vitreoretinal Tuft

Small internal projection of retinal tissue

Noncystic retinal tuft: short, thin (base <0.1 mm) projection of fibroglial tissue; can break off, leaving fragments in vitreous; usually inferonasal; not associated with retinal break; not present at birth

Cystic retinal tuft: chalky white, nodular projection (base 0.1–1.0 mm) of fibroglial tissue; usually nasal; may have pigment at base; increased vitreous adhesion predisposes to tractional tears from PVD; present at birth; occurs in 5% of population; <1%

Ora Serrata Pearl

Glistening opacity over oral tooth

Increased prevalence with age

Resembles drusen

White With/Without Pressure

Geographic areas of peripheral retinal whitening

More common in young individuals, African Americans, and myopes

White with pressure: visible only with scleral depression

White without pressure: visible without scleral depression

Peripheral Microcystoid Degeneration

Typical/"senile" (Blessig-Iwanoff cysts): outer plexiform layer; bubble-like appearance behind ora serrata; lined by Müller's cells; may coalesce and progress to typical degenerative ("senile") retinoschisis

Reticular: nerve fiber layer; linear or reticular pattern, corresponding to retinal vessels; finely stippled internal surface; continuous with and posterior to typical type (therefore, does not reach the ora); may progress to reticular degenerative retinoschisis

Degenerative (Involutional) "Senile" Retinoschisis

Occurs in 7% to 31% of individuals >40 years old, 50% to 80% bilateral, often symmetric; 70% inferotemporal, 25% superotemporal

Usually asymptomatic and nonprogressive; hyperopia in 70%

Findings: splits or cysts within neurosensory retinal layers; typical peripheral cystoid degeneration is precursor
Inner wall: smooth, dome-shaped surface; may be markedly elevated in reticular type; sheathed retinal vessels; holes uncommon (small if present)
Outer wall: pock-marked on scleral depression; holes (16%–23%) are larger and well delineated, more common in reticular type, have rolled margins
Typical: splitting of OPL; bilateral; elderly patients; 1% of adult population; follows coalescence of cavities of microcystoid degeneration; beaten metal appearance; white spots (Müller's cell remnants [Gunn's dots]) in stippled pattern along edge appear as glistening dots or snowflakes; inner layer holes can occur; no risk of RD unless outer layer hole also present; intact outer retinal layer whitens/blanches with scleral depression
Reticular: splitting of NFL; 41% bilateral; 18% of adult population; always posterior to peripheral cystoid; fine delicately stippled surface

Differentiate from RD: no demarcation line, no underlying RPE degeneration, no tobacco dust; absolute scotoma (relative scotoma in RD); laser treatment blanches underlying RPE (RD will not blanch)

Pathology: cavity contains hyaluronic acid, Müller's cell remnants on inner and outer surfaces of cavity, fibrous thickening of vessel walls with patent lumen

Treatment: laser barrier, treat tears and RD

Complications: RD (from outer layer holes; slowly progressive, unless both outer and inner holes), progression (toward posterior pole; rare through fovea), hemorrhage (into vitreous or schisis cavity)

Figure 11-81. Degenerative retinoschisis demonstrating multiple outer layer breaks. (From Tasman WS: Peripheral retinal lesions. In Yanoff M, Duker JS [eds]: *Ophthalmology*. London, Mosby, 1999.)

Pavingstone/Cobblestone Degeneration

Usually inferior; 33% bilateral

Occlusion of choriocapillaris causes loss of outer retinal layers and RPE

Increased incidence with age and myopia (27% in those >20 years old)

No symptoms or complications

Findings: yellow-white spots 1/2 to 2 DD in size adjacent to ora; traverse retinal and choroidal vessels; may have irregular black pigmentation at margins

Pathology: degeneration of choroid and retina; loss of outer retinal layers; RPE absent; firm adhesion between retina and Bruch's membrane/choroid (no predisposition to RD) (Figure 11-82)

Lattice Degeneration

Occurs in 7% of population; more common in myopic eyes; no sex predilection

Often bilateral; usually superotemporal

Present in 20% to 35% of eyes with RD; 0.5% risk that patient with lattice will develop an RD

Findings: peripheral circumferential cigar-shaped atrophic retinal patches; criss-crossing pattern of sclerosed vessels (fine white lines) within lesion in 12%; superficial white dots in 80% (ILM and inner retina); pigmentary disturbance in 82%; firm adhesions of vitreous at margins; clear pockets of vitreous

Figure 11-82. Pavingstone degeneration. (Courtesy of Dr. Ralph Eagle. From Tasman WS: Peripheral retinal lesions. In Yanoff M, Duker JS [eds]: *Ophthalmology*. London, Mosby, 1999.)

fluid over central thin portion; retinal breaks (round or atrophic holes) in 18%, horseshoe tear in 1.4% at posterior or lateral edge due to severe vitreous traction

Pathology: discontinuity of ILM, overlying pocket of liquid vitreous, condensation and adherence of vitreous at margin of lesion, focal area of retinal thinning with loss of inner retinal layers, melanin-laden macrophages, fibrous thickening of retinal vessel walls

Treatment: no proof that prophylactic treatment prevents RD; consider treatment of fellow eye if history of RD from lattice

Figure 11-83. Lattice degeneration showing the typical white lines. (From Tasman WS: Peripheral retinal lesions. In Yanoff M, Duker JS [eds]: *Ophthalmology*. London, Mosby, 1999.)

Retinal Detachments

Rhegmatogenous Retinal Detachment (RD)

Etiology: retinal break allows liquid vitreous access to subretinal space (Figures 11-84 and 11-85)

1 in 10,000/year; retinal break can be found in 97%

Most tears (70%) are located superiorly between 10 and 2 o'clock positions

Types of breaks:
> *Horseshoe tear*
> *Atrophic hole*: myopia, increasing age
> *Dialysis*: splitting of vitreous base (usually infero-temporally, second most common site is supero-nasal); traumatic or idiopathic
> *Giant tear*: greater than 3 clock hours or 90°; trauma (≥90%), myopia; 50% risk of RD in fellow eye
> *Operculated hole*: fragment of retinal tissue found in overlying vitreous

Risk factors: age, history of RD in fellow eye (15%), high myopia/axial length (7%), family history, lattice degeneration, trauma, cataract surgery (1% after ICCE; 0.1% after ECCE with intact posterior capsule), diabetes, Nd:YAG laser posterior capsulotomy

Following blunt trauma dialysis is most common form of tear, followed by giant retinal tear, flap tear, and tear around lattice degeneration

Symptoms: flashes and floaters in 50%

Findings: retinal break; detached retina is opaque, corrugated, and undulates; tobacco dust (pigment in vitreous); decreased IOP; VH; nonshifting subretinal fluid
> *Long-standing RD*: thin retina, small breaks or dialysis, demarcation lines, underlying RPE atrophy, subretinal precipitates, macrocysts; may have increased IOP, PVR

DDx: exudative or traction RD

Treatment:
> *Pneumatic retinopexy*: ideal if RD caused by single break in superior 8 clock hours or multiple breaks within 1 to 2 clock hours; phakic patients tend to do better than aphakic patients
> Injection of inert gas or sterile air into vitreous cavity; strict positioning of patient's head allows gas bubble to contact retinal break and form barrier (RPE pumps subretinal fluid into choroid, allowing retina to reattach), break is sealed with cryo at time of gas injection or sealed with laser once subretinal fluid has resorbed
>> **INTRAOCULAR GASES** (in order of decreasing time gas remains in eye): perfluoropropane (C_3F_8), perfluoroethane (C_2F_8), sulfur hexafluoride (SF_6), air

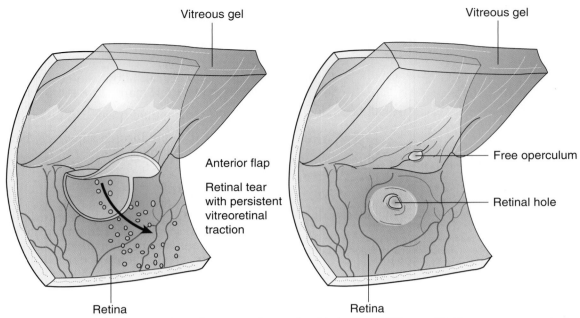

Figure 11-84. Retinal breaks demonstrating horseshoe tear and operculated hole. (From Wilkinson CP: Rhegmatogenous retinal ophthalmology. In Yanoff M, Duker JS [eds]: *Ophthalmology*. London, Mosby, 1999.)

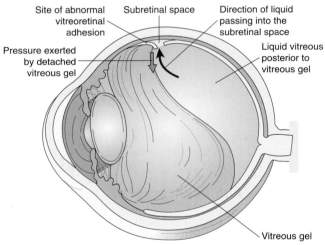

Figure 11-85. Classic pathogenesis of rhegmatogenous retinal detachment. (From Wilkinson CP: Rhegmatogenous retinal ophthalmology. In Yanoff M, Duker JS [eds]: *Ophthalmology*. London, Mosby, 1999.)

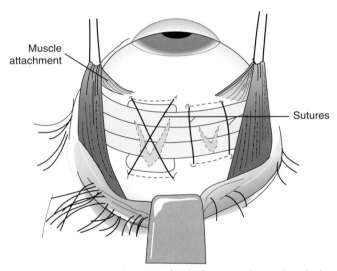

Figure 11-86. Suture placement for both tire and meridional elements. (From Williams GA: Scleral buckling surgery. In Yanoff M, Duker JS [eds]: *Ophthalmology*, 2nd ed, St. Louis, Mosby, 2004.)

Surgery: scleral buckle and/or vitrectomy, with laser therapy or cryotherapy
  GOALS:
  Identify all retinal breaks
  Close all retinal breaks
  Place scleral buckle to support all retinal breaks; retinal tears should be flat on buckle (Figure 11-86)
Complications of cryotherapy: proliferative vitreoretinopathy (PVR), uveitis, CME, intraocular hemorrhage, chorioretinal necrosis
Complications of scleral buckle surgery: ischemia (anterior or posterior segments), infection, perforation, strabismus, erosion or extrusion of explant, change in refractive error (induced myopia from increased axial length), macular pucker, cataract, glaucoma, new retinal tears (1.6%), PVR (4%), failure (5%–10%)
Complications of SRF drainage: hemorrhage, retinal tear, retinal incarceration, hypotony, vitreous loss, infection
Silicone oil: specific gravity less than water; surface tension less than that of all gases; buoyant when placed in eye; therefore, make iridectomy inferiorly; complications: cataract (100%), band

keratopathy (24%), glaucoma (19%), corneal decompensation (8%)

Prognosis: scleral buckle has 91% success rate

Final vision depends on macular involvement: worse prognosis if macular detached; timing of macular detachment is also important: if <1 week, 75% recover vision >20/70; if >1 week, 50% >20/70

Complications: PVR

Proliferative Vitreoretinopathy (PVR)

Retinal break allows cells (RPE, glial, myofibroblasts) to proliferate on inner and outer surfaces of retina along scaffold of detached vitreous

Membranes contract, causing fixed folds and tractional RD

Figure 11-87. Star fold from proliferative vitreoretinopathy. (From Aylward GW: Proliferative vitreoretinopathy, In Yanoff M, Duker JS [eds]: *Ophthalmology*. London, Mosby, 1999.)

Risk of PVR: following ocular perforation = 43%, following rupture = 21%, following penetration = 15%; associated with intraocular foreign body in 11%

Most common reason for failure of retinal reattachment surgery; usually occurs 4 to 6 weeks after initial repair

Classification system: 3 grades (A–C) in order of increasing severity

B-scan ultrasound: detached retina with triangle sign (transvitreal membrane connecting the 2 sides)

Treatment: vitreoretinal surgery is successful in approximately 70% of cases, leading to anatomic success

Exudative RD

Etiology: uveitis (VKH syndrome, sympathetic ophthalmia, pars planitis, viral retinitis), tumors,

glomerulonephritis, hypertension, eclampsia/preeclampsia, hypothyroidism, Coats' disease, nanophthalmos, scleritis, CSR (Figure 11-88)

Findings: shifting fluid, smooth retinal surface, no retinal break, retina behind the lens (pathognomonic)

Traction RD

Etiology: penetrating trauma (PVR), proliferative retinopathies, PHPV, toxoplasmosis, vitreous degenerations

Findings: taut retinal surface, immobile, concave shape, no retinal break

Pathology: subretinal fluid, photoreceptor degeneration, cystoid degeneration, glial membrane formation

Folds of Neurosensory Retina

Due to epiretinal membrane or rhegmatogenous RD

Not visible on FA; can be seen on OCT

Choroidal Disease

Choroidal Folds

Results from shrinkage of inner choroid or Bruch's membrane, causing undulations of overlying RPE and outer retina

Etiology: hypotony, thickened choroid (posterior scleritis, VKH syndrome), orbital pseudotumor, retrobulbar mass

Findings: yellow elevated crests alternating with darker bands between crests

FA: light bands/crests contain thinner RPE, producing prominent choroidal fluorescence; dark bands/troughs contain compressed RPE, producing relative hypofluorescence

Choroidal Detachment

Due to fluid (choroidal effusion) or blood (choroidal hemorrhage) in suprachoroidal space

Etiology: hypotony, uveitis, idiopathic, uremia, nanophthalmos (thickened sclera impedes vortex venous drainage), intraocular surgery (rapid change in IOP shears choroidal perforating arteries), intense PRP

Hemorrhage is caused by rupture of small vessels with sudden decrease of IOP (opening globe for surgery); may be expulsive with loss of intraocular contents through wound

Risk factors: as for suprachoroidal hemorrhage

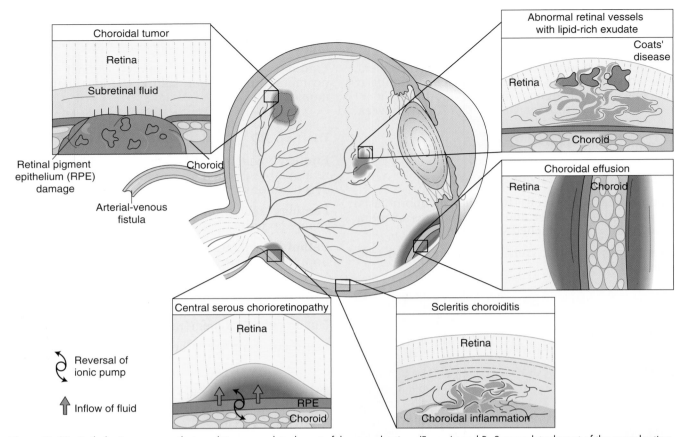

Figure 11-88. Pathologic processes that result in serous detachment of the neural retina. (From Anand R: Serous detachment of the neural retina. In Yanoff M, Duker JS [eds]: *Ophthalmology*, 2nd ed, St. Louis, Mosby, 2004.)

Findings: dark dome-shaped appearance

B-scan ultrasound: echogenic convexity attached at scleral spur and vortex veins (not at optic nerve)

Treatment: treat underlying disorder; consider partial-thickness scleral windows near vortex vein exit sites in 3 or 4 quadrants; if occurs during surgery, immediately close globe and give mannitol IV; may require drainage (sclerotomies)

Choroidal Ischemia

May occur with hypertensive retinopathy

Elschnig's spot: zone of nonperfusion of choriocapillaris, which appears as atrophic area of RPE overlying infarcted choroidal lobule

Siegrist streak: reactive RPE hyperplasia along sclerosed choroidal vessel

Figure 11-89. Hemorrhagic choroidal detachment viewed ophthalmoscopically. (From Kapusta MA, Lopez PF: Choroidal hemorrage. In Yanoff M, Duker JS [eds]: *Ophthalmology*, London, Mosby, 1999.)

Posterior Polypoidal Choroidal Vasculopathy/Posterior Uveal Bleeding Syndrome (PUBS)

Idiopathic peripapillary CNV; may bleed or leak fluid

Miscellaneous

Albinism, Aicardi's syndrome, colorblindness (see Chapter 5, Pediatrics/Strabismus)

Benign Tumors

Choroidal Nevus

Neoplasm of choroidal melanocytes; most common primary intraocular tumor

Can also arise within iris, ciliary body, or optic disc

Usually unilateral and unifocal; increased frequency with age

Multifocal nevi: associated with neurofibromatosis

Findings: flat slate-gray to dark brown choroidal lesion with ill-defined margins; surface drusen common; subretinal fluid and orange clumps of pigment rare

Features that suggest benign nevus may grow and evolve into choroidal melanoma: elevation, orange pigment (lipofuscin), juxtapapillary location, secondary exudative RD, visual symptoms

Pathology: benign spindle cells with pigment (Figure 11-90)

DDx: CHRPE, melanoma, melanocytoma

FA: hyperfluorescence

Figure 11-90. Choroidal nevus showing drusen overlying a heavily pigmented choroidal nevus composed almost completely of plump polyhedral nevus cells. (Modified from Naumann G et al: Arch Ophthalmol 76:784, 1966. From Yanoff M, Fine BS: *Ocular Pathology,* 5th ed, St. Louis, Mosby, 2002.)

Choroidal Cavernous Hemangioma

Congenital, unilateral vascular tumor

2 types:
  Diffuse: associated with Sturge-Weber syndrome
  Circumscribed: not associated with systemic disease

Symptoms: blurred vision, micropsia, metamorphopsia; vision loss due to cystic macular retinal degeneration or adjacent exudative RD

Findings:
  Diffuse type: generalized red-orange choroidal thickening ("tomato catsup" fundus); may have elevated IOP
  Circumscribed type: red-orange dome-shaped choroidal mass within 2 DD of optic disc or fovea

Pathology: lakes of erythrocytes separated by thin, fibrous septa; large-caliber vascular channels lined by mature endothelium. Circumscribed type has sharply demarcated borders and compresses surrounding melanocytes and choroidal lamellae (seen clinically as ring of hyperpigmentation at periphery of lesion and on FA as ring of blockage of underlying choroidal fluorescence)

Figure 11-91. Hemangioma of choroid. (From Yanoff M, Fine BS: *Ocular Pathology,* 5th ed, St. Louis, Mosby, 2002.)

FA: early hyperfluorescent filling of lesion at same time as retinal vessels, and late leakage/staining of entire lesion

ICG: early hyperfluorescent filling of intralesional vessels (Figure 11-92)

Ultrasound: A-scan shows high initial spike with high internal reflectivity; B-scan shows sonoreflective tissue, often with choroidal thickening (Figure 11-93)

Treatment: laser therapy or low-dose external beam XRT for exudative RD

Figure 11-92. Indocyanine green angiography of circumscribed choroidal hemangioma. (From Augsburger JJ, Anand R, Sanborn GE: Choroidal hemangiomas. In Yanoff M, Duker JS [eds]: *Ophthalmology*, London, Mosby, 1999.)

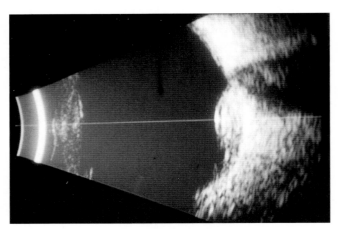

Figure 11-93. B-scan ultrasonography of circumscribed choroidal hemangioma. (From Augsburger JJ, Anand R, Sanborn GE: Choroidal hemangiomas. In Yanoff M, Duker JS [eds]: *Ophthalmology*, London, Mosby, 1999.)

Choroidal Osteoma

Tumor composed of bone

Sporadic, unifocal, bilateral in 20%

Arises in late childhood to early adulthood; women 90%

Symptoms: blurred vision, central scotoma

Findings: yellow-white to pale orange circumpapillary lesion with well-defined pseudopod-like margins; CNV and RPE disruption can cause progressive visual impairment

FA: patchy early hyperfluorescence and late staining of lesion

ICG: hypofluorescence of lesion with hyperfluorescent intralesional vessels, late leakage of lesion

Ultrasound: highly reflective plate-like lesion with orbital shadowing beyond lesion (Figure 11-94)

CT: plate-like thickening of eye wall

Pathology: plaque of mature bone involving full-thickness choroid, usually sparing RPE

Treatment: for CNV if present

Retinal Capillary Hemangioma

Vascular tumor (hemangioblastoma); AD, sporadic, or associated with von Hippel-Lindau disease

Arises in older children and young adults

Symptoms: blurred vision, visual field loss

Findings: red globular mass with prominent dilated tortuous afferent and efferent retinal blood vessels, exudative RD may develop

FA: fills rapidly; leaks into vitreous and subretinal space

Treatment: slowly progressive if untreated; can treat with laser, cryotherapy, or PDT

Retinal Cavernous Hemangioma

Vascular tumor; probably congenital; occasionally associated with similar CNS or skin vascular lesions

Usually unilateral, unifocal; rarely progressive

Findings: cluster of dark red intraretinal vascular sacs ("bunch of grapes" appearance), typically associated with an anomalous retinal vein; associated overlying retinal gliosis; no intraretinal exudates or detachment; may have VH

FA: fluid levels within the vascular sacs

Treatment: vitrectomy for nonclearing VH

Retinal Astrocytoma (Astrocytic Hamartoma)

Glioma arising from retinal glial cells

Occurs in older children and young adults; can be unilateral or bilateral, unifocal or multifocal; usually stable

Figure 11-94. B-scan ultrasonography of choroidal osteoma. A) At 77dB the osteoma appears as an intensely white plate in the posterior eye wall. B) At 55dB the lesion persists but most of the normal tissues are no longer evident. In Yanoff M, Duker JS [eds]: *Ophthalmology*, London, Mosby, 1999.)

Associated with tuberous sclerosis (multifocal, bilateral)

Symptoms: blurred vision, visual field loss, or asymptomatic

Findings: 1 or more yellow-white masses; occasionally exudative RD; calcification in some larger lesions; may have glistening, mulberry appearance or softer, fluffy appearance

Combined Hamartoma of the Retina and RPE

Tumor composed of neurosensory retina and RPE; probably congenital; associated with neurofibromatosis type 2

Usually unilateral, unifocal; minimal progression

Symptoms: blurred vision

Findings: gray juxtapapillary lesion with surface gliosis and prominent intralesional retinal vascular tortuosity; amblyopia (Figure 11-95)

Pathology: cords of proliferated pigment epithelium with excess blood vessels and glial tissue

Treatment: none

Adenoma and Adenocarcinoma

Elevated dark black lesion; may resemble deeply pigmented melanoma; rarely arise from nonpigmented ciliary epithelium

May be associated with iridocyclitis, secondary cataract, subluxated lens

Pathology: massive proliferation of RPE cells

Treatment: excision

Racemose Hemangioma

Congenital AV malformation

Associated with Wyburn-Mason syndrome

No exudate or leakage

Malignant Tumors

Retinoblastoma (RB)

(see Chapter 5, Pediatrics/Strabismus)

Choroidal Malignant Melanoma

Malignant neoplasm of uveal melanocytes; unilateral, unifocal; 75% arise in choroid, less common in CB or iris

Most common primary intraocular malignant tumor in Caucasian adults (1 in 2000)

Uncommon before age 40 years

Risk factors: ocular melanocytosis, sunlight exposure, uveal nevi, race (Caucasian; only 1%–2% in African Americans or Asians), neurofibromatosis, dysplastic nevus syndrome, BDUMP syndrome (bilateral diffuse uveal melanocytic proliferation)

Symptoms: blurred vision, visual field loss, flashes and floaters

Findings: brown, domed-shaped or mushroom-shaped tumor; orange pigment clumps (accumulation of lipofuscin in RPE), adjacent exudative RD, sentinel vessel (dilated tortuous episcleral vessel); secondary glaucoma; may be amelanotic and appear as a pale mass

Pathology: Callender classification (Figures 11-96 to 11-99)

Spindle A cells: slender, cigar-shaped nucleus with finely dispersed chromatin; low nuclear-to-cytoplasmic ratio; absent or inconspicuous nucleolus; no mitotic figures; tumors composed exclusively of spindle A cells are considered benign nevi

Spindle B cells: oval (larger) nucleus with coarser chromatin and prominent nucleolus; mitotic figures; tumors with spindle A and B cells are

A

B

C

D

Figure 11-95. Combined hamartoma of neural retina and retinal pigment epithelium. (C and D, Courtesy Dr. E Howes. From Augsburger JJ, Meyers S: Combined harartoma of retina. In Yanoff M, Duker JS [eds]: *Ophthalmology*, London, Mosby, 1999.)

Figure 11-96. Uveal mushroom melanoma. (From Yanoff M, Fine BS: *Ocular Pathology*, 5th ed, St. Louis, Mosby, 2002.)

Figure 11-97. Callender classification. Spindle A cells, identified by a dark stripe parallel to the long axis of the nucleus, are seen in longitudinal section. They are identified in transverse cross section by the infolding of the nuclear membrane that causes the dark stripe. (From Yanoff M, Fine BS: *Ocular Pathology*, 5th ed, St. Louis, Mosby, 2002.)

called spindle cell melanomas. Spindle A and B cells grow as a syncytium with indistinct cytoplasmic borders

Epithelioid cells: polyhedral with abundant cytoplasm; poorly cohesive; distinct borders; most malignant; large, round-to-oval nucleus with peripheral margination of chromatin; prominent eosinophilic or purple nucleolus (epithelioid cells "look back at you")

Mixed cell melanoma: composed of spindle and epithelioid cells

Gross examination requires identification of vortex veins to rule out tumor extension

Transillumination: most melanomas cast shadow

Figure 11-98. Callender classification. Histologic section of spindle B cells. (From Yanoff M, Fine BS: *Ocular Pathology*, 5th ed, St. Louis, Mosby, 2002.)

Figure 11-99. Callender classification. Histologic section of epithelioid cells. (From Yanoff M, Fine BS: *Ocular Pathology*, 5th ed, St. Louis, Mosby, 2002.)

A

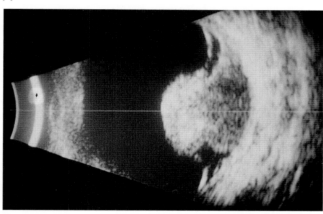

B

Figure 11-100. Ultrasonography of posterior uveal melanoma. (From Augsburger JJ, Damato BE, Bornfield N: Uveal melanoma. In Yanoff M, Duker JS [eds]: *Ophthalmology*, London, Mosby, 1999.)

Ultrasound: A-scan shows low internal reflectivity with characteristic reduction in amplitude from front to back, high amplitude spikes consistent with break in Bruch's; B-scan shows solid tumor with mushroom shape or biconvex shape (Figure 11-100)

FA: "double" circulation (choroidal and retinal vessels), mass is hypofluorescent early, pinpoint leakage late (Figure 11-101)

MRI: bright on T1; dark on T2

Treatment:

Enucleation: large tumor, optic nerve invasion, macular location, painful eye with poor visual potential

Plaque brachytherapy: most eyes with medium-sized tumors with visual potential, or failure of laser

HIGH ENERGY: cobalt-60, iridium-192

LOW ENERGY: Iodine-125 (sphere of radiation), palladium-106 (25% less energy than I-125), Ruthenium-106 (β-particles, travel only 5 mm; therefore, use for small tumors)

Charged particle radiation: proton beam (cylinder of radiation); large anterior segment dose, low macular dose (reverse of plaque)

Resection: most irido and iridociliary tumors; some ciliary body and choroidal tumors

Transpupillary thermotherapy: small tumors

Zimmerman hypothesis: manipulation of tumor during enucleation causes metastasis and increases mortality; not true. Derived from plotting of life table data, which showed Bell-shaped curve for death rate, specifically, mortality rate increased to 8% following enucleation (vs 1% per year in patients with untreated tumors)

Complications of treatment: radiation retinopathy (if severe, treat with PRP to prevent NVG); cataracts (PSC in 42% within 3 years of proton beam therapy); dry eye

Collaborative Ocular Melanoma Study (COMS):

SMALL TUMOR TRIAL (height = 1–3 mm; diameter >5 mm): 1/3 grew; 5-year mortality = 6%

MEDIUM TUMOR TRIAL (height = 2.5–10 mm; diameter <16 mm): survival rates similar between enucleation and iodine-125 plaque brachytherapy; I-125 brachytherapy has a high risk of substantial visual loss (up to 49%)

A

B

Figure 11-101. Fluorescein angiogram of mushroom-shaped choroidal melanoma. (From Augsburger JJ, Damato BE, Bornfield N: Uveal melanoma. In Yanoff M, Duker JS [eds]: *Ophthalmology*, London, Mosby, 1999.)

LARGE TUMOR TRIAL (height >10 mm; diameter >16 mm; without mets): pre-enucleation radiation does not change the survival rate in patients with large choroidal melanomas with or without metastases over enucleation alone

Prognosis:
  Factors:
    CELL TYPE: epithelioid has worst prognosis (5-year survival <30%); presence of epithelioid cells important in survivability; 5-year survival rate for spindle A cell is 95%, 15-year survival rate for mixed tumor is 37%, 15-year survival for pure spindle cell melanoma with no epithelioid cells is 72%
    SIZE: larger and diffuse tumors have a worse prognosis
    LOCATION

VARIABILITY IN NUCLEOLAR SIZE
PRESENCE OF INTRATUMOR VASCULAR NETWORKS
PRESENCE OF NECROSIS
METALLOTHIONEIN LEVELS: may indicate metastatic potential and poor survival
Approximately 50% with large tumors have mets within 5 years
Mean survival after metastasis is 9 months

Metastasis: hematogenous spread via vortex veins; risks include elevation (>2 mm), proximity to optic nerve, visual symptoms, growth; 92% of metastases are to liver, also skin, lungs, other organs; local extension into optic nerve and brain
  Metastatic workup: abdominal (hepatospleno-megaly) examination, LFTs, CXR

MAJOR CLINICAL STUDY

Collaborative Ocular Melanoma Study (COMS)

Objective: to evaluate treatment options for choroidal malignant melanomas

Methods:
  Small tumor study (not large enough for COMS trial) (apical height = 1–3 mm; basal diameter 5–16 mm): not randomized; observation vs treatment at discretion of investigator
  Medium tumor trial (apical height = 2.5–10 mm; basal diameter <16 mm): randomized enucleation vs radiation (I-125 plaque brachytherapy)
  Large tumor trial (apical height >10 mm; basal diameter >16 mm; no mets): randomized enucleation alone vs 20 Gy external beam radiation for 5 days and then enucleation (PERT)
  Primary outcome was survival; secondary outcomes included tumor growth, visual function, time to metastasis, and quality of life

Results:
  Small tumor study: 21% grew by 2 years and 31% by 5 years; 6 deaths were due to metastatic melanoma; 5-year all-cause mortality was 6%, and 8-year was 14.9%; risk factors for growth included initial tumor thickness and diameter, presence of orange pigment, absence of drusen, and absence of adjacent RPE changes
  Medium tumor trial: after 3 years, 43% to 49% of I-125–treated eyes had poor vision outcomes (loss of ≥6 lines of visual acuity or VA of 20/200 or worse), and this was strongly associated with larger tumor apical height and smaller distance from the foveal avascular zone; other risk factors for poor visual outcome included diabetes, tumor-related retinal detachment, and tumors that were not dome-shaped; estimated 5-year survival rates were 81% for the enucleation group and 82% for the I-125 group
  Large tumor trial: 1003 patients enrolled. Estimated 5-year survival rates were 57% for enucleation alone and 62% for radiation followed by

enucleation, and for patients with metastases at the time of death, the 5-year survival was 72% vs 74%; prognostic risk factors were age and basal diameter

Conclusions:

Small tumor study: otherwise healthy patients with small choroidal melanomas have a low risk of death within 5 years

Medium tumor trial: there is a high risk of substantial visual loss from I-125 brachytherapy (up to 49%); I-125 brachytherapy does not change the survival rate (for up to 12 years) in patients with medium choroidal melanomas

Large tumor trial: pre-enucleation radiation does not change the survival rate in patients with large choroidal melanomas with or without metastases

Primary Intraocular Lymphoma (Reticulum Cell Sarcoma)

Non-Hodgkin's B-cell lymphoma, large cell type

Affects elderly patients; usually bilateral and multifocal

No systemic involvement outside of CNS

Increased risk of development of concurrent primary CNS lymphoma

Symptoms (precede CNS signs in 80%): blurred vision, floaters; dementia may occur

Findings: creamy white, diffuse sub-RPE and vitreous infiltrates; AC reaction, hypopyon, vitritis, secondary glaucoma; may have multifocal atrophic or punched-out lesions, and exudative RD; choroidal form manifests with choroidal nodules or detachments of RPE and is associated with systemic lymphoma (Figure 11-102)

Diagnosis: CT scan, LP (positive in 25%), vitreous biopsy (low yield; atypical lymphocytes with prominent nucleoli, mitoses; cellular necrosis) (Figure 11-103)

Treatment: chemotherapy or XRT

Prognosis: poor, mortality often within 2 years (mean survival is 22 months)

Reactive lymphoid hyperplasia of the choroid: benign counterpart

Findings: diffuse or multiple yellow choroidal lesions; overlying RD may occur; often similar infiltrates in conjunctiva and orbit (check conjunctiva for salmon patch)

Associated with systemic lymphoma (vs retinovitreous lymphoma, which is associated with CNS lesions)

Pathology: mass of benign lymphocytes, plasma cells, and Dutcher bodies

Treatment: low-dose XRT

Figure 11-102. Fundus view of yellow-white hemorrhagic retinal infiltrates. (From Burnier MN, Blanco G: Intraocular lymphoma. In Yanoff M, Duker JS [eds]: *Ophthalmology*, London, Mosby, 1999.)

Figure 11-103. Large neoplastic cells in a vitreous specimen. (From Burnier MN, Blanco G: Intraocular lymphoma. In Yanoff M, Duker JS [eds]: *Ophthalmology*, London, Mosby, 1999.)

Intraocular Leukemia

(see Chapter 5, Pediatrics/Strabismus)

Metastases

Most common intraocular tumor (including cases evident only at autopsy)

Most commonly breast carcinoma in women (most have previous mastectomy), lung carcinoma in men (often occult)

Bilateral and multifocal in 20%; 25% have no previous history of cancer

93% to choroid; 2% to ciliary body; 5% to iris; can also metastasize to optic nerve; retina is rare

A   B

Figure 11-104. Ultrasonography of metastic carcinoma to choroid. A) A-scan, B) B-scan. (From Augsburger JJ, Guthoff R: Metastatic cancer to the eye. In Yanoff M, Duker JS [eds]: *Ophthalmology*, London, Mosby, 1999.)

Symptoms: blurred vision, visual field defects, flashes and floaters

Findings: 1 or more golden-yellow, thin, dome-shaped choroidal tumors or creamy yellow amelanotic tumors with placoid or nummular configuration; may produce extensive exudative RD; usually metastasize to macula (richest blood supply)

DDx of amelanotic choroidal mass: amelanotic melanoma, old subretinal hemorrhage, choroidal osteoma, granuloma, posterior scleritis

FA: early hyperfluorescence with late staining of lesions

Ultrasound: A-scan shows medium to high internal reflectivity, minimal to no spontaneous pulsations; B-scan is sonoreflective (Figure 11-104)

Treatment: chemotherapy, external beam XRT, or combination

Cancer-Associated Retinopathy (CAR)

Paraneoplastic syndrome; autoantibodies against retina; CAR antigen (identical to retinal protein recoverin)

Loss of photoreceptors without inflammation

Findings: decreased vision, nyctalopia

ERG: extinguished

Treatment: steroids, treatment of primary cancer (usually small cell lung carcinoma)

Prognosis: poor

Bilateral Diffuse Uveal Melanocytic Proliferation Syndrome (BDUMPS)

Paraneoplastic syndrome

Diffuse uveal thickening

Findings: orange or pigmented fundus spots, iris thickening and pigmentation

ERG: markedly reduced

FA: orange spots hyperfluoresce

Treatment: none

LASER TREATMENT

Thermal burn (photocoagulation) of inner retina will occur with argon blue-green or xenon arc

Retinal structures that absorb laser:
  Melanin: primary site of light absorption and heat emission; absorbs argon blue-green, argon green, and krypton red
  Hemoglobin: absorbs argon blue-green, argon green; does not absorb krypton (used to penetrate hemorrhage)
  Xanthophyll: absorbs blue wavelengths

Wavelengths:
  Blue-green (488 and 514 nm): blue light is absorbed by cornea and lens; heavily absorbed by nuclear sclerotic cataracts and absorbed by xanthophyll pigment
  Green (514 nm): absorbed by blood, melanin; preferred for treatment of CNV in cases in which RPE has little pigment
  Yellow (577 nm): may be better for treatment of microaneurysms; be careful of blood vessels
  Red (647 nm): penetrates cataracts better; not absorbed by blood; causes less inner retinal damage; absorbed by melanin; poorly absorbed by xanthophyll (safer near fovea); passes through mild vitreous hemorrhage and nuclear sclerotic cataracts better than argon
  Infrared (810 nm): similar characteristics as red, but with deeper penetration

Xenon arc: polychromatic white light; not as precisely focused as monochromatic light; emits considerable amount of blue light, which can be harmful to retina and lens

Panretinal Photocoagulation (PRP)

Indications: treatment of NV and peripheral nonperfusion, most commonly in retinal vascular diseases (PDR, CVO, BVO, sickle cell, radiation, and hypertensive retinopathy)

Parameters: 500 μm spot size, 0.1- to 0.5-second duration, 1200 to 2000 spots; moderate white burn, 1 burn-width apart, 2 DD from fovea and 1 DD from optic nerve; 2 or more sessions

Adverse effects: decreased acuity (worsened by 1 line in 11%; worsened by 2 lines in 3%), constricted visual field, loss of color vision in 10%

Retreat at 4 weeks if NVD fails to regress or develops, new NVE develops, iris or angle NV develops, further regression of NV desired

Complications: choroidal effusion, exudative RD, permanent mydriasis and impairment of accommodation (ciliary nerve damage), vitreous hemorrhage, lens or corneal damage, foveal or optic nerve damage, CME, CNV, retinal vascular occlusion, angle closure

Focal Laser

Indication: treatment of macular edema (CSME, BVO, JXT)

Parameters: 50 to 100 μm spot size, 0.1-second duration; burns that slightly blanch the RPE, should be barely visible immediately after treatment, grid pattern 1 burn-width apart, in areas of diffuse edema; focal treatment of leaking vessels and microaneurysms; whiten/darken microaneurysms and/or cause mild depigmentation of RPE; do not treat over hemorrhage; identify leaking microaneurysms by FA

Decreases risk of moderate visual loss over 3 years by 50% in CSME

Retreat at 3 months if CSME still present, or treatable areas seen on repeat FA

Review Questions *(Answers start on page 367)*

1. Which substance does not cause crystalline deposits in the retina?
   a. thioridazine
   b. canthaxanthine
   c. tamoxifen
   d. talc

2. What is the chance that a child of a patient with Best's disease will inherit the disorder?
   a. 25%
   b. 50%
   c. 75%
   d. 100%

3. The MPS showed the best prognosis for laser treatment of CNV in which disorder?
   a. ARMD
   b. myopia
   c. idiopathic condition
   d. POHS

4. Which of the following is not a feature of Stickler's syndrome?
   a. Pierre-Robin malformation
   b. autosomal dominant inheritance
   c. retinoschisis
   d. marfinoid habitus

5. Sites at which the uvea is attached to the sclera include all of the following except
   a. vortex veins
   b. optic nerve
   c. scleral spur
   d. ora serrata

6. The inheritance of gyrate atrophy is
   a. sporadic
   b. X-linked recessive
   c. autosomal dominant
   d. autosomal recessive

7. All 3 types of retinal hemorrhage (preretinal, intraretinal, and subretinal) may occur simultaneously in all of the following conditions except
   a. macroaneurysm
   b. ARMD
   c. diabetes
   d. capillary hemangioma

8. Characteristics of choroidal melanoma include all of the following except
   a. choroidal excavation
   b. high internal reflectivity
   c. double circulation
   d. orbital shadowing

9. Which of the following statements regarding the ETDRS is false?
   a. The ETDRS concluded that PRP reduces the risk of severe visual loss in patients with high-risk PDR
   b. The ETDRS identified the risk factors for development of PDR
   c. The ETDRS defined CSME
   d. The ETDRS showed that aspirin does not affect disease progression

10. The DRVS found that early vitrectomy for vitreous hemorrhage was helpful in
    a. type 1 diabetic patients
    b. type 2 diabetic patients
    c. type 1 and 2 diabetic patients
    d. none of the above

11. Which of the following treatments is a CVOS recommendation?
    a. focal laser for macular edema of >3 to 6 months duration with VA <20/40
    b. PRP for >10 disc areas of nonperfusion
    c. PRP for iris or angle neovascularization
    d. macular grid photocoagulation for CME

12. Which peripheral retinal lesion has the greatest risk of a retinal detachment?
    a. cystic retinal tuft
    b. ayymptomatic retinal hole
    c. senile retinoschisis
    d. lattice degeneration

13. The intraocular structure most commonly affected by leukemia is
    a. iris
    b. choroid
    c. retina
    d. optic nerve

14. Which is not a function of the RPE?
    a. conversion of vitamin A alcohol to aldehyde
    b. concentration of taurine
    c. inactivation of toxic products of oxygen metabolism
    d. phagocytosis of rod outer segments

15. Which of the following best describes the cellular reaction when light strikes a photoreceptor?
    a. increased cGMP, closed Na channel
    b. increased cGMP, open Na channel
    c. decreased cGMP, closed Na channel
    d. decreased cGMP, open Na channel

16. Von Hippel-Lindau disease has been mapped to which chromosome?
    a. 3
    b. 9
    c. 11
    d. 17

17. Which tumor is not associated with von Hippel-Lindau disease?
    a. hepatocellular carcinoma
    b. pheochromocytoma
    c. renal cell carcinoma
    d. cerebellar hemangioblastoma

18. Prognostic factors for choroidal melanoma include all of the following except
    a. size
    b. location
    c. cell type
    d. pigmentation

19. Which of the following does not involve the outer plexiform layer of the retina?
    a. degenerative retinoschisis
    b. cystoid macular edema
    c. Henle's fiber layer
    d. diabetic microaneurysm

20. Which X-linked disorder is not associated with an ocular abnormality in the female carrier?
    a. choroideremia
    b. albinism
    c. juvenile retinoschisis
    d. retinitis pigmentosa

21. All of the following are features of ataxia-telangiectasia except
    a. sinopulmonary infections
    b. thymic hyperplasia
    c. IgA deficiency
    d. autosomal recessive inheritance

22. The best test for distinguishing between a subretinal hemorrhage and a choroidal melanoma is
    a. FA
    b. B-scan
    c. A-scan
    d. ERG

23. Which of the following is the least radiosensitive lesion?
    a. metastases
    b. lymphoma
    c. RB
    d. melanoma

24. Which of the following is not a complication of PRP?
    a. iritis
    b. increased IOP
    c. RD
    d. narrow angle

25. A cluster of pigmented lesions is seen in the peripheral retina of a patient's left eye during routine ophthalmoscopy. Which of the following tests would be most helpful in detecting an associated hereditary disorder?
    a. EKG
    b. colonoscopy
    c. brain MRI
    d. chest CT scan

26. Which of the following is not associated with a typical angiographic appearance of CME?
    a. nicotinic acid
    b. epinephrine
    c. Irvine-Gass syndrome
    d. pars planitis

27. The least likely finding in a patient with a chronic detachment of the inferotemporal retina is
    a. retinal thinning
    b. macrocysts
    c. fixed folds
    d. RPE atrophy

28. All of the following vitreoretinal disorders are inherited in an autosomal dominant pattern except
    a. familial exudative vitreoretinopathy
    b. Wagner's syndrome
    c. Stickler's syndrome
    d. Goldmann-Favre disease

29. In a patient with ARMD, which type of drusen is most associated with development of CNV?
    a. soft
    b. basal laminar
    c. hard
    d. calcific

30. The ERG oscillatory potential is caused by which cell type?
    a. Müller's
    b. amacrine
    c. bipolar
    d. RPE

SUGGESTED READINGS

American Academy of Ophthalmology, vol 12. San Francisco, AAO, 2004.

Bell WJ, Stenstrom WJ: Atlas of the Peripheral Retina. Philadelphia, WB Saunders, 1998.

Byrne SF, Green RL: Ultrasound of the Eye and Orbit, 2nd edition. St. Louis, Mosby, 1992.

Gass J: Stereoscopic Atlas of Macular Diseases: Diagnosis and Treatment, 4th edition. St. Louis, Mosby, 1997.

Guyer DR, Yannuzzi LA, Chang A, Shields JA, Green R: Retina-Vitreous-Macula. Philadelphia, WB Saunders, 1999.

Ryan SJ: Retina, 3rd edition. St. Louis, Mosby, 2001.

Shields JA, Shields CL: Intraocular Tumors: A Text and Atlas. Philadelphia, WB Saunders, 1992.

Wilkinson CP, Rice TA: Michels's Retinal Detachment, 2nd edition. St. Louis, Mosby, 1997.

Yannuzzi LA, Guyer DR, and Green WR: The Retina Atlas. St. Louis, Mosby, 1995.

Answers to Questions

CHAPTER 1   OPTICS

1. Prince's rule is helpful in determining all of the following except
   d. accommodative convergence

2. A myope who pushes his spectacles closer to his face and tilts them is
   d. increasing effectivity, increasing cylinder

3. The Prentice position refers to
   a. glass prism perpendicular to visual axis

4. The purpose of Q-switching a laser is to
   b. decrease energy, increase power

5. A 50-year-old woman with aphakic glasses wants a new pair of spectacles to use when applying make-up. How much power should be added to her distance correction so that she can focus while sitting 50 cm in front of her mirror?
   c. +1.00 D. With a plane mirror, the image is located as far behind the mirror as the object is in front of the mirror; therefore, the distance between her eye and the image of her eye is 100 cm = 1 m, and this requires +1.00 D of extra magnification.

6. How far from a plano mirror must a 6-ft-tall man stand to see his whole body?
   b. 3 feet. To view one's entire body, a plane mirror need be only half one's height.

7. A 33-year-old woman with a refraction of −9.00 +3.00 × 90 OD at vertex distance 10 mm and keratometry readings of 46.00@90/43.00@180 is fit for a rigid gas-permeable (RGP) contact lens 1 D steeper than flattest K. What power lens is required?
   c. −7.00 D. Step 1: change refraction to minus cylinder form (because the tear lake negates the minus cylinder) and use this sphere (−6.00); step 2: adjust to zero vertex distance ($-6 + 0.01[-6]^2 = -5.64$); step 3: adjust for tear lens (SAM-FAP rule) (add −1.00 = −6.64).

8. What is the size of a 20/60 letter on a standard 20-ft Snellen chart (tangent of 1 minute of arc = 0.0003)?
   d. 27 mm. 20/60 letter subtends 5 minutes at 60 ft (18 m); therefore, size of letter = 18 (tan 5′) = 18 (0.0015) = 0.027 m or 27 mm.

9. A Galilean telescope with a +5 D objective and a −20 D eyepiece produces an image with what magnification and direction?
   a. 4×, erect. Magnification = −(−20)/5 = +4, meaning 4× magnification and erect image

10. An object is placed 33 cm in front of an eye. The image formed by reflection from the front surface of the cornea (radius of curvature equals 8 mm) is located
    b. 4 mm behind cornea. Reflecting power of the cornea is −2/0.008 = −250 D; thus, the focal point is 1/−250 = −4 mm, or 4 mm behind the cornea

11. A convex mirror produces what type of image?
    d. virtual, erect, minified. Remember VErMin.

12. In general, the most bothersome problem associated with bifocals is
    a. image jump. Therefore, choose bifocal segment type to minimize jump; flat-top segments minimize image jump because the optical center is near the top; this also reduces image displacement in myopes.

13. A refraction with a stenopeic slit gives the following measurements: +1.00 at 90° and −2.00 at 180°. The corresponding spectacle prescription is
    c. −2.00 + 3.00 × 180. This is the correct spherocylindrical notation for a power cross diagram with +1.00 along the 90° meridian and −2.00 along the 180° meridian.

14. A point source of light is placed 1/3 of a meter to the left of a +7 D lens. Where will its image come to focus?
    a. 25 cm to the right of the lens. The light has vergence of −3 D and encounters a +7 D lens; thus, the exiting light has vergence of +4 D, and the image will come to focus 25 cm to the right of the lens.

15. What is the equivalent sphere of the following cross cylinder: -3.00×180 combined with $+0.50 \times 90$?

    b. -1.25. The cross cylinder has a spherocylindrical notation of $-3.00 + 3.50 \times 90$; so the spherical equivalent is $-3.00 + (3.50/2) = -1.25$.

16. What is the size of a letter on a standard 20-ft Snellen chart if it forms an image of 1/2 mm on a patient's retina?

    d. 18 cm. Using the reduced schematic eye and similar triangles, 0.5/17 mm = object size/6 m; solving for object size yields 18 cm.

17. The image of a distant object is largest in which patient?

    b. hyperope with spectacles

18. What type of image is produced if an object is placed in front of a convex lens within its focal length?

    b. erect and virtual

19. What is the correct glasses prescription if retinoscopy performed at 50 cm shows neutralization with a plano lens?

    a. -2.00. Remember to subtract for working distance (1/0.5 m = 2 D); thus, a plano lens minus 2 D yields a -2.00 D glasses prescription.

20. An anisometropic patient experiences difficulty while reading with bifocals. Which of the following is not helpful for reducing the induced phoria?

    c. progressive lenses. This problem is due to the prismatic effect of the underlying lens and will occur with all bifocal styles, including progressive lenses.

21. A Geneva lens clock is used to measure what?

    d. base curve

22. What is the induced prism when a 67-year-old woman reads 10 mm below the upper segment optical center of her bifocals, which measure $+2.50 + 1.00 \times 90$ OD and $-1.50 + 1.50 \times 180$ OS add $+2.50$ OU?

    c. 2.5 prism diopters. Using Prentice's rule, the induced prism is $(+2.50 \times 1)$ OD and $([-1.50 +1.50] \times 1)$ OS (cylinder power acts in the vertical meridian, so it must be used in the calculation); the total is +2.5 PD BU OD; the effect is due to the underlying lens; the power of the bifocal segment can be ignored because it is the same for both lenses (5 PD BU OD and 2.5 PD BU OS = 2.5 PD BU OD).

23. The optimal size of a pinhole for measuring pinhole visual acuity is approximately

    c. 1.25 mm. Limited by diffraction if smaller than 1.2 mm.

24. A person looking at an object 5 m away through a 10^Δ prism placed base-in over the right eye would see the image displaced

    b. 50 cm to the right. A 10 PD prism displaces light 10 cm/1 m or 50 cm at 5 m, and the image is displaced to the apex.

25. Calculate the soft contact lens power for a 40-year-old hyperope who wears $+14.00$ D glasses at a vertex distance of 11 mm.

    b. $+16.00$ D. Using the simplified formula, new power $= 14 + 0.011 \ (14)^2 = 16.156$.

26. After cataract surgery, a patient's refraction is $-0.75 + 1.75 \times 10$, in what meridian should a suture be cut to reduce the astigmatism?

    d. $10°$. The steep meridian corresponds to the axis of the plus cylinder (plus cylinder acts to steepen the flat meridian, which is $90°$ away from the cylinder axis).

27. What is the appropriate correction in the IOL power if the A constant for the lens to be implanted is changed from 117 to 118?

    b. increase IOL power by 1.0 D. The change in A constant is equivalent to the change in IOL power.

28. An IOL labeled with a power of $+20$ D has a refractive index of 1.5. If this lens were removed from the package and measured with a lensometer, what power would be found?

    d. $+59$ D. Using the formula for calculating the power of a thin lens immersed in fluid $(D_{air}/D_{aqueous}) = (n_{iol} - n_{air})/(n_{iol} - n_{aqueous})$, $D_{air} = 20 \ ([1.5 - 1.0]/[1.5 - 1.33]) = +58.8$ D.

29. The spherical equivalent of a 0.50 D cross cylinder is

    a. plano. By definition, all cross cylinders have a spherical equivalent of zero; this is evident by writing the cross cylinder in spherocylindrical notation.

    EXAMPLE: $+0.50 - 1.00 \times 90$

30. To minimize image displacement in a hyperope, the best type of bifocal segment style is

    c. round top. To minimize image displacement, the prismatic effects of the bifocal segment and the distance lens should be in opposite directions; a round top acts like a base-down prism and the underlying hyperopic lens acts like a base-up prism.

31. The logMAR equivalent to 20/40 Snellen acuity is
    b. 0.3

CHAPTER 2 PHARMACOLOGY

1. Which antibiotic results in the highest intravitreal concentration when administered orally?
   a. ciprofloxacin

2. Which anesthetic agent would most interfere with an intraocular gas bubble?
   d. nitrous oxide

3. Which of the following is not an adverse effect of CAIs?
   c. iris cysts

4. Which β-blocker has the least effect on β_2 receptors?
   b. betaxolol—this is a cardioselective β_1-blocker

5. Which drug has the least effect on uveoscleral outflow?
   d. Trusopt—this is a CAI that decreases aqueous production; Xalatan and atropine increase and pilocarpine decreases uveoscleral outflow.

6. Which enzyme is inhibited by steroids?
   b. phospholipase A_2

7. Which of the following steroid formulations has the best corneal penetrability?
   a. prednisolone acetate—order of corneal penetrability is acetate > alcohol > phosphate

8. Adverse effects of foscarnet include all of the following except
   b. infertility

9. Which glaucoma medication is not effective when IOP is >60 mm Hg?
   c. pilocarpine—because of iris ischemia, which occurs at IOP >40 mm Hg

10. Which medicine is not associated with OCP-like conjunctival shrinkage?
    d. timoptic

11. Which β-blocker is β_1-selective?
    c. betaxolol

12. The most appropriate treatment for neurosyphilis is
    a. penicillin G—IV penicillin is used to treat neurosyphilis

13. The correct mechanism of action of botulinum toxin is
    a. prevents release of acetylcholine

14. Fluoroquinolones are least effective against
    c. anaerobic cocci

15. Hydroxychloroquine toxicity depends most on
    b. cumulative dose

16. Calculate the amount of cocaine in 2 mL of a 4% solution.
    d. 80 mg—a 1% solution indicates 1 g/100 mL; therefore, a 4% solution is 4000 mg/100 mL = 40 mg/mL

17. NSAIDs block the formation of all of the following substances except
    b. leukotrienes—NSAIDs block the conversion of arachidonic acid by cyclooxygenase into endoperoxides (thus inhibiting the formation of prostaglandins, thromboxane, and prostacyclin); leukotrienes are formed from arachidonic acid by lipoxygenase; steroids block the formation of arachidonic acid (and therefore, all subsequent end products) by inhibiting phospholipase A_2

18. Systemic effects of steroids may include all of the following except
    d. renal tubular acidosis

19. Which drug does not produce decreased tear production?
    d. atropine

20. Natamycin is a
    c. polyene

21. Which glaucoma medicine does not decrease aqueous production?
    b. pilocarpine—miotics increase aqueous outflow

22. β-blockers may cause all of the following except
    a. constipation

23. Idoxuridine may cause all of the following except
    c. corneal hypesthesia

24. Which of the following antifungal agents has the broadest spectrum against yeast-like fungi?
    d. amphotericin

25. All of the following medications are combination antihistamine and mast cell stabilizers except
    a. Alomide—is only a mast cell stabilizer

CHAPTER 3   EMBRYOLOGY/PATHOLOGY

1. Which stain is the most helpful in the diagnosis of sebaceous cell carcinoma?

   c. Oil-red-O, which stains lipid

2. Pagetoid spread is most commonly associated with

   c. sebaceous cell carcinoma—this is invasion of intact epithelium by nests of cells and is characteristic of sebaceous cell carcinoma; pagetoid spread can also occur in the rare superficial spreading form of melanoma that occurs on unexposed skin areas (back, legs)

3. A melanoma occurring in which of the following locations has the best prognosis?

   a. iris—often can be completely excised

4. Calcification in retinoblastoma is due to

   a. RPE metaplasia

5. The type of organism that causes Lyme disease is a

   b. spirochete

6. Characteristics of ghost cells include all of the following except

   d. biconcave

7. A moll gland is best categorized as

   b. apocrine

8. Which of the following is not a Gram-positive rod?

   c. *Serratia*—this bacterium is Gram-negative

9. Trantas' dots are composed of what cell type?

   c. eosinophil

10. Types of collagen that can be found in the cornea include all of the following except

    b. II—is found in vitreous; type I is found in normal coneal stroma, III in stromal wound healing, and IV in basement membranes

11. Lens nuclei are retained in all of the following conditions except

    d. Alport's syndrome

12. Vogt-Koyanagi-Harada syndrome is best described by which type of hypersensitivity reaction?

    d. IV

13. Lacy vacuolization of the iris occurs in which disease?

    b. diabetes—lacy vacuolization is a pathologic finding of glycogen-filled cysts in the iris pigment epithelium

14. Antoni A and B cells occur in which tumor?

    a. neurilemmoma (schwannoma)

15. Which tumor is classically described as having a "Swiss cheese" appearance?

    b. adenoid cystic carcinoma

16. Which iris nodule is correctly paired with its pathology

    b. Lisch nodule, neural crest hamartoma—this is correct. JXG nodules are composed of histiocytes and Touton giant cells, Koeppe nodules are collections of inflammatory cells, and Brushfield spots are stromal hyperplasia.

17. Which of the following statements is true concerning immunoglobulin

    a. IgG crosses the placenta

18. A retinal detachment caused by fixation artifact can be differentiated from a true retinal detachment by all of the following except

    a. a fold at the ora serrata—is a fixation artifact found in newborn eyes called Lange's fold. It is not related to an artifactual or true retinal detachment.

19. Which of the following epithelial changes in the eyelid refers to thickening of the squamous cell layer

    b. acanthosis

20. Intraocular hemorrhage may cause all of the following sequelae except

    c. asteroid hyalosis—is calcium soaps suspended in the vitreous and is unrelated to hemorrhage.

21. Intraocular calcification may occur in all of the following except

    b. medulloepithelioma—this tumor may contain cartilage.

22. The histopathology of which tumor is classically described as a storiform pattern of tumor cells

    d. fibrous histiocytoma

CHAPTER 4   NEURO-OPHTHALMOLOGY

1. The visual field defect most characteristic of optic neuritis is

   b. central—all of these may occur in optic neuritis, but a central scotoma is most characteristic

2. Which cranial nerve is most prone to injury in the cavernous sinus?

   d. 6—travels in middle of sinus and is not protected by lateral wall as are CN 3, 4, and 5

3. Which of the following agents is least toxic to the optic nerve?

   b. dapsone

4. Seesaw nystagmus is produced by a lesion located in which area?

   c. suprasellar—also associated with bitemporal hemianopia; chiasmal gliomas can cause spasmus nutans—like eye movements in children; lesions in the posterior fossa cause dissociated nystagmus, and those in the cervicomedullary junction cause downbeat nystagmus

5. What is the location of a lesion that causes an ipsilateral Horner's syndrome and a contralateral CN 4 palsy?

   a. midbrain—this is due to a nuclear/fascicular lesion at the level of the midbrain

6. The least useful test for functional visual loss is

   c. HVF—the other tests can commonly be used to trick the patient

7. Optociliary shunt vessels may occur in all of the following conditions except

   d. ischemic optic neuropathy

8. Which is not a symptom of pseudotumor cerebri?

   b. entoptic phenomena

9. A 63-year-old woman reports sudden onset of jagged lines in the right peripheral vision. She has experienced 3 episodes in the past month, which lasted approximately 10 to 20 minutes. She denies headaches and any history or family history of migraines. The most likely diagnosis is

   c. migraine variant—this is a characteristic visual disturbance that occurs in acephalgic migraines and is called a fortification phenomenon; the other common visual alteration is a scintillating scotoma (appears as flickering colored lights that grow in the visual field)

10. A 60-year-old man with optic disc swelling in the right eye and left optic atrophy most likely has

    a. ischemic optic neuropathy—these findings are consistent with Foster-Kennedy syndrome; however, the most common cause is pseudo–Foster-Kennedy syndrome due to ION

11. Which of the following findings may not be present in a patient with an INO?

    c. absent convergence—this occurs only in an anterior INO, not in a posterior INO (convergence is preserved); thus if the patient has a posterior INO, then absent convergence will not be found; the other 3 findings occur in both anterior and posterior forms of INO

12. A paradoxical pupillary reaction is not found in which condition?

    b. albinism—foveal hypoplasia occurs but pupillary reactivity is normal; paradoxical pupillary response is found in CSNB, achromatopsia, Leber's congenital amaurosis, optic atrophy, and optic nerve hypoplasia

13. Inheritance of Leber's optic neuropathy is

    c. mitochondrial DNA

14. An OKN strip moved to the left stimulates what part of the brain?

    a. right frontal, left occipital

15. The smooth pursuit system does not involve the

    d. frontal motor area—this area is involved with fast eye movements

16. Dorsal midbrain syndrome is not associated with

    a. absent convergence—convergence is present and results in convergence-retraction nystagmus

17. The location of Horner's syndrome is best differentiated by which drug?

    b. paredrine—distinguishes between preganglionic and postganglionic lesions

18. The blood supply to the prelaminar optic nerve is

    c. short posterior ciliary arteries

19. Optic nerve hypoplasia is associated with all of the following except

    d. spasmus nutans

20. A lesion in the pons causes

    b. miosis

21. Which of the following syndromes is characterized by abduction deficit and contralateral hemiplegia?

    c. Millard-Gubler—Foville's and Gradenigo's involve CN 6 but do not cause hemiparesis; Weber's does cause hemiparesis but involves CN 3, not CN 6

22. All of the following are features of progressive supranuclear palsy except

    b. loss of oculovestibular reflex

23. Pituitary apoplexy is characterized by all of the following except

    a. nystagmus

24. Which of the following is most likely to produce a junctional scotoma?

    d. meningioma—a junctional scotoma is caused by a lesion at the junction of the optic nerve and chiasm; this is most commonly due to a meningioma

25. All of the following are characteristics of an optic tract lesion except
    b. decreased vision—visual acuity is not affected

26. The saccade system does not involve the
    a. occipital motor area

27. A 22-year-old man sustains trauma resulting in a transected left optic nerve. Which of the following is true regarding the right pupil?
    c. it is equal in size to the left pupil—because of the intact consensual response in the left eye

28. Characteristics of spasmus nutans include all of the following except
    d. signs present during sleep—spasmus nutans disappears during sleep

29. A congenital CN 4 palsy can be distinguished from an acquired palsy by
    a. vertical fusional amplitude >10 prism diopters

30. Characteristics of a diabetic CN 3 palsy may include all of the following except
    d. aberrant regeneration—this does not occur with vasculopathic causes of CN 3 palsy, only with compression (aneurysm, tumor) or trauma

31. A CN 3 lesion may cause all of the following except
    a. contralateral ptosis—depending on location of the lesion, the ptosis may be ipsilateral (complete or superior division CN 3 paresis), bilateral (nuclear), or no ptosis present (inferior division CN 3 palsy)

32. Optic nerve drusen is associated with all of the following except
    c. CME

33. A lesion causing limited upgaze with an intact Bell's phenomenon is located where?
    a. supranuclear—if Bell's phenomenon is intact, then the lesion must be supranuclear

34. An acute subarachnoid hemorrhage due to a ruptured aneurysm may produce all of the following except
    b. orbital hemorrhage—does not result from a subarachnoid hemorrhage, but vitreous hemorrhage (Terson's syndrome), ptosis, and an afferent pupillary defect (CN 3 palsy) can occur

CHAPTER 5   PEDIATRICS/STRABISMUS

1. The approximate age of onset for accommodative ET is closest to
   b. 3 years old

2. A 15-year-old girl with strabismus is examined, and the following measurements are recorded: distance deviation of 10 prism diopters, near deviation of 35 prism diopters at 20 cm, and interpupillary distance of 60 mm. Her AC/A ratio is
   a. 11 : 1—to calculate the AC/A ratio with this information, use the heterophoria method: IPD + [(N − D)/Diopt] = 6 + [(35 − 10)/5] = 11 (remember to convert IPD to cm, and 20 cm = 5 D)

3. Duane's syndrome is thought to be due to a developmental abnormality of
   d. abducens nucleus

4. The most helpful test in a patient with aniridia is
   b. abdominal ultrasound—to rule out Wilms' tumor in sporadic cases

5. The best test for an infant with a normal fundus and searching eye movements is
   a. VER—can be used to determine acuity

6. The most common congenital infection is
   c. CMV

7. ARC is most likely to develop in a child with
   a. congenital esotropia

8. Which of the following most accurately reflects what a patient with harmonious ARC reports when the angle of anomaly is equal to the objective angle?
   c. simultaneous macular perception

9. The inferior oblique muscle is weakened most by which procedure?
   d. anteriorization

10. The test that gives the best dissociation is
    b. Worth 4 Dot

11. The 3-step test shows a left hypertropia in primary position that worsens on right gaze and with left head tilt. The best surgical procedure is
    d. LIO weakening—this is an LSO palsy, so possible treatments include LIO weakening, RIR recession, LSO tuck, and LIR resection

12. In the treatment of a superior oblique palsy, Knapp recommended all of the following except
    d. resection of the contralateral SR—the contralateral SR should be weakened with a recession, not strengthened with a resection

13. The best results of cryotherapy for ROP occur for treatment of disease in which location?
    b. anterior zone 2

14. Characteristics of congenital ET include all of the following except

   c. amblyopia

15. The contralateral antagonist of the right superior rectus

   a. passes under another muscle—the contralateral antagonist of the right superior rectus is the left superior oblique (the antagonist [LSO] of the yoke muscle [LIO] of the paretic muscle [RSR]); the SO passes under the SR, is an incyclotorter (therefore causes excyclotorsion when paretic), abducts the eye, and is innervated by CN 4

16. With respect to Panum's area, physiologic diplopia occurs at what point?

   c. in front of Panum's area—physiologic diplopia occurs in front of and behind Panum's area; within Panum's area binocular vision occurs with fusion and stereopsis, on the horopter only fusion

17. The best treatment of an A pattern ET with muscle transposition is

   d. LR resection with downward transposition—appropriate surgery for the ET is LR resection or MR recession; to fix the A pattern, the LRs are moved toward the empty space of the pattern (down for ET) or the MRs are moved toward the apex of the pattern (up for ET)

18. A superior rectus Faden suture is used for the treatment of which condition?

   b. dissociated vertical deviation

19. Which medication should be administered to a child who develops trismus under general anesthesia?

   d. dantrolene—because trismus is a sign of malignant hyperthermia

20. Congenital superior oblique palsy is characterized by all of the following except

   d. <10 D of vertical vergence amplitudes—usually, these amplitudes are >10 D

21. Which of the following statements regarding monofixation syndrome is false?

   c. Fusional vergence amplitudes are absent

22. Iridocyclitis is most commonly associated with which form of JRA?

   d. pauciarticular

23. Congenital rubella is most commonly associated with

   a. retinal pigment epitheliopathy

24. The most common cause of proptosis in a child is

   b. orbital cellulitis

25. Which form of rhabdomyosarcoma has the worst prognosis?

   c. alveolar—is the most malignant and has the worst prognosis; embryonal is the most common, botryoid is a subtype of embryonal, and pleomorphic is the rarest and has the best prognosis

26. Which of the following conditions is the least common cause of childhood proptosis?

   a. cavernous hemangioma—this is the most common benign orbital tumor of adults and occurs most commonly in middle-aged women

27. A child with retinoblastoma is born to healthy parents with no family history of RB. The chance of RB occurring in a second child is approximately

   a. 5%

28. The best chronologic age to examine a baby for ROP is

   c. 36 weeks

29. All of the following are associated with trisomy 13 except

   c. epiblepharon

30. Paradoxical pupillary response does not occur in

   d. albinism

CHAPTER 6   ORBIT/LIDS/ADNEXA

1. The most common causitive organism of canaliculitis is

   c. *Actinomyces israelii*

2. Sequelae of a CN 7 palsy may include all of the following except

   b. ptosis—CN 7 palsy causes inability to close the lid and exposure keratopathy; CN 3 palsy causes ptosis

3. Which procedure is the best treatment option for the repair of a large upper eyelid defect?

   a. Cutler-Beard—is a lid-sharing procedure for repair of large upper eyelid defects, Bick is a horizontal lid-shortening procedure, Hughes is a lid-sharing procedure for repair of large lower eyelid defects, and Fasanella-Servat is a tarsoconjunctival resection for ptosis repair

4. The extraocular muscle with the largest arc of contact is the

    b. IO—which is 15 mm; next is LR at 12 mm, then SO at 7–8 mm, and MR at 7 mm

5. The risk of systemic involvement is highest for an ocular lymphoid tumor in which location?

    b. eyelid—67% have systemic involvement; for orbit, it is 35% and for conjunctiva, 20%

6. The rectus muscle with the shortest tendon of insertion is the

    c. MR—the IO has the shortest tendon (1 mm), but of the rectus muscles, the MR has the shortest tendon at 4.5 mm; the others are SR = 6 mm, IR = 7 mm, and LR = 7 mm

7. Which of the following bones does not make up the medial orbital wall?

    d. palatine—is part of the orbital floor; the medial wall is composed of the other 3 bones and the sphenoid

8. Which of the following clinical features is least commonly associated with a tripod fracture?

    a. restriction of the inferior rectus—tripod fractures include disruption of the orbital floor, but entrapment of ocular tissues is rare and is usually associated with large floor fractures (blow-out fracture); the other 3 findings are much more common in a tripod fracture

9. A carotid-cavernous fistula can be differentiated from a dural-sinus fistula by all of the following characteristics except

    a. proptosis—this can occur in both types of AV fistula; the other signs are seen with C-C fistulas

10. Basal cell carcinoma is least likely to occur at which site?

    d. lateral canthus—the order (in decreasing frequency) is as follows: lower lid > medial canthus > upper lid > lateral canthus

11. All of the following are sites of attachment of the limbs of the medial canthal tendon except

    c. orbital process of the frontal bone

12. Which muscle is most commonly responsible for vertical diplopia after 4-lid blepharoplasty?

    b. inferior oblique—because it lies below the IR and is encircled by the capsulopalpebral fascia

13. Congenital and involutional ptosis can be distinguished by all of the following except

    c. width of palprebal fissure

14. Congenital obstruction of the lacrimal drainage system usually occurs at the

    d. valve of Hasner

15. What is the correct order of structures that would be encountered when the upper eyelid is penetrated 14 mm above the lid margin?

    a. preseptal orbicularis muscle, orbital septum, levator aponeurosis, Müller's muscle

16. What is the best treatment option for a child who develops recurrent proptosis after upper respiratory infections?

    a. observation—this scenario is common with an orbital lympangioma, and spontaneous regression often occurs

17. All of the following are features of mucormycosis except

    b. ipsilateral CN 7 palsy—mucor may cause an orbital apex syndrome, but CN 7 is not involved

18. All of the following are associated with blepharophimosis except

    c. AR inheritance—blepharophimosis may be part of an AD syndrome (chromosome 3q), as well as trisomy 18; findings include blepharophimosis, ptosis, telecanthus, ectropion, and epicanthus inversus

19. Which of the following is the most important test to perform in a patient with a capillary hemangioma?

    d. bleeding time—to look for Kassabach-Merritt syndrome (consumptive coagulopathy)

20. For entropion repair, the lateral tarsal strip is sutured

    c. above and anterior to the rim

21. Staged surgery for a patient with severe thyroid-related ophthalmopathy is best done in what order

    a. decompression, strabismus, lid repair—because decompression may affect ocular alignment and lid position, and strabismus surgery may affect lid position

22. Which of the following best explains why when a ptotic lid is lifted, the contralateral lid falls?

    d. Hering's law—equal and simultaneous innervation to synergistic muscles; thus, lifting a ptotic lid decreases the innervation to the levator bilaterally so the contralateral lid will fall slightly

23. Which study is most helpful in the evaluation of a patient with opsoclonus?

    b. MRI—to rule out neuroblastoma or visceral carcinoma

24. What is the most appropriate treatment for a benign mixed tumor of the lacrimal gland?

    b. excision—must excise completely en bloc to prevent recurrence and malignant transformation

25. What is the most appropriate treatment for a biopsy-positive basal cell carcinoma of the lower eyelid?

    d. excision with frozen section control of the margins

26. CT enhancement is most associated with which lesion?

    d. meningioma—produces characteristic railroad track sign

27. Which of the following factors is least likely to contribute to the development of entropion?

    a. preseptal orbicularis override—this can occur but is less common than the other factors

28. A 24-year-old woman presents after blunt trauma to the left orbit with enophthalmos and restriction of upgaze. Which plain film radiographic view would be most helpful?

    c. Waters view—gives best view of orbital floor

29. All of the following may cause enophthalmos except

    b. lymphoma—may cause proptosis but not enophthalmos; breast cancer can cause either, and phthisis and floor fractures may cause enophthalmos

30. All of the following nerves pass through the superior orbital fissure except

    c. CN V_2—passes through the inferior orbital fissure

CHAPTER 7 CORNEA/EXTERNAL DISEASE

1. Which is the least desirable method for corneal graft storage?

    b. glycerin—does not preserve endothelial cells and can be used only for lamellar or patch grafts; moist chamber at 4°C preserves tissue for 48 hours, Optisol for up to 10 days, and cryopreservation potentially for years

2. Presently in the United States, phlyctenule is most commonly associated with

    c. *Staphylococcus*

3. Which blood test is most helpful in the evaluation of a patient with Schnyder's crystalline corneal dystrophy?

    d. cholesterol—may be elevated

4. Which disease has never been transmitted by a corneal graft?

    a. CMV—the others have been transmitted in humans or experimentally in animals

5. Which corneal dystrophy does not recur in a corneal graft?

    d. PPMD

6. A conjunctival map biopsy is typically used for which malignancy?

    c. sebaceous cell carcinoma

7. Corneal clouding does not occur in which mucopolysaccharidosis?

    a. Hunter's

8. All of the following may cause follicular conjunctivitis except

    b. *Neisseria*

9. Which of the following tests is least helpful in determining the etiology of enlarged corneal nerves?

    a. EKG—the others are all helpful in detecting disorders that are associated with enlarged corneal nerves: calcitonin for medullary thyroid carcinoma (MEN 2b), urinary VMA for pheochromocytoma (MEN 2b), acid-fast stain for atypical *Mycobacteria* (leprosy)

10. Corneal filaments are least likely to be present in which condition?

    b. Thygeson's SPK

11. Which of the following is not an appropriate treatment for SLK?

    c. silver nitrate stick—may cause globe perforation; therefore, use only silver nitrate solution

12. In what level of the cornea does a Kayser-Fleischer ring occur?

    d. Descemet's membrane

13. Cornea verticillata—like changes are associated with all of the following except

    b. thorazine

14. The least common location for a nevus is

    a. bulbar conjunctiva

15. All of the following ions move across the corneal endothelium by both active transport and passive diffusion except

    a. Cl^-—moves across endothelium only by passive diffusion

16. Which organism is associated with crystalline keratopathy?

    d. *S. viridans*

17. Which of the following conditions is associated with the best 5-year prognosis for a corneal graft?

    b. Fuchs' dystrophy

18. The best strategy for loosening a tight contact lens is to

    c. decrease the diameter—decreasing the curvature will also loosen a tight lens but not as well; increasing the diameter or curvature will tighten a lens

19. The type of contact lens that causes the least endothelial pleomorphism is

    a. soft daily wear

20. Which of the following conditions is associated with the worst prognosis for a corneal graft?

    c. Reis-Bucklers' dystrophy—this dystrophy commonly recurs in the graft

21. Which is not a treatment of acute hydrops?

    d. corneal transplant—eventually, this may be an option, but short-term treatment is medical only

22. Which organism cannot penetrate intact corneal epithelium?

    c. *P. aeruginosa*—cannot penetrate intact corneal epithelium; the others and *Listeria* can

23. Which organism is most commonly associated with angular blepharitis?

    b. *Moraxella*

24. Which of the following medications would be the best choice in the treatment of microsporidial keratoconjunctivitis?

    a. fumagillin

25. All of the following agents are used in the treatment of *Acanthamoeba* keratitis except

    b. natamycin

26. Goblet cells are most abundant in which location?

    a. fornix

CHAPTER 8   UVEITIS

1. The most effective antibiotic for the treatment of *P. acnes* endophthalmitis is

    c. vancomycin

2. For the diagnosis of granulomatous inflammation, which cell type must be present?

    d. epithelioid histiocyte

3. All of the following are true concerning sarcoidosis except

    a. Touton giant cells are common—sarcoidosis is characterized by Langhans' giant cells

4. Which of the following is not characteristic of Fuchs' heterochromic iridocyclitis?

    c. posterior synechiae

5. The most common organism causing endophthalmitis following cataract surgery is

    d. *S. epidermidis*

6. MEWDS can be differentiated from APMPPE by

    b. female predilection

7. All of the following disorders are correctly paired with their HLA associations except

    a. POHS, B9—POHS is associated with HLA-B7, DR2

8. Decreased vision in a patient with intermediate uveitis is most likely due to

    b. macular edema

9. A 71-year-old woman with a 6-month history of fatigue, anorexia, and 10-pound weight loss is found to have left-sided weakness, visual acuity of 20/80 OD and 20/60 OS, and vitreous cells. The most helpful workup is

    a. LP and vitrectomy—to rule out CNS lymphoma

10. The most common organisms causing endophthalmitis following trauma is

    b. *Bacillus* species and *S. epidermidis*

11. All of the following are features common to both sympathetic ophthalmia and Vogt-Koyanagi-Harada syndrome except

    c. pathology localized to choroid—retina is also involved in VKH

12. Which disorder is more common in males?

    b. uveal effusion syndrome

13. EVS findings include all of the following except

    b. intravitreal corticosteroids were helpful—intravitreal steroids were not evaluated in the EVS

14. Which of the following is not characteristic of MEWDS?

    b. bilaterality

15. The most common cause of posterior uveitis is

    d. toxoplasmosis

16. All of the following are causes of HLA-B27—associated uveitis except

    d. psoriasis—is not associated with uveitis, but psoriatic arthritis is

17. Which of the following is not part of the classic triad of findings in Reiter's syndrome?

    a. iritis—iritis occurs but the classic triad of Reiter's is arthritis, conjunctivitis, and urethritis

18. Which of the following laboratory tests is most commonly found in JRA-related iritis?

    c. RF–, ANA+—which occurs in early-onset pauciarticular JRA

19. Phacoantigenic endophthalmitis is characterized by which pattern of granulomatous inflammation?

    a. zonal

20. Which combination of findings is least likely to occur in rubella?

    b. glaucoma and cataract—each occurs but rarely together

21. A 35-year-old man with decreased vision OD is found to have ON edema and a macular star. The causative organism is most likely

    b. *Bartonella henselae*—which causes cat-scratch disease and a neuroretinitis; *O. volvulus* causes onchocerciasis, *T. pallidum* causes syphilis, and *B. burgdorferi* causes Lyme disease

22. Which is least helpful for the diagnosis of toxocariasis?

    d. stool examination—no ova or parasites are found in the stool

23. A person living in which area of the US would be most likely to develop POHS?

    c. Midwest—in the US, histoplasmosis is most prevalent in the Ohio River valley and Eastern states

24. All of the following are true of birdshot choroidopathy except

    a. more common in males—birdshot choroidopathy is more common in females

25. Which of the following is least commonly associated with *Treponema pallidum* infection?

    d. glaucoma—is not associated with ocular involvement of syphilis

CHAPTER 9   GLAUCOMA

1. Which form of glaucoma is associated with Down's syndrome?

    c. Axenfeld-Rieger

2. What is the most appropriate initial treatment of pupillary block in a patient with microspherophakia?

    d. cyclopentolate—which helps pull the anteriorly displaced lens back to its normal position

3. Which of the following statements is true? Uveoscleral outflow is

    c. increased by atropine—cycloplegics and prostaglandin analogues (Xalatan, Lumigan, Travatan) increase (and miotics decrease) uveoscleral outflow; fluorophotometry measures the rate of aqueous formation; uveoscleral outflow accounts for 15% to 20% of total outflow and is independent of pressure

4. Risk factors for angle-closure glaucoma include all of the following except

    b. myopia—this is a risk factor for open-angle glaucoma, not angle-closure glaucoma

5. Which of the following would cause the greatest elevation in IOP?

    a. blinking—IOP is lowered by decreased blood cortisol levels (reduces aqueous formation) and elevation of the head (changing from supine to sitting position); darkening the room may increase IOP in patients with narrow angles

6. The most likely cause of a large filtering bleb and a shallow chamber is

    d. overfiltration—which causes both findings; a leak would cause a flat or low bleb; pupillary block and aqueous misdirection would not change the size of the blebs

7. A change in Goldmann visual field stimulus from I4E to II4E is equivalent to

    a. 1 log—the Roman numeral indicates the size of the test object in mm² (0 = 1/16, I = 1/4, II = 1, III = 4, IV = 16, V = 64) and is a logarithmic scale; therefore, changing from size I to II is 1 log unit

8. An Amsler grid held at 33 cm measures approximately how many degrees of central vision?

    b. 10

9. The most decreased sensitivity in an arcuate scotoma occurs in which quadrant?

    c. superotemporal

10. The best gonioscopy lens for distinguishing appositional from synechial angle closure is

    b. Zeiss—this is the only lens of the 4 that can be used for indentation gonioscopy (indenting the cornea forces aqueous into the angle pushing the iris backward and allowing one to view the angle)

11. Which is not a risk factor for POAG?

    d. CRAO

12. ALT would be most effective in a patient with which type of glaucoma?

    c. pigmentary—patients with pigmentary glaucoma often respond well to ALT, whereas those with inflammatory, congenital, and aphakic glaucoma do not

13. In which direction should a patient look to aid the examiner's view of the angle during Zeiss gonioscopy?

    b. toward the mirror—this allows for a better view of the portion of the angle being inspected

14. The best parameter for determining the unreliability of a Humphrey visual field is

    a. fixation losses

15. Which of the following does not cause angle-closure glaucoma?

    c. RD—does not cause angle closure; the others do: PHPV and choroidal effusion by a posterior pushing mechanism and ICE syndrome by an anterior pulling mechanism

16. Factors producing increased IOP 2 days postoperatively include all of the following except

    d. steroid drops—steroid response does not occur this quickly (it usually takes at least 7–10 days)

17. Treatment of malignant glaucoma may include all of the following except

    b. pilocarpine—miotics are contraindicated in malignant glaucoma because the aim of medical therapy is to pull the lens/iris diaphragm posteriorly (cycloplegics)

18. The most common organism associated with bleb-related endophthalmitis is

    a. *Streptococcus* species—are most common (~50%) followed by coagulase-negative *Staph* and then *H. flu*

19. Which visual field defect is least characteristic of glaucoma?

    c. central scotoma—central vision is not affected until late in the disease

20. The type of tonometer most greatly affected by scleral rigidity is

    c. Schiøtz—low scleral rigidity yields falsely low readings (i.e., high myopia, thyroid disease, previous ocular surgery, miotic therapy), and high scleral rigidity yields falsely high readings (i.e., high hyperopia, vasoconstrictor therapy)

21. Which of the following conditions is not associated with an increased incidence of glaucoma?

    d. cornea plana

22. As compared with plasma, aqueous has a higher concentration of

    c. ascorbate—has a concentration 15× higher in aqueous than in plasma, whereas the concentrations of sodium, calcium, and protein are lower in aqueous

23. The rate of aqueous production per minute is approximately

    b. 2 μL

24. The location of the greatest resistance to aqueous outflow is

    c. juxtacanalicular connective tissue

25. Facility of aqueous outflow is best measured by

    a. tonography—manometry measures episcleral venous pressure, tonometry measures intraocular pressure, fluorophotometry measures rate of aqueous formation (via decreasing fluorescein concentration)

CHAPTER 10   ANTERIOR SEGMENT

1. The most helpful test for evaluating macular function in a patient with advanced cataract is

    b. 2-light separation—the others test gross function

2. Ectopia lentis is least likely to be associated with

    a. cleft palate—is not associated with lens subluxation; the other abnormalities are pectus excavatum in Marfan's syndrome, short stature in Weill-Marchesani syndrome, and mental retardation in homocystinuria, sulfite oxidase deficiency, and hyperlysinemia

3. Anterior segment signs of ciliary body melanoma include all of the following except

    a. corneal edema—does not occur; however, ciliary body melanoma can cause increased IOP from angle closure (posterior pushing mechanism), and astigmatism and cataract from mechanical effects on the crystalline lens

4. Which of the following is least characteristic of ICE syndrome?

    b. increased IOP

5. The crystalline lens is formed from which embryologic tissue?

    b. ectoderm

6. A stellate anterior subcapsular cataract is most likely to be found in a patient with

    d. electrical injury—the other entities cause different types of cataract: atopic dermatitis (ASC), myotonic dystrophy (Christmas tree cataract), Fabry's disease (spoke-like cataract)

7. The most useful diagnostic test in an infant with an oil-droplet cataract is
   d. urine-reducing substances—to check for galactosemia

8. Which of the following does not occur in siderosis bulbi?
   c. sunflower cataract—is seen in conditions with abnormal copper (not iron) deposition (i.e., Wilson's disease and chalcosis)

9. A patient has a history of increased IOP with exercise; which finding is associated with this condition?
   a. Krukenberg's spindle—these are both signs of pigment dispersion syndrome

10. Separation between the longitudinal and circumferential fibers of the ciliary muscle is called
    b. angle recession—this is the definition; iridoschisis is separation of the iris surface, iridodialysis is separation of the iris root from its insertion, and cyclodialysis is separation of the ciliary body from the scleral spur

11. Characteristics of pigment dispersion syndrome include all of the following except
    c. phacodenesis

12. Genetics of aniridia are best summarized as
    d. 1/3 sporadic, 2/3 AD

13. Blood in Schlemm's canal is not associated with
    a. Fuchs' heterochromic iridocyclitis—there is no blood in Schlemm's canal, but fine-angle neovascularization occurs and may cause spontaneous hyphema

14. A sickle cell patient with a hyphema develops increased IOP; which of the following treatment choices is best?
    d. timoptic—is the safest medication because it does not affect sickling; miotics destabilize the blood-aqueous barrier, CAIs decrease aqueous pH (leading to sickling), and hyperosmotics cause hemoconcentration and sickling

15. A pigmentary retinopathy occurs in which mesodermal dysgenesis syndrome?
    b. Alagille's syndrome

16. Of the following causes of iris heterochromia, the involved iris is hyperchromic in
    a. ICE syndrome—pigmented iris nodules (pseudonevi) can occur; the involved iris is hypochromic in the other 3 conditions

17. Which of the following iris lesions is a true tumor?
    c. Lisch nodule—is an iris hamartoma associated with neurofibromatosis; Kunkmann-Wolffian body is composed of normal iris stroma, Koeppe nodule is composed of inflammatory cells, and nodules in JXG are granulomatous infiltrates

18. At which location is the lens capsule thinnest?
    b. posterior capsule

19. The iris sphincter is derived from what embryologic tissue?
    c. neural ectoderm

20. Which of the following is not associated with sunset syndrome?
    d. hyphema—is not associated with inferior decentration of an IOL; polyopia can occur if the edge of the lens is within the pupil; asymmetric haptic placement and weak zonules (which occur in pseudoexfoliation) are risk factors

CHAPTER 11 POSTERIOR SEGMENT

1. Which substance does not cause crystalline deposits in the retina?
   a. thioridazine

2. What is the chance that a child of a patient with Best's disease will inherit the disorder?
   b. 50%—Best's is autosomal dominant

3. The MPS showed the best prognosis for laser treatment of CNV in which disorder?
   d. POHS—The MPS studied laser treatment of CNV in patients with AMD, POHS, and idiopathic membranes; POHS patients had the best response to laser treatment; patients with CNV secondary to myopia and angioid streaks were not studied

4. Which of the following is not a feature of Stickler's syndrome?
   c. retinoschisis

5. Sites at which the uvea is attached to the sclera include all of the following except
   d. ora serrata

6. The inheritance of gyrate atrophy is
   d. autosomal recessive

7. All 3 types of retinal hemorrhage (preretinal, intraretinal, and subretinal) may occur simultaneously in all of the following conditions except
   c. diabetes—diabetic retinopathy can cause preretinal and intraretinal hemorrhages but does not cause subretinal hemorrhage

8. Characteristics of choroidal melanoma include all of the following except

   b. high internal reflectivity

9. Which of the following statements regarding the ETDRS is false?

   a. The ETDRS concluded that PRP reduces the risk of severe visual loss in patients with high-risk PDR—this conclusion is from the DRS

10. The DRVS found that early vitrectomy for vitreous hemorrhage was helpful in

    a. type 1 diabetic patients

11. Which of the following treatments is a CVOS recommendation?

    c. PRP for iris or angle neovascularization

12. Which peripheral retinal lesion has the most risk of a retinal detachment?

    d. lattice degeneration

13. The intraocular structure most commonly affected by leukemia is

    d. optic nerve

14. Which is not a function of the RPE?

    b. concentration of taurine

15. Which of the following best describes the cellular reaction when light strikes a photoreceptor?

    b. increased cGMP, open Na channel

16. Von Hippel-Lindau disease has been mapped to which chromosome?

    a. 3

17. Which tumor is not associated with von Hippel-Lindau disease?

    a. hepatocellular carcinoma

18. Prognostic factors for choroidal melanoma include all of the following except

    d. pigmentation

19. Which of the following does not involve the outer plexiform layer of the retina?

    d. diabetic microaneurysm

20. Which X-linked disorder is not associated with an ocular abnormality in the female carrier?

    c. juvenile retinoschisis—female carriers have normal fundus; in the other 3 disorders, female carriers have retinal changes: mid-peripheral pigment clusters and mottling in macula in albinism, equatorial pigment mottling in choroideremia, golden reflex in posterior pole in retinitis pigmentosa

21. All are features of ataxia-telangiectasia except

    b. thymic hyperplasia—the thymus is hypoplastic

22. The best test for distinguishing between a subretinal hemorrhage and a choroidal melanoma is

    a. FA—blockage occurs from the hemorrhage, and tumor circulation is visible in the melanoma

23. Which of the following is the least radiosensitive lesion?

    c. RB

24. Which of the following is not a complication of PRP?

    c. RD

25. A cluster of pigmented lesions is seen in the peripheral retina of a patient's left eye during routine ophthalmoscopy. Which of the following tests would be most helpful in detecting an associated hereditary disorder?

    b. colonoscopy—check for polyps (FAP, Gardner's disease)

26. Which of the following is not associated with a typical angiographic appearance of CME?

    a. nicotinic acid—this maculopathy clinically appears like CME, but there is no fluorescein filling of the cysts; other entities that fall into this category are juvenile retinoschisis, Goldmann-Favre disease, and some types of RP

27. The least likely finding in a patient with a chronic detachment of the inferotemporal retina is

    c. fixed folds—may occur from PVR, whereas the other 3 findings are common with chronic RD

28. All of the following vitreoretinal disorders are inherited in an autosomal dominant pattern except

    d. Goldmann-Favre disease—this is autosomal recessive

29. In a patient with AMD, which type of drusen is most associated with development of CNV?

    a. soft

30. The ERG oscillatory potential is caused by which cell type

    b. amacrine

Additional Readings

Albert WM, Jakobiec FA: Principles and Practice of Ophthalmology, 2nd edition. Philadelphia, WB Saunders, 2000.

Kaiser PK, Friedman NJ, Pineda R II: The Massachusetts Eye & Ear Infirmary's Illustrated Manual of Ophthalmology, 2nd edition. Philadelphia, Saunders, 2004.

Kanski JJ: Clinical Ophthalmology, 5th edition. Philadelphia, Butterworth-Heinemann, 2003.

Kaufman PL, Alm A: Adler's Physiology of the Eye, 10th edition. St. Louis, Mosby, 2003.

Mannis MJ, MacSai MS, Huntley AC: Eye and Skin Disease. Philadelphia, Lippincott-Raven, 1996.

Newell FW: Ophthalmology Principles and Concepts, 8th edition. St. Louis, Mosby, 1996.

Pepose JS, Holland GN, Wilhelmus KR: Ocular Infection and Immunity. St. Louis, Mosby, 1996.

Roy FH: Ocular Differential Diagnosis, 7th edition. Philadelphia, Lippincott Williams & Wilkins, 2002.

Spaeth GL: Ophthalmic Surgery Principles and Practice, 3rd edition. Philadelphia, Saunders, 2003.

Spalton DJ, Hitchings RA, Hunter PA: Atlas of Clinical Ophthalmology, 2nd edition. St. Louis, Mosby, 1994.

Tabbara KF: Infections of the Eye, 2nd edition. Boston, Little, Brown, 1995.

Tasman W, Jaeger EA: Duane's Clinical Ophthalmology. Philadelphia, WB Saunders, 2001.

Vaughan D, Asbury T: General Ophthalmology, 16th edition. Norwalk, CT, Appleton & Lange, 2003.

Weingeist TA, Gold DH: Color Atlas of the Eye in Systemic Disease, 3rd edition. Philadelphia, Lippincott Williams & Wilkins, 2001.

Yanoff M, Duker JS: Ophthalmology, 2nd edition. St. Louis, Mosby, 2004.

Index

Note: Page numbers followed by f, t, and b refer to figures, tables, and boxed material, respectively.